HEALTH INSURANCE TODAY

A PRACTICAL APPROACH

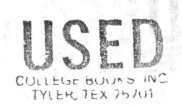

ELSEVIER

evolve

Evolve® Student Resources for *Beik: Health Insurance Today,* offer the following features:

Student Resources

- **Websites to Explore**
  A resource that links the Evolve site to carefully chosen online resources to supplement and reinforce the content of the textbook

- **Content Updates**
  The latest content updates from the author of the textbook to keep you current with recent developments in the area of health insurance billing.

- **Image Collection**
  An assembly of all the figures from this text available for download.

- **Links to Related Resources**
  See what other health insurance billing and coding related resources Elsevier has to offer.

HEALTH INSURANCE TODAY

A PRACTICAL APPROACH

JANET I. BEIK, AA, BA, MEd

Southeastern Community College (retired)
Administrative Instructor
Medical Assistant Program
West Burlington, Iowa

SAUNDERS

ELSEVIER

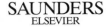

11830 Westline Industrial Drive
St. Louis, Missouri 63146

HEALTH INSURANCE TODAY: A PRACTICAL APPROACH

ISBN-13: 978-1-4160-0054-9
ISBN-10: 1-4160-0054-2

ISBN-13: 978-1-4160-0054-9
ISBN-10: 1-4160-0054-2

Acquisitions Editor: Susan Cole
Developmental Editor: Colin Odell
Publishing Services Manager: Pat Joiner
Project Manager: Jennifer Clark
Designer: Jyotika Shroff

Printed in Canada.

Last digit is the print number: 9 8 7 6 5 4 3 2 1

*• to my husband Lew and daughter Cindy, because
without their help and patience, this endeavor would not have been possible;*

• to my former students, who have taught me as much as I taught them; and

*• to instructors everywhere who are willing to dedicate their time and effort
to instill a desire in students to explore new horizons and promote life-long learning.*

Reviewers

Kay E. Biggs, BS, CMA
Coordinator, Medical Assisting Technology
Columbus State Community College
Columbus, Ohio

Norma Bird, MEd, BS, CMA
Medical Assisting Program Director and Mater
Instructor
Idaho State University College of Technology
Pocatello, Indiana

Michelle Buchman, BSN, RNC
Academic Program Director
Springfield College
Springfield, Missouri

Joyce A. Combs, BS, AAS, CMA
Associate Professor and Program Director,
Medical Assisting
Central Kentucky Technical College
Lexington, Kentucky

Mary Dey, CMA-AC, CPC
Program Director, Medical Assistant Technology
Kalamazoo Valley Community College
Kalamazoo, Michigan

George Fakhoury, MD, DORCP, CMA
Medical Department Director
Silicon Valley College
Walnut Creek, California

Kathryn A Kalanick, CMA, NCPT
Director of Education
Career Academy
Anchorage, Alaska

Jacqueline R. LaForga, CMA
Senior Instructor
Bryman College
San Francisco, California

LaRae P. Lewis, RN
Medical Assisting Program Director
Pamlico Community College
Grantsboro, North Carolina

Elizabeth E. Muniz, CMA, RMA, AHI
Director, Medical Assistant Program
Long Technical College
Phoenix, Arizona

Pamela L. Neu, CMA, MBA
Department Head, Medical Assisting Program
International Business College
Fort Wayne, Indiana

Jane O'Grady, CMA, BS
Adjunct Instructor and Medical Assisting Career
Program Advisory Board
Northwestern Connecticut Community College
Winsted, Connecticut

Linda Scarborough, RN, CMA, BSM
Healthcare Management Technology Program Director
Lanier Technical College
Oakwood, Georgia

Carolyn S. Shankle, LPN, CPC, CCS-P,
CPC, CMC
Adjunct Instructor
South College
Knoxville, Tennessee

Preface

After ten years of teaching medical insurance (and other administrative courses) at a southeastern Iowa community college, I felt a textbook written in a clear, concise format was needed. Health insurance rules and regulations change frequently, almost daily, and although it is difficult to capture all the up-to-date information in a single edition, the use of the Internet along with this text will allow students and instructors to keep current.

Health Insurance Today: A Practical Approach first introduces students to the history of insurance and some general facts regarding its origin; it then shows the *metamorphosis* of health insurance into what we know it to be today.

The textbook and workbook first address completing insurance claims using the universal paper form—the CMS-1500. After students get a grasp of the paper form and its 33 fields, they will be introduced to computerized software, where claims are generated electronically. By approaching claims submission in this manner, students will have a better understanding of the whole picture.

Organization of the Chapters:
- Chapter Objectives
- Chapters Terms
- Opening Scenario
- Summary Check Points
- Closing Scenario
- Websites to Explore

SPECIAL CHAPTER FEATURES

"WHAT DID YOU LEARN?"

The chapters are broken into easy-to-learn sections, after which the students are asked "What Did you Learn?" Several review questions are then presented, which reflect important "focus points" of that section.

Example:

What Did You Learn?

1. To whom do we credit the innovation of the "universal" claim form?
2. List the rules for OCR formatting.
3. Name the two categories of providers who can use the CMS-1500 paper form.

"IMAGINE THIS!"

The "Imagine This!" scenarios allow students to apply information to real-life situations, many of which have been taken from the author's actual healthcare experience. By applying what has been presented in each "Imagine This!" scenario, students can easily relate the importance and how the scenario fits into real life, as well as determine the involved medical setting expectations.

Example:

Imagine This!

Tammy Butler visited Dr. Harold Norton, her family care provider, on February 10 for her yearly wellness examination plus routine diagnostics. Dr. Norton's health insurance professional submitted the claim the day after the visit. A month later, Tammy received an EOB from her health insurer indicating that the services were not covered under her policy. Assuming that her policy did not cover wellness examinations, Tammy forgot about it. During Christmas vacation of that same year, Tammy again visited Dr. Norton for a case of sinusitis. The claim was denied again by her insurer. Puzzled that a second claim had been denied, Tammy contacted Dr. Norton's office and, after some extensive research, learned that they had filed her claims under an old ID number from a previous employer. The problem now was that it was now January of a new year—past the deadline for filing claims for the previous year. The health insurance professional at Dr. Norton's office informed Tammy that she was responsible for the charges.

"STOP AND THINK"

The "Stop and Think" exercises ask the student to read and study a particular paragraph, then apply critical thinking skills to resolve a problem or answer a question. Critical thinking is vital to individuals in the workplace, especially in a medical setting, where members of the health care team are often asked to think "on their feet" to resolve problems.

Example:

● Stop and Think

We learned in this section that two categories of providers are exempt from the ASCA mandate that by October 2003, all claims must be submitted electronically. In your opinion, why are providers falling into these categories allowed to use the CMS-1500 paper form?

HIPAA TIPS

A recent federal law, the Health Insurance Portability and Accountability Act (HIPAA), has presented challenges to both healthcare workers and healthcare patients. Although this book does not attempt to cover all the information included in the HIPAA, it does give periodic applicable tips to help students better understand this very important piece of legislation.

Example:

HIPAA Tip

Any person or organization that furnishes, bills, or is paid for healthcare in the normal course of business falls under HIPAA rules and regulations.

APPENDICES

There are three Appendices: A, B, and C. Appendix A is an example of a CMS-1500 before the National Provider Identifier (NPI) updates. Appendix B presents nine examples of completed claim forms for a variety of payers. Appendix C presents the names of State TANF programs.

STUDENT MATERIALS

A comprehensive student workbook accompanies the textbook and is intended to supplement the material presented in this text. Each chapter follows a precise structure beginning with a short introduction, followed by a review test that allows the student to recall information, and ending with application and enrichment activities that allow students to apply what they have learned to today's health care environment. Most workbook chapters present at least one "Performance Objective." A performance (or learning) objective is a statement of what the students will be expected to do when they have completed a specified course of instruction. It sets the conditions, behavior (action), and standard of task perform-

ance for the training setting. Performance objectives must be mastered to the predetermined criteria set by the instructor, institution, or organization. If the course is competency-based, performance objectives may be repeated up to three times or until the student successfully meets the predetermined grading criteria.

One of the application exercises included in the student workbook involves creating a Health Insurance Professional's notebook. The purpose of this notebook is to allow the student to access information quickly and accurately when preparing insurance claims for some of the major third party payers. If kept current, it will be an excellent resource later on the job.

STUDENT SOFTWARE

In the CD-ROM bound into the Student Workbook, three distinct software offerings support the learning presented in this textbook:

Electronic Forms

Common health insurance forms, such as the CMS-1500, are formatted in Microsoft Word to offer a very simple, straightforward way to electronically complete exercises in the Student Workbook. These files can be saved "mid-exercise" to a disk or hard drive; and, as with any other Microsoft Word document, can be transferred to another computer for continued work. Using the basic forms, students can complete part of an exercise, save their work, and then continue working elsewhere.

Guided Completion

A guided process to completing a CMS-1500, this software element corrects a student as they complete a CMS-1500 form block-by-block. If any incorrect information is provided, the program corrects the student immediately. This software offers both direction and insight to students on how to complete a claim form. This element accompanies select exercises, and serves as an introduction to complete a CMS-1500 form.

Practice Management

This real-life practice management software program simulates a professional environment and works with select claim form completion exercises throughout the workbook. Additionally, the practice management appendix will have instructions and simple exercises that can be applied at the discretion of the student or the instructor.

INSTRUCTOR'S RESOURCE MANUAL

This text is written in such a way so that it can be used in courses that range anywhere from 6 weeks in length to the more traditional 16-week semester. Sample course outlines, as well as syllabi, are included in the Instructor's Resource Manual. If an instructor feels that a particular chapter is not a good fit for his or her class, it can be eliminated from the course outline and substituted with other course material. Also, chapters do not have to be taught in the sequence they are presented.

The Instructor's Resource Manual contains an extensive amount of information and resources for both experienced and newer instructors. The Manual is a culmination of the author's own personal education, work, and teaching experiences over the past 22 years. It will answer questions such as: "Where do I begin?", "How do I assess my students' work?", and "Are the students learning what they need to learn in order to successfully perform out in the real world?" The Manual should be used to supplement the textbook and Student Workbook. The textbook and the Student Workbook have been created for use in the following programs:

- Medical Assisting
- Health Information Management
- Medical Reimbursement Specialist
- Billing and Coding Specialist
- Medical Office Administration

Teaching is a complex task, and this Manual will assist with instructional planning, delivery, and evaluation. A successful instructor must understand the various steps involved in effective teaching. To get the full benefit of this Manual, new and experienced instructors can adopt or adapt various teaching aids from the examples included in the various sections.

TEST BANK

A comprehensive, customizable Test Bank is part of the instructor's material; it includes true and false, multiple choice, matching, and short answer questions. Using ExamView®, instructors can create customized tests or quizzes.

POWERPOINT PRESENTATIONS

PowerPoint slides are included with the instructor's material. These slides are best used as visual summaries of chapter information to supplement oral presentations. Instructors are cautioned against using PowerPoint slides to completely replace lecture and interactive learning.

EVOLVE® LEARNING RESOURCES

The Evolve® site is a free, interactive learning resource that works in coordination with the textbook material. It provides Internet-based course management tools for the instructor and content-related resources for the student. Some of the outstanding features include the ability to:

- Post class syllabi, outlines, and lecture notes
- Set up "virtual office hours" and e-mail communication
- Share important dates and information through the online class calendar
- Encourage student participation through chat rooms and discussion boards

Janet I. Beik, AA, BA, MEd

Acknowledgments

Since this is my first textbook, I initially saw the process as a daunting and tremendous undertaking; however, with the expert help of many people, the experience proved to be both exciting and challenging. I particularly want to express my sincere thanks and heartfelt appreciation to those at Elsevier who assisted me in compiling *Health Insurance Today: A Practical Approach*, especially: Susan Cole, Colin Odell, Pat Joiner, Jennifer Clark, and Jyotika Shroff. Also, I would like to express my gratitude to all the reviewers for their encouragement, suggestions, patience, and helpful guidance. Last, but certainly not least, I would like to thank several of my former students who are now successfully employed by local healthcare facilities (particularly Stephanie Paulus), as well as some of my professional colleagues, for their support and advice.

Janet I. Beik, AA, BA, MEd

Contents

UNIT 1 BUILDING A FOUNDATION

Chapter 4 **TYPES AND SOURCES OF HEALTH INSURANCE**

UNIT 2   HEALTH INSURANCE BASICS

Chapter 5 **THE "UNIVERSAL" CLAIM FORM: CMS-1500**

Chapter 6 TRADITIONAL FEE-FOR-SERVICE/PRIVATE PLANS

Chapter 7 UNRAVELING THE MYSTERIES OF MANAGED CARE

Chapter 8 UNDERSTANDING MEDICAID

Chapter 9 **CONQUERING MEDICARE'S CHALLENGES**

Chapter 10 **MILITARY CARRIERS: TRICARE AND CHAMPVA**

Chapter 11 **MISCELLANEOUS CARRIERS: WORKERS' COMPENSATION AND DISABILITY INSURANCE**

UNIT 3   CRACKING THE CODES

Chapter 12 **DIAGNOSTIC CODING**

Chapter 13 PROCEDURAL, EVALUATION AND MANAGEMENT AND HCPCS CODING

UNIT 4   THE CLAIMS PROCESS

Chapter 14 THE PATIENT

Chapter 15 **THE CLAIM**

UNIT 5   ADVANCED APPLICATION

Chapter 16 **THE ROLE OF COMPUTERS IN HEALTH INSURANCE**

Chapter 17 REIMBURSEMENT PROCEDURES: GETTING PAID

Chapter 18 HOSPITAL BILLING AND THE UB-92

APPENDICES

INDEX

UNIT I

Building A Foundation

Chapter 1

Medical Insurance: Where Did It Come From?

CHAPTER OBJECTIVES

After completion of this chapter, the student should be able to
- Define the terms used in the chapter.
- Explain medical insurance.
- Discuss how medical insurance got its start in the United States.
- Outline the important changes in the evolution of health insurance.
- Describe methods for acquiring health insurance.
- Explore reasons why some Americans can and others cannot get access to health insurance.
- List the reasons why healthcare and health insurance costs have skyrocketed.
- Explain why people buy health insurance.
- Identify the basic types of health insurance.

CHAPTER TERMS

Consolidated Omnibus Budget Reconciliation Act (COBRA)
cost sharing
entity/entities
fee-for-service
group plans
health insurance
Health Insurance Portability and Accountability Act (HIPAA)
Health Maintenance Organization (HMO) Act

indemnify
indemnity insurance
insurance
insured
insurer
managed healthcare
medical insurance
policy
preexisting conditions
premium
preventive medicine

OPENING SCENARIO

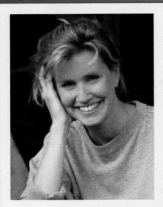

Joy Cassabaum, a single mother of two, has worked at a manufacturing plant in a Midwestern city for nearly 10 years. When the plant closed and moved their facilities out of the country, Joy found herself at the threshold of a new life and a new vocation. Joy decided she wanted a career change—something different from factory work, something more interesting and challenging. When Joy and her friend Barbara decided to attend a college career fair, she was intrigued by a presentation given by the healthcare instructors on medical insurance. Joy was vaguely aware of what healthcare insurance was all about, but never paid a lot of attention to it. Her former employer had provided excellent benefits, and when she or one of her children was ill or injured, they went to the doctor and basically forgot about it. If and when a bill came, she paid it, putting her trust in the doctor's staff. Now that she is unemployed, she not only has to make some smart career moves, but also she has to start thinking about things she had taken for granted before her layoff, and health insurance for her family had not even entered her mind until now.

Joy and Barbara signed up for the insurance billing specialist program at the local community college and eagerly began the first step on the path of their new careers. Let's follow them through their steps toward their goal of becoming health insurance specialists.

WHAT IS INSURANCE?

To understand medical **insurance**, you have to know a little about insurance in general. First, let's look at a typical dictionary definition of insurance:

The act or business, through legal means (normally a written contract), of protecting an individual's person or property against loss or harm arising out of specified circumstances in return for payment, called a **premium**.

The insuring party (called the **insurer**) agrees to **indemnify** (or reimburse) the **insured** for loss that occurs under the terms of the contract.

Now that we know that insurance is basically financial protection against loss or harm, let's break it into smaller pieces. Insurance, as we know it, is a written agreement between two parties (or **entities**), called a **policy**, whereby one entity (the insurance company) promises to pay a specific sum of money to a second entity (often an individual, or it could be another company) if certain specified undesirable events occur. Examples of undesirable events include a windstorm blows a tree over on a house, a car is stolen, or—as in the case of medical insurance— an illness or injury occurs. In return for this promise for financial protection against loss, the second entity (the insured) periodically pays a specific sum of money (premium) to the insurance company in exchange for this protection.

Now that we have a pretty good understanding of what insurance is in general, let's look at **medical insurance** (or **health insurance**, as it is frequently called). Medical insurance narrows down the "undesirable events" mentioned earlier to illnesses and injuries. The insurance

Imagine This!

John and Anna Smith buy a house for $50,000. That's a lot of money, and the Smiths have worked hard to save up for this purchase. Now, they look at the house and wonder, what if a strong wind blows the roof off? Or, worse yet, what if there is an electrical malfunction and the house catches fire? Along comes a neighbor who says, "Hey, I work for Colossus Insurance Company, and I'll write up an agreement saying that if you pay me $500 a year, Colossus will foot the bills for any repair or replacement your house suffers in case of a storm, a fire, or most other bad stuff that can happen." The Smiths think, "Wow! This is great," and agree to the neighbor's offer. So, a contract is drawn up (the insurance policy), John and Anna pay the neighbor $500, their worries about their new house are relieved, and they sleep soundly each night. Homeowners' insurance protects people from having to pay large sums of money out of their own pocket to repair or replace their home in the event of fire, storm, theft, or other hazards.

company promises to pay part (or sometimes all, depending on the policy) of the financial expenses incurred as a result of medical procedures, services, and certain supplies performed or provided by healthcare professionals if and when an individual becomes sick or injured. Some insurance policies also pay medical expenses even if the individual is not sick or injured. Healthcare providers and companies that sell health insurance have determined that it is often less costly to keep an individual well or catch an emerging illness in its early stages when it is more treatable than pay more exorbitant expenses later on should that individual become seriously ill. This is referred to as **preventive medicine**.

Medical insurance may sound a little intimidating to some, but students should not be apprehensive when they hear the term. A good analogy to put medical insurance into perspective might be to compare it with a picture puzzle. When the individual puzzle pieces are dumped onto a table, there is little meaning or continuity to the jumble of pieces lying haphazardly on the table-top. Then slowly, as the pieces are assembled, a picture begins to take shape, and the puzzle starts making sense. Similarly, medical insurance can be perplexing as individual concepts are presented, but when you "look at the whole picture," it becomes clearer and more understandable. As we begin to appreciate how the puzzle pieces fit together, we can understand the whole picture more easily when the puzzle is at last completed. Fig. 1-1 illustrates how the "medical insurance puzzle" is assembled.

● Stop and Think

Read the paragraph again comparing health insurance with a picture puzzle. Can you think of other applicable analogies that would help make the various components of health insurance more understandable at this point?

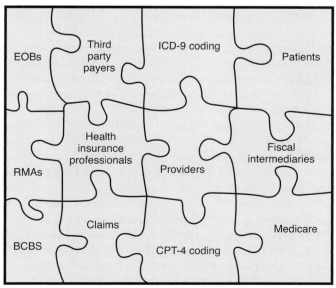

Fig. 1-1 The insurance "puzzle."

What Did You Learn?

1. Give a brief definition of insurance.
2. Medical insurance narrows down "undesirable events" to what two categories?
3. What is the term used when medical services and procedures are performed to keep a person well or prevent a catastrophic illness?

HISTORY

Insurance is not a recent phenomenon. The word "insurance" is derived from the Latin word *securitas*, which translates into the English word, "security."

From the beginning of time, people have looked for ways to ease the misfortunes of existence. It has been common knowledge down through the ages that it has been very difficult for any one individual to survive for long on his or her own. Prehistoric humans quickly learned that to survive, the resources of others must be pooled.

Imagine This!

It's ancient Babylon. Merchants are constantly being robbed or captured for ransom as their caravans cross the desert or as their ships sail off to trade with Egypt, Phoenicia, India, and China. One wealthy businessman, who made loans to the traders—we'll call him Ali-baba Gosmere—conceived a clever plan. As the traders came to him to borrow money for their journeys, he told the merchants, "For two additional gold coins, I will forgive your loan if you are robbed!" The traders thought, "Wow! How can we lose with this deal?" This clever lender, by collecting these "premiums" from many such traders, was able to absorb the losses of the few unfortunate ones who were robbed. And, as these stories go, everyone pretty much lived happily ever after. (According to documented history, this practice was later legalized in the *Code of Hammurabi*.)

Rhodes (an ancient civilization) had an extensive code of sea laws, including the principle of "jettison" or "general average." This law stated that if it becomes necessary to throw goods overboard to lighten the ships in case the safety of the crew became threatened, such sacrifice that benefited all on board should be made good by a common contribution. These laws of the sea, including Solon's Greek laws, found their way into early Roman civil codes and into the laws of the Byzantine Empire. They still exist today as part of our own laws for protection against losses at sea.

The beginnings of modern health insurance occurred in London in 1850, when a company offered coverage for medical expenses for bodily injuries that did not result in death. By the end of that same year in the United States, the Franklin Health Assurance Company of Massachusetts began offering medical expense coverage on a basis resembling health insurance as we know it now. By 1866, many other insurance companies began writing health insurance policies. These early policies were mostly for loss of income and provided health benefits for a few of the serious diseases that were common at that time— typhus, typhoid, scarlet fever, smallpox, diphtheria, and diabetes. People did not refer to these arrangements as "insurance," but the concept was the same.

In the United States, the birth of health insurance came in 1929 when Justin Ford Kimball, an official at Baylor University in Dallas, Texas, introduced a plan to guarantee schoolteachers 21 days of hospital care for $6 a year. Other employee groups in Dallas soon joined the plan, and the idea caught on nationwide. This plan eventually evolved into what we now know as Blue Cross. The Blue Shield concept grew out of the lumber and mining camps of the Pacific Northwest at the turn of the 20th century. Employers, wanting to provide medical care for their workers, paid monthly fees to "medical service bureaus," which were composed of groups of physicians. The Blue Cross and Blue Shield plans traditionally established premiums by community rating—that is, everybody in the community paid the same premium.

 HIPAA Tip

HIPAA amended the Employee Retirement Income Security Act (ERISA) to provide new rights and protections for participants and beneficiaries in group health plans. Understanding this amendment is important in decisions about future health coverage. HIPAA contains protections for health coverage offered in connection with employment (group health plans) and for individual insurance policies sold by insurance companies (individual policies).

Refer to the list of websites at the end of this chapter to explore more interesting and detailed facts related to the history of insurance.

What Did You Learn?

1. What is the Latin word for insurance, and what is its literal English translation?
2. The principle of the "jettison" law was designed for what purpose?
3. What did early insurance policies in the United States typically cover?

METAMORPHOSIS OF MEDICAL INSURANCE

If you ever took a biology course, you may remember how certain insects go through several stages—from the caterpillar to the pupa and from the pupa to the adult butterfly. This is called metamorphosis. By definition, "metamorphosis" is "a profound change in form from one stage to the next in the life history of an organism." The transformation of health insurance from what it was in the beginning to what we know it to be today can be compared with this metamorphosis, although the transformation of health insurance as it was in the beginning into what it has evolved in the 21st century certainly does not resemble a beautiful butterfly—perhaps more that of an ugly duckling into the proverbial swan. To illustrate this changing process, Table 1-1 presents a health insurance timeline.

You should now be familiar with how medical insurance got started and how it developed into what we know as modern health insurance today. It also is important to know how it has changed throughout history and what caused these changes. As you might imagine, politics has played a big role in the development of health insurance in the United States. Support for government health insurance began when Theodore Roosevelt made national health insurance one of the major propositions of the Progressive Party during the 1912 presidential campaign, but the plan was eventually defeated. After 1920, opposition to government-sponsored plans was led by the American Medical Association (AMA) out of concern that government involvement in healthcare would lead to socialized medicine—a public tax–supported national healthcare system. During the middle of the 20th century, it became obvious that something needed to be done to provide medical care for the elderly. In 1965, during President Lyndon B. Johnson's administration, Federal legislation was enacted, resulting in *Medicare* for the elderly and *Medicaid* for the indigent. Since 1966, public and private health insurance has played a key role in financing healthcare costs in the United States. Medicare and Medicaid are examined more closely in later chapters.

Figs. 1-2 and 1-3 illustrate where U.S. health dollars come from and how they are spent.

The structure and system of care that today is known as managed care traces its history to a series of alternative healthcare arrangements that appeared in various communities across the United States in the 19th century. The goal of these arrangements was to help meet the healthcare needs of select groups of people, including rural residents and workers and families in the lumber, mining, and railroad industries. The enrollees paid a set fee to physicians, who delivered care under the terms of their agreement. In urban areas, such groups often were paid by charitable groups to provide care to their members or charges. These prepaid group practices were a

TABLE 1-1   Health Insurance Timeline

	1900s	1910s	1920s	1930s	1940s	1950s	1960s	1970s	1980s	1990s	2000s
Row 1	American Medical Association (AMA) becomes a powerful national force. Membership increases from about 8000 physicians in 1900 to 70,000 in 1910—half of the physicians in U.S. This is the beginning of "organized medicine"	U.S. hospitals now modern scientific institutions, valuing antiseptics, cleanliness, and using medications for the relief of pain	Reformers emphasize the cost of medical care instead of wages lost to sickness—the relatively higher cost of medical care is a new and dramatic development, especially for the middle class	The Depression changes priorities, with greater emphasis on unemployment insurance and "old age" benefits	Penicillin comes into use	Attention turns to Korea and away from health reform; U.S. has a system of private insurance for those who can afford it and welfare services for the poor	In the 1950s, the price of hospital care doubled. Now in the early 1960s, those outside workplace, especially the elderly, have difficulty affording insurance	Prepaid group healthcare plans are renamed health maintenance organizations (HMOs), with legislation that provides federal endorsement, certification, and assistance	Overall, there is a shift toward privatization and corporation of healthcare	Healthcare costs rise at double the rate of inflation	Healthcare costs continue to rise
Row 2	Surgery is becoming more common	American Association for Labor Legislation (AALL) organizes first national conference on "social insurance"	Growing cultural influence of the medical profession—physicians' incomes are higher, and prestige is established	Social Security Act is passed, omitting health insurance	Prepaid group healthcare begins, seen as radical	Federal responsibility for the sick is firmly established	More than 700 insurance companies sell health insurance		Under President Reagan, Medicare shifts to payment by diagnosis (DRG) instead of by treatment. Private plans quickly follow suit	Expansion of managed care helps to moderate increases in healthcare costs	Medicare is viewed by some as unsustainable under the present structure and must be "rescued"

TABLE 1-1   Health Insurance Timeline—cont'd

1900s	1910s	1920s	1930s	1940s	1950s	1960s	1970s	1980s	1990s	2000s
Physicians are no longer expected to provide free services to all hospital patients	Progressive reformers gaining support for health insurance	Rural health facilities are seen by many as inadequate	Against the advice of insurance professionals, Blue Cross begins offering private coverage for hospital care in dozens of states	To compete for workers, companies begin to offer health benefits, giving rise to the employer-based system in place today	Many more medications are available now to treat a range of diseases, including infections, glaucoma, and arthritis, and new vaccines become available that prevent dreaded childhood diseases, including polio. The first successful organ transplant is performed	Major medical insurance endorses high-cost medicine	Healthcare costs escalate rapidly; U.S. medicine is now seen as in crisis	Growing complaints by insurance companies that the traditional fee-for-service method of payment to physicians is being exploited	By the end of the decade, there are 44 million Americans—16% of the nation—with no health insurance at all	Changing demographics of the workplace lead many to believe the employer-based system of insurance cannot last
U.S. lags behind European countries in finding value in insuring against costs of sickness	Opposition from physicians and other interest groups and the entry of the U.S. into World War I in 1917 undermine reform front	Penicillin is discovered, but it will be 20 years before it is widely used to combat infection and disease		Congress is asked to pass an "economic bill of rights," including right to adequate medical care		President signs Medicare and Medicaid into law	Growing complaints by insurance companies that the traditional fee-for-service method of payment to physicians is being exploited	"Capitation" payments to physicians become more common	Human Genome Project to identify all of the >100,000 genes in human DNA gets under way	Human Genome Project to identify all of the >100,000 genes in human DNA is expected to be completed 2 years ahead of schedule, in 2003
Railroads are the leading industry to develop extensive employee medical programs				President offers a single-system, national health program plan that would include all Americans		Number of physicians reporting themselves as full-time specialists grows from 55% in 1960 to 69%	Healthcare costs rise at double the rate of inflation Expansion of managed care helps to moderate increases in healthcare costs		By June 1990, 139,765 people in the U.S. have HIV/AIDS with a 60% mortality rate	Direct-to-consumer advertising for pharmaceuticals and medical devices is on the rise

HIV/AIDS, human immunodeficiency virus/acquired immunodeficiency syndrome.

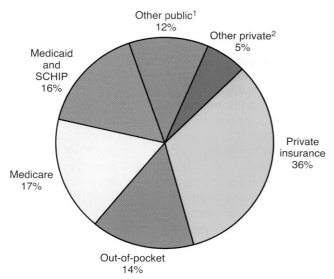

Fig. 1-2 Pie chart of "The Nation's Health Dollar: 2002 (Where It Came From)." (Courtesy of Centers for Medicare and Medicaid Services, Office of the Actuary, National Health Statistics Group.)

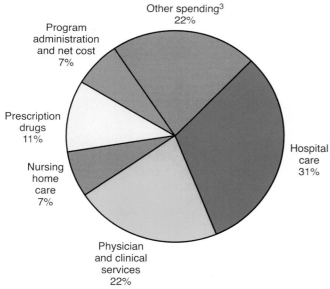

Fig. 1-3 Pie chart of "The Nation's Health Dollar: 2002 (Where It Went)." (Courtesy of Centers for Medicare and Medicaid Services, Office of the Actuary, National Health Statistics Group.)

[1]"Other Public" includes programs such as workers' compensation, public health activity, Department of Defense, Department of Veterans Affairs, Indian Health Service, state and local hospital subsidies, and school health.

[2]"Other Private" includes industrial in-plate, privately funded construction, and nonpatient revenues, including philanthropy.

[3]"Other Spending" includes dentist services, other professional services, home healthcare, durable medical products, over-the-counter medicines and sundries, public health, research, and construction.

model for later entities that came to be known as health maintenance organizations (HMOs).

In 1973, Congress passed the **Health Maintenance Organization (HMO)** Act, which provided grants to employers who set up HMOs. An HMO is a plan that provides healthcare to its enrollees from specific physicians and hospitals that contract with the plan. Usually there are no deductibles to be met, no claim forms to be completed by the enrollee, and a geographically restricted service area. HMOs were intended to be a low-cost alternative to the more traditional **indemnity insurance**, the "standard" type of health insurance individuals can purchase, which provides comprehensive major medical benefits and allows insured individuals to choose any physician or hospital when seeking medical care. By 1997, more than 600 HMOs were in existence providing healthcare to nearly 70 million people in the United States. More detailed information on managed healthcare and HMOs is presented in Chapter 7.

What Did You Learn?

1. How is the transformation of health insurance from what it was in the beginning to what it is today comparable to the metamorphosis of a caterpillar to a butterfly?
2. Why are some people and certain organizations in the United States opposed to the government getting involved in health insurance?
3. What two federal programs got their start in the 1960s during President Johnson's administration?

KEY HEALTH INSURANCE ISSUES

We know that health insurance is a constantly changing industry. At the time of this writing, the factors driving key healthcare issues were confidentiality, patients' rights, and prescription drug coverage for the elderly. Experts predict that lawmakers next will focus their healthcare reform efforts in the following areas:

• Expanding access for the uninsured
• Regulation of managed care plans
• Restrictions on drug formularies and related pharmacy issues
• Stabilizing emergency medical services

In the future, key issues might revolve around safeguarding individuals from the improper use of genetic information, creating precise definitions of "genetic tests" and "genetic information," or perhaps even cloning. Meanwhile, this text focuses on current healthcare issues that affect everyone.

HOW DO PEOPLE GET HEALTH INSURANCE?

Most people who have health insurance get it from one of two major sources—the government or private organizations. As mentioned earlier, the government provides health insurance programs to specific groups, such as the elderly and people who qualify because their income is below the federal poverty level. Most Americans get private health insurance through their employers.

People pay for health insurance in a variety of ways. Many individuals employed full-time (or for a specific number of hours, e.g., 30 or 35, per week) are eligible for a **group plan** and have the cost of insurance premiums (or a certain portion of them) deducted from their paychecks. A group health insurance plan is one insurance policy that covers a group of people. Usually a business entity establishes a group health insurance plan to cover its employees; however, group plans are not limited to employers. Often clubs and organizations, chambers of commerce, special interest groups, trade associations, and church/religious groups organize healthcare for their members.

Until the early 1990s, employers, especially larger ones, commonly paid up to half of their employees' group health insurance premiums as an added benefit. In some cases, employers paid the entire cost of health insurance directly. As healthcare costs increased, however, along with medical insurance premiums, this practice became less common.

Individuals who do not have health insurance benefits through their employment or through government programs can purchase private health insurance policies directly from a commercial insurance company. In the case of the latter, premiums are usually much higher than employer-sponsored plans, and individuals typically must complete a detailed healthcare questionnaire. Often (depending on the person's age and other factors), certain illnesses or injuries that exist before an effective date of the insurance policy are not covered. These are referred to as **preexisting conditions**.

ACCESS TO HEALTH INSURANCE

According to the 2000 census, nearly 40 million people in the United States did not have health insurance coverage. Individuals who are typically without insurance are those who are

1. self-employed,
2. employed only part-time, or
3. work in low-wage jobs that offer no benefits.

These groups typically do not have access to low-cost, employer-sponsored group plans. Most of these individuals cannot afford individual healthcare insurance, and they usually do not qualify for government-sponsored

programs. In 2004, nearly half of all full-time workers in low-paying jobs were uninsured. Part-time workers are often left out because many businesses that operate on a narrow profit margin, specifically businesses in the service industry, try to keep costs to a minimum to compete in the marketplace.

Although millions of Americans lack health insurance because they cannot afford it, many others who can afford it cannot buy it because insurance companies consider them "high risk" owing to the fact that they may need expensive healthcare in the future. Insurance companies assess the chances of whether or not applicants are likely to need expensive future medical care and group them into classes of risk. Individuals who are considered average or better than average risks (basically the young and healthy) usually can purchase insurance policies at a relatively affordable price. If the insurance company thinks an applicant presents too much risk, he or she is put into a high-risk pool; if the individual is allowed to enroll in the healthcare program, he or she is charged a much larger premium. Alternatively the insurance company may refuse to insure a high-risk individual at all.

During the 1980s and 1990s, insurance companies, in an effort to keep costs down, began including a preexisting condition clause in their health insurance policies. This clause often denies access to anyone who already has a medical condition, or at least the insurer would not pay for medical expenses incurred as a result of that particular condition.

Imagine This!

Fred Simmons had been a factory worker at Acme Auto Repair. After 20 years working on the line, Fred decided to open up his own body shop, repairing wrecked automobiles in his garage. Fred had previously been covered under Acme's group insurance plan, but after he became self-employed, he applied for a private policy with Top-Notch Insurance. When the Top-Notch representative asked Fred to fill out an application form, one of the questions was, "Have you ever been treated for, or have had any symptoms of, heart disease?" Fred, honest man that he was, checked "yes," and for an explanatory note, stated, "I went to the emergency room in April of last year with chest pains." Top-Notch, afraid that Fred was in imminent danger of a heart attack, agreed to sell Fred an insurance policy, but excluded payment for any treatment involving his heart, which they determined was a preexisting condition.

As a result of this preexisting condition clause, people found it difficult to change jobs if they, or any of their dependents, had a serious health condition. To get around this problem, Congress introduced the **Health Insurance Portability and Accountability Act (HIPAA)** of 1996, which (among other things) requires most employer-sponsored group health insurance plans to accept transfers from other group plans without imposing a preexisting condition clause. Additional information regarding the HIPAA Act is presented in Chapter 3.

Another provision that serves to prevent people from losing their healthcare coverage is the **Consolidated Omnibus Budget Reconciliation Act (COBRA)**, a health benefit act that Congress passed in 1986. Under COBRA, when an employee quits his or her job or is laid off (or has hours reduced) from a company with 20 or more workers, the law requires the employer to extend group health coverage to the employee and his or her dependents at group rates for 18 months and in some cases up to 36 months. Group health coverage for COBRA participants is usually more expensive than health coverage for active employees because the employer usually pays a part of the premium for active employees, whereas COBRA participants generally pay the entire premium themselves. Coverage under COBRA is less expensive, however, than individual health coverage. More information on COBRA is presented later in this text.

WHY DO HEALTHCARE AND MEDICAL INSURANCE COST SO MUCH?

We all know that the costs of healthcare have increased a lot in recent years. In 1980, Americans spent nearly $250 billion on healthcare. By 1999, that figure had more than quadrupled to $1.2 trillion, and it is projected to total $2.6 trillion (almost 16% of the gross domestic product) by 2010. Fig. 1-4 shows the growth in national health expenditures in the past 2 decades along with the projected expenditure for the present decade.

 HIPAA Tip

The four main provisions of HIPAA are that it
1. allows portability of health insurance coverage;
2. protects workers and their families from pre-existing conditions when they change or lose their jobs;
3. establishes national standards for electronic healthcare transactions and national identifiers for providers, health plans, and employers; and
4. addresses the security and privacy of health data.

Adopting these standards would improve the efficiency and effectiveness of health in the United States.

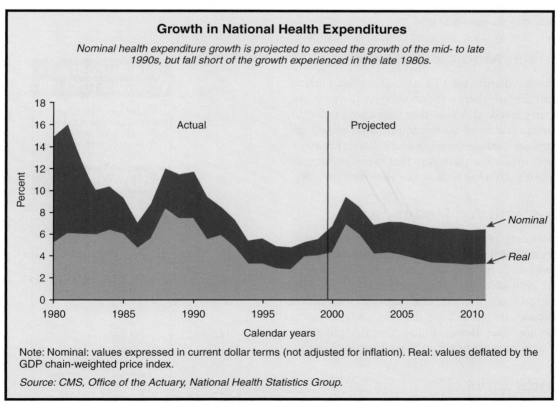

Fig. 1-4 Chart showing growth in national health expenditures. (Courtesy of Centers for Medicare and Medicaid Services, Office of the Actuary, National Health Statistics Group.)

Many factors are to blame for this enormous increase in healthcare costs. Because of the complexity of the problem and the issues involved, it is easy to jump to conclusions that are not based on careful consideration of all the facts. Some blame the insurance companies for these increasing costs, but one of the largest health insurance companies in the United States claims that, contrary to common opinion, administrative costs of processing claims and providing customer service for members amounts to only a small portion of escalating premium dollars. The lion's share goes to pay for the medical care that members receive, and because the cost of this care keeps increasing, members' premiums keep increasing. Some reasons and explanations experts give to try to explain the increasing cost of healthcare are presented in the following paragraphs.

Americans Are Living Longer than Ever Before

In 1900, the average life expectancy of Americans was about 50 years. In 2000, life expectancy was 76 years. You may have heard the phrase, "the graying of America." During the 20th century, the number of people in the United States who were 65 years old or older increased 11-fold. In 1900, only 1 in every 25 Americans made up this age group; however, by the early 1990s, 1 out of every 8 Americans was 65 or older, and elderly people typically require more healthcare. When older Americans join an insured group, the entire group's healthcare risks, along with the costs, increase accordingly.

Advances in Medical Technology

Years ago, when individuals had a serious disease, such as cancer or heart disease, there were no effective ways to treat it, and often they just died. Today, new technology (chemotherapy and organ and bone marrow transplants) and equipment (magnetic resonance imaging and robotics) provide treatments for medical conditions that were previously untreatable, but these new treatments are very expensive.

More Demand for Healthcare

In years past, many people would treat their illnesses at home, reluctant to go to physicians, and many were actually afraid of hospitals. Now, it seems that the trend is to see a physician for even minor medical problems. In the past, people tended to accept certain physical problems, such as sexual dysfunction, attention deficit disorder, and depression as their "lot in life." This increase in the general population's demand for healthcare resulted in higher medical costs.

Media Intervention

The media is partly to blame also. How many of us have watched a commercial on television where someone has

an ache or a pain? A charismatic voice announces that if you are suffering from this or that ailment, some new drug might be the answer, so, "Ask your doctor if Curitall is right for you!" Fig. 1-5 illustrates how the costs of outpatient services and prescription drugs have risen in the last 5 years.

COST SHARING

Cost sharing (a situation where insured individuals pay a portion of the healthcare costs, such as deductibles, coinsurance, or copayment amounts) is one method of curbing the rising cost of health insurance premiums. Most covered workers are in health plans that require a deductible be met before most plan benefits are provided, after which the individual must pay a copayment or a percentage of coinsurance per encounter. In the past, a typical deductible was in the range of $250 to $500 and coinsurance 10% to 20%. Today, to afford premiums, deductibles of $2500 or even $5000 are common. Coinsurance has remained in the 10% to 20% range, however.

What Did You Learn?

1. What four key factors drive healthcare costs up?
2. Explain the importance of creating *precise definitions* of genetic tests and genetic information.

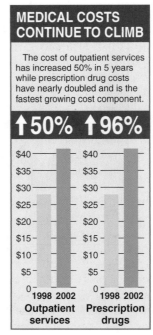

Fig. 1-5 Chart showing how the costs of outpatient services and prescription drugs have risen. (Data from U.S. Department of Health and Human Services.)

REASONS FOR HEALTH INSURANCE

We know why people need health insurance: to protect them from paying out large sums of money, sometimes to the point of bankruptcy, for quality medical care. In some parts of the United States, a 1-day stay in a hospital can cost $1000, and that's just for the room. If surgery is involved, this cost can easily zoom up to $10,000. Most Americans cannot afford to pay these kinds of medical bills out of their own pockets.

Although there is no way to know how much healthcare one individual will need in the future, insurance experts (called actuaries) use statistics to predict the healthcare costs of a large group. Based on these anticipated costs, an insurance company can establish premiums for the members of that group. The basic idea behind insurance is that each person who buys a policy with that particular insurance company technically agrees to pay a share of the group's total losses in exchange for a promise that the group will pay his or her healthcare costs if and when needed. By doing this, the group as a whole shoulders the burden of paying for expensive medical care for the few who may need it.

MEDICAL INSURANCE PLANS

There are basically two categories of private insurance plans—indemnity plans, as we discussed earlier, and managed care plans. The indemnity plan (also called **fee-for-service**) is the type of plan most Americans were covered under until the last 2 decades. Under this type of plan, patients can go to any healthcare provider or hospital they choose, medical bills are sent to the insurance carrier, and the patient (or healthcare provider) is reimbursed according to rules of the policy. Managed care plans function differently.

Any system of healthcare payment or delivery arrangements in which the health plan attempts to control or coordinate use of health services by its enrolled members to contain health expenditures, improve quality, or both falls under the category of **managed healthcare**. Arrangements often involve a defined delivery system of providers with some form of contractual arrangement with the plan. Under managed healthcare plans, patients see designated providers, and benefits are paid according to the structure of the managed care plan. With both types of plans, patients and the insurance company share the cost of services rendered. Lately, many people have become disillusioned with some managed healthcare plans, which has led to changes. Now, some of these plans allow their enrollees to choose from a range of providers who are not employed directly by the plan. Managed care is discussed in detail in Chapter 7.

As mentioned earlier, in addition to private healthcare plans, there are two government-funded plans: Medicare,

which provides healthcare coverage for individuals age 65 and older and individuals with certain disabilities, and Medicaid, which provides healthcare coverage for qualifying low-income individuals. Both of these plans are discussed individually and in more detail in later chapters.

● Stop and Think

Compare the concept of today's health insurance "cost sharing" with the ancient sailors of Babylon.

SUMMARY CHECK POINTS

☑ Medical insurance can be defined as financial protection from loss or harm as a result of medical care and treatment owing to illness and injuries. When an individual purchases an insurance policy, the insuring company promises to pay a portion of the financial expenses incurred (as outlined in the policy) resulting from any medical procedures, services, and certain supplies performed or provided by healthcare professionals if and when the insured or his or her dependents become sick or injured. In return for this financial protection, the insured individual pays a monthly (or periodic) premium.

☑ Medical insurance in the United States began shortly after the turn of the 20th century as a result of a contract between schoolteachers and a hospital in Texas when the hospital agreed to provide certain services for a set number of days for a nominal fee.

☑ Medical insurance has gone through many stages to evolve into what we know it to be today. Politics has played a big role in this growth and change and is responsible for the advent of major government-sponsored plans—Medicare and Medicaid—and HMOs. Important changes include the following:
- Employer-sponsored group health plans
- Creation of Medicare and Medicaid
- Development of managed care
- HIPAA

☑ There are two major sources where people can get access to health insurance: (1) government-sponsored programs and (2) private organizations.

☑ People on both ends of the health insurance spectrum tend to acquire access to medical insurance—individuals who are poor or elderly and individuals who work and are eligible for benefits through an employer-sponsored group plan. Individuals in the middle—part-time workers or workers in low-wage jobs—are often left out.

☑ Healthcare costs and premiums have increased exponentially in recent years as a result of many factors, as follows:
- Americans are living longer than ever before
- Advances in medical technology, leading to more expensive equipment and methods of treatment

- More demand for healthcare
- Media intervention

☑ People buy health insurance to protect them from financial loss or ruin, as just one overnight stay in a hospital coupled with a surgical procedure can cost thousands of dollars.

☑ The two basic types of health insurance plans are indemnity (fee-for-service) and managed care.

CLOSING SCENARIO

After the orientation and the first several class sessions, Joy and Barbara believe they have made the right choice in enrolling in a health careers program in the community college. After completing the first chapter of the text, the women know a health insurance professional career track is right for them. Joy is pleasantly surprised that the topic of insurance can be interesting, especially its history.

One of the most important things the women are experiencing is a growing "camaraderie" with other students in the class and the new friends they are making. During breaks and after class, the women shared ideas, suggestions, and tips and confided worries, concerns, and expectations with their peers.

WEBSITES TO EXPLORE

For live links to the following websites, please visit the Evolve® site at http://evolve.elsevier.com/Beik/today/

- If you are interested in learning more about the evolution of health insurance in the United States, log on to the PBS website and study the Healthcare Timeline table:
http://www.pbs.org/healthcarecrisis/history.htm

- For more information on HIPAA, log on to the following website:
http://www.cms.hhs.gov/hipaa/

- It is important for the health insurance professional to know about COBRA. The following URL will direct your search to an informative website that includes the full text of COBRA:
http://www.cobrainsurance.com/

Chapter 2

Tools of the Trade: A Career as a Health (Medical) Insurance Professional

Chapter Outline

I. Your Future as a Health Insurance Professional
  A. Required Skills and Interests
    1. Education
    2. Preparation
II. Job Duties and Responsibilities

III. Career Prospects
  A. Opportunities
  B. Rewards
IV. Certification Possibilities

CHAPTER OBJECTIVES

After completion of this chapter, the student should be able to

- List the entry-level skills necessary for success in the health insurance professional's career.
- Discuss college courses typically included in a medical insurance billing and coding program.
- Explain the importance of effective study skills and proper preparation to maximize learning.
- Understand the importance of effective time management.
- Identify desirable personality traits and on-the-job skills health insurance professionals should possess to optimize career success.
- Classify various job titles and their corresponding duties included under the general umbrella of "health insurance professional."
- Explore career prospects and job opportunities for health insurance professionals.
- Predict possible rewards of a career in medical related fields.
- Investigate certification possibilities related to the field of insurance billing and coding.

CHAPTER TERMS

application
autonomy
CMS-1500 claim form
certification
communication
comprehension
diligence

initiative
integrity
objectivity
paraphrase
prioritize
professional ethics

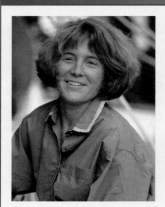

Joy and Barbara, two nontraditional students, are apprehensive about embarking on a new career path. The idea of becoming a health insurance professional sounded important and exciting, and they are willing and eager to learn. They share a common interest in the medical field, but neither one is interested in the clinical side of the profession. When Joy attended the college career fair, she knew immediately that this was an ideal vocation for her. She considered herself an organized person who paid attention to detail. She was treasurer of the PTA at her children's school and took pride in her impeccable bookkeeping. Barbara, too, believed her organizational skills were one of her strong suits, but the idea of detailed, hand-kept records did not appeal to her. Working with computers is what spurred her interest. Was it possible that both women could find their niche as health insurance professionals? Their instructor assured them they could, but it would involve a lot of work and dedication.

YOUR FUTURE AS A HEALTH INSURANCE PROFESSIONAL

Before you begin any college or vocational program, you might want to ask yourself, "Where will this take me, and what career opportunities are available to a graduate of this type of program?" There are several things you should think about. Naturally, the first question in many individuals' minds is, "How much money can I make?" That question is logical, but other factors should be considered when choosing a career. One wise person said, "If you choose a job you love, you'll never have to work a day the rest of your life."

Although there are many different career paths you can choose in the area of healthcare, this chapter refers to the domain of medical expertise of a "health insurance professional," sometimes referred to as a medical insurance specialist. There is not, however, any nationally recognized title or acronym for this broad specialty.

REQUIRED SKILLS AND INTERESTS

Success as a health insurance professional requires a certain degree of competency or knowledge in general educational areas. To increase the potential for success, candidates entering this field should possess college entry-level skills in the following areas:
- Reading and **comprehension** (understanding what you have read)
- Basic business math
- English and grammar
- Oral and written **communication** (sending and receiving information through speech, writing, or signs that is mutually understood)
- Keyboarding and office skills
- Computer **application** skills (ability to use computer hardware and software, including Windows and Microsoft Word [or similar word processing software], and ability to use the Internet)

Education

Many community colleges and career training schools offer programs that provide its graduates with the skills to become specialists in the health insurance field. Typically, students begin the program with core courses that are built on in the later stages of the program. They receive extensive hands-on training and practice in medical insurance billing and coding and computerized patient account management. Table 2-1 lists courses included in a typical insurance billing professional program.

Program length for a health insurance professional is 2 to 4 years at community colleges and technical schools and 4 to 9 months at a career school. Most community colleges offer a 2-year associate degree in this discipline. A 4-year college typically awards a bachelor of science degree in health science, healthcare management, or whatever specific health fields are offered. Diplomas and certificates also can be obtained from correspondence or online courses and home study programs. A graduate of a health insurance professional or billing and coding program has opportunities for entry-level employment as a medical biller, medical coder, or other health insurance–related position in hospitals, nursing homes, physicians' offices, ambulatory care facilities, medical or surgical supply companies, or billing service companies.

Preparation

Another important key for success in any career, besides basic entry-level skills and applicable education, is proper preparation. You might have deduced from the scenario that Joy and Barbara have been out of school for several years. Both women think their study skills need

TABLE 2-1	Courses in a Typical Insurance Billing Professional Program
Core Courses	Anatomy & Physiology Medical Terminology Keyboarding Word Processing Business English Business Math Medical Office Administrative Skills
Specialized Courses	Medical Transcription Medical Records Management Current Procedural Terminology (CPT) Coding International Classification of Diseases (ICD-9-CM) Coding Medical Insurance Billing Computerized Office Management Bookkeeping/Accounting

sharpening. To succeed in any formal college or training program, good study skills are a must.

Schools today encourage "lifelong learning." This means learning will not stop when you graduate from the college or career program you have chosen, but that you will continue to learn for the rest of your career—or, ideally, the rest of your life. In healthcare, this is especially true because this discipline is constantly changing. Many students who have been out of school for several years find that their study skills may be a little rusty. Even if you have been out of school for only a short time, you still may need help to "get back in the groove" of studying. The following is a list of suggestions that may help you develop effective study skills to enhance your chances of success:

1. **Prioritize your life.** Develop a weekly time management schedule in which tasks and activities are **prioritized** (organized by importance). Make sure this schedule
   - allows time for studying each specific subject,
   - spreads out study times throughout the week,
   - permits time for recreation and rest and family, and
   - grants periodic "rewards," such as watching TV or lunch out with friends.

   Make a list of the things you need to do (just as you make a list before you go grocery shopping). Don't create a schedule that is too detailed or rigid. As you progress, make adjustments as needed. Table 2-2 provides an example of a time management schedule.

2. **Learn how to study.** Choose a quiet, suitable area where you
   - can concentrate,
   - will have minimal interruptions,
   - can be comfortable enough to focus on your work, and
   - are close to resources (e.g., computer, reference materials).

3. **Develop positive personality traits.** Not everyone is suited to working in the field of medicine. Following is a list of desirable personality traits and qualities of character that experts believe an individual should possess to be successful in this field:
   - Self-discipline
   - A positive attitude
   - **Diligence** (sticking with a task until it is finished)
   - **Integrity** (having honest ethical and moral principles)
   - **Objectivity** (not influenced by personal feelings, biases, or prejudice)
   - **Initiative** (readiness and ability to take action)
   - Enthusiasm

● Stop and Think

Re-read the personality traits listed. Do you understand what each one means? Jot down a brief definition for each. Do you think you possess each of these personality traits? If there are any that you think you do not have or that you might need to improve on, list them along with ideas on how to develop these traits or make them better.

4. **Prepare for class.** Getting the most out of the courses you take involves effort on your part. The time and effort you invest in your preparation before class and the time you spend in class greatly affect what you get out of your schooling.
   - Attend every class and be on time.
   - Become an active participator—ask questions and take notes.

TABLE 2-2   Time Management Schedule

TIME	SUN	MON	TUES	WED	THUR	FRI	SAT
6:00	Sleep	Shower/eat	Shower/eat	Shower/eat	Shower/eat	Shower/eat	Sleep
7:00	Personal	Personal	Personal	Personal	Personal	Personal	Personal/breakfast
8:00	Breakfast	Bus	Bus	Bus	Bus	Bus	Chores
9:00	Family	Group Discussion Business Policy	Computer Lab Marketing Communications	Group Discussion Business Policy	Computer Lab Marketing Communications	Group Discussion Business Policy	
10:00							
11:00	Self	Marketing Research	Library	Marketing Research	Library	Marketing Research	Self
12:00	Lunch	Lunch		Lunch		Lunch	Lunch
1:00	Group study	Writing Lab	Lunch	Writing Lab	Lunch	Writing Lab	Chores
2:00			Group study/research Business and Professional Speaking		Group study/research Business and Professional Speaking		Shopping
3:00		Expository Writing	Sales Management	Expository Writing	Sales Management	Expository Writing	
4:00	Chores	Bus	Bus	Bus	Bus	Bus	Recreation and rest
5:00		Dinner/recreation and rest	Dinner/recreation and rest	Dinner/recreation and rest	Dinner/recreation and rest	Dinner/recreation and rest	
6:00	Dinner	Chores	Dinner/recreation and rest	Chores	Dinner/recreation and rest	Write paper for Expository Writing	Family
7:00	Study	Study	Bus/shopping	Study	Chores	Recreation and rest	Recreation and rest
8:00			Bus/study		Study		rest

- Learn to recognize important points in the text and from lectures.
- Outline, underline, highlight, or make notes in the text margins.
- Work through questions/examples until you understand them.
- Communicate with your instructor and other students.
- Become a good listener.
- Complete all homework and assigned readings on time.
- Develop the ability to concentrate.
- Enhance your reading comprehension. (After you read a section of the text, stop and ask yourself, "What are they trying to get across to me?")
- **Paraphrase** (write down in your own words) important facts from lectures.

● Stop and Think

Think about each of the bulleted points. Why do you think each one is important to your success as a student and as a career professional? Develop a plan for effective studying. Compare your study plan with those of your peers and share ideas. Keep working on your study plan until you have developed one that works for you.

In addition to the above-listed classroom skills, individuals experienced in working as health insurance professionals suggest that candidates for this field should possess the following on-the-job skills:

- Pay attention to detail
- Follow directions
- Work independently without supervision
- Understand the need for and possess a strong sense of **professional ethics** (moral principles associated with a specific vocation)
- Understand the need for and possess strong people skills (ability to communicate effectively with all types of individuals at all levels)
- Demonstrate patience and an even temperament
- Be empathetic without being sympathetic
- Be organized but flexible
- Be conscientiousness
- Demonstrate a sense of responsibility
- Possess manual dexterity
- Understand and respect the importance of confidentiality
- Demonstrate a willingness to learn

What Did You Learn?

1. List five required classroom skills that help ensure success as a health insurance professional.
2. Why is "preparation" an important key for success?
3. List five "on-the-job" skills that experienced health insurance professionals should possess.

JOB DUTIES AND RESPONSIBILITIES

We mentioned earlier that there are different career options you can choose that fall under the general umbrella of health insurance. The title we have chosen is "health insurance professional," which includes the knowledge and expertise associated with that of medical billing, generating insurance claims, and coding. Table 2-3 lists the various job titles under this specialty and their corresponding duties.

Another positive aspect of the health insurance professional's career is the variety of tasks and responsibilities it offers. These vary from office to office, depending on the number of employees, the degree of job specialization, and the type of practice; however, the variety of roles plus job **autonomy** (working without direct supervision) make this profession attractive to many individuals. Typical duties of health insurance professionals include, but are not limited to, the following:

Imagine This!

Sandra Bence-Franklin works for New Beauty Products, Inc., a large cosmetics firm, where her responsibilities are limited to handling incoming calls on a complicated telephone system and greeting and directing customers. Although the pay and benefits are good, she has quickly become bored and disillusioned with her job. She desires more challenge and variety. Her cousin Lisa, a health insurance professional, has recently been hired at Oceanside Medical Center. Lisa talks constantly about the variety and challenges of her new job. "I'm doing something different every day. I am learning so much, and it's so interesting! I really feel I'm making a difference when I help a patient understand the confusing issues of medical insurance." At first, Sandra paid little attention to Lisa's ramblings, but as time went on, and her job became more and more mundane, she began to pay closer attention to what Lisa was saying. "Maybe," Sandra mused, "I should look into what a career as a health insurance professional has to offer me."

- Scheduling appointments
- Bookkeeping and other administrative duties
- Explaining insurance benefits to patients
- Handling day-to-day medical billing procedures
- Adhering to each insurance carrier's guidelines
- Documenting all activities using correct techniques and medical terminology
- Completing insurance forms promptly and accurately
- Knowing and complying with laws and regulations
- Computer data entry
- Interpreting explanation of benefits (EOBs)
- Posting payments to patient accounts
- Corresponding with patients and insurance companies

What Did You Learn?

1. List at least eight of the various career options that fall under the general umbrella of a health insurance professional.
2. Why do you think autonomy might be attractive to some career-minded individuals?
3. List six typical duties of a health insurance professional.

CAREER PROSPECTS

Individuals who choose a career in the healthcare field such as medical insurance have an opportunity to work in a variety of professional locations, such as the following:

TABLE 2-3 Roles Included Under the Umbrella of the Health Insurance Professional

SPECIALIZED FIELD	ROLE/DUTIES
Claims Assistant Professional (CAP)	Assists patients/consumers in obtaining full benefits from healthcare coverage under private or government health insurance and coordinates with healthcare providers to avoid duplication of payment and overpayment
Medical Coder/Coding Specialist	Possesses expertise in assigning diagnostic and procedural codes using common coding manuals (ICD-9-CM and CPT)
Medical Claims Processor	Prepares and transmits claims by paper and electronically using the computer
Reimbursement Specialist	Checks and verifies records, prepares insurance claims, posts ledger and general journal entries, balances accounts payable and accounts receivable records, and follows up on claims and delinquent reimbursements
Billing Coordinator	Responsible for maintaining patient accounts and for collecting money. A billing coordinator also might create and file insurance claims and handle accounts receivable
Patient Account Representative	Obtains patient insurance information, confirms appointments, verifies insurance eligibility, enters/updates insurance information into the records and computer
Medical Claims Reviewer	Analyzes claims for "medical necessity" and valid policy coverage. Performs audits on charge entry for accuracy and HIPAA and Office of Inspector General compliance. Supports/maintains all forms of billing, payment posting, refunds, and credentialing and system issues
Medical Claims Analyst	Assists with claim rule setup and maintenance, medical claim–related data mapping, claim analysis and other tasks related to supporting client's claims, and medical coding
Electronic Claims Processor	Sets up and implements electronic claims processing (in standardized formats) via electronic modes and transmits claims to third-party payers
Medical Collector	Handles inquiries regarding patient account balances and insurance submission dates. Proficient in collection laws and collection techniques used to settle delinquent accounts and maximize reimbursements

- Physician's or dentist's offices
- Hospitals and urgent care facilities
- Pharmacies
- Nursing homes
- Home health
- Mental health facilities
- Physical therapy and rehabilitation centers
- Insurance companies
- Health maintenance organizations (HMOs)
- Consulting firms
- Health data organizations

Successful completion of a health insurance program gives the student the training and skills to become a health insurance professional, which includes the various subspecialties. If an individual decides to become a medical coder, the education and knowledge of healthcare and disease processes learned during the education process or on the job gives the individual a good background if he or she chooses to become certified in this specialty. In the past, many coders were employed in hospitals; however, the growth of ambulatory care facilities and outpatient clinics has greatly increased the demand for employees with a solid background in coding and excellent computer skills.

 HIPAA Tip

One goal of the administrative simplification provisions of HIPAA is to reduce the number of forms and methods of completing claims and other payment-related documents through the efficient use of computer-to-computer methods of exchanging standard healthcare information.

● **Stop and Think**

The text stated that ambulatory care facilities and outpatient clinics are increasing. What do you think has triggered this growth, and how does it affect health insurance professionals?

OPPORTUNITIES

Advancement opportunities in a health insurance career are virtually unlimited. Employment prospects exist in medical facilities ranging in size from a small staff of one or two healthcare providers to several hundred providers in a multispecialty group practice. An American Hospital Association survey showed that nearly 20% of billing and coding positions are unfilled because of a lack of qualified candidates.

As an alternative to working in a medical office as an employee, health insurance professionals have the option of working independently from a home-based office. Many electronic billing programs are available that can be set up through home office computers. Also, there is the possibility of becoming an independent insurance specialist or consultant who contracts to do coding and claims submission for healthcare providers who do not have the ability or manpower to do it themselves. Another possibility would be to work as a consultant who helps patients understand their insurance bills and what they should be paying.

The Health Insurance Portability and Accountability Act (HIPAA) of 1996 has created an opportunity for the healthcare industry to move from paper claims transactions to electronic transactions using one national standard format. This situation creates tremendous job opportunities for health insurance professionals to help noncompliant providers to achieve HIPAA compliance. More information can be learned about HIPAA by logging onto and studying the websites listed at the end of this chapter.

✓ **HIPAA Tip**

HIPAA, created to reduce healthcare costs and protect patient privacy (through the use of "electronic data interchange"), has established rigorous new standards and requirements for the maintenance and transmission of healthcare information. Healthcare providers, insurers, and clearinghouses need specialists with HIPAA training and HIPAA certification to ensure that medical facilities are in compliance with HIPAA's rules and regulations to avoid federal penalties.

REWARDS

Individuals working as health insurance professionals enjoy many benefits, such as job security, a good income, personal satisfaction, challenges, and other rewarding experiences. One of the biggest rewards is the knowledge that they are helping people. As to earnings, at the turn of the 21st century, a graduate of a medical insurance professional program could expect to earn $20,000 to $30,000 a year on entry into the workforce, depending on the geographic area of the United States in which he or she lives. This base wage typically increases rapidly as the individual gains experience and success in the field. Certified coders, at that same time period, made on average between $24,000 and $60,000 depending on experience, credentials, location, and education.

What Did You Learn?

1. How has HIPAA opened up opportunities for health insurance professionals?
2. What does the text suggest might be the biggest reward for health insurance professionals?

CERTIFICATION POSSIBILITIES

Graduates of a medical insurance professional program can be eligible for many different professional certifications that would enhance their careers. **Certification** is the culmination of a process of formal recognition of the competence possessed by an individual. In many vocational training institutions, certification is handed out as recognition of the successful completion of a vocational training process, based on the time of training and practice and on the evaluated contents. Certification possibilities available to the health insurance professional include following:

- American Academy of Professional Coders (AAPC)
  - Certified Professional Coder (CPC)
  - Certified Professional Coder for Hospitals (CPC-H)
- American Health Information Management Association (AHIMA)
    - Certified Coding Specialist (CCS)
    - Certified Coding Associate (CCA)
    - Certified Coding Specialist for Physicians (CCS-P)

Additional national certifications for the health insurance professional are Nationally Certified Insurance Coding Specialist (NCICS) through the National Center for Competency Testing (NCCT) and Certified Medical Reimbursement Specialist (CMRS) offered by the American Medical Billing Association.

AHIMA also offers certification in the other areas, such as:

- Health Information Management
  - Registered Health Information Administrator (RHIA)
  - Registered Health Information Technician (RHIT)
- Healthcare Privacy and Security
  - Certified in Healthcare Privacy (CHP)
  - Certified in Healthcare Privacy and Security (CHPS)
  - Certified in Healthcare Security (CHS)

For additional possibilities of career-related certifications, explore the websites listed at the end of this chapter.

Individuals who are trained and certified as health insurance professionals, coders, and collection specialists have a basic goal—*to ensure that providers (and patients) get paid correctly the first time, every time, on time.* The ever-increasing complexity of diagnosis and treatment codes, coupled with the confusing and often seemingly contradictory guidelines for what various insurance carriers will accept as a claim, make it almost impossible for healthcare providers to stay on top of the constantly changing healthcare scene and still maintain maximum cash flow.

The U.S. Department of Labor states that continued employment growth for health insurance professionals is spurred by the increased medical needs of an aging population and the number of healthcare practitioners. Federal regulations and confusing health insurance policies also have created a strong demand for professionals who can comprehend and perform successfully the demanding role of compliance and provider education.

After completing this course, you will be able to identify each health insurance payer; its individual rules, guidelines, and procedures; and the relevant information that must be included in each box of the **CMS-1500 claim form**, shown in Fig. 2-1, which is the standard insurance form used by all government and most commercial insurance payers.

Computers have dramatically transformed the medical insurance industry by enabling the health insurance professional to focus on accuracy and efficiency instead of the cumbersome task of manually processing each and every claim. This change has brought medical insurance billing into the limelight as one of the fastest growing disciplines in the workforce today. Health insurance professionals not only are in high demand, but also they have a secure future in the world of medicine.

What Did You Learn?

1. What is the basic goal of the health insurance professional?
2. What two things does the U.S. Department of Labor state is increasing the demand for healthcare professionals?

SUMMARY CHECK POINTS

☑ College entry-level skills necessary for success as a health insurance professional include reading and comprehension, basic business math, English and grammar, oral and written communication, keyboarding and office skills, and computer application skills.

☑ Some college courses typically included in a medical insurance billing and coding program include, but are not limited to, the following:
  - Medical Terminology
  - Anatomy and Physiology
  - Medical Law and Ethics
  - Medical Records Management
  - Current Procedural Terminology (CPT) Coding
  - International Classification of Diseases (ICD-9-CM) Coding
  - Medical Insurance Billing
  - Computerized Office Management

☑ Effective study skills and proper preparation are important components for getting the most out of your education and optimizing your career potential. Success in these areas facilitates "lifelong learning."

☑ An effective plan that organizes and prioritizes study time along with other activities is important to the overall learning process.

PLEASE
DO NOT
STAPLE
IN THIS
AREA

CARRIER

☐☐☐ PICA

HEALTH INSURANCE CLAIM FORM

PICA ☐☐☐

1. MEDICARE	MEDICAID	TRICARE CHAMPUS	CHAMPVA	GROUP HEALTH PLAN	FECA BLK LUNG	OTHER	1a. INSURED'S I.D. NUMBER	(For Program in Item 1)
☐ (Medicare #)	☐ (Medicaid #)	☐ (Sponsor's SSN)	☐ (Member ID#)	☐ (SSN or ID)	☐ (SSN)	☐ (ID)		

2. PATIENT'S NAME (Last Name, First Name, Middle Initial)

3. PATIENT'S BIRTH DATE
MM │ DD │ YY   SEX
M ☐   F ☐

4. INSURED'S NAME (Last Name, First Name, Middle Initial)

5. PATIENT'S ADDRESS (No., Street)

6. PATIENT RELATIONSHIP TO INSURED
Self ☐ Spouse ☐ Child ☐ Other ☐

7. INSURED'S ADDRESS (No., Street)

CITY   STATE

8. PATIENT STATUS
Single ☐   Married ☐   Other ☐

CITY   STATE

ZIP CODE   TELEPHONE (Include Area Code)
(   )

Employed ☐ Full-Time Student ☐ Part-Time Student ☐

ZIP CODE   TELEPHONE (INCLUDE AREA CODE)
(   )

9. OTHER INSURED'S NAME (Last Name, First Name, Middle Initial)

10. IS PATIENT'S CONDITION RELATED TO:

11. INSURED'S POLICY GROUP OR FECA NUMBER

a. OTHER INSURED'S POLICY OR GROUP NUMBER

a. EMPLOYMENT? (CURRENT OR PREVIOUS)
YES ☐   NO ☐

a. INSURED'S DATE OF BIRTH
MM │ DD │ YY   SEX
M ☐   F ☐

b. OTHER INSURED'S DATE OF BIRTH
MM │ DD │ YY   SEX
M ☐   F ☐

b. AUTO ACCIDENT?   PLACE (State)
YES ☐   NO ☐

b. EMPLOYER'S NAME OR SCHOOL NAME

c. EMPLOYER'S NAME OR SCHOOL NAME

c. OTHER ACCIDENT?
YES ☐   NO ☐

c. INSURANCE PLAN NAME OR PROGRAM NAME

d. INSURANCE PLAN NAME OR PROGRAM NAME

10d. RESERVED FOR LOCAL USE

d. IS THERE ANOTHER HEALTH BENEFIT PLAN?
YES ☐   NO ☐   **If yes**, return to and complete item 9 a-d.

READ BACK OF FORM BEFORE COMPLETING & SIGNING THIS FORM.
12. PATIENT'S OR AUTHORIZED PERSON'S SIGNATURE I authorize the release of any medical or other information necessary to process this claim. I also request payment of government benefits either to myself or to the party who accepts assignment below.

SIGNED _____   DATE _____

13. INSURED'S OR AUTHORIZED PERSON'S SIGNATURE I authorize payment of medical benefits to the undersigned physician or supplier for services described below.

SIGNED _____

PATIENT AND INSURED INFORMATION

14. DATE OF CURRENT:
MM │ DD │ YY   ◄ ILLNESS (First symptom) OR INJURY (Accident) OR PREGNANCY(LMP)

15. IF PATIENT HAS HAD SAME OR SIMILAR ILLNESS.
GIVE FIRST DATE MM │ DD │ YY

16. DATES PATIENT UNABLE TO WORK IN CURRENT OCCUPATION
MM │ DD │ YY   MM │ DD │ YY
FROM   TO

17. NAME OF REFERRING PHYSICIAN OR OTHER SOURCE

17a.
17b.

18. HOSPITALIZATION DATES RELATED TO CURRENT SERVICES
MM │ DD │ YY   MM │ DD │ YY
FROM   TO

19. RESERVED FOR LOCAL USE

20. OUTSIDE LAB? $ CHARGES
YES ☐   NO ☐

21. DIAGNOSIS OR NATURE OF ILLNESS OR INJURY. (RELATE ITEMS 1,2,3 OR 4 TO ITEM 24E BY LINE)

1. L___ . ___
2. L___ . ___
3. L___ . ___
4. L___ . ___

22. MEDICAID RESUBMISSION
CODE   ORIGINAL REF. NO.

23. PRIOR AUTHORIZATION NUMBER

24. A. DATE(S) OF SERVICE		B. PLACE OF SERVICE	C. EMG	D. PROCEDURES, SERVICES, OR SUPPLIES (Explain Unusual Circumstances)		E. DIAGNOSIS POINTER	F. $ CHARGES	G. DAYS OR UNITS	H. EPSDT Family Plan	I. ID. QUAL.	J. RENDERING PROVIDER ID. #
From MM DD YY	To MM DD YY			CPT/HCPCS	MODIFIER						
1										NPI	
2										NPI	
3										NPI	
4										NPI	
5										NPI	
6										NPI	

25. FEDERAL TAX I.D. NUMBER   SSN ☐ EIN ☐

26. PATIENT'S ACCOUNT NO.

27. ACCEPT ASSIGNMENT?
(For govt. claims, see back)
YES ☐   NO ☐

28. TOTAL CHARGE
$

29. AMOUNT PAID
$

30. BALANCE DUE
$

31. SIGNATURE OF PHYSICIAN OR SUPPLIER INCLUDING DEGREES OR CREDENTIALS
(I certify that the statements on the reverse apply to this bill and are made a part thereof.)

SIGNED _____ DATE _____

32. SERVICE FACILITY LOCATION INFORMATION

a.   b.

33. BILLING PROVIDER INFO & PH # (   )

a.   b.

PHYSICIAN OR SUPPLIER INFORMATION

Fig. 2-1 Copy of a CMS-1500 form.

☑ Time management schedules are excellent tools to help students develop better study skills, but they should not be too detailed or rigid. Allow for adjustments, as needed, to accommodate not only time for studying, but also for relaxation and rewards.

☑ Some of the personality traits and on-the-job skills health insurance professionals should possess to optimize career success include
- self-discipline,
- a positive attitude,
- diligence,
- integrity,
- objectivity,
- initiative, and
- enthusiasm

☑ There are several different job titles, each with its corresponding duties, included under the general umbrella of "health insurance professional." Job titles and duties vary from office to office, depending on the number of employees, the type of medical practice, and the degree of job specialization.

☑ Career prospects and job opportunities for health insurance professionals include, but are not limited to, physician's or dentist's offices, hospitals, pharmacies, nursing homes, mental health facilities, rehabilitation centers, insurance companies, HMOs, consulting firms, and health data organizations.

☑ Health insurance professionals and similar health-care careers offer job security, good income, personal satisfaction, challenges, and rewarding experiences as possible rewards, plus the most important reward of all—helping people.

☑ Professional certifications that enhance the careers of health insurance professionals include Certified Professional Coder (CPC) certification, the American Health Information Management Association (AHIMA) Certified Coding Specialist (CCS) and Certified Coding Associate (CCA) certifications, and National Center for Competency Testing (NCCT) Nationally Certified Insurance Coding Specialist (NCICS) certification.

CLOSING SCENARIO

Joy and Barbara now have a real feel for not only how to study and prepare for class, but also for what to expect in their future careers as health insurance professionals. It was surprising for them to learn that there was such a demand for specialists trained in this field, and Joy finds the possibility of opening a home-based business particularly attractive because she still has young children at home. Barbara is optimistic that, after she has completed her schooling, job opportunities exist all over the United States. If her family is relocated because of her husband's job, she would be qualified to work in a variety of positions in many different kinds of health-related facilities in the United States. Additionally, Joy and Barbara have decided to begin exploring certification possibilities.

WEBSITES TO EXPLORE

For live links to the following websites, please visit the Evolve® site at http://evolve.elsevier.com/Beik/today/

- For a listing of health-related careers and occupations, go to http://www.bls.gov/oco/

- AHIMA has a good website for health information technology careers. Log on to http://www.ahima.org/careers/intro.asp for more information

- You also might want to explore this website created by coders for coders: http://www.codernet.com/

- For a professional outlook on medical coding and billing, go to http://www.medicalcodingandbilling.com/outlook.htm

- For additional possibilities of career-related certifications, explore these websites:
www.aapc.com
www.phia.cm
www.pmimd.com

- For a complete account of the HIPAA of 1996, log on to and peruse the following websites:
http://www.cms.hhs.gov/hipaa/
http://www.hipaa.org/

Chapter 3

The Legal and Ethical Side of Medical Insurance

Chapter Outline

Chapter Outline

CHAPTER OBJECTIVES

After completion of this chapter, the student should be able to

- Define new terms used in the chapter.
- Discuss the ramifications of medical law and liability as it pertains to health insurance.
- List and explain the elements of a legal contract.
- Name and briefly discuss the important legislative acts affecting health insurance.
- Explain the importance of proper medical ethics and etiquette in the workplace.
- State the requirements and rationalization of proper documentation in patient records.
- Identify the primary objectives of HIPAA.
- Discuss HIPAA's impact on various categories of people involved with healthcare (i.e., health insurance professionals, patients, providers).
- Outline a medical compliance plan.
- List the purposes of a medical record.
- Demonstrate an understanding of confidentiality and privacy laws.
- Critique the various exceptions to confidentiality.
- Analyze cause and effect of fraud and abuse in healthcare.

CHAPTER TERMS

abandoning
abuse
acceptance
accountability
ancillary
binds
breach of confidentiality
competency
confidentiality
consideration
durable power of attorney
emancipated minor
ethics
etiquette
first party (party of the first part)
fraud
implied contract
implied promises
incidental disclosure
litigious
medical ethics
medical etiquette
medical (health) record
negligence
offer
portability
privacy
privacy statement
respondeat superior
second party (party of the second part)
subpoena *duces tecum*
third party

OPENING SCENARIO

Joy and Barbara are well entrenched into their course of study on becoming health insurance professionals. As they progress through the course, they are beginning to identify variations in their interests. Although their basic goals are similar, their individual interests are moving in different directions. Barbara determined early on that she prefers to work in a small facility; she intends to learn all aspects of managing an office. Joy has her heart set on a large, multiprovider office where she will more likely find opportunities to specialize in areas she finds interesting and exciting. One of these areas is the legal and ethical side of health insurance. Before this course, Joy took a class in business law, which gave her a background in various legal processes. Their instructor relates the importance of a good, solid background in medical law and ethics to the class, and both women are convinced it is an important fundamental step in building a solid foundation of knowledge and understanding of health insurance. An in-depth study of how law and ethics affects the world of medical insurance intrigues Joy because a distant relative was involved in a medical lawsuit. For Barbara, law and ethics is a relatively foreign topic, and she is curious to see how it relates to health insurance.

INTRODUCTION

All there is to know about medical law and ethics would fill volumes of books. So as not to overwhelm you, this chapter attempts to zero in on what the author thinks a health insurance professional should know to perform his or her job accurately and efficiently, while maintaining confidentiality and sensitivity to patients' rights.

The practice of medicine is, after all, a business—not unlike an auto body shop. The auto body shop fixes cars; the medical facility fixes people. Although the medical facility may be more altruistic, the bottom line of both (unless supported by tax dollars) is to make a profit.

The primary goals of the health insurance professional is to complete and submit insurance claims and conduct billing and collection procedures that enable him or her to generate as much money for the practice as legally and ethically possible that the medical record will support in the least amount of time. To do this, the health insurance professional must be knowledgeable in the area of medical law and liability.

MEDICAL LAW AND LIABILITY

Medical law and liability can vary widely from state to state; however, some rules and regulations affect medical facilities in the United States as a whole. The health insurance professional should become familiar with the medical laws and liability issues in his or her state and abide by them prudently. The following sections discuss various facets of medical law and liability.

EMPLOYER LIABILITY

In our **litigious** (quick to bring lawsuits) society, people tend more and more to hold physicians to perfection, and the slightest breach of medical care can end up as a malpractice lawsuit. Often, these lawsuits are settled out of court—not because the healthcare provider was afraid he or she would be found negligent and wanted to avoid publicity, but because of cost.

Imagine This!

A well-known medical talk show host tells of a situation where his TV crew was filming a critically ill patient in a California hospital. A woman in Texas saw the episode and, claiming it was her mother who had recently died in a Texas hospital, sued. The film did not show the woman from the front, and the camera clearly showed items that accurately identified the hospital where the actual filming took place. The talk show host won the lawsuit, but it cost nearly $20,000 in court costs and legal fees to clear everything up.

The cost of malpractice insurance premiums for physicians is increasing. In some states (e.g., New Jersey, Pennsylvania, Mississippi, Texas, Nevada, and West Virginia), malpractice insurance premiums for physicians in certain types of specialties cost $200,000 to $400,000 per year. This is more than five times what it cost just a few years ago. Some physicians refuse to perform certain procedures because of the threat of malpractice lawsuits, and individuals who need treatment travel hundreds of miles to find it.

EMPLOYEE LIABILITY

No matter what the employee's position is or how much education he or she has had, direct and indirect patient contact involves ethical and legal responsibility. Although we all know that professional healthcare providers have a responsibility for their own actions, what about the health insurance professional? Can he or she be a party to legal action in the event of error or omission?

You may have heard the Latin term *respondeat superior* (*ree-spond-dee-at superior*). The English translation is "let the master answer." *Respondeat superior* is a key principle in business law, which says that an employer is responsible for the actions of his or her employees in the "course of employment." For instance, if a truck driver for Express Delivery, Inc., hits a child in the street because of **negligence** (failure to exercise a reasonable degree of care), the company for which the driver works (Express Delivery) most likely would be liable for the injuries.

The **ancillary** members of the medical team (e.g., nurses, medical assistants, health insurance professionals, technicians) cannot avoid legal responsibility altogether. They also can be named as a party to a lawsuit. The healthcare provider usually bears the financial brunt of legal action, however, because he or she is what is referred to as the "deep pocket," or the person/corporation who has the most money.

● Stop and Think

Eleanor Stevens is a health insurance professional for Halcyon Medical Clinic. Clara Bartlett, a patient of the clinic, comes in for a physical examination. After the examination, Mrs. Bartlett approaches Eleanor and says, "Hon, my insurance company doesn't pay for doctor visits unless I'm sick or something. Dr. Forrest says I'm perfectly healthy, so I'll have to pay today's charge out of my own pocket. I'm a little short on money this month—the high cost of utilities and all—you understand, don't you? (Sigh.) I'm wondering if you could help me out just a little by fudging something on my claim so that my insurance will pay." How might Eleanor handle this situation?

What Did You Learn?

1. Why are healthcare professionals refusing to perform certain procedures?
2. What does the Latin term *respondeat superior* mean?
3. List members of the healthcare team who would typically make up the "ancillary" staff.

INSURANCE AND CONTRACT LAW

Because a health insurance policy and the relationship between a healthcare provider and a patient are considered legal contracts, it is important that the health insurance professional become familiar with the basic concepts of contract law.

ELEMENTS OF A LEGAL CONTRACT

To understand insurance of any kind, you have to have a reasonable knowledge base of the legal framework surrounding it. In other words, you must learn some basic concepts about the law of contracts. The health insurance policy, being a legal contract, must contain certain elements to be legally binding. These elements are as follows:

1. Offer and acceptance
2. Consideration
3. Legal object
4. Competent parties
5. Legal form (written contracts only)

Let's take a closer look at each of these five contract elements and apply them to the health insurance contract. We'll follow a fictitious character—Jerry Dawson, a self-employed computer consultant—through this process.

Offer and Acceptance

Jerry visits Ned Nelson of Acme Insurance Company and tells him that he wants to purchase a health insurance policy for his family. Jerry completes a lengthy application form detailing his family's medical history. Here, Jerry is making the **offer**—a proposition to create a contract with Ned's company. Ned sends the application to his home office; after verifying the information, someone at the home office might say, "this guy and his family are okay; we'll insure them." This is the **acceptance**; Acme Insurance has agreed to take on Jerry's proposition, or offer. The acceptance occurs when the insurance company **binds** (agrees to accept the individual[s] for benefits) coverage or when the policy is issued.

Consideration

Jerry receives his new insurance contract from Acme. The binding force in any contact that gives it legal status is the **consideration**—the *thing of value* that each party gives to the other. In a health insurance contract, the consideration of the insurance company lies in the promises that make up the contract, for example, the promise to pay all or part of the insured individual's *covered medical expenses* as set forth in the contract. The promise to pay the premium is the consideration of the individual seeking health insurance coverage.

Legal Object

A contract must be *legal* before it can be enforced. If an individual contracts with another to commit murder for a specified amount of money, that contract would be unenforceable in court because its intent is not legal, as murder is against the law. Are we confident that this insurance policy between Jerry, our computer expert, and Acme Insurance Company is legal? We can rest assured a contract is legal if it contains all the necessary elements and whatever is being contracted (the object) is not breaking any laws.

Competent Parties

The parties to the contractual agreement must be capable of entering into a contract in the eyes of the law. **Competency** typically enters into the picture in the case of minors and individuals who are mentally handicapped. The courts have ruled that if individuals in either of these categories enter into a contractual agreement, it is not enforceable because the individuals might not understand all of the legal ramifications involved.

Some minors can enter into a contract, for example, an **emancipated minor**. The term "emancipation" applies to youth older than age 16 and younger than 18 who are
- living separate and apart from their parents,
- not receiving any financial support from them (except by court order or benefits to which they are entitled, i.e., Social Security),
- living beyond the parent's custody and control, and
- not in foster care.

Emancipation involves the renunciation of the legal obligations of a parent and the surrender of parental rights over the child. It may occur when a parent is unwilling or unable to meet his or her obligations to the child, when a child refuses to comply with the reasonable rules of the parent and leaves home, or when a child marries.

Legal Form

Most states require that all types of insurance policies be filed with, and approved by, the state regulatory authorities before the policy may be sold in that state. This procedure determines if the policy meets the legal requirements of the state and protects policyholders from unscrupulous insurance companies that might take advantage of them.

TERMINATION OF CONTRACTS

A contract between an insurance company and the insured party can be terminated on mutual agreement or if either party defaults on the provisions in the policy. The insurance company can terminate the policy for nonpayment of premiums or fraudulent action. The insured individual usually can terminate the policy at his or her discretion.

The contract between a healthcare provider and a patient (referred to as an implied contract, discussed in the next

section) can be terminated by either party; however, when the provider enters into this contractual relationship, he or she must render care as long as the patient needs it and follows the provider's guidelines. The patient can terminate the contract simply by paying all incurred charges and not returning to the practice. The provider must have good reason to discharge a patient, however, and must follow specific guidelines in doing so. Some common reasons for a physician discharging a patient are
- if the patient consistently fails to keep appointments;
- if the patient's account becomes delinquent (typically 90 days), and no effort has been made to arrange for payment; or
- if the patient refuses to follow the physician's advice.

If it is determined that, for a specific reason, the physician desires to withdraw from a particular case, it is prudent that he or she
- notify the patient in writing of such a decision via certified mail with a return receipt to ensure the patient is aware of the decision;
- give the patient the names of other qualified healthcare providers, in the case where the patient needs further treatment;
- explain the medical problems that need continued treatment; and
- state in writing the time (a specific date) of the termination.

It is important that these steps be followed to avoid a lawsuit for abandonment because **abandoning** a patient—ceasing to provide care—is a breach of contract.

What Did You Learn?

1. Name and explain the necessary elements that make a contract legally binding.
2. "Competency" enters into the picture when what two categories of individuals are considered?
3. What governing bodies typically approve insurance contracts?

MEDICAL LAW AND ETHICS APPLICABLE TO HEALTH INSURANCE

Now that some of the fundamentals of contract law have been presented, we'll take a brief look at basic medical law and liability as it applies to health insurance. First, it is important that the health insurance professional understand that the physician-patient relationship is a different kind of contract. The contract (or policy) between our computer guy and Acme Insurance was a written contract. The relationship between a healthcare provider and a patient is an **implied contract**—meaning it is not in writing, but it has all the components of a legal contract and is just as binding. You have *the offer* (the patient enters the provider's office in anticipation of receiving medical treatment) and *the acceptance* (the provider accepts by granting professional services). The *consideration* here lies in the provider's **implied promises** (promises that are neither spoken nor written, but are implicated by the individuals' actions and performance) to render professional care to the patient to the best of his or her ability (this does not have to be in writing), and the patient's consideration is the promise to pay the provider for these services. This implied contract meets the *legal object* requirement because granting medical care and paying for it is within the limits of the law. The healthcare provider, of legal age and sound mind, and the patient (or the patient's parent or legal guardian, in the case of a minor or mentally handicapped individual) would constitute the competent parties—individuals with the necessary mental capacity or old enough to enter into a contract. In an implied contract, however, there would be no *legal form* because it is not in writing.

● Stop and Think

Ned Farnsworth takes a prescription to the local pharmacy. Ned lives in a small town where everyone knows each other, and he frequently plays golf with Archie, the pharmacist. After Archie fills Ned's prescription, Ned says, "Just put this on my bill, Arch. See you next Saturday on the links." Is this transaction a legally binding contract? If so, (1) what kind of a contract took place, and (2) can you identify the four necessary components of this contract?

You might have heard an insurance company referred to as a **third party**. In the implied contract between the physician and patient, the patient is referred to as the **party of the first part (first party)** in legal language, and the healthcare provider is the **party of the second part (second party)**. Because insurance companies often are involved in this contract indirectly, they are considered the party of the third part (**third party**).

● Stop and Think

In our scenario with Ned and Archie, identify the party of the first part and the party of the second part. Would there likely be a "third party" involved in this transaction; if so, who would it be?

What Did You Learn?

1. What is an *implied* contract?
2. True/False: An *implied* contract must be in writing to be enforceable.
3. Explain the function of a *third party* in a contract.

IMPORTANT LEGISLATION AFFECTING HEALTH INSURANCE

Several federal laws have evolved over the past few decades that regulate and act as "watchdogs" over the complicated and confusing world of health insurance.

FEDERAL PRIVACY ACT OF 1974

The Federal Privacy Act of 1974 protects individuals by regulating when and how local, state, and federal governments and their agencies can request individuals to disclose their Social Security numbers (SSN), and if that information is obtained, it must be held as confidential by those agencies. Originally the SSN was supposed to be used only for tax purposes; however, over the years, SSN are being used for other things. With the growing problem of Social Security card fraud, individuals are encouraged to take steps to safeguard their SSN. Many insurance companies use SSN for identification.

FEDERAL OMNIBUS BUDGET RECONCILIATION ACT OF 1980

The Federal Omnibus Budget Reconciliation Act of 1980 (OBRA) states that Medicare is the secondary payer in the case of an automobile or liability insurance policy. If the automobile/liability insurer disallows payment because of a "Medicare primary clause" in the policy, however, Medicare becomes primary. In the event that the automobile/liability insurer makes payment after Medicare has paid, the provider (or the patient) must refund the Medicare payment.

TAX EQUITY AND FISCAL RESPONSIBILITY ACT OF 1982

The Tax Equity and Fiscal Responsibility Act (TEFRA) of 1982 made Medicare benefits secondary to benefits payable under employer group health plans for employees age 65 through 69 and their spouses of the same age group.

CONSOLIDATED OMNIBUS BUDGET RECONCILIATION ACT OF 1986

The Consolidated Omnibus Budget Reconciliation Act (COBRA) of 1986 allows individuals to purchase temporary continuation of group health plan coverage if they are laid off, are fired for any reason (other than gross misconduct), or must quit because of an injury or illness. This coverage is temporary (18 months for the employee and 36 months for his or her spouse) and is available only to companies with more than 20 employees.

FEDERAL FALSE CLAIM AMENDMENTS ACT OF 1986

The Federal False Claim Amendments Act of 1986 expands the government's ability to control fraud and abuse in healthcare insurance. Its purpose is to amend the existing civil false claims statute to strengthen and clarify the government's ability to detect and prosecute civil fraud and to recover damages suffered by the government as a result of such fraud. The False Claims Amendments Act originally was enacted in 1863 because of reports of widespread corruption and fraud in the sale of supplies and provisions to the Union government during the Civil War.

FRAUD AND ABUSE ACT

The Fraud and Abuse Act addresses the prevention of healthcare fraud and abuse of patients eligible for Medicare and Medicaid benefits. It states that any person who knowingly and willfully breaks the law could be fined, imprisoned, or both. Penalties can result from the following:

- Using incorrect codes intentionally that result in greater payment than appropriate
- Submitting claims for a service or product that is not medically necessary
- Offering payment (or other compensation) to persuade an individual to order from a particular provider or supplier who receives Medicare or state health funds

Federal criminal penalties are established for individuals who

- knowingly or purposely defraud a healthcare program or
- knowingly embezzle, steal, or misapply a healthcare benefit program.

FEDERAL OMNIBUS BUDGET RECONCILIATION ACT OF 1987

The Federal Omnibus Budget Reconciliation Act of 1987 allows current or former employees or dependents younger than age 65 to become eligible for Medicare because of end-stage renal disease. When this happens, the employer-sponsored group plan is primary (or pays first) for 12 months. If the individual's condition is due to a disability other than end-stage renal disease, group coverage is primary, and Medicare is secondary. (This applies only if the company has at least 100 full-time employees.)

What Did You Learn?

1. What legislation established that Medicare is the secondary payer in the case of an automobile/liability insurance policy?
2. For OBRA of 1987 to be applicable, how many employees must the employer have?
3. What is the name of the act that allows individuals the option of continuing their group coverage in case they are laid off or quit their job?
4. What did TEFRA of 1982 make Medicare benefits secondary to?

MEDICAL ETHICS AND MEDICAL ETIQUETTE

Most of us are familiar with the Oath of Hippocrates. It is a brief exposition of principles for physicians' conduct, which dates back to the 5th century B.C. Statements in the Oath protect the rights of the patient and oblige the physician voluntarily to behave in a humane and selfless manner toward patients. Although there is no such written or recorded oath for health insurance professionals, certain codes of conduct are expected of all individuals who work in healthcare—referred to as medical ethics and medical etiquette.

MEDICAL ETHICS

The word "ethics" comes from the Greek word *ethos*, meaning "character." **Ethics** are standards of human conduct—sometimes called "morals" (from the Latin word *mores*, meaning "customs")—of a particular group or culture. Although the terms "ethics" and "morals" often are used interchangeably, they are not exactly the same. Morals refer to actions, ethics to the reasoning behind such actions. Ethics are not the same as laws, and if a member of a particular group or culture breaches one of these principles or customs, he or she probably would not be arrested; however, the group can levy sanctions (punishment) against this person, such as fines, suspension, or even expulsion from the group.

Ethics is a code of conduct of a particular group of people or culture; **medical ethics** is the code of conduct for the healthcare profession. The American Medical Association (AMA) has long supported certain principles of medical ethics developed primarily for the benefit of patients. These are not laws, but socially acceptable principles of conduct, which define the essentials of honorable behavior for healthcare providers. Fig. 3-1 provides a list of professional ethics from the AMA website.

The field of medical ethics is a current area of concern for practitioners and consumers. From the time an individual is conceived until death, there are ethical questions regarding healthcare at every juncture, such as:

• birth control,
• abortion,
• experimentation,
• prolongation of life,
• quality of life,
• withholding care,
• euthanasia,
• who makes the medical decisions, and
• who has the knowledge and the right to make these decisions.

It is often difficult to distinguish between absolute right and wrong in controversial medical issues. Although laws are universal rules to be observed by everyone, different cultures follow different moral and ethical codes. Who is to say whether or not these codes are right or wrong? It is sufficient to state here that it is important that all healthcare professionals follow the established standards of conduct issued by these professional organizations to guide their future course of action.

I. A physician shall be dedicated to providing competent medical care, with compassion and respect for human dignity and rights.

II. A physician shall uphold the standards of professionalism, be honest in all professional interactions, and strive to report physicians deficient in character or competence, or engaging in fraud or deception, to appropriate entities.

III. A physician shall respect the law and also recognize a responsibility to seek changes in those requirements, which are contrary to the best interests of the patient.

IV. A physician shall respect the rights of patients, colleagues, and other health professionals, and shall safeguard patient confidences and privacy within the constraints of the law.

V. A physician shall continue to study, apply, and advance scientific knowledge, maintain a commitment to medical education, make relevant information available to patients, colleagues, and the public, obtain consultation, and use the talents of other health professionals when indicated.

VI. A physician shall, in the provision of appropriate patient care, except in emergencies, be free to choose whom to serve, with whom to associate, and the environment in which to provide medical care.

VII. A physician shall recognize a responsibility to participate in activities contributing to the improvement of the community and the betterment of public health.

VIII. A physician shall, while caring for a patient, regard responsibility to the patient as paramount.

IX. A physician shall support access to medical care for all people.

Fig. 3-1 Principles of medical ethics. (From the American Medical Association, www.ama-assn.org, 2006)

Imagine This!

Marian Grube worked in the spinal and brain injuries ward at Blessing Memorial Hospital. Often, she would relate the sad story of patients who lay there in a vegetative state, dying by inches, to close friends and family members. One such patient was a young man who had been severely injured as a result of a motorcycle accident. As a result of her experiences, Marian became an advocate for wearing helmets while riding motorcycles and bicycles. Once, during a public speaking engagement, she referred to this particular patient not by name, but by condition, using him as an example to drive her point home. The patient's family members complained, and Marian lost her job.

Stop and Think

Mary Ann was in the hospital for a dilation and curettage and a tubal ligation. Samantha, the nurse on duty, was preparing Mary Ann for the procedure. "Mary Ann," Samantha began, "do you really think you're doing the right thing?"

"What do you mean?" asked Mary Ann.

"Well," Samantha said, "you're still a young woman, and I notice in the chart that you have only one child. If you go through with this procedure, you will probably never have any more children." Samantha sighed and continued with a note of bitterness, "There are thousands of women in the world who would give anything to become a mother. I know—I'm one of them."

Was Samantha acting ethically? If not, what particular area of ethical conduct was she violating? How do you think this situation should be handled?

MEDICAL ETIQUETTE

The word "etiquette" is derived from a mid 18th century French word for "ticket," very likely from the custom of giving rules for behavior on a soldier's lodging ticket or on cards given out at the royal court. Although etiquette and ethics are closely related, there is a difference in their meaning. **Etiquette** is following the rules and conventions governing correct or polite behavior in society in general or in a particular social or professional group or situation. In our society, etiquette dictates that we do not belch at the table. In the medical office, good etiquette is reflected in how the medical receptionist answers the telephone and greets patients. The health insurance professional can perform his or her duties well within the limits of medical ethics, but this does not mean that it is done so in a mannerly way. If the patient completes the information form incorrectly, causing a delay or rejection in the claim, the healthcare professional can resolve the situation in an ethical manner, but if he or she was rude or impatient with the patient in doing so, a breach of **medical etiquette** has occurred.

Ethics and etiquette are constantly evolving. What is acceptable behavior today might not have been okay 20, or even 10, years ago. In today's healthcare environment, patients are considered "customers," and they should be treated with respect and courtesy.

What Did You Learn?

1. Explain the difference between ethics and laws.
2. Explain the difference between ethics and etiquette.
3. List some current ethical issues facing society today.

DOCUMENTATION OF PATIENT MEDICAL RECORD

A **medical (health) record** is a clinical, scientific, administrative, and legal document of facts containing statements relating to a patient. It incorporates scientific data and scientific events in chronologic order regarding the case history, clinical examination, investigative procedures, diagnosis, treatment of the patient, and patient's response to the treatment. Health records are extremely valuable, not only to healthcare providers and the scientific community, but also to patients and third-party carriers. Properly documented health records expand knowledge and improve the standard of medical care.

Health records are kept for two basic purposes:

1. They document the interaction between the healthcare provider and the patient so that a permanent record of what was said and done exists.
2. They show the ongoing process of patient care.

A health record must be accurate in every detail. It should be identifiable, it should be detailed, and it should

be stored in a safe place. A health record is considered privileged communication, and any information in it should not be disclosed without *written consent* of the patient except if required by law. Records are the property of the healthcare provider and should be preserved for at least 5 years (10 years in legal cases).

It is important that all members of the healthcare team know the correct methods for maintaining health records. Timely, accurate, and complete documentation is crucial to patient care. Thorough and accurate documentation
- facilitates claims review and payment,
- assists in utilization review and quality of care evaluations,
- provides clinical data for research and education, and
- serves as a legal document to be used as verification that care was provided.

Every medical facility should have a policy in place to see that health record entries are accurately documented and signed off in a timely manner. If additional information needs to be added to the record, it should be in the form of an appropriate addendum that has been prepared in accordance with this policy. Fig. 3-2 shows the correct method of correcting an erroneous health record entry.

The physician does not always perform all patient record documentation. Some medical practices assign the task of documenting the chief complaint (CC) and history of present illness (HPI) to ancillary staff members. In such cases, it is important that the staff member understands the process of evaluation and management coding. Adequate and complete documentation helps to establish medical necessity for the visit and the level of service, which justifies the fee charged.

In addition to charting the CC and HPI, documentation that the ancillary medical staff might be responsible for includes the following:
- Patient contact, including office visits and telephone calls
- Routine vital signs: blood pressure, pulse, respirations, weight, and height
- Applicable patient education—verbal instructions and written materials
- Communication or follow-up (either by phone or in writing) to patients who have failed to keep appointments, referrals, or scheduled tests
- Prescription refills authorized by the healthcare provider (some states require the physician's initials in the chart for every prescription refill)

The medical staff also should verify that all laboratory and diagnostic test results are read and signed by the

sprained left ankle FA 12/27/05

12/23/2003   Rachel is seen again in the office today for follow up of her ~~sprained right ankle~~. She is able to put some weight on it, and swelling has subsided. Gradually increase activity. Continue ibuprofen for pain as needed. Recheck in two weeks. (s) Frances Akers, MD

Fig. 3-2 Example of a properly corrected chart entry.

healthcare provider and filed in the patient's chart in a *timely* manner. (The Office of the Inspector General [OIG] interprets "timely" as 24 hours.)

Appropriate documentation serves as the basis for the defense of malpractice claims and lawsuits (Fig. 3-3). Many insurance carriers now conduct record reviews in an effort to ensure proper documentation of services billed. Lack of proper documentation could result in reduced or denied claim payments. A common saying among healthcare professionals is "if it isn't documented, it didn't happen."

What Did You Learn?

1. What is the process of recording information in a patient's health record called?
2. Who shares the responsibility of documentation?
3. List the types of documentation that typically fall into the realm of the ancillary medical staff.
4. What problems can be the result of poorly maintained or inaccurate medical records?

HEALTH INSURANCE PORTABILITY AND ACCOUNTABILITY ACT AND COMPLIANCE

The Health Insurance Portability and Accountability Act (HIPAA) was signed into law in 1996 by the Clinton Administration and congressional healthcare reform leaders. There are four primary objectives to this act:

---

1. All medical record entries should be complete, accurate, and legible and contain the date of when the entry was made.
2. Only authorized individual will make entries into medical records.
3. Entries should be made using a black ink (not felt tip) pen.
4. The author of every medical record entry shall be identified in the entry, and all clinical entries shall be individually authenticated by the responsible practitioner. Other entries will be authenticated as specified by medical staff bylaws or as required by state or federal law or regulation.
5. All authorized individuals who make entries into medical records will make every effort to create such entries in accordance with this policy, applicable medical staff bylaw provisions, and all applicable state and federal laws, regulations, and guidelines. Any questions concerning creation of medical record entries should be directed to appropriate personnel for clarification.
6. All final diagnoses and complications should be recorded without the use of symbols or abbreviations.
7. Only the abbreviations, signs, and symbols approved by the medical staff shall be used in medical records.

Fig. 3-3 Principles of documentation.

1. To ensure health insurance portability
2. To reduce healthcare fraud and abuse
3. To enforce standards for health information
4. To guarantee security and privacy of health information for patients

Let's break this first objective down so that we can understand it better. The word **"portability"** means people with preexisting medical conditions cannot be denied health insurance coverage when moving from one employer-sponsored group healthcare plan to another. This law also helps individuals who need to switch health insurance companies in the event of job termination, job relocation, or quitting a job. Basically, HIPAA states that no one should be denied healthcare coverage. The word **"accountability"** refers to the responsibility the healthcare profession has to others—specifically to patients—so that a feeling of confidence exists between patient and provider. Accountability applies more to patient rights, the billing process, and other aspects of the medical office.

Fig. 3-4 shows a flow chart illustrating who must comply with HIPAA standards. The series of easy "yes" and "no" questions is designed to be a simple test to help providers determine whether or not they must comply with the privacy, security, transactions, and other related standards of HIPAA.

IMPACT OF HEALTH INSURANCE PORTABILITY AND ACCOUNTABILITY ACT

HIPAA's regulations affect more than just the healthcare provider and his or her patients. The impact is felt across the board in professional, business, and private worlds. The following paragraphs discuss some of the more pertinent areas.

Impact on the Health Insurance Professional

Health insurance professionals who work in an office with more than 10 employees are likely to submit insurance claims to major government payers (Medicare and Medicaid) using a standardized electronic format, simplifying and creating efficiency via HIPAA's "Electronic Health Transactions Standards." These standards affect health insurance claims processing, health plan eligibility, payments, and other related transactions. The idea behind these standards is to make processing these records more efficient, more accurate, and less costly. In the past, most health, financial, and insurance records in medical offices were paper documents. Because more and more records are becoming computerized, concern has been raised regarding patient privacy and how it will be maintained in electronic media. It is crucial that a serious effort be made to engage providers and consumers in keeping

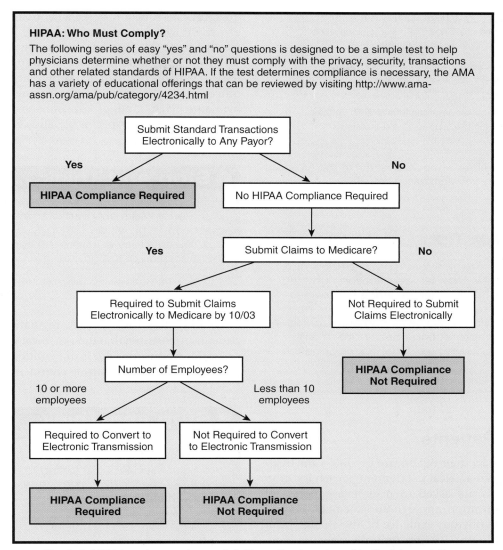

HIPAA: Who Must Comply?

The following series of easy "yes" and "no" questions is designed to be a simple test to help physicians determine whether or not they must comply with the privacy, security, transactions and other related standards of HIPAA. If the test determines compliance is necessary, the AMA has a variety of educational offerings that can be reviewed by visiting http://www.ama-assn.org/ama/pub/category/4234.html

Fig. 3-4 HIPAA—who must comply? (From the American Medical Association, www.ama-assn.org, 2006)

personal health information private. As a result, health insurance professionals have become involved in setting up privacy standards. Patients now have the ability to view their medical records and be informed who else has viewed them and why. For this reason, the "Standards for Privacy"—a set of specific rules to ensure confidentiality—should be considered.

Because HIPAA imposes specific responsibilities on everyone who works in the healthcare field, major changes were required for medical institutions to become HIPAA compliant. Changes were needed on all levels—management of information, patient records, patient care, security, and coding. The health insurance professional must be aware of what these changes are and why they are necessary. Examples of these changes include, but are not limited to, the following:

- Arranging patient charts in the receptacle outside the examination room door in such a way that patient names are not visible
- Locking the physician's office door when confidential laboratory reports and other documents are placed on his or her desk for review
- Closing the window separating the reception area from the waiting room when not in use
- Positioning computer screens so someone standing at the reception desk cannot view them
- Changing computer security passwords routinely
- Avoiding transfer of confidential information via fax or electronic methods to unsecured locations, such as schools, hotel lobbies, or businesses

Fig. 3-5 illustrates "How to HIPAA," a list of the top 10 tips offered by the AMA website.

1. Understand the deadlines and move to compliance.
2. Know your compliance requirements.
3. Prioritize your compliance activities.
4. Ask the right questions.
5. Choose and use consultants wisely.
6. Learn from trusted sources.
7. Separate fact from fiction.
8. Visit Web site resources often for the latest updates.
9. Talk to your patients.
10. Look to the AMA for updates.

Fig. 3-5 How to "HIPAA"—top 10 tips. (From the American Medical Association, www.ama-assn.org, 2006)

 HIPAA Tip

Health insurance professionals need to know how to apply for new provider identification numbers for physicians and other healthcare providers. Health insurance professionals also might be in charge of security measures for computers, which includes virus protection, password mainte-nance, and ensuring confidential information stays secure.

Impact on Patients

When patients go to their healthcare providers for treatment, they are given a **privacy statement** at each location they visit. Patients are asked to read it, ask necessary questions for clarification, and sign the statement. Beyond that, there is little obvious evidence of any change from the patient's standpoint. Patients typically view the statement from both ends of the spectrum. On one end, a patient views it as just one more piece of paper to sign, glances at it, and very likely throws it away. On the other end, a patient reads it word for word, questions areas he or she is not clear on, and files it carefully away for future reference.

The statement not only includes information about who the physician or pharmacy shares health information with and why, but also outlines what rights patients have to access their own health information. The only real change brought about by HIPAA is in presentation. Patients were able to do all those things before HIPAA came into effect, but it was not brought to their attention in this manner and in printed form. Many patients view the ideals behind HIPAA as good, in some cases, but that the implementation of those ideals goes too far. For one thing, the statement tends to be wordy and can be difficult for some people to understand, especially the elderly.

Another way HIPAA has changed patient routines in many offices is that when they sign in at the reception desk, they no longer may see a clipboard with the names of people who have signed in before them (commonly referred to as the "community sign-in sheet"). There are no privacy precautions in the reception room, however, if two patients happen to know each other. In most offices, medical personnel still continue to call the patient by name. That kind of exposure is called **incidental disclosure**, which is specifically allowed under HIPAA.

● Stop and Think

Ellen Porter walks out of an examination room and overhears a physician talking to a patient about treatment as they exit from the adjacent room. Is this a violation of the privacy law?

In the long run, HIPAA regulations will benefit patients by ensuring that their medical information is not accessible by anyone who is not entitled to view it. It also will benefit them by ensuring confidentiality.

● Stop and Think

A patient, waiting at the pharmacy pick-up counter, overhears a pharmacist talking to another patient about her prescription. Is this a violation of HIPAA privacy standards?

Impact on Providers

Providers are required to have business associate agreements with every company they exchange patient information with, including insurance companies, attorneys, financial institutions, and other providers. The idea behind these agreements is to give assurances to providers that the people they do business with also are complying with HIPAA regulations.

Providers no doubt feel HIPAA's impact mostly in their checkbook. Before the implementation of the HIPAA laws, it was estimated that the cost to bring medical facilities

 HIPAA Tip

Healthcare providers are not required to monitor actively the means by which a business associate carries out the safeguards of the contract.

into compliance would be more than $66 billion. Although the final figures are still unavailable, further estimates indicate it is costing each physician practice $10,000 to $250,000, depending on the size of the practice.

Impact on Private Businesses

Businesses have the same obligation to protect medical records as government, medical, and human resource officials. Businesses need to ensure there is uniformity in application of HIPAA requirements. Employees typically receive a letter notifying them of any changes stemming from HIPAA. One of the biggest changes is that health records now must be kept separate from routine personnel records. Some companies already were doing that. Although the average worker might not feel the effects of the new HIPAA privacy requirements on the job, he or she no doubt eventually will feel them indirectly in their wallets.

 HIPAA Tip

Employers should determine what type of computer security, such as a device that blocks unauthorized access, needs to be put into place for risk management purposes, to ensure that health information is not used in the employment process.

What Did You Learn?

1. Name the four primary objectives of the HIPAA act.
2. How does HIPAA affect claims submission and processing?
3. Define *incidental disclosure.*
4. How does HIPAA benefit patients?

ENFORCEMENT OF CONFIDENTIALITY REGULATIONS OF HEALTH INSURANCE PORTABILITY AND ACCOUNTABILITY ACT

One of the primary purposes of HIPAA was continuity of health insurance coverage if an individual changes jobs, but it also provides for standards for health information transactions and confidentiality and security of patient data. This confidentiality portion has had a considerable impact on the day-to-day workflow among medical institutions. HIPAA is complaint driven, however. If no one complains, there probably would not be an investigation. If a deliberate violation of the regulations were found, action would be taken. The Office of Civil Rights will enforce the HIPAA regulations, and there are civil penalties of $100 per violation up to $25,000 per year. Criminal

penalties also are possible, including $50,000 or 1 year in prison or both for wrongful disclosure or $250,000 or 10 years in prison or both for the intent to sell information. As one healthcare worker stated, "HIPAA has teeth, and if you're out of compliance, those teeth will bite you!" For more information about HIPAA, go to their website listed at the end of this chapter.

DEVELOPING A COMPLIANCE PLAN

A written compliance plan can help protect a medical practice and be the best defense against trouble. Compliance programs are a significant tool in reducing the potential for healthcare fraud and abuse; however, they must be adapted and implemented appropriately to be effective. The OIG recommends that the medical facility review its existing standards and procedures to determine if they are in compliance with HIPAA laws and regulations using the following seven steps.

Step 1—Conducting Internal Auditing and Monitoring

Individuals with appropriate billing and medical expertise should conduct internal audits of the practice's actual coding, billing, and documentation performance. These self-audits can be used to determine whether
* services and procedures are accurately coded,
* documentation is complete and correct,
* billed services or other items are reasonable and medically necessary, and
* incentives exist to identify any unnecessary services.

If a problem is discovered, it should be addressed immediately.

Step 2—Establishing Standards and Procedures

The medical facility should have a formal compliance plan in place that includes written standards and procedures that are suitable for dealing with risk areas identified in the practice's internal self-audit. Periodic and regular education of existing and new employees on these standards is crucial. With respect to coding and billing, the most common areas of investigations and audits by the OIG include:
* billing for items or services not performed;
* submitting claims for equipment, supplies, or services that are not reasonable and necessary;
* double billing;
* misuse of provider identification numbers;
* unbundling (billing for components of services that are covered by all-inclusive codes);
* improper use of coding modifiers;
* clustering (exclusive use of middle level Evaluation and Management [E/M] service codes); and

• upcoding (the use of procedure codes that do not match the clinical picture of the patient, but pay at a higher reimbursement amount).

The OIG also advises that every practice develop record retention rules and guidelines for compliance records, business records, and health records. These guidelines should include the time frame for retention of each type of record and should ensure that medical records are not improperly lost, destroyed, or disclosed. The guidelines also should ensure that compliance documents relating to education activities, internal investigations, self-audits, remedial action, and communications with third-party payers and carriers are retained.

Step 3—Designating a Compliance Officer/Contact Person

One or more knowledgeable members of the medical team should be identified who will be responsible for compliance functions. Any new directives should come from this individual.

Step 4—Conducting Appropriate Training and Education

Training and education of all members of the medical team is crucial to the implementation of a successful HIPAA compliance plan. Every employee should understand how to perform his or her job in compliance with the plan and realize that violating any of the standards may result in disciplinary action. Individuals who are directly involved with billing and coding should receive extensive education specific to their responsibilities. Additionally, the OIG recommends at least annual training updates for such employees.

Step 5—Responding to Detected Offenses and Developing Corrective Action Initiatives

The compliance officer should investigate any allegations immediately and take decisive steps to correct any offenses. (*Note:* The Guidelines do not discuss the protocols that should be followed to establish and maintain the attorney/client or work-product privileges to protect the practice during an investigation.) The Guidelines suggest that the practice consider seeking advice from its legal counsel to determine the extent of the practice's liability and to plan the appropriate course of action. The Guidelines recommend that the practice

• develop and monitor "warning indicators," which show significant changes in relevant claims processing information that may signal a violation;
• avoid actions that may compound a violation when it is discovered; and
• promptly identify and return overpayments.

Step 6—Developing Open Lines of Communication

The OIG recommends that the practice implement a clear "open door" policy between healthcare providers and ancillary members of the medical team and post conspicuous notices to provide up-to-date compliance information. The OIG also specifically recommends that physician practices post the Department of Health and Human Services/OIG hotline telephone number. Communication protocols recommended for the practice include the following:

• Require employees to report possible erroneous or fraudulent conduct.
• Create user-friendly processes, such as anonymous drop boxes, for effectively reporting improper conduct.
• Make the failure to report improper conduct a violation of the compliance plan.
• Develop a simple procedure to process reports of improper conduct.
• Coordinate activities with a billing company, if one is used.
• Protect the anonymity of persons who report possible violations and that of the persons to whom the report relates.
• Adopt standards to ensure there will be no retribution for good faith reporting of misconduct.

Step 7—Enforcing Disciplinary Standards Through Well-Publicized Guidelines

As a final step, it is recommended that the practice incorporate measures that ensure employees understand the consequences of noncompliant behavior. These disciplinary actions include verbal warnings, written reprimands, probationary periods, demotion, suspension, termination, restitution of damages, and referral for criminal prosecution. The disciplinary guidelines should be well publicized in the training and procedures manuals.

What Did You Learn?

1. What is the best defense against committing violations against HIPAA guidelines?
2. What entity recommends that all medical facilities review standards and procedures to determine if they are in compliance?
3. State which steps are specifically important steps in developing and maintaining a compliance program.

THE MEDICAL RECORD

The medical record (or health record) is an account of a patient's medical assessment, investigation, and course of treatment. It is a source of information and one component in the quality of patient care. The medical record is a chronologic listing of medical related facts regarding dates of an individual's injuries and illnesses; dates of treatment; and all notes, diagnostic test results, correspondence, and any other pertinent information regarding the medical care and treatment of the patient.

PURPOSES OF A MEDICAL RECORD

The medical record serves several important functions:
• It enables the healthcare provider to render medical care to the best of his or her ability.
• It provides statistical information for research.
• It offers legal protection for the healthcare team.
• It provides support for third-party reimbursement.

COMPLETE MEDICAL RECORD

The Joint Commission on Accreditation of Healthcare Organizations (JCAHO) emphasizes four factors that improve the quality and usefulness of medical records, as follows:
• *Timeliness* (within 24 hours of the encounter)
• *Completeness* (documentation of patient problems and concerns, diagnostic tests performed and their results, diagnosis, treatment or recommended treatment, and prognosis)
• *Accuracy*
• *Confidentiality*
  Typical components of a medical record include the following:
• Demographic information (patient information form, including insurance information)
• Current release of information form (signed and dated)
• Drug or other allergy flags
• Medical/health history
• Physical examination
• Chronologic chart (progress) notes for all subsequent visits
• Medication sheet showing all prescriptions and over-the-counter drugs
• Results of diagnostic tests (x-rays, laboratory tests, electrocardiograms)
• Hospital records (if applicable)
• Correspondence

WHO OWNS MEDICAL RECORDS?

There is still some controversy regarding who actually owns the medical record. It has become an accepted opinion, however, that even though medical records contain a patient's personal and confidential information, medical records are the property of the physician providing the care or the corporate entity where the provider is employed. The information contained in the record is technically the patient's, however, because it cannot be divulged to anyone without the patient's written consent.

● Stop and Think

Dr. Wallace, a long-time family practitioner, decided to retire and sell his practice to another, younger physician. Among the assets were all the medical records of Dr. Wallace's former patients accumulated over the years, which he sold to the new physician for $5 each. Was this legal without the patients' consent?

RETENTION OF MEDICAL RECORDS

It is important that a medical facility have a policy regarding the retention of medical records. According to the AMA, physicians have an obligation to retain patient records that may reasonably be of value to a patient and offer guidelines to assist physicians in meeting their ethical and legal obligations to good patient care.

Several factors may affect time requirements for retaining medical records, including
• expansion rate of records in the practice,
• space available for storage,
• volume of postactive uses,
• statutes of limitation and other federal or state regulations, and
• costs of alternatives.

How long medical records are kept and how they are stored or disposed of vary from practice to practice and state to state. The records of any patient covered by Medicare or Medicaid must be kept at least 5 years.

Imagine This!

Indiana law states that a provider must maintain health records for at least 7 years. A minor younger than 6 years of age has until the minor's eighth birthday to file a claim, however. It is advisable to retain the medical records of a minor younger than age 6 for longer than 7 years.

Some medical facilities go through medical records periodically and pull records that have had no activity for a certain number of years. Often these records are put into storage in another part of the office building. Sometimes the contents are microfilmed, and the actual physical records are destroyed. In all cases, medical records should be kept for at least as long as the length of time of the statute of limitations for medical malpractice claims. The statute of limitations is typically 3 or more years, depending on the state law. State medical associations and insurance carriers are the best resources for this information.

ACCESS TO MEDICAL RECORDS

As governed by JCAHO, access to medical records within an institution or practice is limited to situations involving the following:

1. Treatment
2. Quality assurance
3. Utilization review
4. Education
5. Research

RELEASING MEDICAL RECORD INFORMATION

Under no circumstances should any information from a patient's medical record (or from other sources) be divulged to any third party (including the patient's insurance carrier) without the *written* consent of the patient (parent or guardian in the case of a minor or mentally handicapped adult). Often, there is a place on the patient information form where the patient can sign to release information necessary to complete the insurance claim form so that his or her insurance company can be billed. It is a good idea to advise the patient to specify the name of the insurer on the form. For information to be released to any other third party, a separate release of information should be used. Fig. 3-6 shows a typical information release form that can be used for a range of reasons.

● Stop and Think

You receive a phone call from Abner L. Smith, a local attorney. He is representing Patricia Lane, a patient of your practice, who was recently involved in a rear-end auto collision. Mr. Smith wants to know the results of Ms. Lane's recent MRI of her neck because it is important to the case. He tells you that Ms. Lane is sitting in his office and says it's okay for you to give him this information. What should you do?

● Stop and Think

Sally Sergeant was seen in the office for confirmation of a suspected pregnancy. After Sally left, her husband phones and inquires as to the results of the examination. Can any member of the medical staff give Sally's husband these results?

● Stop and Think

Dr. Smithers, another provider in the same clinic, is seeing Ms. Sergeant for severe acne and needs information to prescribe certain medication. Can this information be provided to Dr. Smithers without Ms. Sergeant signing a release of information?

What Did You Learn?

1. List four purposes of a medical record.
2. According to JCAHO, what are the four factors that improve the quality and usefulness of medical records?
3. What items should be included in a medical record?
4. Who owns medical records?
5. Why is a retention policy important?

CONFIDENTIALITY AND PRIVACY

The words "confidentiality" and "privacy" are sometimes used interchangeably, but there is a distinction between the two. **Privacy** "denotes a zone of inaccessibility" of mind or body, the right to be left alone and to maintain individual autonomy, solitude, intimacy, and control over information about oneself. **Confidentiality** "concerns the communication of private and personal information from one person to another." The key ingredients of confidentiality are trust and loyalty. Professionals rely on the promise of confidentiality to inspire trust in their clients and patients. In the case of healthcare providers, lawyers, and clergy, communications are legally designated "privileged." The following paragraphs examine these two terms separately as they affect healthcare.

CONFIDENTIALITY

Confidentiality is the foundation for trust in the patient-provider relationship. Physicians always have had an ethical

MEDICAL RECORD	Authorization for the Release of Medical Information

INSTRUCTIONS: Complete this form in its entirety and forward the original to the address below:

NATIONAL INSTITUTES OF HEALTH
MEDICAL RECORD DEPARTMENT
ATTN: MEDICOLEGAL SECTION
10 CENTER DRIVE, ROOM 1N208   TELEPHONE: (301) 496-3331
MSC1192   FACSIMILE: (301) 480-9982
BETHESDA, MD 20892-1192

IDENTIFYING INFORMATION:

Patient Name	Daytime Telephone	Date of Birth

REQUEST INFORMATION: Information is to be released to the following individual or party:

Name	Telephone
Address	

The purpose or need for disclosure (charges will be determined based on purpose of disclosure):

Date Range of Information to be Released: from _____ to _____

Please check specific information to be released:

☐ Discharge Summary   ☐ Radiology Reports   ☐ EKG Reports
☐ History & Physical   ☐ Radiology Films   ☐ Echocardiogram Reports
☐ Operative Reports   ☐ Tissue Exam Reports   ☐ Heart Diagnostic Reports
☐ Outpatient Progress Notes ☐ Tissue Slides   ☐ Nuclear Medicine Reports
☐ Length of Stay Verification ☐ Lab Results   ☐ Nuclear Medicine Scans

☐ Other (Please Specify): _____

AUTHORIZATION: Permission is hereby granted to the Warren Grant Magnuson Clinical Center to release medical information to the individual/organization as identified above.
(Note: submission of this form authorizes the release of the information specified within one year from date of signature.)

Patient/Authorized Signature	Print Name	Date

If other than patient, specify relationship: _____

Patient Identification	Authorization for the Release of Medical Information NIH-527 (02-01) P.A. 09-25-0099 File in Section 4: Correspondence

Fig. 3-6 National Institutes of Health (NIH) Release of Information form.

duty to keep their patients' confidences. Even before HIPAA came into being, the AMA's *Code of Medical Ethics* stated that the information disclosed to a physician during the course of the patient-physician relationship or discovered in connection with the treatment of a patient is strictly confidential. The basic reason for this is so that the patient feels comfortable to disclose, fully and frankly, any and all information to the provider. This full disclosure enables the physician to diagnose conditions more effectively and to treat the patient appropriately.

Every healthcare organization and provider must guarantee confidentiality and privacy of the healthcare information they collect, maintain, use, or transmit. Confidentiality means that only certain individuals will have the right to access the information, and that it is secure from others. Confidentiality is at risk when the potential for improper access to information exists.

This obligation of confidentiality extends to health insurance professionals. Every member of the healthcare team has a responsibility to uphold confidentiality for patients. In a busy medical office setting or clinic, maintaining confidentiality might be difficult. Voices carry from the reception work area to waiting patients in chairs and through thin walls of examination rooms. Elevator or cafeteria discussions of Mrs. Brown's cancer or Mr. Lewis' heart attack are common, and this careless practice is prohibited. The person next to you could be a patient's friend, relative, or someone else who is not entitled to this privileged information. Permission must be received from the patient before *any* disclosure.

Any information the health insurance professional learns while caring for a patient or performing administrative duties, such as completing insurance claims, must remain strictly confidential unless authorized in writing by the patient or ordered by law to reveal it. It may seem strange that a written release of information must be obtained from the patient to process an insurance claim for his or her financial benefit, but it is the law.

PRIVACY

As mentioned previously, privacy is different than confidentiality. It refers to an individual's right to keep some information to himself or herself and to have it used only with his or her approval. The American public's privacy concerns are of more recent origin, dating back to events in the 1960s and early 1970s that lead to the Privacy Act of 1974.

Under HIPAA, physicians must use and disclose only the minimum amount of patient information needed for the purpose in question. Patients can request a copy of their medical records and can request amendments to incorrect records. Additionally, patients must receive notification of their privacy rights.

SECURITY

HIPAA also requires administrative procedures for guarding data confidentiality, integrity, and availability with formal procedures for implementation. Physical safeguards are required and include the following:

- Maintaining a system for keeping and storing critical data safe, such as locked, fireproof file cabinets
- Reporting and responding to any attempts to "hack" into the system
- Assessing the security risks of the system
- Developing a contingency plan for data backup and disaster recovery
- Training in security awareness
- Ensuring that the data are secure by monitoring access and protecting the use of passwords or other methods used to ensure security

EXCEPTIONS TO CONFIDENTIALITY

Certain situations and classes of patients do not come under the umbrella of confidentiality. Additionally, certain medical information by law must be reported to state and local governments, where it is maintained in databases for research and public safety. Exceptions to confidentiality include, but are not limited to, the following:

- Treatment of minors
- Human immunodeficiency virus (HIV)–positive patients
- Abuse of a child (or, in most states, an adult)
- Injuries caused by firearms or other weapons
- Communicable diseases

Treatment of Minors

Treatment of minors (patients <18 years old) involves different variables in terms of confidentiality. The AMA states, "Physicians who treat minors have an official duty to promote the autonomy of minor patients by involving them in the medical decision making process to a degree commensurate with their abilities." Minors are categorized as either mature or immature. Maturity is defined most concretely as a patient who is able to undergo a medical examination without his or her parent or guardian present.

Individual state law generally determines whether a minor can consent to medical treatment without parental consent. Virginia law allows minors to make their own medical decisions regarding sexually transmitted diseases and other reportable disease treatment; pregnancy, delivery, and postpartum care; birth control (except for sexual sterilization); outpatient substance abuse; and psychiatric treatment. Special parental notice rules apply to abortion services. A minor mother also can consent to treatment for her child. Married minors and other categories of emancipated minors are able to consent to all types of medical care.

Human Immunodeficiency Virus–Positive Patients

Many states have adopted special statutes to deal with the issue of HIV and disclosure. Maintaining confidentiality is crucial in such cases to guard against discrimination. In certain scenarios involving HIV positivity, however, it is generally legally and ethically acceptable to disclose the fact that a patient is HIV-positive to certain third parties. Some state laws allow disclosure of HIV status to the patient's spouse. Notification of public health authorities is a duty of all physicians caring for an HIV-positive patient and is required by many state laws. Similar laws are in place for hepatitis B and C viruses.

Human Immunodeficiency Virus Confidentiality in Healthcare Workers

A puzzling and controversial situation involves an HIV-positive healthcare worker and whether there is substantial risk to the patient to allow disclosure to maintain informed consent. In other words, is the risk of virus transmission such that the patient needs to know? This situation is often dealt with on a case-by-case basis, taking into account the relative risk of the healthcare worker transmitting the disease. A surgeon has a much higher (albeit relatively low) risk of transmitting HIV compared with a radiology technologist. The U.S. Centers for Disease Control and Prevention has issued guidelines for making such determinations.

Abuse of a Child or Adult

Any healthcare practitioner who has reason to suspect that a child has been abused or neglected must report this immediately to the local Department of Social Services, and all records must be disclosed to Child Protective Services. The reporting individual is protected from liability, unless it is shown that the person making the report acted in bad faith or with malicious intent. In some states, the same rules hold true in cases of suspected abuse of elderly and incompetent adult patients.

Injuries Caused by Firearms or Other Weapons

All healthcare providers are required to report any wound inflicted by a weapon to the police. Failure to do so is a misdemeanor. An individual who reports such an incident is immune from liability. The healthcare professional also has a duty to disclose a patient's threats of imminent physical harm against another identifiable person. In situations in which there is clear evidence of danger to other persons, the healthcare provider must determine the degree of seriousness of the threat and warn the victim, warn the police, or counsel the patient until it has been deter-mined that he or she is no longer believed to be a threat. In extreme cases, the healthcare provider may commit a threatening patient to a mental health facility.

Imagine This!

A California psychologist requested that University of California campus police arrest a patient of his whom he believed was going to kill a woman. The patient was arrested, but subsequently was released after assuring the police that he would stay away from the woman. The woman was never notified of the impending danger, and the patient killed her 2 months later (*Tarasoff vs. Regents of the University of California*).

Communicable Diseases

Communicable disease reporting is so important that written authorization is not required to release this information. Communicable disease reporting is the cornerstone of public health surveillance and disease control. Prompt reporting gives the local health agency time to stop the disease from spreading, locate and treat exposed contacts, identify and contain outbreaks, ensure effective treatment and follow-up of cases, and alert the health community of the problem. The information obtained through disease reporting is used to monitor disease trends over time, identify high-risk groups, allocate resources, develop policy, design prevention programs, and support grant applications. The healthcare facility should contact the state health department for details on which diseases must be reported and the time frame for reporting them. This information should be posted and shared with the entire healthcare team.

AUTHORIZATION TO RELEASE INFORMATION

We discussed earlier in this chapter the importance of obtaining a signed release of information before any information is divulged to any third party, including the patient's insurance carrier. Most states agree on the typical elements of a valid general release of information, which are as follows:

- Patient's name and identifying information
- Address of the healthcare professional or institution directed to release the information
- Description of the information to be released
- Identity of the party to be furnished the information
- Language authorizing release of information
- Signature of patient or authorized individual
- Time period for which the release remains valid

Failure to obtain an appropriate release for disclosing medical records information to a third party can result in serious consequences. Twenty-one states punish disclosure of confidential information by revoking a physician's medical license or taking other serious disciplinary action.

EXCEPTIONS FOR SIGNED RELEASE OF INFORMATION FOR INSURANCE CLAIMS SUBMISSION

In a few situations, a signed release of information is not always required, as discussed in the following paragraphs.

Medicaid-Eligible Patients and Workers' Compensation Cases

When completing an insurance claim form for a Medicaid recipient or a patient being treated as a result of an on-the-job illness or injury (workers' compensation), a written release of information is not usually required. The reason is that the contract in these cases is actually between the healthcare provider and the government agency sponsoring that specific program, and the patient is the third party. In both cases, however, patients cannot be billed for medical procedures or services, unless it is determined that he or she is ineligible for benefits for those particular dates of service. More information is given on Medicaid and Workers' Compensation in later chapters.

Inpatient-Only Treatment

Another group of patients for which the normally required signed release of information for filing insurance claims is waived are patients who are seen in the hospital, but do not come to the office for follow-up care. It is considered that the release of information that the patient signs for hospital services also covers the physician's services, and the health insurance professional can simply insert the phrase, "Signature on file," in block 12 of the CMS-1500 claim form. An example would be when the healthcare provider sees a patient only for consultation purposes.

Court Order

If a patient's record is subpoenaed by a court of law as evidence in a lawsuit, it may be released to the court without the patient's approval. A **subpoena** *duces tecum* is a legal document that requires an individual to appear in court with a piece of evidence that can be used or inspected by the court. The judge determines whether the evidence is relevant to the controversy or issues that must be resolved between the parties of the lawsuit.

BREACH OF CONFIDENTIALITY

When confidential information is disclosed to a third party without patient consent or court order, a **breach of confidentiality** has occurred. The disclosure violation can be oral or written, made by telephone, fax, or transmitted electronically. As mentioned earlier, the release of private health information in a patient's medical record to third parties is allowed only if the patient has consented, in writing, to such disclosure. This rule includes the following categories of individuals:
- Attorneys
- Clergy
- Insurance companies
- Relatives (except in the case where a relative has a **durable power of attorney**, meaning he or she has been named as an agent to handle the individual's affairs if the patient becomes incapacitated)
- Employers (except in the case of workers' compensation cases)
- All other third parties.

State law governs who can give permission to release medical record information. Usually, the authority to release medical information is granted to:
- the patient, if he or she is a competent adult or emancipated minor;
- a legal guardian or parent, if the patient is a minor child or is incompetent;
- an individual to whom the patient has granted power of attorney possessing legal authority to act for the patient in legal and business matters to make such decisions; or
- the administrator or executor of the patient's estate if the patient is deceased.

● Stop and Think

Marcy Knox worked as a health insurance professional in a large medical center where there were many professional offices. One day, as she was delivering some paperwork to a psychiatrist's office on the same floor, she spotted a former teacher waiting in the reception area. At lunch, Marcy met Sherry, a former classmate. "You'll never guess who I saw in Dr. Pilova's office yesterday!" Marcy confided excitedly. Eager to share the news, Marcy didn't wait for her lunch partner to respond. "Our old instructor at Grassland Community College, Mrs. Bitterhaven!" As Marcy was not employed by the psychiatrist's office, was she guilty of a breach of confidentiality in divulging this information to her friend?

HEALTHCARE FRAUD AND ABUSE

Stories about the growing incidence of healthcare fraud and abuse can be found in newspapers and on television. Fraud and abuse in healthcare are widespread and costly to the U.S. healthcare system. Federal investigations have identified fraud and abuse in all areas of healthcare, including physicians' offices and clinics, hospitals, clinical laboratories, durable medical equipment suppliers, hospices, and home health agencies. More recent legislation has enhanced enforcement capabilities, and even more government enforcement activity is expected in the future. Because physicians and members of their healthcare teams are not immune to such government actions, they (and others involved in providing patient care) need to know how to comply with the federal laws to guard against potential liability in fraud enforcement actions.

DEFINING FRAUD AND ABUSE

Fraud can be defined any number of ways. The National Healthcare Anti-Fraud Association (NHCAA) defines fraud as:

> An intentional deception or misrepresentation that the individual or entity makes, knowing that the misrepresentation could result in some unauthorized benefit to the individual, or the entity, or to another party.

Examples of health insurance fraud include billing for services that were not rendered or falsifying a patient's diagnosis to justify tests, surgeries, or other procedures that are not medically necessary.

Abuse, although similar to fraud, is considered less serious when applied to healthcare. Abuse can be defined as improper or harmful procedures or methods of doing business that are contradictory to accepted business practices. Often, it is impossible to establish that the abusive acts were done with intent to deceive the insurance carrier.

Examples of health insurance abuse include charging for services that were not medically necessary, do not conform to recognized standards, or are unfairly priced. Another example of abuse is performing a laboratory test on large numbers of patients when only a few patients should have had the test.

Although no exact dollar amount can be determined, some authorities contend that health insurance fraud and abuse constitutes a $100 billion/year problem. The U.S. General Accounting Office (GAO) estimates that $1 out of every $7 spent on Medicare is lost to fraud and abuse, and that in 1 year, Medicare typically loses nearly $12 billion to fraudulent or unnecessary claims. Private insurers estimate the dollar amount lost to health insurance fraud and abuse to be 3% to 5% of total healthcare dollars spent. When the annual U.S. healthcare expenditure totals $1 trillion, that translates to an estimated annual loss of $30 to $50 billion.

Who Commits Healthcare Insurance Fraud?

Just about anyone can commit health insurance fraud—physicians, hospitals, medical suppliers, pharmacies, nursing homes—the list goes on and on. Dishonest healthcare providers are not the only ones who commit fraud. Patients and insured individuals also commit health insurance fraud and abuse. Most healthcare providers, however, are caring, honest, and ethical professionals.

How Is Healthcare Fraud Committed?

The most popular schemes for committing healthcare fraud include the following:

- Billing for services, procedures, and supplies that were not provided to the patient
  Example: Billing for a diagnostic test that was not performed
- Upcoding—billing for a more expensive service or procedure than what was provided
  Example: Charging for a comprehensive office visit when a shorter, routine visit occurred
- Unbundling of charges or code fragmentation—billing services separately that usually are included in a single service fee
  Example: Making separate charges for each component of a total abdominal hysterectomy; this operation typically has one code, which includes preoperative and postoperative procedures and a lesser fee than coding each component separately
- Misrepresenting services—misrepresenting or falsifying the diagnosis to obtain insurance payment on something that is not covered
  Example: Using a diagnosis of benign cataracts for a routine eye examination with refraction because many insurance policies do not cover this procedure

How Do Consumers Commit Healthcare Insurance Fraud?

The patient can agree or encourage the provider to inflate or misrepresent the services provided. An example might be when a psychiatrist's charge for 1 hour of therapy is $150. The patient, whose policy only covers 50% of psychotherapy charges, might suggest that the therapy session be coded for $1\frac{1}{2}$ or 2 hours so that the insurer pays more of the charges. Other methods consumers use to commit fraud is to create fake receipts and claims or modifying the actual receipt to gain more claim dollars.

PREVENTING FRAUD AND ABUSE

As a health insurance professional, you can do your part to prevent fraud and abuse in the medical office. The following are some general principles to follow:

- Create a file for every major third-party payer your office deals with and keep current providers' manuals, claims completion guidelines, and publications up to date to aid you in generating timely and accurate claims.
- Develop a list of "hot" phone numbers of these carriers to use when questions arise.
- Use the most current coding manuals, and code to the greatest specificity.
- Take advantage of every opportunity to improve your coding skills by attending seminars or continuing education or both.
- Discuss questions or potential problems regarding diagnoses, procedures and services, and fees charged with the physician or other healthcare provider.
- Notify your superior immediately if you suspect fraud or abuse.

What Did You Learn?

1. How does fraud differ from abuse?
2. Who typically commits healthcare fraud?
3. List several common ways that fraud is committed.
4. How can the health insurance professional prevent fraud and abuse?

SUMMARY CHECK POINTS

☑ The health insurance professional should have a basic knowledge of medical law and ethics to aid in accurate claims completion and submission and conduct himself or herself appropriately in and out of the medical facility.

☑ The elements necessary to constitute a legal contract are
  - offer and acceptance,
  - consideration,
  - legal object,
  - competent parties, and
  - legal form (written contracts only).

☑ The relationship between patient and healthcare provider is an *implied* contract, meaning it is not in writing, but it is just as legally binding in the eyes of the law.

☑ The federal laws that regulate health insurance include the following:
  - OBRA (1980)
  - OBRA (1987)
  - COBRA
  - Federal False Claim Amendments Act of 1986
  - Federal Privacy Act of 1974
  - Fraud and Abuse Act
  - TEFRA (1982)

☑ Displaying proper medical ethics and etiquette in the workplace is important for the protection and well-being of the patients and the entire healthcare team. In today's complicated healthcare world, experts recommend that patients be considered as "customers" who are vital to the practice and should be treated with courtesy and respect. When proper medical ethics and etiquette are shown in the workplace, the practice is more likely to avoid potential legal problems.

☑ Accurate, complete, and concise documentation in medical records is essential to the delivery of quality medical care and serves several important purposes:
  - It provides information about the patient's condition, the treatment, the patient's response to this treatment, and the patient's progress.
  - It serves as a legal document, which can protect and defend the provider in the event of legal action.
  - It provides information necessary for third-party reimbursement.
  - It can be used in clinical research under certain circumstances.

☑ The four primary objects of HIPAA are
  - to ensure health insurance portability,
  - to reduce healthcare fraud and abuse,
  - to enforce standards for health information, and
  - to guarantee security and privacy of health information for patients.

☑ HIPAA affects various categories of people involved with healthcare, including
  - health insurance professionals,
  - patients,
  - healthcare providers, and
  - private business entities.

☑ The following are steps recommended by the OIG for developing a HIPAA compliance plan:
- Develop protocols for internal auditing and monitoring of the practice's coding, billing, and documentation performance.
- Establish standards and procedures that identify the practice's self-audit.
- Designate a compliance officer/contact person.
- Conduct appropriate training and education.
- Investigate and respond to compliance offenses and develop corrective action initiatives.
- Develop open lines of communication.
- Enforce disciplinary standards through well-publicized guidelines.

☑ Confidentiality is the foundation for trust in the patient-provider relationship. Every healthcare organization and provider must guarantee confidentiality and privacy of the healthcare information they collect, maintain, use, and transmit. This obligation of confidentiality extends to every member of the healthcare team.

☑ Exceptions to confidentiality include
- minors (under specific circumstances),
- HIV-positive patients and HIV-positive healthcare workers,
- an abused child or adult,
- injuries inflicted by firearms or other weapons, and
- communicable diseases.

☑ Fraud and abuse in healthcare are widespread in the U.S. healthcare system. Not only healthcare providers, but also consumers commit fraud and abuse; however, most providers and consumers are honest and ethical. Fraud and abuse results in millions of wasted healthcare dollars. Health insurance professionals can do their part to prevent fraud and abuse in the medical office in numerous ways, such as
- creating and maintaining a file for each major third-party payer's guidelines,
- developing a list of "hot" phone numbers to use when questions arise,
- using the most current coding manuals and coding to the greatest specificity,
- keeping coding skills by attending seminars or continuing education or both,
- discussing questions or potential problems with healthcare providers, and
- reporting suspected fraud or abuse.

CLOSING SCENARIO

The intricacies of contract law as it applies to health insurance have been an interesting and informative topic for Joy and Barbara. The fact that the relationship between a patient and the healthcare provider is an actual contract and falls under the rules of contract law puts this important relationship in a whole new light. The class Joy previously took in business law had given her a basic background in the legal process, and with the additional information acquired from this chapter, Joy believes she now has an excellent foundation from which she can apply appropriate directives and rules of conduct to the world of health insurance.

Ethics and etiquette, too, have taken on a new meaning for the women. As these terms are applied to becoming a health insurance professional, Joy and Barbara have a better understanding of all the things they should strive for in their careers and professional lives. As Barbara put it, "Ethics and etiquette illustrate not only the *manner* in which we do our jobs, but our *character* while we are on the job."

WEBSITES TO EXPLORE

For live links to the following websites, please visit the Evolve® site at http://evolve.elsevier.com/Beik/today/

- For extensive and up-to-date information on HIPAA, log on to the following websites:
  http://www.hhs.gov/ocr/hipaa/privacy.html
  http://www.cms.hhs.gov/hipaa/

- The activities of the GAO are designed to ensure the executive branch's accountability to Congress under the Constitution and the government's accountability to the American people. You will find many interesting facts and information on medical insurance and healthcare on their website at http://www.gao.gov/

- For more information on the Federal Privacy Act of 1974, research the following websites:
  http://www.info.usda.gov/
  http://www.ftc.gov/foia/privacy_act.htm

- To learn more about healthcare fraud and abuse, log on to the following websites:
  http://www.ama-assn.org/
  http://oig.hhs.gov/publications/hcfac.html

Chapter 4

Types and Sources of Health Insurance

Chapter Outline

CHAPTER OBJECTIVES

After completion of this chapter, the student should be able to

- Describe the two basic types of health insurance plans and how each functions.
- Compare a group insurance contract with an individual policy.
- Discuss the advantages and disadvantages of a group insurance contract.
- List the various sources of health insurance and briefly explain each.
- Explain the purpose and function of a medical savings account (MSA).
- Assess the benefits of a flexible spending account (FSA).
- Discuss the purpose and function of the Consolidated Omnibus Budget Reconciliation Act (COBRA).
- Define terms common to third-party carriers.

CHAPTER TERMS

balance billing
birthday rule
cafeteria plan
CHAMPVA
CMS-1500 form
coinsurance
comprehensive plan
Consolidated Omnibus
  Budget Reconciliation
  Act (COBRA)
coordination of
  benefits (COB)
deductible
disability insurance
enrollees
exclusions
flexible spending
  account (FSA)
group contract
indemnity (fee-for-service)
insured
managed care

Medicaid
medically necessary
medical savings
  account (MSA)
Medicare
Medicare supplement
  plans
Medigap
nonparticipating
  provider (nonPAR)
out-of-pocket maximum
participating provider
  (PAR)
policyholder
preexisting conditions
premium
Social Security Disability
  Insurance (SSDI)
TRICARE
usual, customary, and
  reasonable (UCR)
workers' compensation

OPENING SCENARIO

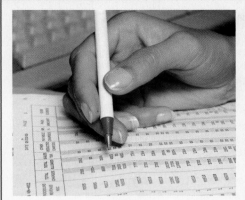

Barbara has volunteered to work two evenings a week for the free clinic in her rural community. Based on Barbara's interest in health insurance and her computer experience from her former job, the physician in charge has agreed to let her assist in the billing and insurance department. Barbara realizes there is still a lot she has to learn about insurance, but the knowledge she has acquired from these few early weeks in class has given her a good foundation on which to begin her volunteer work. She informs the physician that she prefers to watch and learn for a few weeks before actually performing any billing and insurance tasks, and as she gains more confidence, she will begin completing and submitting claims.

At first, the work is challenging, but Barbara becomes more comfortable each day that she works at the clinic. The new terms she's learned take on a much clearer meaning as she applies them to actual situations. Barbara enjoys helping new patients fill out the patient information form and is able to guide them and answer questions relating to primary and secondary insurance coverage. She is especially diligent about each patient having an up-to-date release of information in his or her record and confidently explains the rationale of this important document to patients who inquire. It surprises her that so many patients are willing to put their signature on a document without really knowing the reason why.

Being able to relate her real experiences in the clinic to what she is learning in the classroom allows Barbara to understand better the complexities of health insurance and "puts a face" on many of the issues and topics she is learning. Patient education is quickly becoming her area of special interest because it is obvious that many patients do not know their rights.

TYPES OF HEALTH INSURANCE

Most people in the United States know how important it is to have health insurance in today's world of spiraling medical costs. You may have heard a lot of confusing terms when people speak of health insurance, such as "major medical," "comprehensive," or "managed care." Acronyms such as HMOs, PPOs, and POS make things even more confusing.

In Chapter 1, we learned how insurance got its start. Chapter 2 discussed the education and preparation necessary for becoming a health insurance professional and what job duties and responsibilities are common in this field. Chapter 2 also explained various career opportunities and certification possibilities. Chapter 3 provided a solid background on medical law and ethics. This chapter is the last step in building the foundation in medical insurance. Here, we look at the different types of health insurance and the various ways an individual (and his or her family) may be entitled to or eligible for health insurance benefits. We also explore the different types of health insurance and their sources and things that are common to all carriers. By the end of this chapter, it is hoped that you will begin to make sense of a lot of this medical insurance jargon.

The two basic types of health insurance plans today typically are described as **indemnity** (also called **fee-for-service**) and **managed care**. These two types of plans differ in their basic approach to paying healthcare benefits in three primary ways:

- Choice of providers
- Out-of-pocket costs for covered services
- How bills are paid

INDEMNITY (FEE-FOR-SERVICE)

Indemnity (fee-for-service) is the traditional kind of health-care policy where patients can choose any healthcare provider or hospital they want (including specialists) and change physicians at any time. With indemnity (fee-for-service) plans, the **insured** (or **policyholder**) typically pays a monthly fee called a **premium**. Premiums are based on the policy type and coverage, and the better the coverage, the higher the premium. The patient also pays a certain amount of money up front each year toward his or her medical expenses, known as the **deductible**, before the insurance company begins paying benefits. Historically, this deductible amount was $100 to $500 per year; however, as health insurance costs continue to increase, deductibles of $1000 to $5000 per year commonly are seen. Typically, the higher the deductible, the lower the premiums. In policies that cover whole families, it is common that at least two people in the family must meet this yearly deductible before benefits begin. Additionally, not all medical expenses count toward the deductible, but only those covered in the policy.

After the yearly deductible is met, the patient shares the bill with the insurance company in what is called **coinsurance**. The policy may have an 80/20 coinsurance clause, which means that after the deductible is met, the patient must pay 20% of *covered* medical expenses, and the insurance company pays 80%. This payment is based on what is referred to as **usual, customary, and reasonable (UCR)** rates. UCR rates are the part of a provider's charge that the insurance carrier allows as covered expenses. The UCR value of the provider's service is based on historical data developed from the following criteria:

- How much the provider charges his or her patients for the same or a similar service
- The variance in the charges by most providers for the same service in the same geographic area
- Whether the procedure requires more time, skill, or experience than it usually requires
- The value of the procedure compared with other services

Fee-for-service policies generally have an **out-of-pocket maximum**. This means that when medical expenses reach a certain amount, the UCR fee for covered benefits is paid in full by the insurer. Additionally, there might be lifetime limits as to how much an insurance company pays under the policy (e.g., $1 million).

For the medical bills to be paid, the patient or the healthcare provider must fill out forms and send them to the insurance carrier. The form that is most commonly used is referred to as the **CMS-1500** (Fig. 4-1), a universal form created by the government for Medicare claims and since adopted by most third-party carriers. The CMS-1500 may be submitted in paper form or electronically.

There are two kinds of fee-for-service coverage: basic and major medical. Basic coverage pays toward the costs of room and care while the patient is hospitalized. It also may cover some hospital services and supplies, such as x-rays and prescribed medicine. Basic coverage also pays toward the cost of surgery, whether it is performed in or out of the hospital, and for some physician visits. Major medical takes over where basic coverage leaves off. It covers the cost of long and high-cost illnesses or injuries. Some policies combine basic and major medical coverage into one plan referred to as a **comprehensive plan**. Sometimes the insurance policy does not cover certain medical conditions. These are known as **exclusions** (illnesses or injuries not covered by the policy) and may be due to a **preexisting condition**, which is a physical or mental condition of an insured person that existed before the issuance of a health insurance policy or that existed before issuance and for which treatment was received. Preexisting conditions are excluded from coverage under some policies, or a specified length of time must elapse before the condition is covered.

MANAGED CARE

The term "managed care" is often heard on the news to describe certain medical plans, and many people do not

Imagine This!

Larry Burton, a self-employed carpenter, injured his back in a skiing accident, which involved surgery and extensive treatment and therapy. Larry's medical expenses were covered through an individual policy with HealthNet Insurance Company. Several years later, because of HealthNet's rising premiums, Larry decided to apply for coverage under American Carpenter's Indemnity (ACI), which had lower premiums. ACI required Larry to complete an application form, which included an extensive questionnaire regarding his medical history. Eventually, ACI granted Larry coverage, but excluded payment for treatment of future medical services or procedures involving his back and spine.

know what this phrase means. Managed care is medical care that is provided by a corporation established under state and federal laws. This corporation makes medical decisions for its **enrollees** (people who are covered under the managed care plan). A managed care provider tells patients which physicians they can see, monitors the medications and treatments prescribed, and ensures enrollees that their costs will remain as low as possible. For these services, enrollees pay a set insurance premium each year and a small copayment with each visit. To perform these services satisfactorily, the corporation typically hires a medical staff (physicians, nurses, and other healthcare providers). These "employees" are under contract and, to some degree, take their orders from corporate management. There are many types of managed care organizations. For more detailed information on managed care, see Chapter 7.

What Did You Learn?

1. Name the two basic types of health insurance plans today.
2. List the three primary ways these two types of insurance are different.

SOURCES OF HEALTH INSURANCE

There are several ways to obtain healthcare coverage in today's insurance markets. Many individuals are eligible for coverage through their employers. Self-employed individuals and individuals who are ineligible for coverage through their employer should contact a professional health insurance agent and apply for a private policy. Additionally, government programs, such as Medicare and Medicaid, are available for qualifying individuals.

PLEASE
DO NOT
STAPLE
IN THIS
AREA

CARRIER

HEALTH INSURANCE CLAIM FORM

PICA   PICA

1. MEDICARE   MEDICAID   TRICARE   CHAMPVA   GROUP   FECA   OTHER
              CHAMPUS   HEALTH PLAN   BLK LUNG
   (Medicare #) (Medicaid #) (Sponsor's SSN) (Member ID#) (SSN or ID) (SSN) (ID)

1a. INSURED'S I.D. NUMBER   (For Program in Item 1)

2. PATIENT'S NAME (Last Name, First Name, Middle Initial)

3. PATIENT'S BIRTH DATE   SEX
   MM   DD   YY   M   F

4. INSURED'S NAME (Last Name, First Name, Middle Initial)

5. PATIENT'S ADDRESS (No., Street)

6. PATIENT RELATIONSHIP TO INSURED
   Self   Spouse   Child   Other

7. INSURED'S ADDRESS (No., Street)

CITY   STATE

8. PATIENT STATUS
   Single   Married   Other

CITY   STATE

ZIP CODE   TELEPHONE (Include Area Code)
                (   )

   Employed   Full-Time   Part-Time
               Student   Student

ZIP CODE   TELEPHONE (INCLUDE AREA CODE)
                (   )

9. OTHER INSURED'S NAME (Last Name, First Name, Middle Initial)

10. IS PATIENT'S CONDITION RELATED TO:

11. INSURED'S POLICY GROUP OR FECA NUMBER

a. OTHER INSURED'S POLICY OR GROUP NUMBER

a. EMPLOYMENT? (CURRENT OR PREVIOUS)
   YES   NO

a. INSURED'S DATE OF BIRTH   SEX
   MM   DD   YY   M   F

b. OTHER INSURED'S DATE OF BIRTH   SEX
   MM   DD   YY   M   F

b. AUTO ACCIDENT?   PLACE (State)
   YES   NO

b. EMPLOYER'S NAME OR SCHOOL NAME

c. EMPLOYER'S NAME OR SCHOOL NAME

c. OTHER ACCIDENT?
   YES   NO

c. INSURANCE PLAN NAME OR PROGRAM NAME

d. INSURANCE PLAN NAME OR PROGRAM NAME

10d. RESERVED FOR LOCAL USE

d. IS THERE ANOTHER HEALTH BENEFIT PLAN?
   YES   NO   If yes, return to and complete item 9 a-d.

READ BACK OF FORM BEFORE COMPLETING & SIGNING THIS FORM.

12. PATIENT'S OR AUTHORIZED PERSON'S SIGNATURE I authorize the release of any medical or other information necessary to process this claim. I also request payment of government benefits either to myself or to the party who accepts assignment below.

SIGNED _____   DATE _____

13. INSURED'S OR AUTHORIZED PERSON'S SIGNATURE I authorize payment of medical benefits to the undersigned physician or supplier for services described below.

SIGNED _____

14. DATE OF CURRENT: ILLNESS (First symptom) OR
    MM   DD   YY   INJURY (Accident) OR
                        PREGNANCY(LMP)

15. IF PATIENT HAS HAD SAME OR SIMILAR ILLNESS.
    GIVE FIRST DATE   MM   DD   YY

16. DATES PATIENT UNABLE TO WORK IN CURRENT OCCUPATION
    MM   DD   YY   MM   DD   YY
    FROM   TO

17. NAME OF REFERRING PHYSICIAN OR OTHER SOURCE
    17a.
    17b.

18. HOSPITALIZATION DATES RELATED TO CURRENT SERVICES
    MM   DD   YY   MM   DD   YY
    FROM   TO

19. RESERVED FOR LOCAL USE

20. OUTSIDE LAB? $ CHARGES
    YES   NO

21. DIAGNOSIS OR NATURE OF ILLNESS OR INJURY. (RELATE ITEMS 1,2,3 OR 4 TO ITEM 24E BY LINE)

1. ___ . ___   3. ___ . ___

2. ___ . ___   4. ___ . ___

22. MEDICAID RESUBMISSION
    CODE   ORIGINAL REF. NO.

23. PRIOR AUTHORIZATION NUMBER

24. A. DATE(S) OF SERVICE						B. PLACE OF SERVICE	C. EMG	D. PROCEDURES, SERVICES, OR SUPPLIES (Explain Unusual Circumstances) CPT/HCPCS	MODIFIER	E. DIAGNOSIS POINTER	F. $ CHARGES	G. DAYS OR UNITS	H. EPSDT Family Plan	I. ID. QUAL.	J. RENDERING PROVIDER ID. #
From MM	DD	YY	To MM	DD	YY										
1															NPI
2															NPI
3															NPI
4															NPI
5															NPI
6															NPI

25. FEDERAL TAX I.D. NUMBER   SSN EIN

26. PATIENT'S ACCOUNT NO.

27. ACCEPT ASSIGNMENT?
    (For govt. claims, see back)
    YES   NO

28. TOTAL CHARGE
    $

29. AMOUNT PAID
    $

30. BALANCE DUE
    $

31. SIGNATURE OF PHYSICIAN OR SUPPLIER INCLUDING DEGREES OR CREDENTIALS
    (I certify that the statements on the reverse apply to this bill and are made a part thereof.)

SIGNED _____   DATE _____

32. SERVICE FACILITY LOCATION INFORMATION

a.   b.

33. BILLING PROVIDER INFO & PH # (   )

a.   b.

PATIENT AND INSURED INFORMATION

PHYSICIAN OR SUPPLIER INFORMATION

EXAMPLE ONLY

Fig. 4-1 Copy of a blank CMS-1500 form (both sides).

BECAUSE THIS FORM IS USED BY VARIOUS GOVERNMENT AND PRIVATE HEALTH PROGRAMS, SEE SEPARATE INSTRUCTIONS ISSUED BY APPLICABLE PROGRAMS.

NOTICE: Any person who knowingly files a statement of claim containing any misrepresentation or any false, incomplete or misleading information may be guilty of a criminal act punishable under law and may be subject to civil penalties.

REFERS TO GOVERNMENT PROGRAMS ONLY

MEDICARE AND CHAMPUS PAYMENTS: A patient's signature requests that payment be made and authorizes release of any information necessary to process the claim and certifies that the information provided in Blocks 1 through 12 is true, accurate and complete. In the case of a Medicare claim, the patient's signature authorizes any entity to release to Medicare medical and nonmedical information, including employment status, and whether the person has employer group health insurance, liability, no-fault, worker's compensation or other insurance which is responsible to pay for the services for which the Medicare claim is made. See 42 CFR 411.24(a). If item 9 is completed, the patient's signature authorizes release of the information to the health plan or agency shown. In Medicare assigned or CHAMPUS participation cases, the physician agrees to accept the charge determination of the Medicare carrier or CHAMPUS fiscal intermediary as the full charge, and the patient is responsible only for the deductible, coinsurance and noncovered services. Coinsurance and the deductible are based upon the charge determination of the Medicare carrier or CHAMPUS fiscal intermediary if this is less than the charge submitted. CHAMPUS is not a health insurance program but makes payment for health benefits provided through certain affiliations with the Uniformed Services. Information on the patient's sponsor should be provided in those items captioned in "Insured"; i.e., items 1a, 4, 6, 7, 9, and 11.

BLACK LUNG AND FECA CLAIMS

The provider agrees to accept the amount paid by the Government as payment in full. See Black Lung and FECA instructions regarding required procedure and diagnosis coding systems.

SIGNATURE OF PHYSICIAN OR SUPPLIER (MEDICARE, CHAMPUS, FECA AND BLACK LUNG)

I certify that the services shown on this form were medically indicated and necessary for the health of the patient and were personally furnished by me or were furnished incident to my professional service by my employee under my immediate personal supervision, except as otherwise expressly permitted by Medicare or CHAMPUS regulations.

For services to be considered as "incident" to a physician's professional service, 1) they must be rendered under the physician's immediate personal supervision by his/her employee, 2) they must be an integral, although incidental part of a covered physician's service, 3) they must be of kinds commonly furnished in physician's offices, and 4) the services of nonphysicians must be included on the physician's bills.

For CHAMPUS claims, I further certify that I (or any employee) who rendered services am not an active duty member of the Uniformed Services or a civilian employee of the United States Government or a contract employee of the United States Government, either civilian or military (refer to 5 USC 5536). For Black-Lung claims, I further certify that the services performed were for a Black Lung-related disorder.

No Part B Medicare benefits may be paid unless this form is received as required by existing law and regulations (42 CFR 424.32).

NOTICE: Any one who misrepresents or falsifies essential information to receive payment from Federal funds requested by this form may upon conviction be subject to fine and imprisonment under applicable Federal laws.

NOTICE TO PATIENT ABOUT THE COLLECTION AND USE OF MEDICARE, CHAMPUS, FECA, AND BLACK LUNG INFORMATION
(PRIVACY ACT STATEMENT)

We are authorized by CMS, CHAMPUS and OWCP to ask you for information needed in the administration of the Medicare, CHAMPUS, FECA, and Black Lung programs. Authority to collect information is in section 205(a), 1862, 1872 and 1874 of the Social Security Act as amended, 42 CFR 411.24(a) and 424.5(a) (6), and 44 USC 3101;41 CFR 101 et seq and 10 USC 1079 and 1086; 5 USC 8101 et seq; and 30 USC 901 et seq; 38 USC 613; E.O. 9397.

The information we obtain to complete claims under these programs is used to identify you and to determine your eligibility. It is also used to decide if the services and supplies you received are covered by these programs and to insure that proper payment is made.

The information may also be given to other providers of services, carriers, intermediaries, medical review boards, health plans, and other organizations or Federal agencies, for the effective administration of Federal provisions that require other third parties payers to pay primary to Federal program, and as otherwise necessary to administer these programs. For example, it may be necessary to disclose information about the benefits you have used to a hospital or doctor. Additional disclosures are made through routine uses for information contained in systems of records.

FOR MEDICARE CLAIMS: See the notice modifying system No. 09-70-0501, titled, 'Carrier Medicare Claims Record,' published in the Federal Register, Vol. 55 No. 177, pages 37549, Wed. Sept. 12, 1990, or as updated and republished.

FOR OWCP CLAIMS: Department of Labor, Privacy Act of 1974, "Republication of Notice of Systems of Records," Federal Register Vol. 55 No. 40, Wed. Feb. 28, 1990, See ESA-5, ESA-6, ESA-12, ESA-13, ESA-30, or as updated and republished.

FOR CHAMPUS CLAIMS: PRINCIPLE PURPOSE(S): To evaluate eligibility for medical care provided by civilian sources and to issue payment upon establishment of eligibility and determination that the services/supplies received are authorized by law.

ROUTINE USE(S): Information from claims and related documents may be given to the Dept. of Veterans Affairs, the Dept. of Health and Human Services and/or the Dept. of Transportation consistent with their statutory administrative responsibilities under CHAMPUS/CHAMPVA; to the Dept. of Justice for representation of the Secretary of Defense in civil actions; to the Internal Revenue Service, private collection agencies, and consumer reporting agencies in connection with recoupment claims; and to Congressional Offices in response to inquiries made at the request of the person to whom a record pertains. Appropriate disclosures may be made to other federal, state, local, foreign government agencies, private business entities, and individual providers of care, on matters relating to entitlement, claims adjudication, fraud, program abuse, utilization review, quality assurance, peer review, program integrity, third-party liability, coordination of benefits, and civil and criminal litigation related to the operation of CHAMPUS.

DISCLOSURES: Voluntary; however, failure to provide information will result in delay in payment or may result in denial of claim. With the one exception discussed below, there are no penalties under these programs for refusing to supply information. However, failure to furnish information regarding the medical services rendered or the amount charged would prevent payment of claims under these programs. Failure to furnish any other information, such as name or claim number, would delay payment of the claim. Failure to provide medical information under FECA could be deemed an obstruction.

It is mandatory that you tell us if you know that another party is responsible for paying for your treatment. Section 1128B of the Social Security Act and 31 USC 3801-3812 provide penalties for withholding this information.

You should be aware that P.L. 100-503, the "Computer Matching and Privacy Protection Act of 1988", permits the government to verify information by way of computer matches.

MEDICAID PAYMENTS (PROVIDER CERTIFICATION)

I hereby agree to keep such records as are necessary to disclose fully the extent of services provided to individuals under the State's Title XIX plan and to furnish information regarding any payments claimed for providing such services as the State Agency or Dept. of Health and Human Services may request.

I further agree to accept, as payment in full, the amount paid by the Medicaid program for those claims submitted for payment under that program, with the exception of authorized deductible, coinsurance, co-payment or similar cost-sharing charge.

SIGNATURE OF PHYSICIAN (OR SUPPLIER): I certify that the services listed above were medically indicated and necessary to the health of this patient and were personally furnished by me or my employee under my personal direction.

NOTICE: This is to certify that the foregoing information is true, accurate and complete. I understand that payment and satisfaction of this claim will be from Federal and State funds, and that any false claims, statements, or documents, or concealment of a material fact, may be prosecuted under applicable Federal or State laws.

According to the Paperwork Reduction Act of 1995, no persons are required to respond to a collection of information unless it displays a valid OMB control number. The valid OMB control number for this information collection is 0938-0008. The time required to complete this information collection is estimated to average 10 minutes per response, including the time to review instructions, search existing data resources, gather the data needed, and complete and review the information collection. If you have any comments concerning the accuracy of the time estimate(s) or suggestions for improving this form, please write to: CMS, N2-14-26, 7500 Security Boulevard, Baltimore, Maryland 21244-1850.

Fig. 4-1—cont'd

GROUP CONTRACT

A **group contract** is a contract of insurance made with a company, a corporation, or other groups of common interest wherein all employees or individuals (and their eligible dependents) are insured under a single policy. The group policy is issued to the company or corporation, and everyone receives the same benefits. Often, when you think of a group healthcare plan, the first thing that comes to mind is coverage that is acquired through an individual's employment.

Group healthcare plans through an employer or other group has many advantages and some disadvantages.
Advantages
- Group policies are usually less expensive than individual policies.
- Everyone is usually eligible for coverage regardless of health status.
- Coverage is typically comprehensive.
- Premiums can be deducted from paychecks (if it is the policy of the employer).
- Coverage generally cannot be terminated because of frequent claims.
- Protection under the Health Insurance Portability and Accountability Act (HIPAA) allows an individual to move from one job to another without the fear of exclusions owing to preexisting conditions.

Disadvantages:
- Individuals have little or no choice in the type of coverage provided under the group contract.
- Individuals must accept whatever coverage the group policy provides; modifications are not optional.
- Individuals often lose comprehensive coverage when they no longer belong to the "group," even though they may have "conversion" privileges (see the section on COBRA).
- Premiums for conversion policies tend to be much higher.

Some professions, such as the American Association of Professional Engineers, and individuals sharing a common occupation (e.g., farmers or labor union members) offer group health insurance plans for their members.

INDIVIDUAL POLICIES

If a person is self-employed or if the company with whom he or she is employed does not offer a group policy, the individual may need to buy individual health insurance. Individual health insurance policies can be purchased from most commercial insurers and companies such as Blue Cross and Blue Shield. As with group policies, there are advantages and disadvantages of having an individual health insurance policy.
Advantages:
- The individual can select the type of policy that best fits the individual's (and his or her dependents') situation.

- The policy can be "individualized" to the individual's (or family's) needs.
- The individual controls the insurance contract.
- The individual usually does not lose coverage if he or she changes occupations.

Disadvantages:
- Requirements are usually more restrictive.
- Premiums are typically higher and often depend on the individual's age and health risk.
- There are lower limits for certain coverages (e.g., mental health, substance abuse).
- Preexisting conditions are often excluded, or there is a waiting period before coverage begins.
- Exclusions are more common.
- The insurer can terminate some individual healthcare policies under certain circumstances.

MEDICARE

Medicare is a federal health insurance program that provides benefits to individuals 65 years old or older and individuals younger than 65 with certain disabilities. In many parts of the United States, Medicare-eligible patients now have a choice between managed care and indemnity plans. For individuals who enroll in the traditional Medicare plan, private insurance options help cover some of the gaps in Medicare coverage. These supplemental policies are sometimes called **Medigap** or **Medicare Supplement plans**. These policies must cover certain expenses, such as deductibles and the daily coinsurance amount for hospitalization. Some policies may offer additional benefits, such as coverage for preventive medical care, prescription drugs, or at-home recovery, that Medicare does not cover. For more details on Medicare, Medigap, and Medicare Supplement plans, see Chapter 9.

MEDICAID

Medicaid covers some low-income individuals (particularly children and pregnant women) and certain disabled individuals. Medicaid is a joint federal-state health program that is administered by the individual states. Medicaid coverage differs from state to state. See Chapter 8 for more extensive information on Medicaid.

TRICARE/CHAMPVA

TRICARE is the U.S. military's comprehensive healthcare program for active duty personnel and eligible family members, retirees and family members younger than age 65, and survivors of all uniformed services (i.e., Army, Air Force, Marines, Navy). The TRICARE program is managed by the military in partnership with civilian hospitals and clinics. It is designed to expand access to care, ensure high-quality care, and promote medical readiness. All military hospitals and clinics are part of the TRICARE program.

The Civilian Health and Medical Program of the Department of Veterans Affairs (**CHAMPVA**), is a health benefits program in which the Department of Veterans Affairs (VA) shares the cost of certain healthcare services and supplies with eligible beneficiaries. CHAMPVA is managed by the VA's Health Administration Center in Denver, Colorado, where applications are processed, eligibility is determined, benefits are authorized, and medical claims are processed. Military insurance programs are discussed in detail in Chapter 10.

DISABILITY INSURANCE

Disability insurance is a form of health insurance that pays the policyholder a specific sum of money in place of his or her usual income if the policyholder cannot work because of illness or accident. Usually, policies begin paying after a waiting period stipulated in the policy and pay a certain percentage of the policyholder's usual income. Sometimes disability insurance is provided by employers, but it also is available as a separate coverage. There are several types of disability insurance.

Private

An individual can purchase a private disability insurance policy or can be covered by a disability policy offered by his or her employer. Disability insurance does not cover illnesses or injuries related to one's employment. It is designed to replace 45% to 60% of an individual's gross income on a tax-free basis should an illness unrelated to the job prevent him or her from earning an income. Disability insurance policies vary from one insurance company to another, and each can be very different. Disability insurance can provide short-term or long-term benefits, depending on the stipulations of the policy. Private disability insurance can be costly; however, some employers offer it to their employees at more reasonable rates. There is often a waiting period (e.g., 30 days) before benefits begin.

Social Security Disability Insurance

Social Security Disability Insurance (SSDI) is an insurance program for individuals who become unable to work. It is administered by the Social Security Administration (SSA), funded by Federal Insurance Contributions Act (FICA) tax withheld from workers' pay and by matching employer contributions. SSDI pays qualifying disabled workers cash and healthcare benefits. Workers who have worked and paid FICA tax for at least 5 of the 10 years before the date they become disabled typically are covered by SSDI. In other words, applicants must have worked 20 out of the 40 calendar quarters immediately preceding the onset date of disability to be covered. Younger workers can qualify with fewer years of work. A person can apply

for SSDI benefits at any SSA office. A free booklet entitled *Social Security Disability Benefits* (SSA Publication No. 05-10029) is available at any Social Security office or by calling the SSA toll-free at 800-772-1213. Individuals can apply via the Internet, at www.ssa.gov, but the procedure is relatively new, and there are still some "bugs" in the system.

The supplemental security income (SSI) disability program has marked similarities to SSDI. Both programs are run by the SSA, both offer disability benefits, and both use the same legal definition of "disability." The programs differ significantly, however, in their financial qualifications and benefits.

Workers' Compensation

Workers' compensation insurance pays workers who are injured or disabled on the job or have job-related illnesses. Laws governing workers' compensation are designed to ensure that employees who are injured or disabled on the job are provided with fixed monetary awards, eliminating the need for litigation. These laws also provide benefits for dependents of workers who die as a result of work-related accidents or illnesses. Some laws also protect employers and fellow workers by limiting the amount an injured employee can recover from an employer and by eliminating the liability of coworkers in most accidents. State workers' compensation statutes establish this framework for most employment and differ from state to state. Federal statutes are limited to federal employees or workers employed in some significant aspect of interstate commerce.

The Federal Employment Compensation Act provides workers' compensation for nonmilitary, federal employees. Many of its provisions are typical of most workers' compensation laws. Awards are limited to "disability or death" sustained while in the performance of the employee's duties, but not caused willfully by the employee or by intoxication. The act covers medical expenses resulting from the disability and may require the employee to undergo job retraining. In other words, if the employee is unable to return to his or her original position because of a particular disability, the employee is trained to perform in a different position, ideally at an equal level of pay. A disabled employee receives two thirds of his or her normal monthly salary during the disability period and may receive more for permanent physical injuries or if he or she has dependents. The act provides compensation for survivors of employees who are killed. The Office of Workers' Compensation Programs administers the act.

The Federal Employment Liability Act, although not a workers' compensation statute, provides that railroads engaged in interstate commerce are liable for injuries to their employees if they have been negligent. Disability insurance and workers' compensation are discussed in Chapter 11.

MEDICAL SAVINGS ACCOUNT

A **medical savings account (MSA)** is a special tax shelter set up for the purpose of paying medical bills. Known as the Archer MSA, it is similar to an IRA (a retirement account that allows individuals to make tax-deferred contributions to a personal retirement fund) and works in conjunction with a special low-cost, high-deductible health insurance policy to provide comprehensive health-care coverage at the lowest possible net cost for individuals who qualify. MSAs currently are limited to self-employed individuals and employees of small businesses comprising fewer than 50 employees where a small group MSA health plan is in place.

Here's how an MSA works. Instead of buying high-priced health insurance with low copays and a low deductible, the individual or business purchases a low-cost policy with a high deductible for the big bills and saves the difference in the MSA to cover smaller bills. Money deposited into the MSA account is 100% tax deductible (similar to a traditional IRA) and can be easily accessed by check or debit card to pay most medical bills tax-free (even expenses not covered by insurance, such as dental and vision). The funds that are not used for medical bills stay in the MSA account and keep growing on a tax-favored basis to cover future medical bills or to supplement retirement. An MSA plan offers (1) lower premiums, (2) lower taxes, (3) freedom of choice, and (4) more cash at retirement.

> **✓ HIPAA Tip**
>
> Medical savings accounts under HIPAA provide federal tax deductions for contributions to multi-year savings accounts established for medical purposes.

FLEXIBLE SPENDING ACCOUNT

The **flexible spending account (FSA)** is an IRS Section 125 **cafeteria plan**. A plan falls under the cafeteria category when the cost of the plan (premium) is deducted from the employee's wages before withholding taxes are deducted. This allows employees the option of pretax payroll deduction for some insurance premiums, unreimbursed medical expenses, and child/dependent care expenses. Cafeteria plans are among the fastest growing employee benefits. Employers use plans such as the FSA to retain "quality employees" and as an incentive to help hire new employees. Employers save when employees elect for pretax payroll deduction because lower adjusted gross income also reduces matching FICA and federal unemployment tax. Employees benefit because expenses for such items as health insurance premiums and unreim-

bursed medical, vision, dental, and child/dependent care expenses paid pretax result in immediate tax savings. When employees switch expenses to "before tax," they save on Social Security tax, federal income tax, and state and local tax (in most states).

There are obvious advantages associated with FSAs. Consequently, the government has placed certain restrictions on plans of this type in exchange for the favorable tax treatment. One such restriction is the "use it or lose it" rule. At the beginning of each plan year, individuals designate a certain portion of their before-tax salary to the FSA for dependent care and medical expenses. Any funds left over in either category at the end of the year are forfeited. During the year, you may change the amount of your contribution designation only if there is a change in the health premium or your family status, which includes

- marriage,
- divorce,
- change of employment by spouse,
- birth or adoption of a child,
- death of a spouse or a child, and
- change in employment status (i.e., from full-time to part-time)

> **✓ HIPAA Tip**
>
> HIPAA mandates that when an employee's health-care coverage is terminated, the employer automatically sends the employee, on the coverage's cancellation, a Certificate of Creditable Coverage.

LONG-TERM CARE INSURANCE

When we are healthy, it is easy to take activities of daily living (ADLs), such as bathing, dressing, and feeding ourselves, for granted. When an individual is stricken with a degenerative condition, however, such as a stroke or Alzheimer's disease, performing these ADLs becomes impossible without the assistance of another person. This type of care is referred to as long-term care; it is ongoing and quickly becomes very expensive. Long-term care is not medical care, but rather custodial care. Custodial care involves providing an individual with assistance or supervision or both with ADLs that he or she no longer can perform. Long-term care can be provided in many settings, including nursing homes, one's own home, assisted living facilities, and adult day care.

Today, long-term care insurance typically covers a broad range of services, including nursing home care, assisted living facilities, certain types of home healthcare, and adult day care. Similar to any insurance product, long-term care insurance allows the insured to pay an affordable premium to protect himself or herself in case of an unaffordable catastrophic event.

HIPAA Tip

The Health Insurance Reform Act, incorporated within HIPAA, includes consumer protections for purchasers of long-term care insurance and clarifications that make treatment of private long-term care insurance identical to that of health insurance coverage.

CONSOLIDATED OMNIBUS BUDGET RECONCILIATION ACT

Congress passed the **Consolidated Omnibus Budget Reconciliation Act (COBRA)** health benefit provisions in 1986. The law amends the Employee Retirement Income Security Act, the Internal Revenue Code, and the Public Health Service Act to provide continuation of group health coverage that otherwise would be terminated when an individual leaves his or her place of employment. The law generally covers group health plans maintained by employers with 20 or more employees in the prior year. It applies to plans in the private sector and plans sponsored by state and local governments. The law does not apply, however, to plans sponsored by the U.S. government and certain church-related organizations. Under COBRA, a group health plan ordinarily is defined as a plan that provides medical benefits for the employer's own employees and their dependents through insurance or otherwise (e.g., a trust, health maintenance organization, self-funded pay-as-you-go basis, reimbursement, or combination of these).

COBRA contains provisions that give certain former employees, retirees, spouses, and dependent children the right to temporary continuation of health coverage at group rates. Events that can cause workers and their family members to lose group health coverage that may result in the right to COBRA coverage include the following:

- Voluntary or involuntary termination of the covered employee's employment for reasons other than gross misconduct
- Reduced hours of work for the covered employee
- Covered employee becoming entitled to Medicare
- Divorce or legal separation of a covered employee
- Death of a covered employee
- Loss of status as a dependent child under plan rules

Group health coverage for COBRA participants is typically more expensive than health coverage for active employees because the employer usually formerly paid a part of the premium. It is often less expensive, however, than individual health coverage.

Medical benefits provided under the terms of the plan and available to COBRA beneficiaries may include the following:

- Inpatient and outpatient hospital care
- Physician care
- Surgery and other major medical benefits
- Prescription drugs
- Any other medical benefits, such as dental and vision care

 HIPAA Tip

HIPAA does not set premium rates, but it does prohibit plans and issuers from charging an individual more than similarly situated individuals in the same plan because of health status. Plans may offer premium discounts or rebates for participation in wellness programs.

What Did You Learn?

1. Who qualifies for a medical savings account?
2. Explain how a medical savings account operates.
3. What are the benefits of a flexible spending account?
4. What happens to leftover funds in a flexible spending account at the end of the year?
5. What type of healthcare typically falls under the category of long-term care?
6. To whom does the COBRA law generally apply?
7. List the various events that qualify an employee for COBRA coverage.
8. What medical benefits are included under COBRA?

OTHER TERMS COMMON TO THIRD-PARTY CARRIERS

There are many commonly used terms in the medical provider, hospital, and healthcare industries. A few of the more commonly used term are discussed here. In the Websites to Explore at the end of this chapter, several URLs for accessing a comprehensive list of health insurance terms and their definitions are given.

BIRTHDAY RULE

The **birthday rule** is an informal procedure used in the health insurance industry to help determine which health plan is considered "primary," when individuals (usually children) are listed as dependents on more than one health plan. This scenario occurs frequently among divorced parents. Often, parents include their children on each other's insurance plan to maximize coverage and to ensure that the child will be covered when visiting the other parent. The insurance plans need to coordinate benefits so that the claim is paid properly. To prevent overpayment, one parent's plan is designated as the primary plan and the other as a secondary plan. The birthday rule determines which plan is primary. It states that *the health plan of the parent whose birthday comes first in the calendar year will be considered the primary plan*.

Exceptions to the birthday rule are as follows:
- Parents who share the same birthday
- Divorced or separated parents
- Active employees
- Different plan types

When parents have the same birthday, the parent who has had his or her plan longer pays first. When parents are divorced or separated, the plan of the parent who has legal custody is considered primary. If the custodial parent remarries, the new spouse's plan would be considered secondary. The plan of the parent without custody would pay any additional expenses not covered. If one spouse is currently employed and has insurance and the other spouse has coverage through a former employer (COBRA), the plan of the currently employed spouse would be primary. Group plans are considered primary over individual plans.

These are generally accepted rules, not laws. A prudent health insurance professional should discuss this situation with the patient's parent or guardian as it arises.

● Stop and Think

Helen and Paul Jackson are recently divorced. Hunter, their 7-year-old son, comes to the office with a broken wrist. Helen informs the health insurance professional that she is the custodial parent, but that the court has named Paul as the party responsible for all medical bills. After the divorce, Helen quit her job to become a stay-at-home mom, and she and Hunter are still covered on a COBRA policy through Packers United; Paul is covered by a Blue Cross/Blue Shield PPO group plan. Helen's birth date is listed on the patient information form as May 24, 1964. Hunter's father's birth date is September 5, 1959. To which third-party insurer should the insurance claim be sent first?

COORDINATION OF BENEFITS

Coordination of benefits (COB) came into being several years ago when it was common for a husband and wife to each have the same or similar group health insurance benefits but on different policies. This was commonly referred to as "overinsurance." Possible sources of overinsurance include:
- The husband and the wife are employed and eligible for group health coverage, and each lists the other as a dependent.

- A person is employed in two jobs, both of which provide group health insurance coverage.
- A salaried or professional person who has group health insurance coverage with an employer also has an association group health plan.

The historical concept of COB has been to limit the total benefits an insured individual can receive from both group plans to not more than 100% of the allowable expenses. This prevents the policyholders from making a profit on health insurance claims.

Under COB, the primary plan pays benefits up to its limit, then the secondary plan pays the difference between the primary insurer's benefits and the total incurred allowable (historically 100% of the allowed expenses) up to the secondary insurer's limit. Each state may have different COB regulations based on the National Association of Insurance Commissioners and variations in the language used to facilitate consistent claim administration. When this situation arises, the health insurance professional must rely on the patient (or his or her parent or guardian if a minor) to state which policy is primary. It is not the health insurance professional's responsibility to make this determination.

MEDICAL NECESSITY

Most third-party payers do not pay for medical services, procedures, or supplies unless
- they are proper and needed for the diagnosis or treatment of a patient's medical condition;
- they are provided for the diagnosis, direct care, and treatment of a medical condition;
- they meet the standards of good medical practice in the local area; and
- they are not mainly for the convenience of the patient or the healthcare provider.

When medical services, procedures, or supplies meet these criteria, they are said to be **medically necessary** or meet the standards of "medical necessity." When treating Medicare patients, it is sometimes necessary to complete a certificate of medical necessity (Fig. 4-2).

USUAL, REASONABLE, AND CUSTOMARY

We learned earlier in this chapter that usual, reasonable, and customary (UCR) is a calculation of what certain third-party payers (e.g., Medicare) believe is the appropriate fee for healthcare providers to charge for a specific service or procedure in a certain geographic area. The fee is based on a consensus of what most local hospitals, physicians, or laboratories are charging for a similar procedure or service in the geographic area in which the provider practices. The state and federal governments do not regulate UCR charges, but Medicare publishes their own UCR charges.

Fig. 4-2 Certificate of medical necessity. (Courtesy U.S. Department of Health & Human Services, Centers for Medicare & Medicaid Services.)

SECTION A: **(May be completed by the supplier)**

CERTIFICATION TYPE/DATE: If this is an initial certification for this patient, indicate this by placing date (MM/DD/YY) needed initially in the space marked "INITIAL." If this is a revised certification (to be completed when the physician changes the order, based on the patient's changing clinical needs), indicate the initial date needed in the space marked "INITIAL," and also indicate the recertification date in the space marked "REVISED." If this is a recertification, indicate the initial date needed in the space marked "INITIAL," and also indicate the recertification date in the space marked "RECERTIFICATION." Whether submitting a REVISED or a RECERTIFIED CMN, be sure to always furnish the INITIAL date as well as the REVISED or RECERTIFICATION date.

PATIENT INFORMATION: Indicate the patient's name, permanent legal address, telephone number and his/her health insurance claim number (HICN) as it appears on his/her Medicare card and on the claim form.

SUPPLIER INFORMATION: Indicate the name of your company (supplier name), address and telephone number along with the Medicare Supplier Number assigned to you by the National Supplier Clearinghouse (NSC).

PLACE OF SERVICE: Indicate the place in which the item is being used; i.e., patient's home is 12, skilled nursing facility (SNF) is 31, End Stage Renal Disease (ESRD) facility is 65, etc. Refer to the DMERC supplier manual for a complete list.

FACILITY NAME: If the place of service is a facility, indicate the name and complete address of the facility.

HCPCS CODES: List all HCPCS procedure codes for items ordered that require a CMN. Procedure codes that do not require certification should not be listed on the CMN.

PATIENT DOB, HEIGHT, WEIGHT AND SEX: Indicate patient's date of birth (MM/DD/YY) and sex (male or female); height in inches and weight in pounds, if requested.

PHYSICIAN NAME, ADDRESS: Indicate the physician's name and complete mailing address.

UPIN: Accurately indicate the ordering physician's Unique Physician Identification Number (UPIN).

PHYSICIAN'S TELEPHONE NO: Indicate the telephone number where the physician can be contacted (preferable where records would be accessible pertaining to this patient) if more information is needed.

SECTION B: **(May not be completed by the supplier. While this section may be completed by a non-physician clinician, or a physician employee, it must be reviewed, and the CMN signed (in Section D) by the ordering physician.)**

EST. LENGTH OF NEED: Indicate the estimated length of need (the length of time the physician expects the patient to require use of the ordered item) by filling in the appropriate number of months. If the physician expects that the patient will require the item for the duration of his/her life, then enter 99.

DIAGNOSIS CODES: In the first space, list the ICD9 code that represents the primary reason for ordering this item. List any additional ICD9 codes that would further describe the medical need for the item (up to 3 codes).

QUESTION SECTION: This section is used to gather clinical information to determine medical necessity. Answer each question which applies to the items ordered, circling "Y" for yes, "N" for no, "D" for does not apply, a number if this is offered as an answer option, or fill in the blank if other information is requested.

NAME OF PERSON ANSWERING SECTION B QUESTIONS: If a clinical professional other than the ordering physician (e.g., home health nurse, physical therapist, dietician), or a physician employee answers the questions of Section B, he/she must print his/her name, give his/her professional title and the name of his/her employer where indicated. If the physician is answering the questions, this space may be left blank.

SECTION C: **(To be completed by the supplier)**

NARRATIVE DESCRIPTION OF EQUIPMENT & COST: Supplier gives **(1)** a narrative description of the item(s) ordered, as well as all options, accessories, supplies and drugs; **(2)** the supplier's charge for each item, option, accessory, supply and drug; and **(3)** the Medicare fee schedule allowance for each item/option/accessory/supply/drug, if applicable.

SECTION D: **(To be completed by the physician)**

PHYSICIAN ATTESTATION: The physician's signature certifies **(1)** the CMN which he/she is reviewing includes Sections A, B, C and D; **(2)** the answers in Section B are correct; and **(3)** the self-identifying information in Section A is correct.

PHYSICIAN SIGNATURE After completion and/or review by the physician of Sections A, B and C, the physician must sign and date the CMN in Section D, verifying the Attestation appearing in this Section. The physician's signature also certifies the items ordered are medically necessary for this patient. Signature and date stamps are not acceptable.

According to the Paperwork Reduction Act of 1995, no persons are required to respond to a collection of information unless it displays a valid OMB control number. The valid OMB control number for this information collection is 0938-0679. The time required to complete this information collection is estimated to average 15 minutes per response, including the time to review instructions, search existing resources, gather the data needed, and complete and review the information collection. If you have any comments concerning the accuracy of the time estimate(s), or suggestions for improving this form, write to: CMS, 7500 Security Blvd., N2-14-26, Baltimore, Maryland 21244-1850.

Fig. 4-2—cont'd

Healthcare providers' actual charge may be different from the UCR (allowable) charge of the third-party payer. When an insurance carrier has a UCR charge that is below the actual provider's charge, the patient may be responsible for paying this difference. This is called **balance billing**.

PARTICIPATING VERSUS NONPARTICIPATING PROVIDERS

A **participating provider (PAR)** is one who contracts with the third-party payer and agrees to abide by certain rules and regulations of that carrier. In doing so, the provider usually must accept the insurance carrier's UCR (allowable) fee as payment in full (after patient deductibles and coinsurance are met) and may not balance bill the patient. Some insurance companies offer certain incentives to providers if they agree to become PAR, such as processing claims more quickly and furnishing claims with pre-identifying information. Another advantage of becoming a PAR is that payment from the insurer is paid directly to the provider, rather than to the patient.

A **nonparticipating provider (nonPAR)** has no contractual agreement with the insurance carrier; the provider does not have to accept insurance company's reimbursement as payment in full. Patients can be billed for the difference between the insurance carrier's allowed fee and the provider's actual fee. (Medicare limits how much a nonPAR can charge, however.) One disadvantage of being nonPAR is that, typically, insurance payments are sent to the patient, rather than to the provider.

What Did You Learn?

1. When a child is listed on both parents' health plan, which one pays first?
2. List some exceptions to the birthday rule.
3. What are some possible sources of over-insurance?
4. Name the four stipulations that determine medical necessity.

SUMMARY CHECK POINTS

☑ The two basic types of health insurance plans are indemnity (fee-for-service) and managed care. Under the indemnity type of plan, the patient may visit any healthcare provider, such as a physician or hospital. The patient or the medical provider sends the bill to the insurance company, which typically pays a certain percentage of the fee after the patient meets the policy's annual deductible. A fee-for-service plan might pay 80% of a medical bill. The patient would pay the remaining 20% of the bill—an amount

often called coinsurance. Managed care organizations finance medical care in a way that provides incentives for patients to maintain good health. Most managed care plans designate which healthcare providers and facilities patients can receive treatment from. Managed care plans also attempt to make patients and physicians aware of the costs associated with their healthcare decisions. Advocates of managed care claim that by emphasizing health maintenance and illness prevention, managed care organizations reduce the number of expensive medical treatments in the long run.

☑ **Group health insurance** is one insurance policy covering a group of people. Usually a company establishes a group health insurance plan to cover its employees; however, health insurance plans are not limited to employers. Many different specialized groups can obtain a group health insurance plan for their members, such as clubs/organizations, special interest groups, trade associations, and church/religious groups. An individual health insurance policy covers one person, or a family, on one plan.

☑ The advantages of group health insurance include:
  • Group policies usually are less expensive than individual policies.
  • Everyone usually is eligible for coverage regardless of health status.
  • Coverage is typically comprehensive.
  • Premiums can be deducted from paychecks (if it is the policy of the employer).
  • Coverage generally cannot be terminated because of frequent claims.
  • Protection under HIPAA allows an individual to move from one job to another without the fear of exclusions because of preexisting conditions.

☑ The disadvantages of group health insurance include:
  • Individuals have little or no choice in the type of coverage provided under the group contract.
  • Individuals must accept whatever coverage the group policy provides; modifications are not optional.
  • Individuals often lose comprehensive coverage when they no longer belong to the "group," even though they may have "conversion" privileges (see the section on COBRA).
  • Premiums for conversion policies tend to be much higher.

☑ The various sources of health insurance are as follows:
  • *Medicare*—a federal health insurance program for individuals 65 years old and older and

individuals younger than 65 with certain disabilities.

- *Medicaid*—a joint federal-state health insurance program that is run by the individual states. Medicaid covers some low-income individuals and certain categories of disabled individuals.
- *TRICARE/CHAMPVA*—TRICARE is the U.S. military's comprehensive healthcare program. TRICARE covers active duty personnel and their eligible family members and retirees and their qualifying family members. CHAMPVA is a healthcare benefits program for the spouse or widow (or widower) and children of certain qualifying categories of veterans.
- *Disability insurance*—insurance that is designed to replace a portion of an individual's gross income in the case of an accident or illness that is unrelated to his or her employment.
- *Social Security Disability Insurance (SSDI)*—an insurance program administered by the SSA and funded by a combination of FICA taxes withheld from employees' pay and matching contributions of the employer. SSDI pays healthcare benefits to qualifying disabled workers.
- *Workers' Compensation*—this type of insurance pays workers who are injured or disabled on the job or suffer from job-related illnesses.
- *Medical savings account*—a health insurance option for certain qualifying self-employed individuals and small businesses consisting of two components—a low-cost, high-deductible insurance policy and a tax-advantaged savings account. Individuals pay for their own healthcare up to the annual deductible by withdrawing from the savings

account or paying medical bills out of pocket. The insurance policy then pays for most or all costs of covered services after the deductible is met.

- *Flexible spending account*—offers advantages to the employer and the employee.

☑ Advantages of a flexible spending account to the employer include the following:
- Offers benefits that employees desire, such as medical reimbursement and child care reimbursement
- Incurs little or no cost; in some cases, you generate a positive cash flow through tax savings
- Controls the cost of medical and insurance benefits by passing along premium increases to employees
- Attracts and retains quality employees desiring benefit coverage

☑ Advantages of a flexible spending account to the employee include the following:
- Saves taxes on applicable expenses, such as uninsured medical, dental, and vision services; contributory insurance premiums; and dependent care
- Has a low risk because contributions are determined before participating
- Provides a higher spendable income

☑ COBRA gives workers and their dependents who lose their health insurance benefits the right to continue group coverage temporarily under the same group health plan sponsored by their employer in certain instances where coverage under the plan would otherwise end. The law generally covers group health plans maintained by employers with 20 or more employees in the prior year.

CLOSING SCENARIO

Barbara and Joy have learned much about the fundamentals of medical insurance. The first four chapters have given them a good foundation of knowledge regarding health insurance in general. The legal and ethical side of health insurance has been particularly informative, and the women are aware of the importance of having a sound footing in this area. On their own, they have researched the HIPAA rules and regulations extensively. Joy is considering enrolling in a business law course evenings to enhance her understanding of law as it pertains to healthcare.

The two women have become involved in the Student Health Careers Club and developed an "activity board" to encourage other students to take part in a health fair being sponsored by the free clinic where Barbara volunteers. The main theme they have chosen is, "Educating Patients About Their Rights." They intend to apply what they have learned in class and through their research to a short presentation to clinic visitors.

WEBSITES TO EXPLORE

For live links to the following websites, please visit the Evolve® site at http://evolve.elsevier.com/Beik/today/

- For a comprehensive list of health insurance terms and their definitions, log on to the following websites:
  http://www.cms.hhs.gov/glossary/
  http://www.bcbs.com/glossary/glossary.html
  http://www.valleyhealth.biz/glossary.html

- For more information on healthcare in general, explore these websites
  http://www.cms.hhs.gov/
  http://www.ahima.org/
  http://www.hiaa.org/

- Browse this CMS website to learn more about HIPAA
  http://www.cms.hhs.gov/hipaa

UNIT II

Health Insurance Basics

Chapter 5

The "Universal" Claim Form: CMS-1500

Chapter Outline

I. Universal Insurance Claim Form
  A. CMS-1500 Paper Form
    1. Format of the Form
    2. Optical Character Recognition
    3. Using Optical Character Recognition Format Rules
  B. Who Uses the Paper CMS-1500 Form
II. Documents Needed When Completing the CMS-1500 Claim Form
  A. Patient Information Form
    1. New Patient Information
    2. Insurance Section
    3. Additional Insurance
    4. Insurance Authorization and Assignment
  B. Patient Insurance Identification Card
C. Patient Health Record
D. Encounter Form
E. Patient Ledger Card
III. Completing the CMS-1500 Paper Form
  A. Patient/Insured Section
  B. Physician/Supplier Section
IV. Preparing the Claim Form for Submission
  A. Proofreading
  B. Claim Attachments
  C. Tracking Claims
V. Generating Claims Electronically
VI. Claims Clearinghouses
  A. Using a Clearinghouse
  B. Direct Claims
  C. Clearinghouses versus Direct

CHAPTER OBJECTIVES

After completion of this chapter, the student should be able to

- Explain how the CMS-1500 "universal" insurance claim form was developed.
- Discuss the format of the form.
- List the major rules necessary for optical character recognition.
- Identify the necessary criteria for using the paper CMS-1500 form.
- Describe each of the five documents needed for completion of the CMS-1500 form.
- Apply general guidelines for completing a CMS-1500 paper form.
- Discuss the importance of proofreading claims.

CHAPTER TERMS

abstract
ASCII (American Standard Code for Information Interchange)
assign benefits
beneficiary
claims clearinghouse
clean claims
CMS-1500 (form)
demographic information
encounter form
mono-spaced fonts
OCR scannable
optical character recognition (OCR)
patient ledger card
release of information
small provider
waiver

CHAPTER OBJECTIVES

- Explain the function of claims clearinghouses.
- Compare and contrast the use of a clearinghouse versus direct claims submission.

OPENING SCENARIO

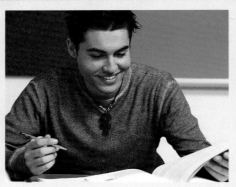

Emilio Sanchez and Latisha Howard are enrolled in a health insurance course at a career school in their area. Emilio graduated from high school just last year and knew immediately what career path he wanted to pursue—health insurance administration. Latisha has worked in the healthcare field for 5 years as a nursing assistant, but she injured her back lifting a patient and had to give up her job at a long-term care facility. Because her experience lies in healthcare, she decided to stay in this discipline, but pursue a different avenue that did not involve physical exertion.

In the class in which they are enrolled, the facilitator allows students to progress at their own speed, and Emilio and Latisha found that they not only work well together, but also they work at about the same pace. Both students feel comfortable that they know the material covered in Unit I well enough to move on to Unit II and continue with their learning experience in health insurance.

After reading over the outline for Chapter 5, Emilio and Latisha agree that the idea of using a universal form for all health insurance claims makes good sense, but knowing what information to enter in each of the 33 blocks is, at this point, puzzling. They also are curious to learn how information from a patient's health record can be adapted to this form. They reassure one another, however, that completing the CMS-1500 should become routine with practice.

UNIVERSAL INSURANCE CLAIM FORM

A major innovation that made the process of health insurance claims submission simpler was the development of a universal form. Before the emergence of this universal form, every insurance carrier had its own specialized type of paperwork for submitting claims. Imagine the frustration a health insurance professional must have felt trying to figure out how to complete all these different forms properly. In the mid-1970s, the Health Care Financing Administration (HCFA, pronounced "hick-fa") created a new form for Medicare claims, called the HCFA-1500. The form was approved by the American Medical Association Council on Medical Services and was subsequently adopted by all government healthcare programs. Although the HCFA-1500 originally was developed for submitting Medicare claims, it eventually was accepted by most commercial/private insurance carriers to facilitate the standardization of the claims process. Because HCFA is now called the Center for Medicare and Medicaid Services (CMS), the name of the form has been changed to **CMS-1500**; however, it is basically the same document.

The National Uniform Claim Committee (NUCC) and the National Uniform Billing Committee (NUBC) have revised the CMS-1500 universal form. The original form, initiated in 1990, was referred to as CMS-1500 (12-90). The revised version is called the CMS-1500 (08-05). The new form is very similar to the original form, but there are new areas to place national provider identifier (NPI) numbers for the Referring Provider (Box 17), Service Facility Location Information (Box 32), and the Billing Provider Information (Box 33). NUCC has established the following timeline for transition to the revised version of the CMS-1500 as follows:

October 1, 2006: Health plans, clearinghouses, and other vendors should be ready to handle and accept the revised CMS-1500 Claim Form.

October 1, 2006- February 1, 2007: Providers can use either the current version (CMS-1500 [12-90]) or the revised version of the claim form (CMS-1500 [08-05]).

February 1, 2007: The CMS-1500 (12-90) will be discontinued and only the revised form should be used. All rebilled claims should use the revised form even if earlier submissions were on the discontinued form. A February 2007 transition is being used to ensure the functioning of the revised form prior to the May 23, 2007 deadline for reporting NPI numbers.

Providers should contact health plans prior to submitting claims on the revised form to ensure they are prepared to accept it. Once the new form is implemented, claims submitted on the CMS-1500 (12-90) form will be rejected.

The front and back sides of the official CMS-1500 (08-05) are shown in Fig. 5-1. Additional information regarding the revised form is available at the NUCC website listed under "Websites to Explore" at the end of this chapter.

☑ HIPAA Tip

Any person or organization that furnishes, bills, or is paid for healthcare in the normal course of business falls under HIPAA rules and regulations.

CMS-1500 PAPER FORM

Format of the Form

The CMS-1500 form is an 8½ × 11–inch, two-sided document. The front side is printed in **OCR scannable** red ink; the back side contains instructions for various government and private health programs. There are two sections to the CMS-1500; the top portion is for the patient/insured information (Blocks 1-13); the bottom portion is for the physician/supplier information (Blocks 14-33). In the later section entitled "Completing the CMS-1500," the student learns what typically goes in each block. Keep in mind, however, that there are some minor differences from one major payer to another; these are pointed out in the individual chapters pertaining to the particular major carrier.

Optical Character Recognition

In most instances, when the paper CMS-1500 claim form is prepared for submission, **Optical Character Recognition (OCR)** formatting guidelines should be used. OCR is the recognition of printed or written *text characters* by a computer. This involves photo scanning of the text character by character, analysis of the scanned-in image, and translation of the character image into character codes, such as **ASCII (American Standard Code for Information Interchange)**. ASCII is the most common *format* used for *text files* in computers and on the Internet.

In OCR processing, the scanned-in image is analyzed for light and dark areas to identify each alphabetic letter or numeric digit. When a character is recognized, it is converted into an ASCII code. Special circuit boards and computer chips designed expressly for OCR are used to speed up the recognition process. The CMS-1500 is printed in a special red ink to optimize this OCR process. When the form is scanned, everything in red "drops out," and the computer reads the information printed within the blocks.

Using Optical Character Recognition Format Rules

Because many third-party carriers use OCR scanning for reading health insurance claims, the health insurance professional should complete all paper CMS-1500 forms using the specific rules for preparing a document for OCR scanning. OCR works best with originals or very clear copies and **mono-spaced fonts** (where each character takes up exactly the same amount of space); standard mono-spaced type fonts (such as Courier or Times New Roman) in 12-point font size and black text are recommended. No special formatting, such as bold, italics, or underline, should be used, and extreme care should be taken when keying the information. Type should be lined up so that all entries and characters fall within the spaces provided on the form.

The following are specific guidelines for preparing OCR scannable claims:
- Use all uppercase (capital) letters.
- Omit all punctuation.
- Use the MM DD YYYY format (with a space—not a dash—between each set of digits) for dates of birth.
- Use a *space* instead of the usual punctuation or symbols for each of the following situations:
  - dollar signs and decimal points in fee charges and ICD codes
  - dash preceding a procedure code modifier
  - parentheses around the telephone area code
  - hyphens in Social Security and employer identification numbers
- Omit titles and other designations, such as Sr., Jr., II, or III, unless they appear on the patient's identification (ID) card.
- Use two zeros in the cents column when the charge is expressed in whole dollars.
- Do not use lift-off tape, correction tape, or whiteout.

A section of the CMS-1500 form showing the proper OCR format is shown in Fig. 5-2.

When the health insurance professional has completed the claim form, it is important that the form is thoroughly examined for errors and omissions. If you are new to the profession, it is recommended that you ask a coworker or supervisor to proofread forms before submission until you acquire the necessary proficiency in the claims process. The most important task the health insurance professional is responsible for is to obtain the maximal amount of reimbursement in the minimal amount of time that the medical record supports. Fig. 5-3 shows common CMS-1500 claim form errors and omissions.

If a claim is being resubmitted, most carriers require a new one using the original (red print) CMS-1500 form. Additional tips for submitting paper claims include the following:
- Do not include any handwritten data (other than signatures) on the forms.
- Do not staple anything to the form.

PLEASE
DO NOT
STAPLE
IN THIS
AREA

CARRIER

HEALTH INSURANCE CLAIM FORM

| | PICA | | | | | | | PICA | |

1. MEDICARE	MEDICAID	TRICARE CHAMPUS	CHAMPVA	GROUP HEALTH PLAN	FECA BLK LUNG	OTHER	1a. INSURED'S I.D. NUMBER	(For Program in Item 1)
(Medicare #)	(Medicaid #)	(Sponsor's SSN)	(Member ID#)	(SSN or ID)	(SSN)	(ID)		

2. PATIENT'S NAME (Last Name, First Name, Middle Initial)

3. PATIENT'S BIRTH DATE MM DD YY   SEX   M   F

4. INSURED'S NAME (Last Name, First Name, Middle Initial)

5. PATIENT'S ADDRESS (No., Street)

6. PATIENT RELATIONSHIP TO INSURED   Self   Spouse   Child   Other

7. INSURED'S ADDRESS (No., Street)

CITY   STATE

8. PATIENT STATUS   Single   Married   Other   Employed   Full-Time Student   Part-Time Student

CITY   STATE

ZIP CODE   TELEPHONE (Include Area Code) (   )

ZIP CODE   TELEPHONE (INCLUDE AREA CODE) (   )

9. OTHER INSURED'S NAME (Last Name, First Name, Middle Initial)

10. IS PATIENT'S CONDITION RELATED TO:

11. INSURED'S POLICY GROUP OR FECA NUMBER

a. OTHER INSURED'S POLICY OR GROUP NUMBER

a. EMPLOYMENT? (CURRENT OR PREVIOUS)   YES   NO

a. INSURED'S DATE OF BIRTH MM DD YY   SEX   M   F

b. OTHER INSURED'S DATE OF BIRTH MM DD YY   SEX   M   F

b. AUTO ACCIDENT?   PLACE (State)   YES   NO

b. EMPLOYER'S NAME OR SCHOOL NAME

c. EMPLOYER'S NAME OR SCHOOL NAME

c. OTHER ACCIDENT?   YES   NO

c. INSURANCE PLAN NAME OR PROGRAM NAME

d. INSURANCE PLAN NAME OR PROGRAM NAME

10d. RESERVED FOR LOCAL USE

d. IS THERE ANOTHER HEALTH BENEFIT PLAN?   YES   NO   *If yes*, return to and complete item 9 a-d.

READ BACK OF FORM BEFORE COMPLETING & SIGNING THIS FORM.
12. PATIENT'S OR AUTHORIZED PERSON'S SIGNATURE I authorize the release of any medical or other information necessary to process this claim. I also request payment of government benefits either to myself or to the party who accepts assignment below.

SIGNED _____   DATE _____

13. INSURED'S OR AUTHORIZED PERSON'S SIGNATURE I authorize payment of medical benefits to the undersigned physician or supplier for services described below.

SIGNED _____

PATIENT AND INSURED INFORMATION

14. DATE OF CURRENT: MM DD YY   ILLNESS (First symptom) OR INJURY (Accident) OR PREGNANCY(LMP)

15. IF PATIENT HAS HAD SAME OR SIMILAR ILLNESS. GIVE FIRST DATE MM DD YY

16. DATES PATIENT UNABLE TO WORK IN CURRENT OCCUPATION MM DD YY   FROM   TO   MM DD YY

17. NAME OF REFERRING PHYSICIAN OR OTHER SOURCE

17a.
17b.

18. HOSPITALIZATION DATES RELATED TO CURRENT SERVICES MM DD YY   FROM   TO   MM DD YY

19. RESERVED FOR LOCAL USE

20. OUTSIDE LAB? $ CHARGES   YES   NO

EXAMPLE ONLY

21. DIAGNOSIS OR NATURE OF ILLNESS OR INJURY. (RELATE ITEMS 1,2,3 OR 4 TO ITEM 24E BY LINE)

1. ____ . ____   3. ____ . ____
2. ____ . ____   4. ____ . ____

22. MEDICAID RESUBMISSION CODE   ORIGINAL REF. NO.

23. PRIOR AUTHORIZATION NUMBER

24. A. DATE(S) OF SERVICE		B. PLACE OF SERVICE	C. EMG	D. PROCEDURES, SERVICES, OR SUPPLIES		E. DIAGNOSIS POINTER	F. $ CHARGES	G. DAYS OR UNITS	H. EPSDT Family Plan	I. ID. QUAL.	J. RENDERING PROVIDER ID. #
From MM DD YY	To MM DD YY			CPT/HCPCS	MODIFIER						
1											NPI
2											NPI
3											NPI
4											NPI
5											NPI
6											NPI

25. FEDERAL TAX I.D. NUMBER   SSN   EIN

26. PATIENT'S ACCOUNT NO.

27. ACCEPT ASSIGNMENT? (For govt. claims, see back)   YES   NO

28. TOTAL CHARGE $

29. AMOUNT PAID $

30. BALANCE DUE $

31. SIGNATURE OF PHYSICIAN OR SUPPLIER INCLUDING DEGREES OR CREDENTIALS (I certify that the statements on the reverse apply to this bill and are made a part thereof.)

SIGNED _____   DATE _____

32. SERVICE FACILITY LOCATION INFORMATION

a.   b.

33. BILLING PROVIDER INFO & PH # (   )

a.   b.

PHYSICIAN OR SUPPLIER INFORMATION

Fig. 5-1 Front and back of a blank CMS-1500 (red ink) form.

BECAUSE THIS FORM IS USED BY VARIOUS GOVERNMENT AND PRIVATE HEALTH PROGRAMS, SEE SEPARATE INSTRUCTIONS ISSUED BY APPLICABLE PROGRAMS.

NOTICE: Any person who knowingly files a statement of claim containing any misrepresentation or any false, incomplete or misleading information may be guilty of a criminal act punishable under law and may be subject to civil penalties.

REFERS TO GOVERNMENT PROGRAMS ONLY

MEDICARE AND CHAMPUS PAYMENTS: A patient's signature requests that payment be made and authorizes release of any information necessary to process the claim and certifies that the information provided in Blocks 1 through 12 is true, accurate and complete. In the case of a Medicare claim, the patient's signature authorizes any entity to release to Medicare medical and nonmedical information, including employment status, and whether the person has employer group health insurance, liability, no-fault, worker's compensation or other insurance which is responsible to pay for the services for which the Medicare claim is made. See 42 CFR 411.24(a). If item 9 is completed, the patient's signature authorizes release of the information to the health plan or agency shown. In Medicare assigned or CHAMPUS participation cases, the physician agrees to accept the charge determination of the Medicare carrier or CHAMPUS fiscal intermediary as the full charge, and the patient is responsible only for the deductible, coinsurance and noncovered services. Coinsurance and the deductible are based upon the charge determination of the Medicare carrier or CHAMPUS fiscal intermediary if this is less than the charge submitted. CHAMPUS is not a health insurance program but makes payment for health benefits provided through certain affiliations with the Uniformed Services. Information on the patient's sponsor should be provided in those items captioned in "Insured"; i.e., items 1a, 4, 6, 7, 9, and 11.

BLACK LUNG AND FECA CLAIMS

The provider agrees to accept the amount paid by the Government as payment in full. See Black Lung and FECA instructions regarding required procedure and diagnosis coding systems.

SIGNATURE OF PHYSICIAN OR SUPPLIER (MEDICARE, CHAMPUS, FECA AND BLACK LUNG)

I certify that the services shown on this form were medically indicated and necessary for the health of the patient and were personally furnished by me or were furnished incident to my professional service by my employee under my immediate personal supervision, except as otherwise expressly permitted by Medicare or CHAMPUS regulations.

For services to be considered as "incident" to a physician's professional service, 1) they must be rendered under the physician's immediate personal supervision by his/her employee, 2) they must be an integral, although incidental part of a covered physician's service, 3) they must be of kinds commonly furnished in physician's offices, and 4) the services of nonphysicians must be included on the physician's bills.

For CHAMPUS claims, I further certify that I (or any employee) who rendered services am not an active duty member of the Uniformed Services or a civilian employee of the United States Government or a contract employee of the United States Government, either civilian or military (refer to 5 USC 5536). For Black-Lung claims, I further certify that the services performed were for a Black Lung-related disorder.

No Part B Medicare benefits may be paid unless this form is received as required by existing law and regulations (42 CFR 424.32).

NOTICE: Any one who misrepresents or falsifies essential information to receive payment from Federal funds requested by this form may upon conviction be subject to fine and imprisonment under applicable Federal laws.

NOTICE TO PATIENT ABOUT THE COLLECTION AND USE OF MEDICARE, CHAMPUS, FECA, AND BLACK LUNG INFORMATION
(PRIVACY ACT STATEMENT)

We are authorized by CMS, CHAMPUS and OWCP to ask you for information needed in the administration of the Medicare, CHAMPUS, FECA, and Black Lung programs. Authority to collect information is in section 205(a), 1862, 1872 and 1874 of the Social Security Act as amended, 42 CFR 411.24(a) and 424.5(a) (6), and 44 USC 3101;41 CFR 101 et seq and 10 USC 1079 and 1086; 5 USC 8101 et seq; and 30 USC 901 et seq; 38 USC 613; E.O. 9397.

The information we obtain to complete claims under these programs is used to identify you and to determine your eligibility. It is also used to decide if the services and supplies you received are covered by these programs and to insure that proper payment is made.

The information may also be given to other providers of services, carriers, intermediaries, medical review boards, health plans, and other organizations or Federal agencies, for the effective administration of Federal provisions that require other third parties payers to pay primary to Federal program, and as otherwise necessary to administer these programs. For example, it may be necessary to disclose information about the benefits you have used to a hospital or doctor. Additional disclosures are made through routine uses for information contained in systems of records.

FOR MEDICARE CLAIMS: See the notice modifying system No. 09-70-0501, titled, 'Carrier Medicare Claims Record,' published in the Federal Register, Vol. 55 No. 177, pages 37549, Wed. Sept. 12, 1990, or as updated and republished.

FOR OWCP CLAIMS: Department of Labor, Privacy Act of 1974, "Republication of Notice of Systems of Records," Federal Register Vol. 55 No. 40, Wed. Feb. 28, 1990, See ESA-5, ESA-6, ESA-12, ESA-13, ESA-30, or as updated and republished.

FOR CHAMPUS CLAIMS: PRINCIPLE PURPOSE(S): To evaluate eligibility for medical care provided by civilian sources and to issue payment upon establishment of eligibility and determination that the services/supplies received are authorized by law.

ROUTINE USE(S): Information from claims and related documents may be given to the Dept. of Veterans Affairs, the Dept. of Health and Human Services and/or the Dept. of Transportation consistent with their statutory administrative responsibilities under CHAMPUS/CHAMPVA; to the Dept. of Justice for representation of the Secretary of Defense in civil actions; to the Internal Revenue Service, private collection agencies, and consumer reporting agencies in connection with recoupment claims; and to Congressional Offices in response to inquiries made at the request of the person to whom a record pertains. Appropriate disclosures may be made to other federal, state, local, foreign government agencies, private business entities, and individual providers of care, on matters relating to entitlement, claims adjudication, fraud, program abuse, utilization review, quality assurance, peer review, program integrity, third-party liability, coordination of benefits, and civil and criminal litigation related to the operation of CHAMPUS.

DISCLOSURES: Voluntary; however, failure to provide information will result in delay in payment or may result in denial of claim. With the one exception discussed below, there are no penalties under these programs for refusing to supply information. However, failure to furnish information regarding the medical services rendered or the amount charged would prevent payment of claims under these programs. Failure to furnish any other information, such as name or claim number, would delay payment of the claim. Failure to provide medical information under FECA could be deemed an obstruction.

It is mandatory that you tell us if you know that another party is responsible for paying for your treatment. Section 1128B of the Social Security Act and 31 USC 3801-3812 provide penalties for withholding this information.

You should be aware that P.L. 100-503, the "Computer Matching and Privacy Protection Act of 1988", permits the government to verify information by way of computer matches.

MEDICAID PAYMENTS (PROVIDER CERTIFICATION)

I hereby agree to keep such records as are necessary to disclose fully the extent of services provided to individuals under the State's Title XIX plan and to furnish information regarding any payments claimed for providing such services as the State Agency or Dept. of Health and Human Services may request.

I further agree to accept, as payment in full, the amount paid by the Medicaid program for those claims submitted for payment under that program, with the exception of authorized deductible, coinsurance, co-payment or similar cost-sharing charge.

SIGNATURE OF PHYSICIAN (OR SUPPLIER): I certify that the services listed above were medically indicated and necessary to the health of this patient and were personally furnished by me or my employee under my personal direction.

NOTICE: This is to certify that the foregoing information is true, accurate and complete. I understand that payment and satisfaction of this claim will be from Federal and State funds, and that any false claims, statements, or documents, or concealment of a material fact, may be prosecuted under applicable Federal or State laws.

According to the Paperwork Reduction Act of 1995, no persons are required to respond to a collection of information unless it displays a valid OMB control number. The valid OMB control number for this information collection is 0938-0008. The time required to complete this information collection is estimated to average 10 minutes per response, including the time to review instructions, search existing data resources, gather the data needed, and complete and review the information collection. If you have any comments concerning the accuracy of the time estimate(s) or suggestions for improving this form, please write to: CMS, N2-14-26, 7500 Security Boulevard, Baltimore, Maryland 21244-1850.

Fig. 5-1—cont'd

1.   MEDICARE   MEDICAID   TRICARE CHAMPUS   CHAMPVA   GROUP HEALTH PLAN   FECA BLK LUNG   OTHER

1.   MEDICARE   MEDICAID   TRICARE CHAMPUS   CHAMPVA   GROUP HEALTH PLAN   FECA BLK LUNG   OTHER
   (Medicare #)   (Medicaid #)   (Sponsor's SSN)   (Member ID #)   [X]   (SSN or ID)   (SSN)   (ID)

2. PATIENT'S NAME (Last Name, First Name, Middle Initial)
SMITH JOHN Q

3. PATIENT'S BIRTH DATE   MM   DD   YY   SEX
01 | 06 | 1934   M [X]   F [ ]

5. PATIENT'S ADDRESS (No., Street)
1000 WEST ACORN DRIVE

6. PATIENT RELATIONSHIP TO INSURED
Self [X]   Spouse [ ]   Child [ ]   Other [ ]

CITY
GOODTOWN

STATE
XY

8. PATIENT STATUS
Single [X]   Married [ ]   Other [ ]

ZIP CODE
23456

TELEPHONE (Include Area Code)
(555) 292 4444

Employed [X]   Full-Time Student [ ]   Part-Time Student [ ]

Fig. 5-2 Section of the CMS-1500 form illustrating proper OCR format.

- Improper identification of patient, either the insurance identification number or name
- Missing or invalid subscriber's name and/or birth date
- Missing or incomplete name, address, and identifier of an ordering provider, rendering, or referring provider (or others)
- Invalid provider NPI identifier (when needed) for rendering providers, referring providers or others
- Missing "insurance type code" for secondary coverage (This information, such as a spouse's payer, is important for filing primary claims in addition to secondary claims.)
- Preauthorization codes missing
- Missing payer name and/or payer identifier, required for both primary and secondary payers.
- Invalid diagnostic and/or procedure code(s)
- Missing or invalid admission date for inpatient services
- Missing or incomplete service facility name, address, and identification for services rendered outside the office or home, including invalid ZIP codes or two-letter state abbreviations
- Failing to include necessary documentation when needed
- Filing the claim after the deadline date

Fig. 5-3 List of common errors/omissions on the CMS-1500 claim form.

WHO USES THE PAPER CMS-1500 FORM

To improve the efficiency and effectiveness of the healthcare system, the Health Insurance Portability and Accountability Act (HIPAA) includes a series of administrative simplification provisions that require the Department of Health and Human Services to adopt national standards for electronic healthcare transactions. By ensuring consistency throughout the industry, these national standards presumably make it easier for healthcare carriers, physicians, hospitals, and other healthcare providers to submit claims and other transactions electronically.

The HIPAA Administrative Simplification Compliance Act (ASCA) set the deadline for compliance with the HIPAA Electronic Healthcare Transactions and Code Set standards as October 2003, meaning that providers' offices must be computerized and capable of submitting all claims electronically by that date. ASCA prohibits the Department of Health and Human Services from paying Medicare claims that are not submitted electronically after this date,

unless the Secretary grants a **waiver** for this requirement. A waiver, in this case, would be if the Secretary formally tells a provider (usually in writing) that he or she does not have to comply with this regulation. ASCA further stated that the Secretary must grant such a waiver if a provider had no method available for the submission of claims in electronic form or if the facility submitting the claim was a **small provider** of services or supplies. ASCA, according to the Centers for Medicare and Medicaid Services' website, defines a small provider or supplier as *a provider of services with fewer than 25 full-time equivalent employees or a physician, practitioner, facility, or supplier (other than a provider of services) with fewer than 10 full-time equivalent employees.*

This provision does not prevent providers from submitting paper claims to other health plans. It also states that if a provider transmits *any* claim electronically, it is subject to the HIPAA Administrative Simplification requirements, regardless of size. In other words, if a provider's office submits any claims electronically, ASCA says it must submit all claims electronically. It cannot submit some claims on paper and some electronically.

So, who uses the paper CMS-1500 form? If the provider falls into one of the two following categories, the paper CMS-1500 form can be used—but, remember, it has to be used exclusively with all carriers that have the capability of receiving electronic transmissions:

1. Providers who are not computerized and do not have the capability of submitting claims electronically can still use the paper version of the form.
2. "Small providers" who fit the previous italicized description can still use the paper version of the form.

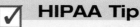

✓ HIPAA Tip

The "under 10" rule applies only to Medicare/Medicaid. If a medical facility has only one employee but is doing *anything* electronic, the office must be in compliance with HIPAA's privacy rules and regulations.

● **Stop and Think**

We learned in this section that two categories of providers are exempt from the ASCA mandate that by October 2003, all claims must be submitted electronically. In your opinion, why are providers falling into these categories allowed to use the CMS-1500 paper form?

What Did You Learn?

1. To whom do we credit the innovation of the "universal" claim form?
2. List the rules for OCR formatting.
3. Name the two categories of providers who can use the CMS-1500 paper form.

DOCUMENTS NEEDED WHEN COMPLETING THE CMS-1500 CLAIM FORM

Several documents are needed when completing the CMS-1500 claim form.

PATIENT INFORMATION FORM

A patient information form, sometimes referred to as a patient registration form, is a document (typically one page) that patients seeking care at a healthcare facility are asked to complete for the following reasons:

1. to gather all necessary demographic information to aid the healthcare professional in providing appropriate treatment,
2. to have a record of current insurance information for claim preparation and submission, and
3. to keep health records up to date.

When the form is completed, it becomes an integral part of the patient's health record. This information form is considered a legal document and should be updated at least once a year. It is a good idea to ask returning patients if there have been any changes since they were last in the office. A typical patient information is shown in Fig. 5-4.

New Patient Information

Look at this section in the example patient information form in Fig. 5-4. Note that it asks for general **demographic information**, such as name, address, Social Security number, and employment.

Insurance Section

The second section contains questions regarding the patient's insurance. Having the patient fill out the blanks in this section is important, but it is necessary also to request and make photocopies of the front and the back of the patient's insurance ID card. The ID card often lists additional information that patients might not routinely include on the form, such as telephone numbers for preauthorization or precertification. Also, it is common for patients to transpose or omit identifying alpha characters or numbers or both.

Additional Insurance

In some cases, patients may be covered under more than one insurance policy. Most patient information forms have a separate section where additional insurance is listed. Information from a secondary insurance policy should be included in this section, including the name of the policy, the policyholder's name, and the policy numbers. It is important for the health insurance professional to confirm that the "additional insurance" is secondary. Some patients, particularly elderly patients, can become confused over the technicalities of dual insurance coverage. If the patient is uncertain which of the policies is primary and which is secondary, the health insurance professional may have to do some detective work, such as telephoning one or both of the insuring agencies, to find out.

Insurance Authorization and Assignment

The section on insurance authorization and assignment should be completed and signed by the patient or responsible party, in the case of a minor or mentally disabled individual. This section gives the healthcare professional the authorization to release the information necessary to complete the insurance claim form. It also "**assigns benefits**"—that is, it authorizes the insurance company to send the payment directly to the healthcare professional. This authorization should be updated at least once a year, unless it is a "lifetime" release of information worded specifically for Medicare claims.

PATIENT INSURANCE IDENTIFICATION CARD

Every insurance company has a unique identification card that it issues to its subscribers. With Medicare, every individual (referred to as a **beneficiary**) has his or her own individual card. Other insurers, such as Blue Cross and Blue Shield, may issue a card that covers not only the subscriber, but also his or her spouse and any dependents included on the policy. This is referred to as a family plan.

ACCOUNT # _____

PATIENT # _____

NEW PATIENT INFORMATION DATE _____

PATIENT'S NAME (PLEASE PRINT)	S.S. #	MARITAL STATUS					SEX		BIRTH DATE	AGE
		S	M	W	D	SEP	M	F		

STREET ADDRESS PERMANENT TEMPORARY	CITY AND STATE	ZIP CODE	HOME PHONE#

PATIENT'S EMPLOYER	OCCUPATION (INDICATE IF STUDENT)	HOW LONG EMPLOYED	BUS. PHONE # EXT. #

EMPLOYER'S STREET ADDRESS	CITY AND STATE	ZIP CODE

DRUG ALLERGIES, IF ANY	PHARMACY	PHARMACY PHONE #

SPOUSE OR PARENT'S NAME	S.S. #	BIRTH DATE

SPOUSE OR PARENT'S EMPLOYER	OCCUPATION (INDICATED IF STUDENT)	HOW LONG EMPLOYED	BUS. PHONE #

EMPLOYER'S STREET ADDRESS	CITY AND STATE	ZIP CODE

*SPOUSE'S STREET ADDRESS, IF DIVORCED OR SEPARATED	CITY AND STATE	ZIP CODE	HOME PHONE #

PLEASE READ: ALL CHARGES ARE DUE AT THE TIME OF SERVICES. IF HOSPITALIZATION IS INDICATED, THE PATIENT IS RESPONSIBLE FOR FURNISHING INSURANCE CLAIM FORMS TO THE OFFICE PRIOR TO HOSPITALIZATION.

REFERRED BY	STREET ADDRESS, CITY, STATE	ZIP CODE	PHONE #
BLUE SHIELD (GIVE NAME OF POLICYHOLDER) ☐	☐ ALLIANCE ☐ OTHER ☐ ALLIANCE SELECT	BIRTH DATE	POLICY #
OTHER (WRITE IN NAME OF INSURANCE COMPANY) ☐	NAME OF POLICYHOLDER	BIRTH DATE	POLICY #
OTHER (WRITE IN NAME OF INSURANCE COMPANY) ☐	NAME OF POLICYHOLDER	BIRTH DATE	POLICY #

MEDICARE # ☐	RAILROAD RETIREMENT # ☐	MEDICAID # ☐

INDUSTRIAL ☐	WERE YOU INJURED ON THE JOB? ☐ YES ☐ NO	DATE OF INJURY	INDUSTRIAL CLAIM #
ACCIDENT ☐	WAS AN AUTOMOBILE INVOLVED? ☐ YES ☐ NO	DATE OF ACCIDENT	NAME OF ATTORNEY

WERE X-RAYS TAKEN OF THIS INJURY OR PROBLEM? ☐ YES ☐ NO	IF YES, WHERE WERE X-RAYS TAKEN? (HOSPITAL, ETC.)	DATE X-RAYS TAKEN

HAS ANY MEMBER OF YOUR IMMEDIATE FAMILY BEEN TREATED BY OUR PHYSICIAN(S) BEFORE? INCLUDE NAME OF PHYSICIAN AND FAMILY MEMBER.

NEAREST RELATIVE OR FRIEND NOT RESIDING WITH YOU	STREET ADDRESS, CITY, STATE	ZIP CODE	PHONE #

ALL PROFESSIONAL SERVICES RENDERED ARE CHARGED TO THE PATIENT. NECESSARY FORMS WILL BE COMPLETED TO HELP EXPEDITE INSURANCE CARRIER PAYMENTS. HOWEVER, THE PATIENT IS RESPONSIBLE FOR ALL FEES, REGARDLESS OF INSURANCE COVERAGE. IT IS ALSO CUSTOMARY TO PAY FOR SERVICES WHEN RENDERED UNLESS OTHER ARRANGEMENTS HAVE BEEN MADE IN ADVANCE WITH OUR OFFICE BOOKKEEPER.

INSURANCE AUTHORIZATION AND ASSIGNMENT

Name of Policy Holder _____   HIC Number _____

I request that payment of authorized Medicare/Other Insurance company benefits be made either to me or on my behalf to _____ for any services furnished me by that party who accepts assignment/physician. Regulations pertaining to Medicare assignment of benefits apply.
I authorize any holder of medical or other information about me to release to the Social Security Administration and Health Care Financing Administration or its intermediaries or carriers any information needed for this or a related Medicare claim/other Insurance Company claim. I permit a copy of this authorization to be used in place of the original, and request payment of medical insurance benefits either to myself or to the party who accepts assignment. I understand it is mandatory to notify the health care provider of any other party who may be responsible for paying for my treatment. (Section 1128B of the Social Security Act and 31 U.S.C. 3801-3812 provides penalties for withholding this information.)

Signature _____   Date _____

Accounts past 60 days will accrue an interest charge.   **NEW PATIENT INFORMATION**

Fig. 5-4 A typical patient information form.

As mentioned previously, at the same time the patient completes the information form, the health insurance professional should ask to see his or her insurance ID card and make a photocopy of it to keep in the health record.

It is important to always make sure you copy the front and the back of the ID card, if there is information on the back. On subsequent visits, ask the patient if there is any change in coverage. If so, ask for and make a copy of the new card. The rationale for this procedure is to have complete and correct insurance information on file for the purpose of completing the CMS-1500 claim. It also is helpful for obtaining telephone numbers to contact for preauthorization/precertification from the carrier if certain procedures or inpatient hospitalization is required. Fig. 5-5 shows the front and back sides of a typical insurance ID card.

PATIENT HEALTH RECORD

After the patient information form is completed, the health insurance professional should examine it to ensure that all necessary information has been entered, and that the entries are legible. The form is customarily placed in the patient's health record near the front so that the health insurance professional has easy access to it when it is time to complete and submit a claim. Details of the patient medical record are discussed in Chapter 3. To review, a medical record is an account of a patient's medical assessment, investigation, and course of treatment. It is a source of information and a vital component in quality patient care. A complete medical record should

- outline the reason for the patient's visit to the health-care professional,
- document the healthcare professional's findings,
- include a detailed discussion of the recommended treatment,
- provide information to any referring physician or other healthcare provider,
- serve as a teaching or research tool (or both), and
- provide a means for assessing the quality of care by the practitioner or other healthcare provider.

The clinical chart note illustrated in Fig. 5-6 is a typical example taken from a patient's health record.

Imagine This!

Tammy Butler visited Dr. Harold Norton, her family care provider, on February 10 for her yearly wellness examination plus routine diagnostics. Dr. Norton's health insurance professional submitted the claim the day after the visit. A month later, Tammy received an EOB from her health insurer indicating that the services were not covered under her policy. Assuming that her policy did not cover wellness examinations, Tammy forgot about it. During Christmas vacation of that same year, Tammy again visited Dr. Norton for a case of sinusitis. The claim was denied again by her insurer. Puzzled that a second claim had been denied, Tammy contacted Dr. Norton's office and, after some extensive research, learned that they had filed her claims under an old ID number from a previous employer. The problem now was that it was now January of a new year—past the deadline for filing claims for the previous year. The health insurance professional at Dr. Norton's office informed Tammy that she was responsible for the charges.

Stop and Think

In the scenario in Imagine This!, do you agree with Dr. Norton's health insurance professional that Tammy is responsible for the charges on the two visits in question? What should the health insurance professional have done to prevent this?

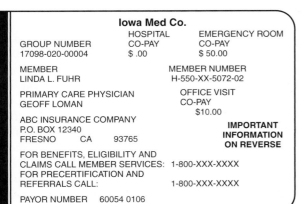

Fig. 5-5 Insurance ID card.

BROWN, SARA J.   DOB 11/27/1989   CURRENT DATE: 12/03/2001

HX: This 12-year-old white female presents to the clinic today for chief complaint of fever, chills, sweats, temperature recorded up to 101.5°, mild earache, stuffy nose, sinus pain and pressure, and an episodic cough that is worse in the evening, wheezing, shortness of breath, or dyspnea that started approximately five days ago.
    PAIN ASSESSMENT: Scale 0-10, zero.
    ALLERGIES: NKA.
    CURRENT MEDS: None.

PE: NAD. Ambulatory. Appears well.
    VS: **T:** 98.2°
    ENT: **TMs:** The TMs appear dull, primarily on the left as opposed to the right but without erythema, bulging, or retraction.
    NOSE: Minimal nasal congestion, slightly inflamed nasal mucosa.
    SINUS: Mild tenderness in the maxillary and frontal sinus areas to palpation and percussion.
    THROAT: Clear without tonsillar enlargement, inflammation, or exudate.
    NECK: Supple, not rigid, without adenopathy or thyropathy.
    LUNGS: CTA all fields with good breath sounds heard throughout. No wheezes or rales. Occasional upper bronchial rhonchi noted on examination that clear with cough. Respiratory excursion is symmetric and equal. No respiratory stridor or costal retractions. Normal vocal fremitus without egophony change. Peak flow 300, 350, 350. O2 saturation 98%.
    SKIN: Warm to touch, good turgor, without viral-like exanthemas, petechiae, or purpura.

IMP: URI with mild sinusitis, possibly allergy-related.

PLAN: The patient was started on Allegra 60 mg 1 p.o. b.i.d., given samples for 10 days, Septra DS 1 p.o. b.i.d. #20 given. Regular diet and activity as tolerated, force fluids. Recommended that they humidify the room. Routine follow up in 10 days or sooner if her symptoms worsen.
    RTN PRN

Frank O. McDermott
Frank O. McDermott, M.D./jj

Fig. 5-6 Clinical (chart) notes from a patient's health record.

ENCOUNTER FORM

We have discussed three of the items necessary for completing the CMS-1500 form. Now we look at a document used by most medical practices, which is often referred to as the **encounter form**. This multipurpose billing form is known by many names (e.g., superbill, routing form, patient service slip). The encounter form can be customized to medical specialties and preprinted with common diagnoses and procedures for that particular specialty. Fig. 5-7 shows an example of an encounter form.

Typically, this form is clipped to the front of the patient's medical record before the patient is seen in the clinical area. Note the variety of information included on the form shown in Fig. 5-7:

- demographic,
- accounting,
- professional services rendered,
- CPT and ICD-9 codes,
- professional fees, and
- return appointment information

It is important that the sections dealing with professional services, diagnostic, and procedure codes be updated annually so that revised codes are changed, new codes are added, and old codes are deleted.

The following is a typical routine in many medical offices. Each morning, the medical records clerk (or whichever member of the healthcare team is in charge of this task) prepares the health records for the patients who are to be seen that day. An encounter form is attached to the front of each record, and any areas on the form regarding the date of service, patient demographics, and accounting information is filled out. (If computerized patient accounting software is used, this is printed automatically on the form.) Each encounter form has a number (usually at the top), which serves as an identifier for that particular patient visit.

As each patient is seen in the clinical area, the healthcare provider indicates on the form what services or procedures were performed along with the corresponding fees. The provider signs the encounter form and indicates if and when the patient needs to return or have any follow-up tests. It is important that the encounter form is checked for accuracy, after which the medical receptionist totals the day's charges, enters any payment received, and calculates the balance due. The patient receives a copy of the completed encounter form, and a copy is retained in the medical office for accounting purposes and future reference in case any question comes up regarding that particular visit. Many offices file these forms by number within files that are separated into months and days. Medical offices are subject to accounting and insurance audits. The original encounter form can be requested by auditors to verify services rendered on any patient or on any date of service. A few insurance companies still accept the original encounter form for claim payment; in some cases, an insurer asks that a copy of the encounter form be included with the CMS-1500 claim form.

Tri-State Medical Group

008112

400 North 4th Street • Anytown, Iowa 50622
Phone: 319-555-5734 • Fax: 319-555-5758
Fed. Tax I.D. # 42-1435XXX

ACCOUNT NO.		DOB		DATE OF SERVICE	
PATIENT NAME			PROVIDER		
INSURANCE ID #-PRIMARY			SECONDARY		

DESCRIPTION	CODE		FEE	DESCRIPTION	CODE	FEE	DESCRIPTION	CODE	FEE
OFFICE VISIT	NEW	ESTAB.		DT, Pediatric	90702		Removal Skin Tags up to 15 Lesions	*11200	
Minimum	99201	99211		MMR	90707		Exc. Malignant Lesion, Trunk, Arm or Leg		
Brief	99202	99212		Oral Polio	90712		Exc. Malignant Lesion, Face, Ear, Eyelid, Nose		
Limited	99203	99213		IVP Polio	90713		Exc. Malignant Lesion, Scalp, Hand, Neck, Feet		
Extended	99204	99214		Varicella	90716		Lacer, Repair 2.5cm or Less/Location:	*12001	
Comprehensive	99205	99215		Td, Adult	90718		Scalp, Nk, Axille, Ext. Genitalia, Trk, Hands/Feet		
Prenatal Care		59400		DTP & HIB	90720		Lacer, Repair 2.5cm or Less/Location:	*12011	
Global		99024		Influenza	90659		Face, Ears, Eyelids, Nose, Lips & Mucous Mem.		
PREVENTIVE	NEW	ESTAB.		Hepatitis B, Newborn to 11 Years	90744		Burn w/Dressing, w/o Anesth. Small	16020	
Infant	99381	99391		Hepatitis B, 11-19 Years	90747		Wart Removal	*17110	
Age 1-4	99382	99392		Hepatitis B, 20 Years & Above	90746		Removal FB Conjunct. Ext. Eye	*65205	
Age 5-11	99383	99393		Pneumococcal	90732		Removal FB Ext. Auditory Canal	69200	
Age 12-17	99384	99394		Hemophilus Infl. B	90645		Ear Lavage	69210	
Age 18-39	99385	99395		Therapeutic:	90782		Tympanometry	92567	
Age 40-64	99386	99396		Allergy Inject Single	95115		EKG Tracing Only w/o Interp. & Rept	93005	
Age 65 & Over	99387	99397		Allergy Inject Multiple	95117		Nebulizer Therapy (x)	94640	
OFFICE CONSULTATION				B-12	J3420		Pulse Oximetry	94760	
Limited		99241		Injection / Aspiration	20600		Cryosurgery		
Intermediate		99242		Small joint-Finger, Toes, Ganglion			Debridement	11041	
Extended		99243		Injection / Aspiration	20605		Excise Ingrown Toenail	11730	
Comprehensive		99244		Intermediate jt-Wrist, Elbow, Ankle			Colposcopy w/Biopsy	57454	
Complex		99245		Injection / Aspiration	20610		Leep	57460	
LABORATORY PROCEDURES				Major jt. - Shoulder, Hip, Knee			Endometrial Bx	58100	
Venipuncture		36415		Inject Tendon/Ligament	20550		Cryotherapy	57511	
Routine Urinalysis w/o Microscopy		81002		Aristacort	J3302		Peak Flow Measurement	94160-52	
Hemoccult		82270		Depo Provera	J1055		Intradermal Tests CMI # Doses =	95025	
Glucose Blood Reagent Strip		82948		Rocephin	J0696		Intradermal Tests/Allergens	95024	
Wet Mount		87210		**OFFICE PROCEDURE / MINOR SURGERY**			Intravenous Access	36000	
PAP Smear		88155		I & D Abscess	10060		Immunotherapy/Single Injection	95120	
Urine Pregnancy		81025		Removal FB Subcutaneous	*10120		Immunotherapy/Double Injection	95125	
Other:		99000		I & D Hematoma	10140		Regular Spirometry	94010	
X-RAY				Puncture Aspiration Abscess	10160		Spirometry Read by Physician	94010-26	
X-ray Cervical Spine		75052		Exc. Ben. Lesion #:			Spirometry w/pre & Post Bronchodilator	94060	
X-ray Thoracic Spine		72070		Location:			Spirometry/Bronchodilator read by Doctor	94060-26	
X-ray Lumbar Spine (2)		72100		Exc. Ben. Lesion #:			Skin Prick Test: # of Tests =	95004	
X-ray Lumbar Spine (Comp)		72110		Location:			Vial Preparation	95165	
X-ray Pelvis (1 view)		72170							
X-ray Sacrum & Coccyx		72220							

HOSPITAL ORDERS		
OB Non-Stress Test	Cystogram	Physical Therapy
OB Ultrasound-Diagnostic	MRI	
OB Ultrasound-Routine	CT Scan_____	
Biophysical Profile	Chest X-ray	Diet Consultation
Mammogram-Diagnostic	X-ray_____	
Mammogram-Routine	Bone Densitometry	
	EKG	Laboratory
Ultrasound _____	Holter Monitor	_____
Gallbladder Ultrasound	Echocardiogram	_____
Pelvic Ultrasound	Treadmill _____	_____
Doppler Studies _____	Thallium Stress Test	_____
	Doppler Studies_____	_____
IVP	PFT-Partial	_____
Upper GI	PFT-Complete	_____
Lower GI	Cardiac Rehab	_____
Barium Enema		
Barium Swallow		

X-ray table continued:

DESCRIPTION	CODE
X-ray Clavicle (Complete)	73000
X-ray Shoulder (2) or	73030
X-ray Humerus (2 views)	73060
X-ray Elbow (AP & LATE)	73070
X-ray Forearm (AP & LA)	73090
X-ray Wrist (AP & LATE)	73100
X-ray Wrist (3 Views)	73110
X-ray Hand (2 Views)	73120
X-ray Hand (3 Views)	73130
X-ray Finger (2 Views)	73140
X-ray Hip (2 Views)	73510
X-ray Hips (Bilateral)	73520
X-ray Scoliosis (2 AP & LA)	72069
X-ray Femur (AP & LATE)	73550
X-ray Knee (AP & LATE)	73560
X-ray Knee (3 Views)	73564
X-ray Tibia & Fibula	73590
X-ray Ankle (3 Views)	73610
X-ray Foot (AP & LATER)	73620
X-ray Foot (AP. LA.,)	73630
X-ray Calcaneus (2 Views)	73650
X-ray Toes	73660
X-ray Pelvis & Hip Inf	73540
Elbow, Minimum of 3 Views	73080
IMMUNIZATIONS & INJECTIONS	
PPD Intradermal TB Tine	86580
DTaP	90700

AUTHORIZATION TO PAY BENEFITS AND RELEASE INFORMATION TO TRI-STATE MEDICAL GROUP: I hereby authorize payment directly to the undersigned Physician of all Surgical and / or Medical Benefits, if any, otherwise payable to me for his / her services as described above. I have read and understand the Financial Policy and that I am financially responsible for charges not covered by this insurance. I also authorize the undersigned Physician to release any information acquired in the course of my examination or treatment.

Signed: _____

Date: _____

Provider's Signature   Date

PREVIOUS BALANCE	
CHARGES TODAY	
TOTAL	
AMOUNT PAID	
BALANCE DUE	

DX or Other Information

Samples:

Your next appointment is:

BILLING COPY

Fig. 5-7 Sample encounter form.

PATIENT LEDGER CARD

In offices that do not use computerized patient accounting software, patient charges and payments are kept track of on a **patient ledger card** (Fig. 5-8). A ledger card is an accounting form on which professional service descriptions, charges, payments, adjustments, and current balance are posted chronologically. Although many medical professional offices are becoming computerized, there are still some offices that are not, so to become a well-rounded healthcare professional, you must be familiar with manual accounting methods.

 HIPAA Tip

A medical office can use sign-in sheets and announce names; however, reasonable safeguards still need to be used. This decision has been added to HIPAA's rules and regulations to address incidental disclosures of protected health information. Examples of safeguards used by some medical offices include the following:
1. Covering sign-in sheet with a separate, non-transparent sheet of paper
2. Using a heavy black marking pen to cross through names after the chart is verified, copay is collected (if applicable), and patient is seated

---

A patient ledger card is prepared for each new patient. In some medical offices, particularly family practice facilities, one ledger card is set up for the head of household, and all dependent family members are included on it. This makes sense because it not only saves time and space in the ledger file, but also minor children usually are not responsible for their own bills, and statements are normally not addressed directly to them. Be cautious, however, in the case of divorced parents because it is important that the parent who is financially responsible for the child is billed. More information is given on the maintenance of the patient ledger card as we proceed through the chapters on third-party payers and process insurance claims and reimbursements.

What Did You Learn?

1. List the documents needed for filing a paper CMS-1500 claim.
2. Explain why it is important to photocopy both back and front of the ID card.
3. What types of information are typically included on an encounter form?

COMPLETING THE CMS-1500 PAPER FORM

Before filling in any of the blocks, type the name and address of the insurance carrier to whom the form will be mailed. This information should appear in the upper right hand corner of the form as illustrated in Fig. 5-9.

The following instructions for completing the CMS-1500 are relatively nonspecific. For the most part, they do not include details specific to any one major carrier, such as Medicare or Medicaid. More detailed guidelines applicable to each of the major carriers are presented in later chapters under the particular carrier's name. In these generic guidelines, we assume that the patient is covered by a private (commercial) insurance policy and has no secondary insurance coverage.

PATIENT/INSURED SECTION

Information required in many of the blocks varies from claim to claim and from one insurance carrier to another. Blocks 9 through 9d are examples of this. For a patient who has no secondary coverage, blocks 9 through 9d are left blank. More detailed information is given as to how these blocks should be completed as each major carrier is discussed later in the text.

Block 1—Indicate the type of health insurance coverage applicable to the claim by checking the appropriate box. Usually, only one box is checked except when the claim involves dual coverage, in which case more than one box is checked.

Block 1a—Enter the patient's health insurance claim number exactly as it appears on his or her ID card including any alpha characters.

Block 2—Enter the patient's last name, first name, and middle initial (if any). Do not use shortened names or nicknames. (Remember to use upper case letters and no punctuation.)

Block 3—Enter the patient's 8-digit birth date, using the MM DD YYYY format, and check the appropriate box for sex. It is important to use this exact formatting style (the 4-digit year) for a birth date so that it is clear when the patient was born. Entering a birth date of 05 10 03 could represent a centenarian or a young child.

Block 4—Enter the policyholder's (subscriber's) name here exactly as it is listed on the insurance card. If the patient and the policyholder is one and the same, enter the word "SAME."

Note: On Medicare claims, the patient (referred to as the beneficiary) and the policyholder are the same. Sometimes there is insurance primary to Medicare, through the patient's or spouse's employment or some other source. If this is the case, list the insured's name here. If Medicare is primary, leave blank. (Instructions on how to fill out the CMS-1500 claim form for Medicare secondary claims are discussed in Chapter 9.)

STATEMENT

Tri-State Medical Group
400 North 4th Street
Anytown, Iowa 50622
Phone: 319-555-5734
Fax: 319-555-5758

Mrs. Samantha Taylor
6345 Elm
Ames, Iowa 50010

DATE	PROFESSIONAL SERVICE DESCRIPTION	CHARGE		CREDITS		CURRENT BALANCE	
				PAYMENTS	ADJUSTMENTS		
12-15-xx	Init OV, D hx/exam, LC decision making.	95	00			95	00
12-15-xx	EKG c̄ interpret & report.	55	00			150	00

Due and payable within 10 days.   **Pay last amount in balance column**   ⇧

Key: PF: Problem-focused   SF: Straightforward   CON: Consultation   HCD: House call (day)
     EPF: Expanded problem-focused   LC: Low complexity   CPX: Complete phys exam   HCN: House call (night)
       D: Detailed   MC: Moderate complexity   E: Emergency   HV: Hospital visit
       C: Comprehensive   HC: High complexity   ER: Emergency dept.   OV: Office visit

Fig. 5-8 Sample patient ledger card (Modified from Fordney MT: Insurance handbook for the medical office, ed 9, St Louis, 2006, Saunders).

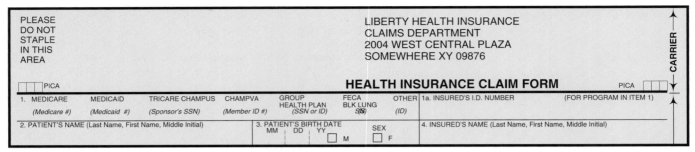

Fig. 5-9 How and where name and address of carrier should appear on the CMS-1500 form.

Block 5—Enter the patient's mailing address (city, state, and Zip Code) and telephone number as the form indicates. Remember, do not separate the telephone number groups with dashes.

Block 6—Check the applicable box for the patient's relationship to the insured when Block 4 is completed. (Do not use the box for "other.")

Block 7—Enter the policyholder's address and telephone number. If the address is the same as the patient's, enter "SAME." (Usually, this item is completed only when Blocks 4 and 11 are completed.)

Block 8—Check the appropriate box for the patient's marital status and whether employed or a student. Checking the "married" or "student" boxes is not mandatory for all carriers.

Blocks 9-9d—Rather than try to explain what information to enter here for various third-party carriers, these blocks are left blank for this generic run-through, and they are addressed individually in later chapters.

Blocks 10-10c—This is a crucial area of the form. You must check "yes" or "no" to indicate whether the services or procedures listed in Block 24 are the result of an accident or illness resulting from employment, an auto accident, or other accident. If auto accident is checked, enter the 2-letter code for the state in which the accident occurred. An item checked "yes" indicates that there may be another insurance carrier that is primary, such as workers' compensation or an auto insurance carrier.

Block 10d—This block is used for Medicaid claims. If the patient is a Medicaid recipient, enter the patient's Medicaid ID number preceded by the letters "MCD." Otherwise, leave blank. (Verify this with your state Medicaid office.)

Block 11—The completion of this item, similar to Blocks 9 through 9d, depends on the guidelines of the carrier to whom the claim is being sent or whether or not the patient is covered under another insurance policy. If there is a second health insurance policy, go back and complete Blocks 9 through 9d. In our generic case, the "patient" is covered by a private insurance company with no secondary coverage. In this case, Blocks 11 through 11c are left blank.

On Medicare claims, completion of this item acknowledges that the physician/supplier has made a good faith effort to determine whether Medicare is the primary or secondary carrier. More detailed information is given in the sections of the text that deal with the various major carriers.

Block 11a—Enter the insured's 8-digit birth date and sex, *if different from Block 3.*

Block 11b—If this is an employer-sponsored group insurance, enter the employer's name. For Medicare claims, if the beneficiary is retired, enter the 8-digit retirement date preceded by the word "RETIRED."

Block 11c—For most claims, this item is left blank. For Medicare claims, enter the 9-digit PAYERID number of the primary insurer. If no PAYERID number exists, enter the program or plan name of the primary payer.

Block 11d—Check "yes" or "no," whichever is applicable. Leave blank on Medicare claims.

Block 12—The patient (or his or her authorized representative) must sign and enter the date in this block. If there is a current release of information retained in the patient's health record, a physical signature is not required, and the words "SIGNATURE ON FILE" or the letters "SOF" can be entered. (Remember, for a release of information to be valid, it should not be more than one year old. On Medicare claims, a properly worded "lifetime" release of information is acceptable.) An example of a HIPAA-compliant release of information is shown in Fig. 5-10. A Medicare-approved lifetime release of information is shown in Chapter 9.

Block 13—A signature here tells the insurance carrier that the patient (or insured) authorizes them to **assign benefits** (send reimbursement check directly to the healthcare provider). If a separate signed authorization to assign benefits exists elsewhere (it is often included on a patient information form), the letters "SOF" can be entered here. In certain instances, a signature here is unnecessary, but there are some exceptions, as in the case of Medicaid and Medigap. (This information is discussed in more detail in later chapters.)

Authorization for Release of Information

I hereby authorize the use or disclosure of my individually identifiable health information as described below. I understand that this authorization is voluntary and that I may revoke it at any time by submitting my revocation in writing to the entity providing the information.

Participant Name: _____   ID Number: _____

Person(s) authorized to provide information:

_____

_____

Person(s) authorized to receive information:

_____

_____

Description of information to be used or disclosed:

_____

_____

(Facility Name) will not receive financial or in-kind compensation in exchange for using or disclosing the health information described above.

This authorization will expire _____ . (Indicate date, or an event relating to you personally or to the purpose of the authorization).

IMPORTANT INFORMATION ABOUT YOUR RIGHTS

I have read and understood the following statements about my rights:

• I may revoke this authorization at any time prior to its expiration date by notifying (Facility Name) in writing, but the revocation will not have any affect on any actions the entity took before it received the revocation.

• I may see and copy the information described on this form if I ask for it.

• I am not required to sign this form to receive my benefits.

• The information that is used or disclosed pursuant to this authorization may be redisclosed by (Facility Name). I have the right to seek assurances from the above-named person(s) authorized to receive the information that they will not redisclose the information to any other party without my further authorization.

_____   _____
Signature of Participant   Date

_____   _____
Printed Name of Participant's Personal Representative   Relationship to the Participant

Fig. 5-10 Form for authorization for release of information.

What Did You Learn?

1. What is the rationale for using the MM DD YYYY date format?
2. When is it necessary to complete Blocks 9 through 9d?
3. Why is it important to check "yes" or "no" in all three boxes in Blocks 10 through 10c?

PHYSICIAN/SUPPLIER SECTION

We now turn our attention to the part of the CMS-1500 form that contains information the health insurance professional must **abstract**, from the health record or the encounter form or both. Learning how to abstract, or pull out, information from the health record that is necessary for completing the CMS-1500 claim form takes some level of expertise, which the novice health insurance professional might not possess. This skill develops with experience and practice, however.

The new CMS-1500 form (08-05) accommodates the National Provider Identifier (NPI) numbers that all health care providers or organizations defined as "covered entities" under HIPAA must obtain. This unique 10-digit numeric identifier is considered permanent and, once assigned, will be assigned for life. The NPI will replace all other provider identifiers previously used by health care providers, e.g. UPIN, Medicare/Medicaid numbers, etc.

When completing the CMS-1500 form, date fields (other than date of birth), should be one or the other format, 6-digit (MM/DD/YY) or 8-digit (MM/DD/CCYY). Intermixing the two formats on the claim is not allowed. The date of birth must be in the 8-digit format.

Block 14—Enter the date of the first symptom of the current illness, injury, or pregnancy in this block (if one is documented in the health record) or the date of the last menstrual cycle if the claim is related to a pregnancy. Use caution here because an incorrect date could indicate a preexisting condition, and the claim could be rejected.

Example: If a patient was treated for a back injury before the effective date of his or her existing healthcare policy, this policy might not cover charges stemming from this same back injury.

Block 15—Enter the date the patient was first treated for this condition. (Leave blank for Medicare claims).

Block 16—Enter the date (or date range) that the patient was unable to work in his or her current occupation if it is a workers' compensation claim. Completion of this block is not required for most other carriers.

Block 17—Enter the name of the referring or ordering physician, if applicable. For laboratory and x-ray claims, enter the name of the physician who ordered the diagnostic services.

For example, if Dr. Madigan orders an electrocardiogram, which is performed by a medical assistant but interpreted by Dr. Madigan, his name is entered into Block 17. Completion of this box also is required if billing for a consultation.

Blocks 17a and 17b—An entry in Block 17a and/or 17b is required when a listed service on the form was ordered or referred by a physician. The provider's unique provider identification number (UPIN) can be used until May 22, 2007. The UPIN should appear in Block 17a. Effective May 23, 2007, the UPIN in 17a is *not* to be reported. Instead, the NPI must be reported in 17b when a service was ordered or referred by a physician. *Note:* If a claim involves multiple referring and/or ordering physicians, a separate form should be used for each ordering/referring physician.

Block 18—If the claim is related to a hospital stay, enter the dates of hospital admission and discharge. If the patient has not yet been discharged, leave the "to" box blank.

Block 19—Enter either a 6-digit or an 8-digit date when the patient was last seen and the UPIN (NPI when it becomes effective) of his/her attending physician when an independent physical or occupational therapist submits claims or a physician providing routine foot care submits claims.

Block 20—Leave this block blank if no laboratory or diagnostic tests were performed. If any diagnostics are listed in Block 24, and these services were performed in the provider's facility, check "No" or leave blank. If any diagnostic tests shown on the claim were performed by an outside laboratory and *billed to the provider,* check "Yes," then enter the total amount of the charges in the space provided.

Block 21—Enter the patient's diagnosis using ICD-9-CM code number, listing the primary diagnosis first. There is space for up to four codes (listed in priority order) in Block 21.

Block 22—This block is used only for Medicaid replacement claims.

Block 23—This block is conditionally required. Consult the specific guidelines for the payer to whom the claim is being submitted.

Block 24a—Submit each date of service on a separate line. Enter the month, day, and year (in the MM DD YYYY format) for each procedure, service, or supply. When "from" and "to" dates are shown for a series of identical services, enter the number of days or units in 24G. *Note:* Only one procedure may be billed on each line. If there are more than six procedures, a second claim form will need to be used.

Block 24b—Enter the applicable *place of service* code (Table 5-1).

Block 24c—This block is conditionally required. Enter an "X" or an "E" as appropriate for services performed as a result of a medical emergency. Leave blank for Medicare claims.

Block 24d—Enter the procedure, service, or supply code using appropriate 5-digit CPT or HCPCS procedure code. Enter the 2-digit modifier when applicable. If using an unlisted procedure code (codes ending in "...99"), a complete description of the procedure must be provided as a separate attachment.

Block 24e—Link the procedure/service code back to the diagnosis code in Block 21 by indicating the applicable number of the diagnosis code (1, 2, 3, or 4).

Block 24f—Enter the amount charged for each listed procedure, supply, or service.

Block 24g—Enter the number of days or units. If only one service is performed, enter the number 1. Do not leave blank.

Block 24h—This is required only on certain Medicaid claims. EPSDT is an acronym for Medicaid's *Early and Periodic Screening Diagnosis and Treatment* Program. If this is applicable, enter the appropriate code. The annual EPSDT report (*Form CMS-416*) (*PDF-47K*) provides

TABLE 5-1	Place-of-Service Codes

11　Office
12　Home
21　Inpatient hospital
22　Outpatient hospital
23　Emergency department—hospital
24　Ambulatory surgical center
25　Birthing center
26　Military treatment facility
31　Skilled nursing facility
32　Nursing facility
33　Custodial care facility
34　Hospice
41　Ambulance—land
42　Ambulance—air or water
50　Federally qualified health center
51　Inpatient psychiatric facility
52　Psychiatric facility partial hospitalization
53　Community mental health center
54　Intermediate care facility/mentally retarded
55　Residential substance abuse treatment facility
56　Psychiatric residential treatment center
60　Mass immunization center
61　Comprehensive inpatient rehabilitation facility
62　Comprehensive outpatient rehabilitation facility
65　End stage renal disease treatment facility
71　State or local public health clinic
72　Rural health clinic
81　Independent laboratory
99　Other unlisted facility

basic information on participation in the Medicaid child health program.

Block 24i—Enter the ID qualifier 1C in the shaded portion for Medicare claims. Contact the third party payer for ID qualifiers for non-Medicare claims.

Block 24j—Prior to May 23, 2007, enter the rendering provider's PIN in the shaded portion. After May 23, 2007, do not use the shaded portion. Instead, enter the rendering provider's NPI number in the lower portion. In the case of a service-provided incident to the service of a physician or non-physician practitioner, when the person who ordered the service is not supervising, enter the PIN of the supervisor into the shaded position.

Block 25—Enter the 9-digit federal tax identification number assigned to that provider (or group), and check the appropriate box in this field. In the case of an unincorporated practice, enter the provider's Social Security number.

Block 26—This block is conditionally required. Enter the patient's account number as assigned by the provider's accounting system.

Block 27—Check the appropriate block to indicate whether the provider accepts assignment of benefits. If the supplier is a participating provider, assignment must be accepted for all covered charges. For nonparticipating providers, this can be left blank. For Medicare and Medicaid claims, check "yes."

Block 28—Enter the total charges for services listed in column 24f.

Block 29—Enter the total amount, if any, that the patient has paid. Leave blank if no payment has been made.

Block 30—This block is conditionally required. Enter the balance owing (Block 28 minus Block 29).

Block 31—Enter the signature of the provider, or his or her representative and his or her initials, and the date the form was signed. The signature may be typed, stamped, or handwritten; however, no part of the signature should fall outside of the block.

☑ **HIPAA Tip**

If providers choose to use electronic signatures, the signatures must comply with HIPAA standards.

Block 32— Enter the word "SAME" in this block, if the individual carrier's guidelines allow it. Medicare requires the name, address, and zip code of the facility regardless of where services were performed and does not allow "SAME."

Block 32a—Enter the NPI of the service facility in Block 32.

Block 32b—Enter the appropriate ID qualifier followed by one blank space and then the PIN of the service facility. After May 23, 2007, 32b is not to be reported. *Note:* Providers of service (namely physicians) must identify the supplier's PIN when billing for purchased diagnostic tests.

Block 33—Enter the provider's billing name, address, zip code, and telephone number.

Block 33a—Effective May 23, 2007, the NPI of the billing provider or group must be reported here.

Block 33b—Enter the appropriate ID qualifier followed by one blank space and then the PIN of the billing provider or group. Effective May 23, 2007, 33b is not to be reported. Enter the group UPIN, including the two-digit location identifier, for the performing practitioner/supplier who is a member of a group practice.

The physician/supplier portion of the CMS-1500 form is the most challenging part. There is so much to learn, and the fact that all major payers' guidelines are slightly different complicates the process. Be patient, however, because you will not be expected at this point to know everything.

Refer to "Websites to Explore" at the end of this chapter for more detailed instructors for completing the new CMS-1500 (08-05) claim form.

PREPARING THE CLAIM FORM FOR SUBMISSION

PROOFREADING

After the form has been completed according to the applicable payer guidelines, it should be meticulously proofread for accuracy. The goal is always to submit **clean claims**—claims that can be processed for payment quickly without being returned. Returned or rejected claims delay the payment process and cost the practice and the patient money. On average, nearly one quarter of the claims submitted by medical practices to insurers are rejected because they contain some type of error. One national professional association estimates that resubmitting a paper claim could cost a medical practice between $24 and $41.67.

A claim that is rejected for missing or invalid information must be corrected and resubmitted by the provider. Common examples of claim rejections include the following:

- Incomplete/invalid patient diagnosis code
- Diagnosis code that does not justify the procedure code
- Missing or improper modifiers
- Omitted or inaccurately entered the referring/ordering/supervising provider's name or NPI
- Performing physician/supplier is a member of a group practice; however, you did not complete or enter accurately their carrier-assigned PIN
- Insured's subscriber or group number missing or incorrect
- Charges not itemized
- Provider signature missing

CLAIM ATTACHMENTS

Under certain circumstances, it may be necessary to include certain supporting documentation with a claim, as in the case where an unlisted procedure code (a code ending in "99") is used or to justify certain procedures or charges or both. Attachments also might include laboratory reports, physician notes, and other documents, which further explain the medical appropriateness for the claim. When it is necessary to include an attachment with the claim, a complete description of the procedure must be provided as a separate document and included with the completed CMS-1500 claim form. Every carrier has specific guidelines for how to handle attachments. A carrier's guidelines may state that "all attachments must be at least 3-5 inches in size and clearly readable." Under most circumstances for paper claims, the attachment is paper-clipped behind each claim form when submitted. (Most carriers prefer that attachments not be stapled to the claim form.)

One last thing you must remember to do before mailing the claim is to make a copy of the completed form for your files. Some carriers require making and keeping copies of paper claims for a certain length of time (e.g., 5 years). Consult your carrier's guidelines to find out how long you must retain copies of paper claims.

TRACKING CLAIMS

Many practices use some sort of claims follow-up system so that claims can be tracked and delinquent claims resolved before it is too late to resubmit (as in the case of a lost claim). An example of a claims follow-up system is an insurance log or insurance register. The insurance log or register should include various entries, such as the patient's name, insurance company's name, date claim filed, status of the claim (e.g., paid, pending, denied), date of explanation of benefits (EOB) or payment receipt, and resubmitted date. A claims follow-up system can be set up manually or electronically. It is a helpful tool for the health insurance professional and the provider because it ultimately leads to an increase in payments to the practice. Insurance claims can be overlooked if a tracking system is not in place, which can lead to lost revenue. Fig. 5-11 shows an example of an insurance log.

GENERATING CLAIMS ELECTRONICALLY

Many practices submit their claims electronically because of the time and money savings that result. Experts tell practitioners that processing insurance claims electronically (1) improves cash flow, (2) reduces the expense of

Insurance Claims Tracking Form (Sample)

Patient Name	Carrier Name	Date Filed	Claim Amount	Date of Payment/EOB	Payment Amount	Claim Status	Action Taken/Date
Anderson, Joseph L.	Metropolitan Life	01/12/XX	1450.00			Pending	Telephone call to Met Life 2/12/XX
Siverly, Penelope R.	Medicare	01/23/XX	125.00	02/13/XX	64.50		
Loper, Michael C.	Medicaid	01/25/XX	65.00			Denied	Appeal Letter to Medicaid 2/16/XX
Carpenter, Susan	BCBS	01/27/XX	255.00			Lost Claim	Resubmitted on 2/22/XX

Fig. 5-11 Sample insurance claim tracking form.

claims processing, and (3) streamlines internal processes, allowing them to focus more on patient care. On average, a paper insurance claim typically takes 30 to 45 days for reimbursement, whereas the average payment time for electronic claims is approximately 10 to 14 days. This reduction in insurance reimbursement time results in a significant increase in cash available for other practice expenses. As with everything, however, there is a tradeoff because often the expense of setting up for an electronic process is not taken into account. First, the office has to purchase adequate equipment—computers, printers, and software programs. Additionally, everyone involved in the claim process must become computer literate. Depending on the size and needs of the practice, computer hardware and software can cost from $10,000 to $250,000. Also, an intensive training program may be needed to teach staff how to use the equipment and become adept at operating the software.

There are basically two ways to submit claims electronically: through an electronic claims clearinghouse or directly to an insurance carrier. Many large practices can be set up to support both methods. Whether a practice chooses to use a clearinghouse or to submit claims directly to the carrier, it usually must go through an enrollment process before submitting electronic claims. The enrollment process is required so that the company the practice has hired can "set up" information about the practice on their computer system. Most government and many commercial carriers require such an enrollment. Some also require that the practice sign a contract with them. The enrollment process typically takes 6 to 7 weeks to complete. The largest obstacle in getting set up for electronic claims processing is the time that it takes for approval from state, federal, and, in some cases, commercial/health maintenance organization carriers.

 HIPAA Tip

For entities that choose to transmit claims electronically, practice management software or a clearinghouse is needed to handle the conversion of data to meet the requirements of HIPAA.

CLAIMS CLEARINGHOUSES

A **claims clearinghouse** is a company that receives claims from healthcare providers and specializes in consolidating the claims so that they can send one transmission to each third-party payer containing batches of claims. A clearinghouse typically is an independent, centralized service available to healthcare providers for the purpose of simplifying medical insurance claims submission for multiple carriers. HIPAA defines a healthcare clearinghouse as *"a public or private entity that processes or facilitates the processing of nonstandard data elements of health information into standard data elements."* The clearinghouse acts as a simple point of entry for paper and electronic claims from providers. Clearinghouse personnel edit the claims for validity and accuracy before routing the edited claim on to the proper third-party carrier for payment. A medical practice can send *all* completed claims to one central location, rather than to multiple payers. If the clearinghouse finds errors on the claim that would cause the claim to be rejected or denied, it sends the claim back to the provider for correction and resubmission.

Clearinghouses also are capable of translating data from one format to another (e.g., electronic to paper or vice versa). Many private clearinghouses are available to healthcare providers and payers that facilitate electronic and paper claims processing. Payers also can act as clearinghouses for claims of other payers.

Most clearinghouses have the ability to meet the requirements of each insurance company using their specific computer formats. They can submit electronic claims to any insurance company in a format that exactly matches that of the insurance company's computers. This clearinghouse task is essential for electronic claims because it is usually too complex and costly for independent billing services to perform on each claim. Clearinghouse services are not free, however. Charges for paper claims vary from 25 to 75 cents each, but some providers feel the advantages outweigh the disadvantages. Electronically submitted claims are less costly (some cost only 5 cents each), and many clearinghouses do not charge for claims submitted in certain standard electronic formats.

USING A CLEARINGHOUSE

Here is how using a clearinghouse typically works. The medical practice subscribes to a clearinghouse. After this process is completed, the health insurance professional enters the practice's billing information in a preformatted template, and a file is created from this template that contains that practice's specific claim information. This file is transmitted through the modem to the clearinghouse using the clearinghouse's specific built-in functionality.

As the clearinghouse receives claims from the medical practice, they are checked for completeness and accuracy. If an error has been made, the practice is notified that there is a problem with a claim. Ideally, the claim information is quickly corrected, and the claim is resubmitted to the clearinghouse. This validation process normally takes just minutes, eliminating the costly delays associated with submitting "dirty" claims directly to the insurer. When submitted and validated for accuracy, claims are forwarded electronically (in most cases overnight) to the specific insurance carriers for reimbursement.

DIRECT CLAIMS

Submitting electronic claims directly to an insurance carrier is a little more complicated. As explained previously, you first must enroll with the carrier. Most government carriers and many commercial carriers require that you enroll with them before submitting claims electronically to them. You also need some additional software from each insurance carrier to whom you wish to submit claims. Many carriers have their own software or can refer the health insurance professional to someone who supports direct transmissions in the area.

The most common direct claims submission method is done by creating a "print image" file of the claim and using the applicable direct claims software to send the claim to the proper insurance carrier. Printing claims to a file is as easy as printing claims to paper. The first step is to set up a printer properly that has the capability to designate "print to file." After completing the printer setup and entering the billing information, claims can be printed to the carrier transmission file. The health insurance professional would select an option such as "print insurance claims" and select which claims to send to a particular insurance carrier. When prompted to select a printer to print claims, you simply select the printer that has been set up to print to file. A prompt screen appears requesting that you enter a filename. Enter the filename that was given to you by the direct claims software product. Then using the direct claims software, transmit the file to the carrier. Some carriers may "edit" claims; the health insurance professional needs to work with that particular insurance carrier to determine how to identify and resubmit claims that contain errors.

CLEARINGHOUSES VERSUS DIRECT

When deciding whether to send claims electronically through a clearinghouse or direct to the carrier, there are several things to consider. Carrier direct is usually less expensive if the medical practice submits most claims to just one carrier. When multiple carriers are used, however, a clearinghouse is generally less expensive. With a clearinghouse, the health insurance professional needs to dial into only one location. If the decision is made to go direct, there will be multiple dialups. When using a clearinghouse, all claims can be submitted in one transmission, and the convenience of sending all claims to one location should not be underestimated. Submitting claims to multiple insurance carriers requires members of the health insurance team to become experts in each of the claims submission software applications used. Because each one is unique, the health insurance professional must be adequately trained and available to submit all variety of claims. Clearinghouses typically generate a separate confirmation report for each carrier where claims are submitted directly.

Insofar as which method of electronic claims submission is better, if a medical practice submits insurance claims to only multiple carriers and has someone who is well trained technically to handle the task of electronic claims submission, an electronic claims clearinghouse might be the better choice. If claims are sent primarily to one carrier, the practice should consider using *direct submission* to that carrier. Whichever method is selected, it is a proven fact that claims are processed much faster and reimbursement time is shortened using electronic claims submission.

What Did You Learn?

1. What is a claims clearinghouse?
2. List two advantages of submitting claims electronically.
3. Explain the process for submitting direct claims.

SUMMARY CHECK POINTS

☑ In the mid-1970s, HCFA created a form for Medicare claims, which was approved by the American Medical Association Council on Medical Services. All government healthcare programs and most commercial/private carriers subsequently adopted this form, now referred to as the CMS-1500, to standardize the claims process.

☑ The CMS-1500 is an $8\frac{1}{2} \times 11$–inch, two-sided form printed in OCR scannable red ink. The top section of the form is for patient/insured information; the bottom section is for provider/supplied data.

☑ For the CMS-1500 form to be OCR "readable," certain rules must be followed. Some of the more important ones are
  • use all uppercase letters,
  • omit all punctuation, and
  • use the MM DD YYYY format (with a space—not a dash—between each set of digits) for dates of birth.

☑ HIPAA mandates that all providers must submit claims electronically unless the provider falls into either of the following categories:
  • The healthcare provider has no method available for submitting claims in electronic format.
  • The "small provider" criteria are met, which are defined as *a provider of services with fewer than 25 full-time equivalent employees or a physician, practitioner, facility or supplier*

(other than a provider of services) with fewer than 10 full-time equivalent employees.

☑ In either of these cases, the Secretary may grant a waiver from the mandatory electronic submission rule.

☑ The five documents needed for completion of the CMS-1500 include the following:
  • The *patient information form*, which supplies demographic and insurance information and provides the necessary signed release of information
  • The *patient's insurance ID card*, which contains current subscriber numbers and other information necessary for preauthorization of certain procedures and inpatient hospitalization
  • The *patient's health record*, which contains detailed documentation of the reason for the patient's visit, the physician's findings, and a discussion of the recommended treatment
  • The *encounter form*, which includes the professional services rendered and corresponding CPT and ICD-9 codes
  • The *patient ledger card*, which documents the fees charged for the services listed on the claim form

☑ The primary objective in submitting claims is to submit "clean" claims. For this reason, thorough proofreading of each claim form is crucial to prevent claim rejection or denial.

☑ A claims clearinghouse is a company that receives multiple claims from healthcare providers, edits each for validity and accuracy, and routes the edited claims on to the proper carrier for payment.

☑ Studies have shown that a clearinghouse is the best method of submitting electronic claims if the provider submits claims to multiple carriers. Direct claim submission is the method of choice if most claims are being sent to a single carrier.

CLOSING SCENARIO

Studying the information in Chapter 5 one topic at a time and reviewing each main point proved helpful to Emilio and Latisha in comprehending the new material. The chapter contained a lot of information that could have proved difficult had they not adopted a structured method for studying. At the beginning of the chapter, the CMS-1500 form presented a challenging picture, as did the concept of OCR. The students worked through the "generic" guidelines many times, however, until they felt they understood them thoroughly. To get a better grasp on the OCR rules, they practiced lining up the forms and keying information into the blocks using the all caps, no punctuation OCR format.

Emilio preferred to learn how to generate claims using a computer; however, he realized it was important to understand what information should appear in each of the 33 blocks of the form, why that particular piece of datum needed to be there, and how it was derived. Emilio and Latisha agree now that the best way to understand the intricacies of the CMS-1500 form is to abstract information from the five documents explained in the chapter and generate a paper claim. After completing this chapter, Latisha believes she is now ready to begin completing paper forms at the clinic where she volunteers.

WEBSITES TO EXPLORE

For live links to the following websites, please visit the Evolve® site at http://evolve.elsevier.com/Beik/today/

- For students who are interested in learning more about OCR technology, log on to the following website, key "OCR Technology" into the search block, and peruse articles of interest: http://www.eric.ed.gov/

- For tips on keeping up-to-date on CMS-1500 completion guidelines for Medicare and Medicaid, log on to the CMS website and type "CMS-1500 Guidelines" into the search block: http://www.cms.hhs.gov/

- For specific instructions on completing a new CMS-1500 form for Medicare, refer to the Medicare Claims Processing Manual searchable by visiting this address: http://www.cms.hhs.gov/

- For additional information on the revised CMS-1500 form, visit the NUCC website at http://www.nucc.org

- More information on electronic claims and/or clearinghouses is available on the Federal Register. Use the following web address, then key applicable words, such as "claims clearinghouse" or "electronic claims." http://www.gpoaccess.gov/fr/index.html

- Specific and detailed instructions for completing claims using the new CMS-1500 form are given in the National Uniform Claim Committee's instruction manual, which is searchable at this address: http://www.nucc.org/

Chapter 6

Traditional Fee-for-Service/Private Plans

Chapter Outline

CHAPTER OBJECTIVES

After completing this chapter, the student should be able to
- Describe fee-for-service (indemnity) insurance.
- List the various levels of coverage available under a fee-for-service plan.
- Discuss how a fee-for-service plan works.
- Define commercial/private insurance.
- Explain self-insurance.
- Relate the functions of third-party administrators and administrative services organizations to self-insured organizations.
- Summarize the Blue Cross and Blue Shield health insurance program.

CHAPTER TERMS

administrative services organization (ASO)
autonomy
basic health insurance
BlueCard Program
BlueCard Worldwide
Blue Cross and Blue Shield Federal Employee Program (FEP)
coinsurance
commercial health insurance
comprehensive insurance
covered expenses
deductible
Employee Retirement Income Security Act (ERISA) of 1974
explanation of benefits (EOB)
Federal Employee Health Benefits (FEHB) Program

CHAPTER TERMS

fee-for-service (FFS)/indemnity plan	participating provider (PAR)
fiscal intermediary	point-of-service (POS) plan
group insurance	policyholder
Healthcare Service Plans	preferred provider organization (PPO)
health insurance policy premium	reasonable and customary fee
health maintenance organization (HMO)	self-insured/self-insurance
insurance cap	single or specialty service plans
lifetime maximum cap	stop loss insurance
major medical insurance	supplemental coverage
managed care plan	third-party payer
Medicare supplement plans	third-party administrator (TPA)
nonforfeitable interest	

OPENING SCENARIO

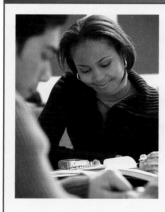

The subject matter of Chapter 6 is traditional fee-for-service insurance, sometimes referred to as indemnity, private, or commercial insurance. Traditional, indemnity, fee-for-service, private, commercial, self-insurance—Emilio and Latisha are amazed that so many different terms can be interrelated. Blue Cross and Blue Shield is a type of insurance they are both familiar with. As Emilio put it, "Who hasn't heard of 'The Blues'?" Emilio's parents currently have a Blue Cross and Blue Shield health insurance policy, and Emilio is still covered on it. Latisha's husband has a family plan with Liberty Value Insurance Company, a commercial carrier, through his employer. The term "commercial" did not have much meaning to Latisha until now, and she is looking forward to learning more about it.

TRADITIONAL FEE-FOR-SERVICE/INDEMNITY INSURANCE

Fee-for-service (FFS), or indemnity, insurance is a traditional type of healthcare policy where the insurance company pays fees for the services provided to the individuals covered by the policy. As discussed in an earlier chapter, this type of health insurance offers the most choices of physicians and hospitals. Typically, patients can choose any physician they want and can change physicians at any time. Additionally, they can go to any hospital in any part of the United States and still be covered.

To review, we know why people need health insurance. Today's healthcare costs are continually increasing, and individuals need to protect themselves from catastrophic financial losses that result from serious illnesses or injuries. If you have health insurance, a **third-party payer** covers a major portion of your medical expenses. A third-party payer is any organization (e.g., Blue Cross and Blue Shield, Medicare, Medicaid, or commercial insurance company) that provides payment for specified coverages provided under the health plan. Many Americans obtain health insurance through their employment, through what is referred to as **group insurance**. Group insurance is a contract between an insurance company and an employer (or other entity) that covers eligible employees or members. Group insurance is generally the least expensive kind. In many cases, the employer pays part or, in some cases, all of the cost.

If an employer does not offer group insurance, or if the insurance offered is very limited, a wide variety of individual, private policies are available. There are two basic categories available in individual health insurance—FFS plan or some type of **managed care plan**. A managed care plan typically involves the financing, managing, and delivery of healthcare services and is composed of a group of providers who share the financial risk of the plan or who have an incentive to deliver cost-effective, but quality, service. It is important that options are weighed carefully when choosing an individual healthcare plan because coverage and costs and how comprehensive the coverage is vary considerably from one insurance company to another.

☑ HIPAA Tip

Although HIPAA makes it much easier to get health insurance from a new employer when switching jobs, it does not guarantee the same level of benefits, deductibles, and claim limits the individual might have had under the former employer's health plan.

Looking more closely at these two broad categories of insurance, we find four basic types of plans, as follows:

1. Traditional **FFS/indemnity plans**
2. **Preferred provider organizations (PPOs)**
3. **Point-of-service (POS) plans**
4. **Health maintenance organizations (HMOs)**

No one type of healthcare plan is universally better than the other. It depends on an individual's (or group's) needs and preferences. FFS health plans can cover everything, but the tradeoff is the cost. The **autonomy**, or freedom to choose what medical expenses will be covered, offered by FFS plans is attractive to some, whereas others prefer the lower costs associated with most types of managed care.

Traditional FFS insurance is gradually becoming less popular as managed care moves to the forefront in healthcare. For individuals who value autonomy and flexibility of choices and can afford to spend a little extra money for the type of coverage they prefer, however, an individual health insurance policy may be the best policy for them.

FFS healthcare offers unlimited choices. The **policyholder** (the individual in whose name the policy is written) controls the choice of physician and facility, from primary caregiver to specialist, surgeon, and hospital. Flexible coverage offered by the FFS usually allows immediate treatment for medical emergencies or unexpected illness. FFS health plans do have restrictions, however. Often, they do not cover preventive medicine, so checkups, routine office visits, and injections (among a few other services)

Imagine This!

Maria Solaris is 52 years old and has worked for Olympia Products for 10 years. Her husband Alonzo is a self-employed auto mechanic. Olympia offers a comprehensive group health plan to its employees and pays half of their health insurance premium costs. Maria's share of the family plan premium through Olympia is $240 per month. (They have no children eligible for the plan.) Maria and Alonzo decided to purchase a private policy from a company that offers a husband and wife only plan with basically the same benefits as the group plan with Olympia at a monthly premium rate of $265. Although this private policy is more costly, Maria and Alonzo feel more secure with their new healthcare plan. If Maria loses her job at Olympia or retires, she and her husband don't have to worry about loss of benefits or preexisting conditions.

are likely to be the patient's responsibility. This can make FFS insurance impractical for a large family that requires many routine visits and preventive care.

Choice does not come cheap. Although it is hard to predict the annual cost of healthcare under a FFS insurance plan, there are a few costs that are relatively standard, as follows:
- A monthly (or quarterly) fee, called a **health insurance policy premium**
- A yearly **deductible** (out-of-pocket payment) before the health insurance carrier begins to contribute
- A per-visit **coinsurance**, or percentage of healthcare expenses

As a rule, healthcare services that are not covered by the health insurance policy (e.g., checkups) do not count toward satisfying the deductible. FFS health plans are not all created equal. There are three levels of coverage available:

1. **Basic health insurance,** which includes:
   - Hospital room and board and inpatient hospital care
   - Some hospital services and supplies, such as x-rays and medicine
   - Surgery, whether performed in or out of the hospital
   - Some physician visits

2. **Major medical insurance,** which includes:
   - Treatment for long, high-cost illnesses or injuries
   - Inpatient and outpatient expenses

3. **Comprehensive insurance,** which is a combination of the two

The cost of the FFS plan varies with the level of coverage chosen—the better the coverage, the higher the premiums. Although indemnity health insurance plans offer choice and security, these advantages are reflected in the cost of the coverage.

HOW A FEE-FOR-SERVICE PLAN WORKS

With a FFS type of plan, the policyholder pays a periodic fee, referred to as a premium. In addition to the premium, a specific amount of money must be paid up front each year as costs are incurred before the insurance payments begin. This is called the deductible. In a typical plan, the deductible might be anywhere from $100 to $10,000. Most family plans require the deductible be paid on at least two people in the family. The deductible requirement applies each year of the policy, and not all healthcare expenses count toward the deductible—only the expenses specifically covered by the policy. After the deductible for the year has been met, the policyholder (or dependents) shares the cost of services with the insurance carrier. The patient might pay 20% of **covered expenses**—charges incurred that qualify for reimbursement under the terms of the policy contract—whereas the insurer pays 80%. This type of cost sharing is referred to as coinsurance.

Most FFS plans have an **insurance cap**, which limits the amount of money the policyholder has to pay out-of-pocket for any one incident or in any one year. The cap is reached when out-of-pocket expenses for deductibles and coinsurance total a certain amount. This amount may be $1000 or $5000. After the "cap" is reached, the insurance company pays the reasonable and customary amount in excess of the cap for the items the policy says it will cover and coinsurance provision does not apply. (The cap does not include the premiums.)

Also, many FFS policies have a **lifetime maximum cap** the insurer pays. This cap is an amount after which the insurance company would not pay any more of the charges incurred. Often this cap is quite high—$500,000 to $1 million. This can be a "per incident" cap or a "lifetime" cap, depending on the policy.

Most insurance plans pay the **reasonable and customary fee** for a particular service. The term "reasonable and customary" is used to refer to the commonly charged or prevailing fees for health services within a geographic area. A fee is generally considered to be reasonable if it falls within the parameters of the average or commonly charged fee for the particular service within that specific community. If the healthcare provider charges $1000 for a specific procedure, whereas most other providers in the same geographic area charge only $600, the policyholder may be billed for the $400 difference. If the provider is a **participating provider (PAR)**, one who participates through a contractual arrangement with a healthcare service contractor in the type of health insurance in question, he or she agrees to accept the amount paid by the carrier as payment in full. The policyholder does not have to pay the $400 difference—it is adjusted off, which means the provider absorbs this difference in cost.

COMMERCIAL OR PRIVATE HEALTH INSURANCE

WHAT IS COMMERCIAL INSURANCE?

Commercial health insurance (also called "private" health insurance) is any kind of health insurance paid for by someone other than the government. Medicare, Medicaid, TRICARE, and CHAMPVA are all government programs and do not fall into the category of commercial or private plans. There is also one kind of commercial insurance that the government does pay for, the **Federal Employee Health Benefit (FEHB) Program**, which is a government health insurance coverage for its own civilian employees.

Government health insurance is standard for each program it sponsors, but commercial health insurance includes many variations in price and the kinds of benefits that the policy covers. The rules about a health insurance policy, such as what benefits are received and what rights the individuals covered under the policy have, depend on two things: the type of insurance (e.g., HMO, FFS) and who is paying for the insurance.

 HIPAA Tip

HIPAA protects millions of American workers by offering portability and continuity of health insurance coverage when changing jobs.

WHO PAYS FOR COMMERCIAL INSURANCE?

Commercial health insurance usually is paid for by an employer, a union, an employee and employer sharing the cost, or an individual. When the cost of health insurance is shared, the cost is much less than if he or she is buying health insurance as an individual. Not all jobs come with health insurance, and sometimes individuals are between jobs and not eligible for coverage. In these situations, it may be necessary to consider a private insurance policy to maintain healthcare coverage.

 HIPAA Tip

Under HIPAA, *group* health plans cannot deny an application for coverage based solely on the individual's health status. It also limits exclusions for preexisting conditions.

WHAT IS SELF-INSURANCE?

Some employers are **self-insured**, which means that when an employee needs healthcare, the employer—not an insurance company—is responsible for the cost of medical services. Most organizations that are self-insured are large entities, which can draw from hundreds or thousands of enrollees. Self-insured plans usually do not have to obey traditional laws governing insurance because they are technically not considered insurance companies.

Employee Retirement Income Security Act of 1974

Self-insured plans are sometimes called ERISA plans. The only law that governs self-insured plans is the federal law known as ERISA, an acronym for the **Employee Retirement Income Security Act (of 1974)**. ERISA sets minimum standards for pension plans in private industry, which is how most self-insured employers fund their programs.

Self-insured employers typically set up employee benefit plans that provide benefits to employees in the form of life insurance, disability insurance, health insurance, severance pay, and pensions. These benefits are funded through the purchase of insurance policies or through the establishment of trusts, paid for by the employer or the employer and employee. When the money is put into a trust, the employer takes a tax deduction for its contribution to the trust. The trust money is then invested. If an employer maintains a pension plan, ERISA specifies

1. when an employee must be allowed to become a participant,
2. how long an employee has to work before acquiring a **nonforfeitable interest** (an amount employees do not have to give up when quitting or retiring) in their pension,
3. how long an employee can be away from the job before it affects benefits, and
4. whether a spouse has a right to part of an employee's pension in the event of death.

Most of these ERISA provisions are effective for plan years beginning on or after January 1, 1975.

Third-Party Administrators/Administrative Services Organizations

Many self-insured groups, such as employers and union trusts, hire **third-party administrators (TPAs)** or **administrative services organizations (ASOs)** to manage and pay their claims. A TPA is a person or organization who processes claims and performs other contractual administrative services. An ASO, similar to a TPA, provides a wide variety of health insurance administrative services for organizations that have chosen to self-fund their health benefits. TPAs and ASOs are neither health plans nor insurers, but organizations that provide claims-paying functions for the clients they service. Although historically TPAs and ASOs only paid claims, their functions are expanding. Now, these organizations typically perform some or all of the following functions:

• General administrative functions
• Planning
• Marketing
• Human resources management
• Financing and accounting

Many self-insured groups were pioneers in PPO development. As a result, a TPA or ASO may pay claims based on discounted rates negotiated by a PPO on behalf of a self-insured group. A self-insured group may contract directly with providers, or it may use the services of a managed care organization.

Instead of paying premiums to health insurers (who would charge group premiums to pay for the healthcare services rendered to the group's enrollees), self-insured groups assume the risk of providing such services on their own, usually with some kind of **stop loss insurance**. Stop loss insurance is protection from the devastating effect of exorbitant medical claims. Examples are claims resulting from prolonged or intense medical services resulting from premature births, multiple trauma, transplant, or any other extended care that can result in catastrophic medical fees. Stop loss insurance limits the amount the insurer has to pay to a specified amount.

Single or Specialty Service Plans

Single or specialty service plans are health plans that provide services only in certain health specialties, such as mental health, vision, or dental plans. These health plans developed as people realized that eliminating a specific category of healthcare (e.g., mental health services) might slow the rate of increasing costs for healthcare in general and facilitate the management of care within these specialties. Eliminating a certain specialty of health services from coverage under the healthcare policy is referred to as a **carve out**. Employers wanting to include these special carved-out coverages for their employees can contract with one of these single or specialty service plans that focus on the desired specialty service.

Vision and dental plans and prescription drug coverage have often been add-on or **supplemental coverage** to health plans. Supplemental coverage varies greatly in the benefit services that they offer and represent another example of single specialty service plans.

BLUE CROSS AND BLUE SHIELD

OVERVIEW oldest

Blue Cross and Blue Shield is probably the best-known commercial insurance company in the United States. The Blue Cross and Blue Shield Association, created in 1982, is the result of a merger of the Blue Cross Association and National Association of Blue Shield Plans. This national organization coordinates and oversees more than 40 independent local programs that provide healthcare coverage to more than 80 million Americans through indemnity insurance, HMOs, PPOs, POS plans, and FFS plans. Some Blue Cross and Blue Shield Association chapters also administer (are fiscal intermediaries for) Medicare plans for the federal government.

Blue Cross policies cover inpatient hospital care, and Blue Shield policies cover physicians' services. Blue Cross and Blue Shield plans, often referred to as "Blue Plans" or "The Blues," offer health insurance coverage in all 50 states, the District of Columbia, Puerto Rico, and Canada. These plans cover all sectors of the population, including large employer groups, small businesses, and individual consumers and their families. Most healthcare providers accept Blue Cross and Blue Shield cards.

As mentioned, Blue Cross and Blue Shield offers indemnity and managed care plans. One of their more popular types of managed care plans is referred to as a preferred provider organization (PPO). Under this plan, members have the freedom to select any provider they choose, but they are encouraged to receive care from PPO network providers. The incentive to use PPO plan providers is that the out-of-pocket costs the member pays are typically less if they choose a provider within the network. Similar to Medicare, Blue Cross and Blue Shield plans have provider identification (ID) numbers and PAR and nonparticipating (nonPAR) provider arrangements. Most plans pay participating providers directly, and the providers agree not to bill the patient for the difference between the plan's allowable charge and the actual fee charged.

HISTORY OF BLUE CROSS

In 1929, Justin Ford Kimball, an official at Baylor University in Dallas, introduced a plan to guarantee schoolteachers 21 days of hospital care for $6 a year. Other groups of employees in Dallas soon joined the plan, and the idea quickly attracted nationwide attention. By 1939, the Blue Cross symbol was officially adopted by a commission of the American Hospital Association as the national emblem for plans that met certain guidelines. In 1960, the commission was replaced with the Blue Cross Association, and all formal ties with the American Hospital Association were severed in 1972.

HISTORY OF BLUE SHIELD

The Blue Shield concept grew out of the lumber and mining camps of the Pacific Northwest early in the 20th century. Employers wanted to provide medical care for their workers, so they paid monthly fees to "medical service bureaus" composed of groups of physicians. These pioneer programs led to the first Blue Shield Plan, which was founded in California in 1939. The Blue Shield symbol was informally adopted in 1948 by a group of nine Plans known as the Associated Medical Care Plans. This group eventually became the National Association of Blue Shield Plans.

BLUE CROSS AND BLUE SHIELD PROGRAMS

Local chapters of the independent Blue Plans offer products and services uniquely tailored to meet community and individual consumer needs. At the same time, their membership in the Blue Cross and Blue Shield Association enables them to serve large regional and national employers effectively. Although healthcare coverage options differ from region to region, they typically include FFS and managed FFS plans and PPO plans.

BlueCard and BlueCard Worldwide

The **BlueCard and BlueCard Worldwide program** links independent Blue Plans so that members and their families can obtain healthcare services while traveling or working anywhere in the United States, receiving the same benefits they would receive if they were at home. To help identify members who participate in the BlueCard Program, the health insurance professional should look for the suitcase logo on the ID card. If the member belongs to a BlueCard PPO, the initials PPO appear inside the suitcase logo (Fig. 6-1).

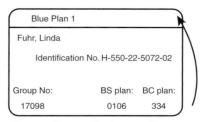

Fig. 6-1 Location on the card where suitcase can be found.

BlueCard Worldwide provides Blue Plan members inpatient and outpatient coverage at no additional cost in more than 200 foreign countries. BlueCard Worldwide participating hospitals are located in major travel destinations and business centers around the world. When plan members travel or live outside the United States and require inpatient hospital care, all they have to do is show their ID card to any of these participating hospitals, and their claim is handled just as if they were at home. Plan members have the choice of using a nonparticipating hospital; however, they may have to pay the hospital directly and then file a claim with Blue Cross and Blue Shield for reimbursement of covered expenses. The preferred form to file for BlueCard Worldwide claims is shown in Fig. 6-2.

Federal Employees Health Benefits

Congress instituted the FEHB Program in 1960. FEHB is the largest employer-sponsored group health insurance program in the world, covering more than 9 million federal civilian employees, retirees, former employees, family members, and former spouses. Under this program, eligible members of the participating insurance companies (of which Blue Cross and Blue Shield is one) have access to a wide variety of health plans. Choices include various types of plans, as follows:
- FFS
- PPOs
- POS plans
- HMOs (if the individual works within an area serviced by an HMO plan)

Federal Employee Program

The Federal Employees Health Benefits Act is the law governing the FEHB Program. This program provides health benefits coverage for federal employees. The Office of Personnel Management has overall administration responsibility for the FEHB Program. The Office of Personnel Management also receives and deposits payments to the FEHB Program and remits payment to the carriers. Each carrier is responsible for furnishing ID cards to enrollees, adjudicating claims, and maintaining and reconciling operational and enrollment records. The **Blue Cross and**

Please see the instructions on the reverse side of this form before completing. Please type or print.

1. Patient Information – 1A. Alpha prefix   Identification number   *Copy this from your Blue Cross Blue Shield identification card.*

1B. Patient's name (First, middle initial, last)	1C. Patient's date of birth MM/DD/YY / /	1D. Patient's sex ☐ Male ☐ Female
1E. Name of subscriber (First, middle initial, last)	1F. Subscriber's date of birth MM/DD/YY / /	1G. Patient's relationship to subscriber ☐ Self ☐ Spouse ☐ Child

2. Other Health Insurance – Is the patient covered under other health insurance, including Medicare A or B? ☐ Yes ☐ No
If yes, complete 2A through 2K below.

2A. Name and address of insuring company

2B. Type of policy ☐ Family ☐ Individual	2C. Effective date MM/DD/YY / /	2D. Termination date MM/DD/YY / /	2E. Policy or identification number of other coverage

3. Diagnosis – 3A. Describe illness, injury, or symptoms requiring treatment | 3B. Was patient's treatment due to a work-related accident or condition? ☐ Yes ☐ No

3C. Complete for care related to accidental injuries
Date of accident _____   Location: ☐ At home ☐ Auto ☐ Other _____
Time of accident _____   *If the accident was caused by someone else, attach a statement describing the accident.*

4. Charges – Use a separate line to list each type of service or provider and attach itemized bills for all services.

4A. Type of provider	4B. Name of provider making charge	4C. Description of service	4D. Dates of service or purchase	4E. Charges

5. Payee – Select one of the following payment options:
5A. ☐ Make payment to subscriber; provider has been paid.
Currency– Do you want the check issued in the currency reflected on the itemized bill(s) or in U.S. dollars? ☐ Currency on itemized bill(s) ☐ U.S. dollars
Please specify subscriber name as it appears on bank account: _____

5B. ☐ Make payment to provider (hospital, doctor). Please complete and sign.
Authorization for Assignment of Benefits
I, the undersigned, authorize and request Blue Cross and Blue Shield to make payment for benefits due herein to:
Name of provider _____   Signature of subscriber or spouse _____   Date _____

6. Signature – I certify the above is complete and correct and that I am claiming benefits only for charges incurred by the patient named above.

Signature of subscriber or patient _____   Date _____

N20-00-155

Fig. 6-2 Sample International Claim form.

General Information

The International Claim Form is to be used to submit institutional and professional claims for benefits for covered services received outside the United State, Puerto Rico, Jamaica and the U.S. Virgin Islands. For filing instructions for other claim types(e.g., dental, prescription drugs, etc.) contact your carrier.

The International Claim Form must be competed for each patient in full, and accompanied by fully itemized bills. It is not necessary for you to provide an English translation or convert currency.

Since the claim cannot be returned, please be sure to keep photocopies of all bills and supporting documentation for your personal records.

International Claim Form Instructions

Please complete all items on the claim form. If the information requested does not apply to the patient, indicate N/A (Not Applicable). Special care should be taken when completing the following items:

2. Other Health Insurance

If the patient holds other insurance coverage, please complete items A through K as completely as possible. It is especially important to indicate the name and address of the other insurance company and the policy or identification number of that coverage, as well as the name and birth date of the person who holds that policy.

In addition, if the patient is someone other than the subscriber and has received benefits from any other health insurance plan held by reason of law or employment, the Explanation of Benefits Form furnished by the other carrier pertaining to these charges must be included with the claim. A clear photocopy of the other carrier's Explanation of Benefits Form is acceptable in place of the original document.

Itemized Bill Information

Each provider's original itemized bill must be attached and must contain:

- The letterhead indicating the name and address of the person or organization providing the service
- The full name of the patient receiving the service
- The date of each service
- A description of each service
- The charge for each service

This completed claim form, together with itemized bills and supporting documentation, should be submitted to:

Smith & Co. Insurance
113 Waverton
Springfield, XY 33142 USA

Fig. 6-2—cont'd

Blue Shield Federal Employee Program (FEP) enrolls several million federal government employees, retirees, and their dependents. FEP has covered federal workers and their families since the FEHB act was adopted in 1960. Today, Blue Cross and Blue Shield FEP covers nearly half of all people eligible for FEHB program benefits. To examine sample BCBS FEP ID cards, refer to *Websites to Explore* at the end of this chapter.

Medicare

Blue Cross and Blue Shield plans have partnered with the U.S. government in administering the Medicare program since its beginning in 1966. Blue Plans helped design the original infrastructure for tracking and processing Medicare payments. Today, the Blue System is the largest single processor (**fiscal intermediary**) of Medicare claims—handling most Part A claims (hospitals and institutions) and more than half of Part B claims from physicians and other healthcare practitioners. Blue Cross and Blue Shield is not the fiscal intermediary for Medicare in all states, however. A fiscal intermediary is a commercial insurer or agent (e.g., Blue Cross) that contracts with the Department of Health and Human Services (Centers for Medicare and Medicaid Services) for the purpose of processing and administering Part A Medicare claims for reimbursement of healthcare coverage. In addition to handling financial matters, a fiscal intermediary may perform other functions, such as providing consultative services or serving as a center for communication with providers and making audits of providers' needs.

Healthcare Service Plans

Healthcare Service Plans, typically operated by Blue Cross and Blue Shield Plans throughout the United States, have provided healthcare coverage for many years. Although they were initially involved in paying claims for indemnity carriers, many Healthcare Service Plans have developed managed care products to compete with companies offering managed care plans.

Because the individual member Blue Cross and Blue Shield organizations no longer are governed at a national level, each has its own specific guidelines for completing the CMS-1500 claim form. Although guidelines are similar, there may be subtle differences from one plan to the next. To make absolutely certain that you follow the correct claims completion guidelines for the Blue Cross and Blue Shield plan in your area, log on to the Blue Cross and Blue Shield main website http://www.bcbs.com/ and insert the appropriate area code.

Medicare Supplement Plans

In addition to indemnity and managed care plans, Blue Cross and Blue Shield offers **Medicare supplement plans**.

Medicare supplement insurance is designed specifically to provide coverage for some of the costs that Medicare does not pay, such as Medicare's deductible and coinsurance amounts, and for certain services not allowed by Medicare. If Medicare-eligible patients do not have supplemental coverage, they must pay the deductibles and coinsurance amounts themselves.

What Did You Learn?

1. What type of services does Blue Cross cover?
2. Explain the BlueCard program.
3. List the various programs offered under the Blue Cross and Blue Shield system.
4. What role does Blue Cross and Blue Shield play in the FEP program?

PARTICIPATING VERSUS NONPARTICIPATING PROVIDERS

We discussed PAR providers and nonPAR providers in Chapter 4. A PAR provider enters into a contractual agreement with a carrier and agrees to follow certain rules involving claims and payment in turn for advantages granted by the carrier. Not all insurance companies offer such contracts to healthcare providers, but Blue Cross and Blue Shield does. A healthcare provider who is PAR with Blue Cross and Blue Shield agrees to

• file claims for all Blue Cross and Blue Shield patients and
• accept the Blue Cross and Blue Shield "allowed" fee as payment in full and write off (adjust) any differences between the fee charged and that which is allowed by Blue Cross and Blue Shield.

In turn, under this contractual agreement, Blue Cross and Blue Shield agrees to

• send payments directly to the provider,
• host periodic staff training seminars,
• offer guides and newsletters at no charge,
• provide assistance with claim problems, and
• publish the practice's information in the Blue Cross and Blue Shield PAR directory.

Providers who are not a part of the above-described contractual agreement are referred to as nonPAR providers. In this case, providers do not have to file patient claims and can balance bill the difference between their charges and Blue Cross and Blue Shield–allowed charges. The downside is that Blue Cross and Blue Shield mails payments to the patient rather than the provider, however, and the health insurance professional must collect the fees directly from the patient unless the patient agrees to assign benefits (in writing).

Imagine This!

Dr. Mueller is nonPAR with Blue Cross and Blue Shield. The medical receptionist neglected to ask new patient Agnes Blank to assign benefits, so Blue Cross and Blue Shield sent the payment for Agnes' medical services directly to her. Agnes cashes the insurance check, but fails to pay Dr. Mueller's bill. Statements mailed to Agnes are returned stamped "moved; no forwarding address."

What Did You Learn?

1. Name two things a Blue Cross and Blue Shield PAR provider must agree to.
2. What special benefits does Blue Cross and Blue Shield extend to PAR providers?

COMPLETING THE CMS-1500 FORM FOR A COMMERCIAL PLAN

Guidelines for completing the CMS-1500 form for commercial claims, as shown in Fig. 6-3, are basically the same for all carriers with a few subtle differences in certain blocks. Health insurance professionals should be familiar with the guidelines of common carriers that their patients use. These guidelines should be kept handy in a file or portfolio and updated periodically to ensure any changes are noted. When a patient is covered by an insurance company with which the health information professional is unfamiliar, the carrier should be called and guidelines requested to facilitate claim submission and to avoid claim delays and rejections.

For an example of how to complete the CMS-1500 claim for a commercial carrier, the Blue Cross and Blue Shield step-by-step guidelines are used in Fig. 6-3.

What Did You Learn?

1. In what block should the patient's insurance ID number appear?
2. What is the POS code for services rendered in the provider's office?
3. What information might appear in Blocks 17 and 17a and/or b?
4. How do you relate Block 24e with Block 21?

SUBMITTING COMMERCIAL CLAIMS

Blue Cross and Blue Shield member offices publish specialty-specific billing guides to help practitioners code and bill specific services, such as physical medicine, eye care, and home medical equipment. These guides can be viewed online under "Provider Guides" on most member websites. Paper copies also are available on request.

TIMELY FILING

Providers contracting with Blue Cross and Blue Shield must file claims within 365 days following the last date of service provided to the patient. If a claim is not filed within this timely filing period, Blue Cross and Blue Shield normally does not allow benefits for the claim. If payment on the claim is denied for this reason, the provider cannot collect payment from the patient.

FILING COMMERCIAL PAPER AND ELECTRONIC CLAIMS

Filing CMS-1500 paper claims for commercial carriers is similar to filing claims with all other carriers. If up-to-date guidelines for claims completion for the specific carrier are not on file, the health insurance professional should contact the carrier and request these guidelines. If the provider's office is set up for electronic claims filing, the health insurance professional should contact the carrier before submitting the claims directly to find out what format to use to be compatible. If the provider uses a claims clearinghouse, the clearinghouse manages this process. The Health Insurance Portability and Accountability Act-Administrative Simplification (HIPAA-AS) was passed by Congress in 1996 to set standards for the electronic transmission of healthcare data and to protect the privacy of individually identifiable health-care information.

What Did You Learn?

1. What is the filing deadline for submitting Blue Cross and Blue Shield claims?
2. If the provider's office is set up for electronic claims filing, how can the health insurance professional find out if his or her facility is compatible with the carrier's electronic standards?

Block	Block Name	Explanation
1	Type of Insurance	Place an "X" in the proper box indicating the type of insurance
1a	Insured's ID Number	Enter the policyholder's alpha-prefix and ID number as shown on his/her identification card.
2	Patient's Name	Enter the patient's full "given" name.
3	Patient's Date of Birth	Enter the correct date of birth (MM/DD/YYYY) and sex of the patient.
4	Insured's Name	Enter the policyholder's name. (If the policyholder and the patient are one and the same, enter "SAME."
5	Patient's Address	Required if it is not the same as the policyholder's address.
6	Patient Relationship to Insured	Check the appropriate box. Do not use the box for "Other."
7	Insured's Address	Enter the complete address of the policyholder.
8	Patient Status	Check the appropriate box.
9	Other Insurance information	Required if 11d is marked "yes." If you determine the patient has other coverage, enter the name of the other insured.
9a	Other insured's policy or group number.	Enter the other insured's policy or group number in this field.
9b	Other insured's date of birth	Enter the other insured's date of birth and sex.
9c	Employer's name or school name.	Enter the employer's (or school's) name.
9d	Insurance plan	Enter the insurance plan name or program. Block 9d may be used to indicate that a Medicare eligible patient elected not to purchase Medicare art A or Part B coverage. Enter "No Medicare Part A and/or Part B Coverage," depending on the patient's situation.
10	Is Patient's Condition Related to	Check the appropriate box if the patient's condition is related to employment or an author accident or check "other."
11d	Another Health Benefit Plan	Request this information from the member. If the answer is "yes," go back and complete blocks 11 through 11c.
12	Patient's authorization to release information	Patient (or his/her authorized representative) should sign in this block. If a current release of information is on file, the words "SIGNATURE ON FILE," OR "SOF" is acceptable.
13	Assign Benefits	Not required
14	Date of Current Illness/ Injury/Pregnancy	Enter the date (MM/DD/YY) that applies to accident and medical emergency situations. If you submit services that relate to more than one accident or medical emergency, submit separate claims for each accident or medical emergency.

Fig. 6-3 Step-by-step claims completion guidelines for Blue Cross and Blue Shield.

COMMERCIAL CLAIMS INVOLVING SECONDARY COVERAGE

It is not unusual for a patient to be covered under a second insurance policy. A typical situation would be when a husband and wife are employed with companies who offer a paid, or partially paid, group insurance plan. Because of the rising costs of health insurance, however, dual coverage is becoming less common. When a situation such as this arises, it is important to find out which policy is primary and submit the CMS-1500 claim to that carrier first. Usually, the best way to determine primary coverage is to ask the patient. Normally, when a husband and wife are covered under separate policies, primary coverage follows the patient. If the patient is unsure, call his or her employer or contact the third-party payer directly.

Block	Block Name	Explanation
15	Same or similar illness.	Not required.
16	Dates unable to work.	Not required.
17	Name of Referring Physician or other source	Enter the name of the referring physician. For lab and x-ray claims, enter the physician's name that ordered the diagnostic services.
17 a and b	ID Number of Referring Provider or other source	Until May 23, 2001, enter the referring physician's UPIN. Effective May 23, 2007, the NPI must be reported in 17b.
18	Related hospitalization	Enter the dates of any related inpatient hospitalization.
19	Reserved for local use.	Enter either a 6-digit or an 8-digit date when the patient was last seen and the UPIN (NPT) when it becomes effective of the attending physician.
20	Outside lab	Not required.
21	Diagnosis or Nature of Illness/Injury	Enter an ICD-9-CM code. List the primary diagnosis first. If there is more than one diagnosis, indicate in field 24E which diagnoses apply to the procedure being billed on each line item of the claim. (Narrative descriptions are not accepted.)
22	Medicaid resubmission	Not required.
23	Prior authorization number	Not required.
24a	Date of Service From/To	If you submit office or hospital outpatient services, submit each service and/or each date of service on a separate line with the same "from" and "to" dates. The only exceptions in which date spanning is allowed on a line is if when billing inpatient services or monthly rental of home medical equipment (HME) For inpatient practitioner visits, date spanning is acceptable as long as the following is true: • The service provided is the same procedure code • The dates of service are consecutive • Services are submitted with the same month.
24b	Place of Service	Enter the place of service code by using the 2-digit codes. Electronic Submitters: Enter the standard 2-digit place of service codes. Paper Submitters: If the place of service code does not match the procedure code, or if you leave this field blank, the claim will be returned.
24c	Type of Service Codes	Enter an "X" or and "E" as appropriate for services performed as a result of a medical emergency.

Fig. 6-3—cont'd

In the case of dual coverage, a CMS-1500 claim should be submitted to the primary carrier first. When the primary carrier has processed the claim and payment is determined, a new claim is sent to the secondary carrier with the **explanation of benefits (EOB)** from the primary carrier attached. An EOB, also called a remittance notice, is a document prepared by the carrier that gives details of how the claim was adjudicated. It typically includes a comprehensive listing of patient information, dates of service, payments, or reasons for nonpayment (Fig. 6-5).

● **Stop and Think**

Carol Bolton is a computer programmer for American Commuter Services (ACS), Inc. She and her dependents are covered under an employer-sponsored group policy, and ACS pays the entire premium. Jim Bolton, her husband, is employed by ESI Repairs and is covered under a similar family plan through his employer. How might it be determined which policy is primary when Carol is seen in the office for her yearly physical?

Block	Block Name	Explanation
24d	Procedure Codes/Modifiers	Enter CPT or HCPCS code(s). Enter a current two-digit CPT or HCPCS modifier when applicable.
24e	Diagnosis Code	Link the diagnostic code for the listed service back to Block 21, using numbers 1, 2, 3 or 4, whichever is applicable.
24f	Total Charge	Enter a charge for each service billed on a line.
24g	Days or Units	Enter the number of services (in whole numbers) based on the time period or amount designated by the procedure code. To bill anesthesia, submit the actual time in minutes spent administering anesthesia services.
24h	EPSDT Family Plan	Not applicable to BCBS claims
24i	EMG	Enter the ID qualifier 1C in the shaded portion.
24j	COB	Prior to May 23, 2007, enter the rendering provider's PIN in the shaded portion. After May 23, 2007, do not use the shaded portion. Enter the provider's NPI number in the lower portion.
25	Federal Tax ID Number	Enter the practice's 9-digit federal taxpayer ID number (EIN). For sole proprietors, use the provider's Social Security number.
26	Patient's Account No.	Required for electronic submissions only
27	Accept Assignment	This is required for Medicare-related claims only
28	Total Charges	Enter the total of all charges from Block 24f.
29	Amount Paid	Leave blank
30	Amount Due	Leave blank
31	Signature of Provider	In addition to the physician/supplier's signature, a computer generated name, a stamp facsimile, or the signature of an authorized person is acceptable in this block.
32 a and b	Facility Information	Enter NPI of service facility in Block 32a. Enter the appropriate ID qualifier followed by one blank space and the PIN of the facility. After May 23, 2007, 32b is not to be reported.
33 a and b	Billing Provider Information	Effective May 23, 2007, the NPI of the billing provider must be reported in 33a. Enter the appropriate ID qualifier followed by one blank space and then the PIN of the facility. After May, 23, 2007, 33b is not to be reported.

Fig. 6-3—cont'd

What Did You Learn?

1. What is the best way to determine primary coverage for a patient who has two insurance policies?
2. What is the purpose of an EOB?

SUMMARY CHECK POINTS

☑ FFS, or indemnity, insurance is a traditional kind of healthcare policy where the insurance company pays fees for the services provided to the insured individuals covered by the policy. This type of health insurance offers the most choices of healthcare providers.

PLEASE
DO NOT
STAPLE
IN THIS
AREA

CARRIER

| | PICA | | | | | | **HEALTH INSURANCE CLAIM FORM** | | PICA | |

1. MEDICARE	MEDICAID	TRICARE CHAMPUS	CHAMPVA	GROUP HEALTH PLAN	FECA BLK LUNG	OTHER	1a. INSURED'S I.D. NUMBER	(For Program in Item 1)
(Medicare #)	(Medicaid #)	(Sponsor's SSN)	(Member ID#)	(SSN or ID)	(SSN)	(ID)		

2. PATIENT'S NAME (Last Name, First Name, Middle Initial)

3. PATIENT'S BIRTH DATE MM | DD | YY   SEX   M   F

4. INSURED'S NAME (Last Name, First Name, Middle Initial)

5. PATIENT'S ADDRESS (No., Street)

6. PATIENT RELATIONSHIP TO INSURED Self   Spouse   Child   Other

7. INSURED'S ADDRESS (No., Street)

CITY   STATE

8. PATIENT STATUS Single   Married   Other

CITY   STATE

ZIP CODE   TELEPHONE (Include Area Code) (   )

Employed   Full-Time Student   Part-Time Student

ZIP CODE   TELEPHONE (INCLUDE AREA CODE) (   )

9. OTHER INSURED'S NAME (Last Name, First Name, Middle Initial)

10. IS PATIENT'S CONDITION RELATED TO:

11. INSURED'S POLICY GROUP OR FECA NUMBER

a. OTHER INSURED'S POLICY OR GROUP NUMBER

a. EMPLOYMENT? (CURRENT OR PREVIOUS) YES   NO

a. INSURED'S DATE OF BIRTH MM | DD | YY   SEX   M   F

b. OTHER INSURED'S DATE OF BIRTH MM | DD | YY   SEX   M   F

b. AUTO ACCIDENT?   PLACE (State) YES   NO

b. EMPLOYER'S NAME OR SCHOOL NAME

c. EMPLOYER'S NAME OR SCHOOL NAME

c. OTHER ACCIDENT? YES   NO

c. INSURANCE PLAN NAME OR PROGRAM NAME

d. INSURANCE PLAN NAME OR PROGRAM NAME

10d. RESERVED FOR LOCAL USE

d. IS THERE ANOTHER HEALTH BENEFIT PLAN? YES   NO   **If yes,** return to and complete item 9 a-d.

READ BACK OF FORM BEFORE COMPLETING & SIGNING THIS FORM.

12. PATIENT'S OR AUTHORIZED PERSON'S SIGNATURE I authorize the release of any medical or other information necessary to process this claim. I also request payment of government benefits either to myself or to the party who accepts assignment below.

SIGNED _____   DATE _____

13. INSURED'S OR AUTHORIZED PERSON'S SIGNATURE I authorize payment of medical benefits to the undersigned physician or supplier for services described below.

SIGNED _____

PATIENT AND INSURED INFORMATION

14. DATE OF CURRENT: MM | DD | YY ILLNESS (First symptom) OR INJURY (Accident) OR PREGNANCY(LMP)

15. IF PATIENT HAS HAD SAME OR SIMILAR ILLNESS. GIVE FIRST DATE MM | DD | YY

16. DATES PATIENT UNABLE TO WORK IN CURRENT OCCUPATION MM | DD | YY FROM   TO   MM | DD | YY

17. NAME OF REFERRING PHYSICIAN OR OTHER SOURCE

17a.
17b.

18. HOSPITALIZATION DATES RELATED TO CURRENT SERVICES MM | DD | YY FROM   TO   MM | DD | YY

19. RESERVED FOR LOCAL USE

20. OUTSIDE LAB? $ CHARGES YES   NO

21. DIAGNOSIS OR NATURE OF ILLNESS OR INJURY. (RELATE ITEMS 1,2,3 OR 4 TO ITEM 24E BY LINE)

1. ____.____   3. ____.____

2. ____.____   4. ____.____

22. MEDICAID RESUBMISSION CODE   ORIGINAL REF. NO.

23. PRIOR AUTHORIZATION NUMBER

24. A. DATE(S) OF SERVICE						B. PLACE OF SERVICE	C. EMG	D. PROCEDURES, SERVICES, OR SUPPLIES (Explain Unusual Circumstances)		E. DIAGNOSIS POINTER	F. $ CHARGES	G. DAYS OR UNITS	H. EPSDT Family Plan	I. ID. QUAL.	J. RENDERING PROVIDER ID. #
From MM	DD	YY	To MM	DD	YY			CPT/HCPCS	MODIFIER						
1														NPI	
2														NPI	
3														NPI	
4														NPI	
5														NPI	
6														NPI	

PHYSICIAN OR SUPPLIER INFORMATION

25. FEDERAL TAX I.D. NUMBER   SSN   EIN

26. PATIENT'S ACCOUNT NO.

27. ACCEPT ASSIGNMENT? (For govt. claims, see back) YES   NO

28. TOTAL CHARGE $

29. AMOUNT PAID $

30. BALANCE DUE $

31. SIGNATURE OF PHYSICIAN OR SUPPLIER INCLUDING DEGREES OR CREDENTIALS (I certify that the statements on the reverse apply to this bill and are made a part thereof.)

SIGNED _____   DATE _____

32. SERVICE FACILITY LOCATION INFORMATION

a.   b.

33. BILLING PROVIDER INFO & PH # (   )

a.   b.

Fig 6-4 CMS-1500 "Template" with shaded blocks.

Explanation of Health Care Benefits

THIS IS NOT A BILL

Page Number
1

|||||||||||||||||||||||||||||||||||||||||||

MURRAY L. WHITE
3434 West Covington Place
Somewhere, XY 12345

Identification No.:	111-23-4567
Patient Name:	Sarah M. White
Provider Name:	Dean P. Locks, MD

Benefits Summary

Billed Charges	Provider Savings	Other Insurance Settlement	Blue Cross Blue Shield Settlement	Amount You Owe
136.00				136.00

Claim Details

			Notes		Notes		Notes		Notes
Place of Service	OFFICE			OFFICE		OFFICE		OFFICE	
Description of Service	MEDICAL CARE			LABORATORY		LABORATORY		LABORATORY	
Service Date: From/To	12/11	12/11/03		12/11 12/11/03		12/11 12/11/03		12/11 12/11/03	
Billed Charge	90.00			18.00		18.00		10.00	
Provider Savings (-)									
Contract Limitations (-)				11.00		11.00		6.25	
Copayment (-)									
Deductible (-)	90.00			7.00		7.00		3.75	
Sub-Total					1		1		1
Coinsurance									

Please see the back of this form for the "Definition of Terms."

Group Number	Claim Number	Account Number	Provider Number	Date Received	Date Processed
000059999–2104	05040190981500	A–0000960	17437	01–19–04	01–20–04

NOTES

1– YOU MAY BE MISSING OUT ON SAVINGS THAT YOU WOULD RECEIVE IF SERVICES HAD BEEN PERFORMED BY A BLUE CROSS AND BLUE SHIELD PARTICIPATING PROVIDER. (Z183)

$107.75 OF THIS CLAIM HAS BEEN APPLIED TO YOUR BASIC BLUE CROSS AND BLUE SHIELD DEDUCTIBLE. FOR THE PERIOD BEGINNING ON 10/01/02 THROUGH 12/31/03, THIS PATIENT HAS SATISFIED $2969.42 OF THE $5000.00 DEDUCTIBLE. (Z551)

530-409 C-5356 (MD) 7/02

Fig. 6-5 Sample Explanation of Benefits.

NOTES KEY

A. Your benefit plan covers accidental injury, medical emergency and surgical care. Other medical care received in the hospital's outpatient department or practitioner's office is not covered by your benefit plan.

B. The services identified on this claim do not meet the criteria of a medical emergency as defined in your benefit plan.

C. These services and/or supplies are not a benefit for the diagnosis, symptom or condition given on the claim.

D. These services are not covered by your benefit plan as described in the **Services Not Covered** section.

E. Routine physical exams and related services are not covered by your benefit plan as described in the **Services Not Covered** section.

F. These services were not performed within the time limit for treatment of accidental injury.

G. Routine vision examinations, eyeglasses, or examinations for their prescription or fittings are not covered by your benefit plan as described in the **Services Not Covered** section.

H. The services of this provider are not covered by your benefit plan.

I. These services exceed the maximum allowed by your benefit plan as described in the **Summary of Payment** section.

J. These services were received before you satisfied the waiting period required by your benefit plan as described in **Your Payment Obligations** section.

K. These services were not submitted within timely filing limits. Timely filing requires that we receive claims within 365 days after the end of the calendar year you receive services.

L. Using the identification number provided, we are unable to identify you as a member.

M. These services were performed before your benefit plan became effective.

N. These services were performed after your benefit plan was cancelled.

O. This individual is not covered by your benefit plan.

P. This individual may be eligible for Medicare. File this claim first with Medicare, if the individual has no other group health coverage as primary.

Q. The Plan in the state where these services were received will process this claim. Your claim has been sent to that Plan for processing.

R. These services have been billed to the wrong plan. Please forward your claim to the plan named on your identification card for processing.

S. These services are a duplication of a previously considered claim.

T. All or part of these services were paid by another insurance company or Medicare.

U. We have received no response to our request for additional information. Until this information is received, the claim is denied.

V. Personal convenience items or hospital-billed non-covered services are not covered by your benefit plan as described in the **Services Not Covered** section.

W. Services covered by Worker's Compensation are not covered by your benefit plan as described in the **Services Not Covered** section.

X. These services should be billed to the carrier that provides your hospital or medical coverage.

DEFINITION OF TERMS

Billed Charge: The total amount billed by your provider. *(If your coverage is Select and you receive covered services in the office of a Select provider, your coinsurance is based on this amount).*

Coinsurance: The amount, calculated using a fixed percentage, you pay each time you receive certain covered services.

Copayment: The fixed dollar amount you pay for certain covered services.

Deductible: The fixed dollar amount you pay for covered services before benefits are available.

Sub-Total: The amount reached by subtracting from the billed charge the following applicable amounts: provider savings; contract limitations; copayment and deductible. Your coinsurance is calculated on this amount *(unless your coverage is Select and you receive covered services in the office of a Select provider. In this case, your coinsurance is based on billed charge).*

Settlement: The total amount fulfilled by us as a result of our agreement with the provider; or the amount we pay directly to you.

Other Insurance Settlement: The total amount settled by another carrier (or us) because you are covered by more than one health plan.

Provider Savings: The amount saved because of our contracts with providers. For some inpatient hospital services, this amount may be an estimate. See explanation of payment arrangements in your benefits certificate.

Contract Limitations: Amounts for which you are responsible based on your contractual obligations with us. Examples of contract limitations include all of the following:
- Amounts for services that are not medically necessary.
- Amounts for services that are not covered by this certificate.
- Amounts for services that have reached contract maximums.
- If you receive services from a nonparticipating provider, any difference between the billed charge and usual, customary, and reasonable (UCR) amount.
- Penalty amounts for services that are not properly precertified.
- Penalty amounts for receiving inpatient hospital services from a nonparticipating hospital.

NOTICE OF RIGHT TO APPEAL AND ERISA RIGHTS

If you disagree with the denial, or partial denial of a claim, you are entitled to a full and fair review.

1. Submit a WRITTEN request for a review within 180 days OF THE DATE OF THIS NOTICE. Your request should include:

   - Date of your request;
   - Your printed name and address (and name and address of authorized representative if you have designated one);
   - The identification number and claim number from your Explanation of Health Care Benefits;
   - The date of service in question.

2. Send your request to:

Fig. 6-5—cont'd

☑ FFS insurance offers three levels of coverage:
1. *Basic health* includes
   - hospital room and board and inpatient hospital care;
   - some hospital services and supplies, such as x-rays and medicine;
   - surgery, whether performed in or out of the hospital; and
   - some physician visits.
2. *Major medical* includes
   - treatment for long, high-cost illnesses or injuries and
   - inpatient and outpatient expenses.
3. *Comprehensive* is a combination of the two.

☑ With FFS, the insurance company pays for part of the physician and hospital bills. The patient pays the following:
   - A monthly fee, called a *premium*
   - A certain amount of money each year, known as the *deductible*, before the insurance payments begin (deductible amounts vary with choice, typically from $100 to $5000, and apply to each year of the policy; not all health expenses count toward the deductible)
   - A portion of each charge, called *coinsurance*. After the *deductible* amount for the year has been met, the patient shares the bill with the insurance company based on certain percentages spelled out in the policy— typically 90/10 or 80/20.

☑ Commercial (or private) health insurance is any kind of health insurance paid for by somebody other than the government.

☑ A self-insured health plan is one for which an employer or other group sponsor, rather than an insurance company, is financially responsible for paying plan expenses, including claims made by group plan members.

☑ TPAs and ASOs are administrative entities that typically perform some or all of the following functions for self-insured plans:
   - General administrative
   - Planning
   - Marketing
   - Human resources management
   - Financing and accounting

☑ Blue Cross and Blue Shield is a nonprofit agency that offers a wide variety of healthcare plans to all sectors of the population in all 50 states, the District of Columbia, Puerto Rico, and Canada. The 41 independent local chapters are able to tailor their products and services to meet community and individual needs. Plan choices include
   - FFS,
   - PPOs,
   - POS plans, and
   - HMOs.

☑ More than 80% of healthcare providers in the United States accept Blue Cross and Blue Shield patients.

☑ Blue Cross and Blue Shield underwrites or administers many plans, including
   - BlueCard and BlueCard Worldwide Programs,
   - FEHB Program,
   - FEP,
   - Healthcare Service Plans, and
   - Medicare Supplemental Plans.

☑ Blue Cross and Blue Shield claims must be filed within 365 days following the last date of service provided to the patient.

CLOSING SCENARIO

Some of the topics in this chapter turned out to be a little more challenging than Emilio and Latisha had anticipated, especially the concept of self-insurance. Both students found the information on Blue Cross and Blue Shield particularly interesting, and they were already aware that it was a large and well-known organization. They had seen TV commercials on "The Blues," but they were unaware of how the organization got its start. Compared with today's costs, the idea of hospital room and board costing $6 a day was difficult to comprehend.

Emilio recalls changing physicians 2 years ago because the practice from which his family received most of their medical care discontinued their participating provider contract with Blue Cross and Blue Shield. He was unaware at the time, however, of the ramifications of a provider being either PAR or nonPAR. Now, he realizes how this difference can affect the patient directly.

Latisha is focusing her attention on the Blue Cross and Blue Shield guidelines for completing the CMS-1500 claim form. Many of the patients in the healthcare facility where she previously worked were covered under a Blue Cross and Blue Shield preferred provider plan, and she was familiar with how that plan functioned.

WEBSITES TO EXPLORE

For live links to the following websites, please visit the Evolve® site at http://evolve.elsevier.com/Beik/today/

- A wealth of information about Blue Cross and Blue Shield can be found on their website http://www.bluecares.com/

- For more information on HIPAA-AS, log on to http://www.hipaadvisory.com

Chapter 7

Unraveling the Mysteries of Managed Care

Chapter Outline

CHAPTER OBJECTIVES

After completion of this chapter, the student should be able to
- Explain the concept of managed care.
- Discuss the structure of the two major types of managed care organizations.
- List and briefly explain the various health maintenance organization models.

CHAPTER TERMS

capitation
closed panel HMO
consultation
copayment
direct contract model
enrollees
grievance
group model

health maintenance organization (HMO)
iatrogenic effects
individual practice association (IPA)
managed care
network
network model

OPENING SCENARIO

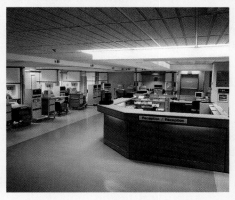

Emilio and Latisha had heard a lot about managed care before they enrolled in the course, but they did not think they fully understood the term and its effect on healthcare in general. Both students remember hearing stories on the news of medical cases gone wrong because of an HMO's refusal to pay for certain services; however, they are determined to remain open-minded regarding these controversial issues. They are prepared to learn the pros and cons of all facets of medical insurance and realize that there is a lot to learn in this particular area of healthcare.

Latisha has gotten a part-time job at Isis Healthcare. She is certain her new job will offer a great deal of insight into managed care because many of the patients visiting the facility are enrolled in a preferred provider organization. She admits that she does not fully understand the ramifications of this type of managed care.

Emilio has decided to volunteer at the free clinic in his neighborhood, which he hopes will foster his understanding of health insurance and what it means to be a health insurance professional. His mentor at the clinic has explained how their HMO functions. Similar to Latisha, Emilio still has a lot of unanswered questions. Both students are anticipating the information this chapter offers and are confident their questions will be answered and their uncertainty put to rest.

WHAT IS MANAGED CARE?

No doubt you have heard the term **managed care**. Managed care is on television news broadcasts nearly every day; it's in the papers; it's everywhere you go! But exactly what is managed care? We learned what traditional fee-for-service (indemnity) insurance was in Chapter 6. In this chapter, we attempt to unravel the mysteries of managed care.

The cost of healthcare is increasing rapidly. In the 1970s, there was a growing concern within the general population with how much individuals in the United States had to pay for good healthcare. Experts came up with some ideas for controlling, or "managing," these costs. Some of these ideas were considered good and some not so good. Whether it is good or not, managed care has changed the face of healthcare in the United States today, and it is no doubt here to stay.

Managed care is a complex healthcare system in which physicians, hospitals, and other healthcare professionals organize an interrelated system of people and facilities that communicate with one another and work together as a unit, commonly referred to as a **network**. This network coordinates and arranges healthcare services and benefits for a specific group of individuals, referred to as **enrollees**, for the purpose of managing cost, quality, and access to healthcare. A managed care organization (MCO) typically performs three main functions (Fig. 7-1):

- MCOs set up the contracts and organizations of the healthcare providers who furnish medical care to the enrollees.
- MCOs establish the list of covered benefits tied to managed care rules.
- MCOs oversee the healthcare provided by the MCO.

Managed care has strongly influenced the practice of medicine. The principles of managed health care shown in Fig. 7-1 represent key components in promoting effective managed care techniques that are fair and equitable

1. Managed care organizations should encourage access to health coverage - including those individuals with the greatest health risk.
2. Managed care organizations must recognize physicians' principal role in making medical decisions and guarantee strong physician leadership.
3. Managed care organizations should promote members' health by ascertaining that health plans and providers have incentives to provide high quality medical care.
4. Managed care organizations should be accountable for the health of members by preventing, as well as managing, diseases and illnesses.
5. Managed care organizations are ultimately accountable for the health of the enrollees, and for the outcomes of the treatment they receive.
6. Managed care organizations should communicate the outcomes of their services based on valid measures of medical quality.
7. To fulfill their responsibility to society and the communities they serve, managed care organizations should work together with public sector agencies to resolve gaps between commercial insurance and "safety net" programs.
8. Managed care organizations can help the government fulfill its responsibility to ensure health care for all through the provision of a more cost-effective and comprehensive system of care.

Fig. 7-1 Principles of managed healthcare.

to physicians in ensuring that high quality health care services are delivered to patients. MCOs and third party payers are strongly encouraged to use these guidelines in developing their own policies and procedures. In addition, any public or private entities that evaluate managed care organizations or their contracted entities for purposes of certification or accreditation are encouraged to use these principles in conducting their evaluations.

Imagine This!

Managed care is not a new idea or even a recent one. Its origins can be traced back to the 1880s, when German Chancellor Otto Van Bismarck developed a form of prepaid health insurance for his workers as a means of warding off plans for a government-run insurance program in Germany. Here in the United States, the original form of managed care dates back to 1933, when a young California surgeon accepted the invitation of Henry Kaiser to provide his workers healthcare on a prepaid basis, and the Permanente Foundation Hospital was established. The hospital was named after the Permanente River, which never ran dry (*permanente* means "everlasting" in Spanish.) Today, Kaiser Permanente is the largest HMO in the United States.

What Did You Learn?

1. Explain the concept of managed care.
2. How did managed healthcare get started in the United States?
3. What main functions do MCOs perform?

COMMON TYPES OF MANAGED CARE ORGANIZATIONS

Although there are many forms of managed healthcare (Fig. 7-2), we are going to concentrate on the two most common types:
- Preferred provider organization (PPO)
- Health maintenance organization (HMO)

PREFERRED PROVIDER ORGANIZATION

PPOs are very popular throughout the United States. PPOs typically provide a high level of healthcare and a variety of medical facilities to everyone who chooses to participate in the PPO.

Here's how a PPO functions: A group of healthcare providers works under one umbrella—the PPO—to provide medical services at a discount to the individuals who participate in the PPO. The PPO contracts with this network of providers, who agree to offer medical services to the PPO members at lower rates (smaller copayments and coinsurance limits) in exchange for being part of the network. This agreement allows the PPO to reduce overall healthcare costs. Two things about PPOs make them popular:
- PPO members do not have to choose a **primary care physician** (PCP), which is a specific provider who oversees the member's total healthcare treatment.
- Participants do not need authorization from the PCP, commonly referred to as a **referral**, to visit any physician, hospital, or other healthcare provider who belongs to the network.

Plan members also can visit physicians and hospitals outside of the network. Visits to healthcare providers who do not belong to the PPO network do not have the same coverage, however, as visits to providers within the network, and the amount of money the patient has to pay out of his or her own pocket, the **copayment**, is higher. The deductible normally does not change if and when a PPO member sees a provider outside the network.

Other advantages of PPOs include the following:
- PPO networks are not as tightly controlled by laws and regulations as HMOs.
- Many PPOs offer a wider choice of treatments to members with fewer restrictions than HMOs.

Disadvantages include the following:

- Loosely controlled PPOs are often not much better at controlling costs than traditional fee-for-service (indemnity) health insurance, which results in higher premiums over time.
- More tightly controlled PPOs come at the expense of the patients' ability to manage their own healthcare treatments.
- The fact that an individual belongs to a PPO may lead the individual to believe that he or she is paying lower premiums than he or she would for traditional healthcare, when this may not be the case at all.

● Stop and Think

Ellen Comstock's health insurance carrier is a PPO. Soon after her second child was born, Ellen learned that Dr. Wallingford, her obstetrician, severed her contractual affiliation with the PPO network. Ellen wants to continue seeing Dr. Wallingford. What ramifications should Ellen consider in seeing a provider outside of her PPO network?

HEALTH MAINTENANCE ORGANIZATION

Under the federal HMO Act, an entity must have three characteristics to call itself an HMO, as follows:

- An organized system for providing healthcare or otherwise ensuring healthcare delivery in a geographic area
- An agreed-on set of basic and supplemental health maintenance and treatment services
- A voluntarily enrolled group of people

HMOs provide members with basic healthcare services for a fixed price and for a given period of time. In return, the participant receives medical services, including physician visits, hospitalization, and surgery, at no additional cost other than a small per-encounter copayment—typically less than $25 per visit and sometimes only $5.

Each HMO has a network of physicians who participate in the HMO system. When an individual first enrolls in the HMO, he or she chooses a PCP from the HMO network. This PCP serves as *caretaker* for the enrollee's future medical needs and is the first person the patient calls when he or she needs medical care. PCPs are usually physicians who practice family medicine, internal medicine, or pediatrics. The PCP determines whether or not the patient's problem warrants a referral to a **specialist**, a physician who is trained in a certain area of medicine (e.g., a cardiologist, who specializes in diseases and conditions of the heart). If an enrollee sees a specialist without the PCP's approval, the HMO normally does not pay specialist's fees, even if the specialist practices within the network. Figure 7-2 is a comparison of three common types of health care plans.

HMOs are more tightly controlled by government regulations than PPOs. Members must use the HMO's healthcare providers and facilities, and medical care outside the system usually is not covered except in emergencies. HMOs typically have no deductibles or plan limits. As mentioned earlier, the member pays only a small fee, called a copayment, for each visit or sometimes nothing at all. Because the HMO provides all of a member's healthcare

PLAN COST	PROVIDER SELECTION	CONSULTS/SPECIALIST	MEMBER OUT-OF-POCKET COSTS
Traditional Insurance	Patient can select any physician, hospital or health care provider (HCP).	Patient can use any specialist. However, some plans require pre-approval for certain procedures performed by specialists.	Patient may have to pay an annual deductible usually ranging from $250 to $1000 (depending on what they choose). Patient may also be responsible for co-insurance payments (typically 20%). Coverage for routine care & drugs vary with the policy.
PPO	Patient may select any HCP in the network. If they use a provider outside of the network, they pay a larger portion (up to 50%) of the fee.	Patients may use any specialist in the network, but if they use a provider outside of the network, they will pay a larger portion of the fee.	Patients may have to pay copayments for network doctor visits and drugs. When using a provider outside the network, there may be a deductible and then the plan will reimburse at 70% of the costs.
HMO	Patients may only select providers in the network. If they select a provider outside the network without the HMO approval, they will pay the entire bill.	The PCP determines the need for a specialist—if approval is not received for the patient is responsible for the entire bill.	Patients may have to pay copayments for doctor visits and drugs. May be charged co-payments for hospital stays and ER visits. Usually there are no deductibles.

Fig. 7-2 Comparison of types of healthcare plans, providers, consultants, and costs.

for one set monthly premium, it is considered in everyone's best interest to emphasize preventive healthcare.

Some HMOs operate their own facilities, staffed with salaried physicians; others contract with individual physicians and hospitals to be part of the HMO. A few do both. An HMO can be a good choice for some individuals; however, there are many restrictions. If its facilities are convenient, and the individual wants to avoid most out-of-pocket expenses and paperwork, an HMO might be a good healthcare option. One problem exists, however, and that is that some states, especially states that are predominantly rural, offer few HMO choices. Iowa, for instance, had only 4 functioning HMOs in 2002 compared with 27 in New York.

Several types of managed care come under the HMO umbrella. We look at some of the more common types in the following paragraphs.

Staff Model

A **staff model** HMO is a multispecialty group practice in which all healthcare services are provided within the buildings owned by the HMO. The staff model is a **closed panel HMO**, meaning other healthcare providers in the community generally cannot participate. Participating providers are salaried employees of the HMO who spend their time providing services only to the HMO enrollees. All routine medical care is furnished, or authorized, by the member's PCP. Preauthorization is necessary for referrals to specialists. In a staff model HMO, the HMO bears the financial risk for the entire cost of healthcare services furnished to the HMO's members.

Group Model

In a **group model**, the HMO contracts with independent, multispecialty physician groups who provide all healthcare services to its members. Physician groups usually share the same facility, support staff, medical records, and equipment. Group physicians receive reimbursement in the form of **capitation**, a reimbursement system in which healthcare providers receive a fixed fee for every patient enrolled in the plan, regardless of how many or few services the patient uses. (The word "capitation" comes from the Latin phrase *per capita,* meaning "each head.") For example, the managed care insurer negotiates with the provider and agrees to pay him or her $100 a month to care for each of its subscribers, regardless of the amount of services each subscriber uses. Generally, the financial risk (whether or not the capitation amount is enough for the HMO to make a profit) falls on the shoulders of the group practice.

Individual Practice Association

In an **individual practice association (IPA)**, services are provided by outpatient networks composed of individual healthcare providers (the IPA) who provide all the needed healthcare services for the HMO. The providers maintain their own offices and identities and see patients who belong to the HMO and non-HMO patients. This is an **open panel plan** because healthcare providers in the community may participate, if they meet certain HMO/IPA standards. IPA reimbursement methods vary from plan to plan.

Network Model

The **network model** HMO has multiple provider arrangements, including staff, group, or IPA structures. This model usually allows the healthcare provider to be paid on a fee-for-service basis, whereas the group practices in the network might receive a capitation payment by the healthcare plan.

Direct Contract Model

The **direct contract model** HMO is similar to an IPA except the HMO contracts directly with the individual physicians. The HMO recruits a variety of community healthcare providers, including PCPs and specialists.

Point of Service

The **point of service (POS)** model is a "hybrid" type of managed care (also referred to as an open ended HMO) that allows patients to use the HMO provider or go outside the plan and use any provider they choose. Using healthcare providers outside the plan is discouraged, however, because copayments and deductibles are higher.

What Did You Learn?

1. Name the two most common types of managed care.
2. Explain how a PPO works.
3. List the main differences between PPOs and HMOs.
4. What is the function of a PCP?
5. List four types of managed care.

ADVANTAGES AND DISADVANTAGES OF MANAGED CARE

There are advantages and disadvantages to managed care.

ADVANTAGES

- *Preventive care*—HMOs pay for programs aimed at keeping their members healthy (e.g., yearly wellness checkups) to avoid paying for more costly services if and when they get sick.

- *Lower premiums*—Because they limit which physicians their members can see and when they can see them, HMOs are able to charge lower premiums.
- *Prescriptions*—As part of their preventive approach, HMOs typically cover most prescriptions for a low copayment (e.g., $2).
- *Fewer unnecessary procedures*—HMOs give physicians financial incentives to provide only necessary care, so physicians are less likely to order tests or operations their patients might not need.
- *Limited paperwork*—Although physicians and hospitals have more paperwork under some types of managed care, HMO members usually only have to show their membership card and pay a relatively low copayment.

DISADVANTAGES

- *Limited provider pool*—To keep costs down, many HMO models tell their members which physicians they can see, including specialists.
- *Restricted coverage*—Often, members cannot expect treatment on demand because the PCP first must justify the need based on what benefits the plan covers.
- *Prior approval needed*—If a member wants to see a specialist, authorization is needed from the PCP.
- *Possibility of undertreatment*—Because HMOs typically give physicians financial incentives to limit care, some physicians have been known to hold back on the treatment they give their patients.
- *Compromised privacy*—HMOs use patient records to monitor physicians' performance and efficiency, so details of members' medical histories are seen by other people, which may breach their right to privacy.

● Stop and Think

Imagine you are employed as a health insurance professional with a multispecialty medical group. Mr. Washburn, a new patient, says to you, "I hear a lot of bad things about HMOs. Are they all true?" What would you tell him?

What Did You Learn?

1. List and explain the advantages of managed care.
2. List and explain disadvantages of managed care.

MANAGED CARE CERTIFICATION AND REGULATION

HMOs receive their accreditation from two organizations: The National Committee on Quality Assurance (NCQA) and the Joint Commission on Accreditation of Healthcare Organizations (JCAHO).

NATIONAL COMMITTEE ON QUALITY ASSURANCE

NCQA, a private, nonprofit organization, accredits healthcare plans based on careful evaluation of the quality of care members receive and member satisfaction rates. Its membership includes about 90% of all MCOs nationwide. NCQA is committed to improving the quality of healthcare throughout the United States. NCQA provides healthcare information through the World Wide Web and the media to help consumers and employers make more informed healthcare choices.

In addition to accrediting and certifying a wide range of healthcare organizations, NCQA manages the development of the Health Plan Employer Data and Information Set (HEDIS), the performance measurement tool used by most health plans in the United States. MCOs must collect and report HEDIS data to earn NCQA accreditation.

For a particular managed healthcare plan to become accredited by NCQA, it first must undergo a survey and meet certain standards designed to evaluate the facility's clinical and administrative systems. These standards fall into five broad categories, as follows:
- Access and service
- Qualified providers
- Staying healthy
- Getting better
- Living with illness

To evaluate these five categories, NCQA reviews health plan records and providers' credentials, conducts surveys, and interviews health plan staff. A national committee of physicians assigns one of five possible accreditation levels (excellent, commendable, accredited, provisional, or denied) based on the plan's level of compliance with NCQA standards.

Access and Service

NCQA evaluates how well a health plan provides its members with access to needed care and with good customer service. Evaluative questions might include: Are there enough PCPs and specialists to serve the number of people in the plan? What kind of problems do patients report in getting needed care? Does the health plan follow up effectively on grievances?

Qualified Providers

NCQA evaluates health plan activities that ensure each physician is licensed and trained to practice medicine, and that the health plan's members are satisfied with their physicians' performance. Things NCQA might ask include: Does the health plan check whether physicians have had sanctions or lawsuits against them? How do health plan members rate their personal physicians or nurses?

Staying Healthy

NCQA evaluates health plan activities that help people maintain good health and avoid illness. For example: Does the health plan give its practitioners guidelines about how to provide appropriate preventive healthcare? Are members receiving appropriate tests and screenings?

Getting Better

To make an appraisal in this category, NCQA looks at health plan activities that help people recover from illness. For example: How does the health plan evaluate new medical procedures, drugs, and devices to ensure that patients have access to the most up-to-date care? Do physicians in the health plan advise smokers to quit?

Living with Illness

NCQA evaluates health plan activities that help people manage chronic illness. For example: Does the plan have programs in place to assist patients in managing chronic conditions such as asthma? Do diabetics, who are at risk for blindness, receive eye examinations as needed?

NATIONAL COMMITTEE ON QUALITY ASSURANCE AND HEALTH INSURANCE PORTABILITY AND ACCOUNTABILITY ACT

The 2003 standards also make NCQA's privacy and confidentiality requirements reflect key elements of the Health Insurance Portability and Accountability Act (HIPAA). In particular, NCQA has strengthened standards requiring members to be notified at the time of enrollment of their MCO's policies on the use of their personal health information (e.g., treatment records, claims data). Since the new standards went into effect in July 2003, an organization must inform members about its privacy policies, along with the members' rights and options for accessing their own medical information. The 2003 *Standards and Guidelines for the Accreditation of Managed Care Organizations* that went into effect in July 2003 have been made available as printed or electronic publications.

JOINT COMMISSION ON ACCREDITATION OF HEALTHCARE ORGANIZATIONS

JCAHO is the second entity that evaluates and accredits healthcare organizations. Similar to NCQA, JCAHO is an independent, not-for-profit organization and is considered the predominant standards-setting and accrediting body in healthcare in the United States. JCAHO is governed by a 29-member Board of Commissioners that includes nurses, physicians, consumers, medical directors, administrators, providers, employers, a labor representative, health plan leaders, quality experts, ethicists, a health insurance administrator, and educators.

Since 1951, JCAHO's standards have been used to evaluate the compliance of healthcare organizations. Their evaluation and accreditation services are provided for all types of healthcare organizations, including
- hospitals,
- managed care plans,
- home care organizations,
- nursing homes and other long-term care facilities,
- assisted living facilities,
- behavioral healthcare organizations,
- ambulatory care providers, and
- clinical laboratories.

JCAHO accreditation is nationally recognized as a symbol of quality that reflects an organization's commitment to meeting quality performance standards. To earn and maintain accreditation, an organization must undergo an on-site survey by a JCAHO survey team every 2 to 3 years, depending on the type of facility.

JCAHO developed its standards in consultation with healthcare experts, providers, measurement experts, purchasers, and consumers. The standards address an organization's level of performance in key functional areas, such as patient rights, patient treatment, and infection control. The standards focus not only on an organization's ability to provide safe, high-quality care, but also on its actual performance. JCAHO's standards outline performance expectations for activities that affect the safety and quality of patient care. These standards include
- the rights of patients,
- the assessment and treatment of patients,
- a safe environment for patients and healthcare employees,
- the quality of patient care,
- the management of patients' records, and
- the organizational responsibilities of leadership and staff.

Both the Joint Commission on Accreditation of Healthcare Organizations (JCAHO) and the National Committee for Quality Assurance (NCQA) have incorporated the HIPAA standards into their own accreditation criteria.

UTILIZATION REVIEW

Utilization review, sometimes referred to as utilization management, is a system designed to determine the medical necessity and appropriateness of a requested medical service, procedure, or hospital admission prior, concurrent, or retrospective to the event. A utilization review may include ambulatory review, case management, certification, concurrent review, discharge planning, prospective review, retrospective review, or second opinions. The utilization review is generally accomplished by the third-party payer's professional staff (nurses and physicians) using standardized medical research data from across the United States and reviewing patient health records in an attempt to make fair and reasonable decisions on behalf of the patients and the third-party payers. Deciding whether or not a service, procedure, or hospital admission is "appropriate" also can be influenced by what is covered in the individual's health insurance plan.

Utilization review is used in managed care plans to reduce unnecessary medical inpatient or outpatient services. An individual or individuals within the plan or a separate organization on behalf of the insurer reviews the necessity, use, appropriateness, efficacy, or efficiency of healthcare services, procedures, providers, or facilities.

COMPLAINT MANAGEMENT

If a particular medical service or procedure is determined not to be medically necessary by the payer or by an independent utilization review organization, it will not be paid for by the insurer. If the patient disagrees, he or she may file a **grievance** protesting the decision. A grievance is a written complaint submitted by an individual covered by the plan concerning any of the following:

1. An insurer's decisions, policies, or actions related to availability, delivery, or quality of healthcare services
2. Claims payment or handling or reimbursement for services
3. The contractual relationship between a covered individual and an insurer
4. The outcome of an appeal

Some states have enacted laws that allow residents to air their complaints to the state insurance commissioner's office when certain medical payments are denied by their health insurer. If a complaint is accepted, an independent review organization (IRO) looks into the situation and determines whether or not the claim should have been paid under the guidelines of the medical policy. The IRO decision is generally final, and if the IRO sides with the insurer, the individual's only remaining alternative is to pursue remediation through the court system. Fig. 7-3 shows an example of one state's insurance complaint system.

A Review of Michigan's Insurance Complaint System, May 2002

Michigan's Office of Financial and Insurance Services (OFIS) contracted with two organizations to act as independent review organizations to review residents' complaints. The system was put into effect in May of 2002. The external review process followed strict policies and procedures; the independent review organizations had 14 days to process the review request. The independent review panel was staffed with qualified, trained, and licensed clinicians as well as other health professionals who are experts in the treatment of the medical condition that is the subject of the external review.

Findings: During the first sixteen months of the insurance complaint program, 418 requests for claim reviews were filed with Michigan's OFIS. From the initial 418 requests, there were 309 cases that went to internal review organizations for adjudication. Of these 309 cases, 143 cases were resolved in favor of the patient. A total of 36 cases were dismissed, resulted in a split decision, or have yet to be decided. The OFIS staff resolved the remaining 72 cases internally, thus avoiding the need for external review. One request for external review was withdrawn.

Fig. 7-3 A review of Michigan's insurance complaint system, May 2002.

Imagine This!

Texas is the first state to post information about complaints filed against HMOs and other insurers on the Internet. The Internet Complaint Information System, launched by the state's Department of Insurance, also includes complaints against auto and property insurers. The information is updated quarterly, and only complaints that have been investigated and resolved are included. The most common complaints from members concerned prescription coverage, reimbursement, and denial or nonpayment for emergency care. Most provider complaints were related to denial or delay of payment.

What Did You Learn?

1. MCOs receive their accreditation from what two organizations?
2. List NCQA's five evaluative categories.
3. What types of healthcare facilities does JCAHO evaluate?
4. What is a utilization review?

PREAUTHORIZATION, PRECERTIFICATION, AND REFERRALS

A common method many healthcare payers use to monitor and control healthcare costs is by evaluating the need for a medical service *before* it is performed. Most commercial healthcare organizations and MCOs now request that they be made aware of and consent to certain procedures and services before their enrollees acquire them. Preauthorization and precertification are two cost-containment features whereby the insured must contact the insurer before a hospitalization or surgery and receive prior approval for the service.

PREAUTHORIZATION

Preauthorization is a procedure required by most managed healthcare and indemnity plans before a provider carries out specific procedures or treatments for a patient—typically inpatient hospitalization and certain diagnostic tests. Preauthorization typically works as follows: The healthcare provider or a member of his or her staff contacts the healthcare plan by phone, by fax, or in writing and requests permission to perform the treatment or service proposed. The plan's representative authorizes the service or procedure or not, depending on what the plan covers and whether the procedure or service is considered medically necessary and appropriate. Often, when a procedure or service is authorized, the MCO or carrier assigns a specific identifying number or code.

☑ HIPAA Tip

Before faxing any patient information, make sure that the individual on the receiving end of the transmission has a "medical right to know," and that the destination location has a security system in place.

Preauthorization pertains to medical necessity and appropriateness only and does not, in all instances, guarantee payment. It is not a treatment recommendation or a guarantee that the patient will be insured or eligible for benefits when services are performed.

Preauthorization also is used to identify members for case management or disease management programs. Approval or denial of requests for services is determined by review of all available related medical information and possibly a discussion with the requesting physician (Fig. 7-4).

● Stop and Think

You overhear a patient telling another that she is going to be admitted to the hospital for an operation. "They have to get permission from my HMO before I can be admitted," the woman says. "If my HMO says it's okay," she continues, "they'll pay all of my hospital bills." Should you, as a health insurance professional interrupt the conversation to clarify what impact a preauthorization has on her hospitalization? If so, what would you say?

PRECERTIFICATION

Precertification is a process used by health insurance companies to control healthcare costs and is similar to preauthorization. The Internet's popular search engine "Google" defines precertification as "a formal assessment of the medical necessity, efficiency or appropriateness of a medical provider's treatment plan for a specific illness or injury." The treatment plan needs to be consistent with the diagnosis or condition; rendered in a cost-effective manner; and in line with national medical practice guidelines regarding type, frequency, and duration of treatment.

Precertification involves collecting information before inpatient admissions or performance of selected ambulatory procedures and services (Fig. 7-5). The process permits advance eligibility verification, determination of coverage, and communication with the physician or plan member or both. It also allows the insurance company to coordinate the patient's transition from the inpatient setting to the next level of care (discharge planning) or to register patients for specialized programs, such as disease management, case management, or a prenatal program.

In some instances, precertification is used to inform physicians, members, and other healthcare providers about cost-effective programs and alternative therapies and treatments. Typically, the things the plan's representative takes into consideration when precertifying a service or procedure include the following:

- Verifying the member's eligibility and benefits in accordance with applicable plan documents
- Determining coverage for inpatient admissions and selected ambulatory services
- Assessing appropriateness of the proposed site of service
- Identifying alternatives to proposed care or site of service when appropriate
- Identifying and referring to case management programs when appropriate
- Identifying any quality-of-care issues and refer for review
- Identifying and documenting potential coordination of benefits, subrogation, or workers' compensation information

Tri-State Medical Group

PREAUTHORIZATION REQUEST FORM

PATIENT INFORMATION

Last Name: _____   First Name: _____

DOB: _____   Member #: **R**_____   Group #: _____

PREAUTHORIZATION REQUEST INFORMATION

Please list *both* procedure/product code <u>and</u> narrative description:

CPT / HCPCS Code(s): _____   Durable Medical Equipment: ☐ Rental ☐ Purchase

Description: _____
_____

Date of Service: _____   Length of Stay (if applicable): _____

Place of Service or Vendor Name: _____

Assistant Surgeon Requested? ☐ Yes ☐ No **Please list *both* diagnosis(es) code <u>and</u> narrative description:**

1. ICD-9 Code: _____
   Description: _____

2. ICD-9 Code: _____
   Description: _____

Ordering Physician/Provider: _____   Office Location: _____
FIRST <u>AND</u> LAST NAMES PLEASE

Referring Physician/Provider: _____
FIRST <u>AND</u> LAST NAMES PLEASE; REQUIRED FOR PRIME PLANS

Date: _____   Contact Person: _____   Phone: _____

> ***Please Note: Incomplete forms will delay the preauthorization process.***
> **Requests received after 3:00 PM are processed the next working day.**
>
> **PacificSource responds to preauthorization requests within 2 working days.**
> **A determination notice will be mailed to the requesting provider, facility, and patient.**
>
> **Please attach pertinent chart notes as appropriate.**

FOR INTERNAL OFFICE USE ONLY:

STATUS: APPROVED / DENIED / PENDING / EXPLANATION

DATE: _____   ACUITY: _____   INITIALS: _____

Reason/Status _____
_____

Field 11 Notes _____   LOS Approved _____

☐ Chart notes filed with preauthorization

Notes _____

Field 10 Facility Copy _____

PO Box 5555 • Somewhere OR 00908 • (541) 555-5584 • (800) 555-6052 x 2584

| MEDICAL AFFAIRS DEPARTMENT CONFIDENTIAL FAX: (541) 555-2051 |

9/8/2003

Fig. 7-4 Generic preauthorization form.

Tri-State Medical Group

FAX Request Form for Precertification Review

To:______________________________ Date:______________________________

(Area Code) Fax:______________________________

(Area Code) Phone:______________________________

Attn:______________________________

From:______________________________ Fax:______________________________

Number of Pages (Including Cover Sheet):__________
If there is problem with the receipt of this fax, please call ____________________.Thank you.

Recipient/Patient Name:______________________________
Complete Recipient
Address ______________________________

____

ID Number:______________________________ CAMA ☐ Yes ☐ No

Requested Admit Date:____________________ Diagnosis Code(s):____________________

Procedure Date(s): ______________________________

Days Requested: ____________________ Procedure Code(s)____________________

New Admit? ( ) Transfer ( )

Recertification Review? Y( ) If So, Par/Reference #______________________________

Setting: ☐ Inpatient ☐ Outpatient ☐ Physician Office ☐ Out of State

Admit Type: ☐ Non-urgent/Emergent ☐ Urgent/Emergent

Physician Name:______________________________ Phone:____________________
Fax:____________________

Facility:______________________________ Phone:____________________
Fax:____________________

Clinical Information:______________________________

____

____

____

____

____

This message is intended for the use of the individual entity to which it is transmitted and may contain information that is privileged, confidential and exempt from disclosure under applicable laws. If the reader of this communication is not the intended recipient, you are hereby notified that any dissemination, distribution or copying of this communication is strictly prohibited. If you have received this communication in error, please notify us immediately by telephone and return the original communication to us at the address below via U.S. Postal Service. We will reimburse you for the mailing costs.

Thank you.
400 North 4th Street Anytown, Iowa 50622
Phone: 319-555-5734 Fax: 319-555-5758

Fig. 7-5 Generic precertification form.

REFERRALS

A **referral** is a request by a healthcare provider for a patient under his or her care to be evaluated or treated by another provider, usually a specialist. The purpose of a referral by a PCP to a specialist is to

- inform a specialist that the patient needs to be seen for care (or second opinion) in his or her field of specialty and
- inform the insurance company that the PCP has approved the visit to a specialist because most managed care companies would not pay for care that has not been authorized with a referral.

How a Patient Obtains a Referral

The patient schedules a visit with the PCP, who evaluates the problem. If the PCP decides that the patient's condition or symptoms warrant a specialist's opinion, a referral form is completed (Fig. 7-6). In most managed care situations, for the insurance company to recognize the referral, it must come from the patient's designated PCP or a provider who is covering for the PCP. If an orthopedic physician refers a patient to a physical therapist, the patient also must obtain a referral from his or her PCP to process through the insurance company.

Imagine This!

Velda Smith, a 34-year-old HMO enrollee, injured her knee in an ice skating accident. Dr. Mazzio, Velda's PCP, referred her to an orthopedist for evaluation, who subsequently performed arthroscopy of her knee. After the surgical procedure, the orthopedist recommended physical therapy four times a week for 6 weeks. Velda was instructed by her HMO that she must return to Dr. Mazzio for proper authorization procedures before beginning physical therapy.

Referrals Versus Consultations

There is a significant difference between a **referral** and a **consultation**. A consultation is when the PCP sends a patient to another healthcare provider, usually a specialist, for the purpose of the consulting physician rendering his or her expert opinion regarding the patient's condition. The intent of a consultation usually is for the purpose of an expert opinion only, and the PCP does not relinquish the care of the patient to the consulting provider. In the case of a referral, the PCP typically relinquishes care of the patient—at least a specific portion of care—to the specialist.

Imagine This!

Daniel Bowers visited Dr. Adler, his PCP, with complaints of back pain and numbness in his left leg radiating down to his left foot. Dr. Adler x-rayed Daniel's spinal column and discovered a degenerative disk condition and subsequently referred him to Dr. Langford, who specialized in degenerative disk disease.

Susan Lane, another patient of Dr. Bowers, complained of heart palpitations during an office visit for treatment of a severe case of poison ivy. After performing an electrocardiogram, Dr. Bowers informed Susan he was sending her to Dr. Woodley for a stress electrocardiogram and an echocardiogram to determine if her palpitations represented a serious cardiac problem.

While in the hospital for a hip replacement, Evelyn Conner was diagnosed with diabetes. Dr. Blake, her surgeon, asked Dr. Martin, a specialist in endocrinology, to manage Mrs. Conner's diabetic condition.

● Stop and Think

Study the three cases in Imagine This! Decide whether each one is a consultation or a referral.

What Did You Learn?

1. Explain the difference between preauthorization and precertification.
2. List some of the typical things that a plan's representative takes into consideration when precertifying a procedure or service.
3. What is a referral?

HEALTH INSURANCE PORTABILITY AND ACCOUNTABILITY ACT AND MANAGED CARE

The Health Insurance Portability and Accountability Act (HIPAA) of 1996 was intended to improve the efficiency of healthcare delivery, reduce administrative costs, and protect patient privacy. Health plan compliance with these regulations was required by October 2003. Previously, we discussed the fact if an insured person lost insurance coverage for some reason (e.g., losing a job), he or she could

---

FLORIDA DEPARTMENT OF HEALTH

Florida WIC Program Medical Referral Form

Shaded areas must be completed.   See instructions for completing this form on the reverse side.

Is this client eligible for Healthy Start? ❑ Yes ❑ No   For WIC Office Use Only:
Date of WIC Certification Appointment _____

Client's Name _____ Birth Date _____ Sex M F

Address _____ Phone Number (_____) _____-_____

City _____ Zip Code _____ Social Security # _____-_____-_____

Parent's/Guardian's Name _____ (for infants and children only)

❑ For Pregnant Women
Height _____ Weight _____ Date Taken _____ (no older than 60 days)
Hemoglobin _____ OR Hematocrit _____ Date Taken_____ (must be taken during current pregnancy)
Expected Date of Delivery _____ Date of First Prenatal Visit _____ Prepregnancy Weight _____

❑ For Breastfeeding and Postpartum (Non-Breastfeeding) Women
Height _____ Weight _____ Date Taken _____ (no older than 60 days)
Hemoglobin _____ OR Hematocrit _____ Date Taken_____ (must be taken in postpartum period)
Date of Delivery _____ Date of First Prenatal Visit _____ Weight at Last Prenatal Visit _____

❑ For Infants and Children less than 24 months of age
Birth Weight _____ lb _____ oz   Birth Length _____inches
Current Height _____ Current Weight _____ Date Taken _____ (no older than 60 days)
Hemoglobin _____ OR Hematocrit _____ Date Taken_____ (required once between 6 to 12 months
                                                                AND once between 12 to 24 months)

❑ For Children 2 to 5 years of age
Current Height _____ Current Weight _____ Date Taken _____ (no older than 60 days)
Hemoglobin _____ OR Hematocrit _____ Date Taken_____ (once a year unless value < 11.1 Hgb or
                                                              < 33% Hct, then required in 6 months)

✓ **Check all that apply. Please refer your client to WIC, even if nothing is checked below.** This information assists the WIC nutritionist in determining eligibility, developing a nutrition care plan, and providing nutrition counseling. WIC staff may need to contact you or your staff to obtain more detailed medical information prior to providing WIC services.

❑ Medical condition (specify)
_____
❑ High venous lead level (10 μg/dl or more)
   Lead level _____ Date taken _____
❑ Recent major surgery, trauma, burns (specify)
_____
❑ Food allergy (specify) _____
❑ Current or potential breastfeeding complications
   (specify) _____

❑ Failure to Thrive
❑ **Special Formula Needed** (diagnosis/signature required)
   Type of formula _____
   Number of months _____ (not to exceed 6 months)
   Diagnosis _____
   Signature of physician, PA, or ARNP required for
   special formula _____
❑ Other (specify) _____

❑ **Nutrition Counseling Requested** – specify diet prescription/order _____

WIC Local Agency Address:

I refer this client for WIC eligibility determination:
Signature/Title of Health Professional _____
Date _____ **PLEASE PLACE OFFICE STAMP BELOW:**
Address:

Phone Number:

| ***Parent or Guardian: Please bring a copy of your baby's/child's shot record to the WIC office.*** |

DH Form 3075, 12/03 (Stock Number: 5744-000-3075-5) (Replaces 1/01 edition, which may be used.)   *WIC is an equal opportunity provider.*

Fig. 7-6 Referral form (Courtesy Florida Department of Health).

Instructions for Completing the Florida WIC Program Medical Referral Form
All shaded areas must be completed in order for the form to be processed.

1. Check (✔) YES if the client has been screened and is eligible for Healthy Start. Check (✔) NO if the client is not eligible for Healthy Start. Leave blank if the client has not been screened. <u>Note</u>: Eligibility for Healthy Start does <u>not</u> affect a client's eligibility for WIC.

2. Complete the **client's name and birth date.**

3. Optional Information: the client's sex, mailing address, phone number, city, zip code, social security number, and the parent's or guardian's name for infants and children.

4. Complete the appropriate shaded section for the client.

    Pregnant Women: Complete the height and weight measurements and the date they were taken. These measurements are to be taken no more than 60 days before the client's WIC appointment. (The WIC appointment may be recorded at the top of the form.) Complete the hemoglobin or hematocrit value and the date the value was taken. There is no limit on how old the bloodwork data can be, as long as the measurement was taken during the current pregnancy. Complete the expected date of delivery, the date of the client's first prenatal visit, and the prepregnancy weight.

    Breastfeeding Women (eligible up to one year after delivery) **and Postpartum Women—Non-Breastfeeding** (eligible up to 6 months after delivery/termination of pregnancy)**:** Complete the height and weight measurements and the date they were taken. These measurements are to be taken no more than 60 days before the client's WIC appointment. (The WIC appointment may be recorded at the top of the form.) Complete the hemoglobin or hematocrit value and the date the value was taken. There is no limit on how old the bloodwork data can be, as long as the bloodwork is taken after delivery of the most recent pregnancy. Complete the actual date of delivery, the date of the first prenatal visit, and the weight measurement at the last prenatal visit.

    Infants and Children less than 24 months of age: Complete the infant's birth weight and birth length. Complete the current height and weight measurements and the date they were taken. These measurements are to be taken no more than 60 days before the client's WIC appointment. (The WIC appointment may be recorded at the top of the form.) Complete the hemoglobin or hematocrit value and the date the value was taken. <u>A bloodwork value is required once during infancy between 6 to 12 months of age (preferably between 9 to 12 months of age) and once between 1 to 2 years of age (preferably 6 months from the infant bloodwork value).</u>

    Children 2 to 5 years of age: Complete the current height and weight measurements and the date they were taken. These measurements are to be taken no more than 60 days before the client's WIC appointment. (The WIC appointment may be recorded at the top of the form.) Complete the hemoglobin or hematocrit value and the date the value was taken. A bloodwork value is required once a year unless the value is abnormal (< 11.1 hemoglobin or < 33% hematocrit), then a bloodwork value is required in 6 months.

5. Check (✔) any health problem that you have identified. **Even if you have not identified a health problem, refer the client to the WIC program.**

6. **Special Formula Needed**: This form may be used to order special formula as long as the type of formula, number of months that the special formula is needed, and the diagnosis are completed. Also, the signature of a physician, PA, or ARNP is required in order to accept the prescription.

7. If you would like a nutritionist to counsel your client on a specific diet, check the box and specify the diet prescription or diet order requested.

8. If possible, please provide a copy of the immunization record for infant and child clients.

9. Complete the shaded area at the bottom of the form with the **signature** of the health professional taking the measurement or his/her designee and the office address and phone number. **Stamp** the form with the office stamp or the health professional's stamp.

10. Give this completed form to the client or parent/guardian to bring to the WIC certification appointment or mail/fax the form to the local WIC agency address shown in the bottom left corner of the form.

Fig. 7-6—cont'd

be required to prove insurability before obtaining new coverage. For most individuals, this was not a problem; however, for individuals with chronic or preexisting health problems or whose health deteriorated while they were covered, it was a serious problem. Such individuals frequently lived in fear of losing their jobs or stayed in "dead end" jobs so that they would not lose their health-care coverage. Now, under HIPAA regulations, if an individual has been insured for the past 12 months, a new insurance company cannot refuse to cover the individual and cannot impose preexisting conditions or a waiting period before providing coverage.

HIPAA regulations affect other areas of healthcare, too, including

• maintaining patient confidentiality,
• implementing standards for electronic transmission of transactions and code sets,
• establishing national provider and employer identifiers, and
• resolving security and privacy issues arising from the storage and transmission of healthcare data.

How do these regulations affect managed healthcare? Some experts claim the cost of complying with HIPAA would exceed the $9 billion cost of Y2K preparations. The repercussions of this added cost likely would affect all healthcare, not just managed care. Large medical facilities for the most part were able to shoulder the expense of becoming HIPAA compliant; however, many small one- or two-physician practices found it very difficult. HIPAA zeros in on electronic health information. Even if a solo practitioner has all paper records, as soon as he or she starts dealing electronically with billing of third-party payers, he or she encounters HIPAA's strict regulations.

Imagine This!

Elliot Larson was the sole proprietor of a small podiatry practice in south-central Iowa. He employed two full-time staff members—a receptionist and an assistant who was a licensed practical nurse. When the HIPAA law was enacted, his office was already computerized and submitting claims electronically to a certain major carrier. Dr. Larson's financial advisor calculated that it would cost approximately $50,000 to upgrade his office to HIPAA compliancy. Dr. Larson did not want to revert back to a manual accounting system, plus he was under contract to submit claims electronically to the major carrier under whom most of his patients had coverage. To justify the cost to upgrade to HIPAA's regulations, he would have to raise his fees. The socioeconomic area where he practiced was predominantly agricultural-related—farmers and rural people—who could not afford increased charges. Dr. Larson closed his practice in the small, rural town where he'd been practicing for 10 years and joined a multispecialty group in Des Moines.

The consequences of noncompliance are the legal penalties HIPAA provides for failure to adopt its standards. Fines range from $100 for violating a general requirement to $50,000 or more for more serious offenses, such as wrongful disclosure of individually identifiable health information.

 HIPAA Tip

HIPAA impact on MCOs is the same as that for fee-for-service–type structures. HIPAA does not have a separate set of rules and regulations for MCOs.

What Did You Learn?

1. List four areas of healthcare affected by HIPAA regulations.
2. What are the consequences of HIPAA noncompliance?

IMPACT OF MANAGED CARE

Since the 1990s, the United States has witnessed a transformation in all phases of the healthcare system, from financing to the way healthcare services are organized and delivered. The driving force in this transformation, experts say, is the shift from traditional fee-for-service systems to managed care networks. These changes in the U.S. healthcare system are in response to market forces for cost control, to regulatory initiatives on cost and quality, and to consumer demands for quality care and greater flexibility in provider choice. Because these changes occurred so rapidly and extensively, little is known about the long-term effects of managed care on access to care, cost, and quality of care.

The Agency for Healthcare Policy and Research (AHCPR) is the leading federal agency charged with supporting and conducting health services research. Their studies are designed to produce information that ultimately will improve consumer choice, improve the quality and value of healthcare services, and support and improve the healthcare marketplace. Most research on managed care has been conducted in HMOs.

IMPACT OF MANAGED CARE ON THE PHYSICIAN-PATIENT RELATIONSHIP

Managed care can affect relationships between physicians and patients in a variety of ways. First, it may change the way in which such relationships begin and end. The typical

HMO pays only for care provided by its own physicians. Preferred provider groups restrict access to physicians by paying a smaller percentage of the cost of care when patients go outside the network. These restrictions can limit patients' ability to establish a relationship with the physician of their choice. Termination of physician-patient relationships also can occur without patients' choosing. When employers shift managed care health plans that mandate the determination of PCPs, employees may have no choice but to sever ties with the PCP of the previous plan and establish a relationship with a new one.

Imagine This!

Arnold Talbott is a fabrication specialist with Jones Implement. Employees were covered under a group health insurance contract with Superior Healthcare Systems, an HMO, when Arnold first started working for Jones Implement in 1993. Over the years, Arnold and his family established a mutually satisfying patient-provider relationship with Dr. VanHorn, their PCP. In 2004, Jones changed carriers and switched their group coverage to Ideal Health Maintenance Group. Because Dr. VanHorn was not a part of Ideal's network, Arnold and his family had to choose a new PCP and have all of their health records transferred.

Some forms of managed care create a financial incentive for physicians to spend less time with each patient. Under preferred provider arrangements, physicians may compensate for reduced fees for services by seeing more patients. This compensation ultimately reduces the time available to discuss patients' problems, explore alternative treatment options, and maintain a meaningful relationship with established patients.

Managed care arrangements often control patients' access to medical specialists, restricting patients' freedom to choose providers and obtain the medical services they desire. In HMOs, PCPs function as "gatekeepers" who authorize patient referrals to medical specialists. Critics of managed care claim that this gatekeeping lowers the quality of care, whereas supporters believe that gatekeeping yields benefits such as reducing **iatrogenic effects** (a symptom or illness brought on unintentionally by something that a physician does or says), promoting rigorous review of standards of care, and emphasizing low-technology, care-oriented services.

The physician—and the practice as a whole—is the main experience of their plan for most patients. If that experience is difficult or substandard, the patient is likely to blame the practice. Whatever help a practice can give its patients in navigating the waters of managed care can reduce problems for everybody.

IMPACT OF MANAGED CARE ON HEALTHCARE PROVIDERS

Most healthcare providers believe that the shift within the healthcare industry from fee-for-service toward managed care is requiring providers to

1. become participants in larger provider practice structures (e.g., single-specialty or, preferably, multi-specialty group practices, or independent practice associations);
2. become participants in integrated delivery systems, which may include acquisition of physician practices by a hospital system; or
3. become employees and service providers for large insurance organizations or HMOs or both.

With the advent of managed care, such acquisitions are being considered necessary more often by smaller scale healthcare providers (e.g., sole practitioners and small partnerships and group practices) to satisfy the increasing demands of managed care contracting. Large employers, insurance organizations, and HMOs view as appealing—and seek to contract with—healthcare providers who can offer a complete package of "seamless" healthcare services, which satisfies most medical needs within a single integrated delivery system. Providers within these more integrated medical organizations are likely to experience increasing economic viability as managed care continues to transform the medical environment.

The PCP is considered by most within the medical sector of the healthcare industry to be the future controller of patient flow and revenue-generating potential of fellow practitioners. Functioning in the role of gatekeeper, the PCP is likely to be required to perform an increased level of services—services that formerly were referred to specialists—to control healthcare costs in capitation model heath care plans.

On a more positive note, in a study of 20,000 subjects that examined variations in healthcare delivery systems, AHCPR-supported research indicated the following:

- *HMO physicians spent more time* with their patients than fee-for-service physicians, and their patients received more preventive care, asked more questions, and were more involved in treatment planning.
- *Managed care patients spent 2 fewer days* in an intensive care unit (ICU) than patients with fee-for-service health insurance, with the average stay for managed care patients costing less. (There was no difference, however, in mortality or ICU readmission between the two groups.)
- *HMO patients were hospitalized 40% less* than patients with fee-for-service plans and treated in solo practices. Group practice outpatient clinic patients had shorter stays and incurred lower costs at a hospital in the study, but received the same quality of care as traditional clinic patients at the hospital.

• *Chronically ill patients in managed care plans had better access to care* than patients in fee-for-service plans, but (in a study of 1200 patients in three cities) their care was not as comprehensive, they waited longer for care, and physician-patient continuity was less.

Most patients and healthcare providers agree the theory of managed care is a good one: Patients receive care through a single, "seamless" system as they move from wellness to sickness back to wellness again. Continuity of care, prevention, and early intervention are stressed.

What Did You Learn?

1. What is AHCPR, and how does it relate to managed care?
2. How does managed care affect the patient-physician relationship?
3. List ways that managed care affects healthcare providers.

FUTURE OF MANAGED CARE

Many people think that managed care is more a principle than a structure. This principle says that a healthcare system should work to keep people healthy, and when they are sick or injured, a well-run system should work to ensure the right treatment in the right setting by the right people. At its core, managed care places healthcare providers as the individuals responsible for the health of the community. Managed care exists in different forms, with different benefit structures, financing mechanisms, and provider configurations. Managed care is still evolving and is very much a work in progress.

The future of managed care is not clear-cut. Statistics show that the public and private sector movement from fee-for-service systems to managed care has slowed in recent years. Surveys have indicated that there is also a shift from staff-model HMOs toward less centralized systems, such as PPOs and POS plans. Public concerns about managed care have influenced many healthcare providers and integrated delivery systems to back away from strongly capitated plans in favor of discounted fee-for-services structures.

Experts predict, however, that despite the alleged problems and negative implications voiced in regard to managed healthcare, it will continue to be a popular choice for the delivery of healthcare in the United States. As stated earlier, managed care for the most part focuses on quality, choice, and access—not just cost cutting. It is predicted that any future cost-cutting will come from innovation, especially in the area of information technology. Computers will help MCOs do exactly what their name implies—*manage care* and costs. Huge databases of information on patients' and providers' use of healthcare delivery and outcomes will help to determine optimal treatment programs. With an aging population and increasingly sophisticated and expensive medical technology, healthcare costs no doubt will continue to increase, and managed care will play an important role in helping curb these rising costs. It already has shown real progress in the area of preventive health.

What Did You Learn?

1. What is the principle behind managed healthcare?
2. What effect will managed care have on the future of healthcare in general?
3. In what ways will information technology affect the future of healthcare?

SUMMARY CHECK POINTS

☑ Managed care is a healthcare system where insurance companies attempt to control the cost, quality, and access of medical care to individuals enrolled in their plan by limiting the reimbursement levels paid to providers, by reducing utilization, or both.

☑ A PPO is a group of hospitals and physicians that agree to render particular services to a group of people, generally under contract with a private insurer. These services may be furnished at discounted rates if the members receive their healthcare from member providers. Services received from providers outside the organization may result in larger out-of-pocket expenses.

☑ In HMOs, enrollees receive comprehensive preventive and hospital and medical care from specific medical providers who receive a prepaid fee. Members select a PCP or medical group from the HMO's list of affiliated physicians. PCPs coordinate the patient's total care, which is normally free from hassles involving deductibles or claim forms. When using medical services, members pay a small copayment, usually between $5 and $25. There are several types of plans under the HMO umbrella, as follows:
  • *Staff model*—a closed panel HMO in which a multispeciality group of physicians are contracted to provide healthcare to HMO members and are compensated by the contractor via salary and incentive programs.
  • *Group model*—a managed healthcare model involving contracts with physicians organized as a partnership, professional corporation,

or other association. The health plan compensates the medical group for contracted services at a negotiated rate, and that group is responsible for compensating its physicians and contracting with hospitals for care of their patients.

- *IPA*—a type of HMO in which enrollees' healthcare is arranged through contracting physicians in the community, who practice in their own offices and who also may see patients from other HMOs or non-HMO patients on a fee-for-service basis. Physicians may be paid on a capitated or discounted fee-for-service basis.

- *Network model*—a type of HMO that contracts with two or more independent group practices to care for their members. Compensation is specific to the contract between the medical groups and the physicians. Participating groups maintain their independent practices and serve their own patients and HMO patients.

- *Direct contract model*—similar to an IPA except the HMO contracts directly with individual physicians.

- *POS*—a managed care plan (also called an open ended model HMO) that allows enrollees to use the HMO providers or to go outside the plan and use a provider of their choice; however, when non-HMO providers are used, enrollees typically pay larger out-of-pocket expenses.

☑ Advantages of managed care include
  - preventive care,
  - lower premiums,
  - prescription coverage,
  - fewer unnecessary procedures, and
  - limited paperwork

☑ Disadvantages of managed care include
  - limited physician pool,
  - restricted coverage,
  - prior approval needed for specialists,
  - possibility of undertreatment, and
  - compromised privacy

☑ Managed care organizations (MCOs) receive their accreditation from two organizations: NCQA and JCAHO.

☑ NCQA is a private, not-for-profit organization dedicated to improving healthcare quality and is frequently referred to as a watchdog for the managed care industry. NCQA has been accrediting MCOs since 1991 in response to the need for standardized, objective information about the quality of these organizations. Although the MCO accreditation program is voluntary, it has been well received by the managed care industry. For an organization to become accredited by NCQA, it must undergo a rigorous survey and meet certain standards designed to evaluate the health plan's clinical and administrative systems. In particular, NCQA evaluates health plans in the areas of patient safety, confidentiality, consumer protection, access, service, and continuous improvement.

☑ JCAHO is a private, independent, nonprofit organization that evaluates medical facility compliance based on a focused set of standards that are long known as essential to the delivery of good patient care. JCAHO standards are guidelines for achieving "quality" patient care. These standards include
  - the rights of patients,
  - the assessment and treatment of patients,
  - a safe environment for patients and healthcare employees,
  - the quality of patient care,
  - the management of patients' records, and
  - the organizational responsibilities of leadership and staff

☑ The *utilization review* process is a method of tracking, reviewing, and giving opinions regarding care provided to patients. Utilization review evaluates the necessity, appropriateness, and efficiency of the use of healthcare services, procedures, and facilities to control costs and manage care. Utilization review is one of the primary tools used by MCOs and other health plans.

☑ *Preauthorization* is the process whereby certain tests, procedures, or inpatient hospitalization is ascertained as "medically necessary" before the service or procedure is performed. Preauthorization does not guarantee payment.

☑ *Precertification* is a process whereby the provider (or a member of his or her staff) contacts the patient's managed care plan before inpatient admissions and performance of certain procedures and services to verify the patient's eligibility and coverage for the planned service.

☑ A *referral* is when the PCP requests another provider (usually a specialist) to render a second opinion or to perform a more extensive evaluation or treatment of a patient's problem.

☑ The future of managed care is not clear-cut, but the movement from fee-for-service systems to managed care has slowed, and managed care choices tend to be moving away from the tighter controlled staff model HMOs toward less centralized systems, such as PPOs and POS plans. Experts predict, however, that managed healthcare will overcome its problems and will have a prominent place in the future of healthcare.

CLOSING SCENARIO

There was a lot of information to assimilate in this chapter regarding managed care, especially because Emilio and Latish knew so little about it before they began the course. They now think they understand the concepts much better, however. Latisha was surprised to learn that there were so many different types of HMOs—she thought an HMO was an HMO. She and Emilio, similar to so many others, had heard a lot of negative reports regarding managed care, and they assumed it was inferior healthcare. They now realize that not all MCOs are bad; there are many good ones and a few inferior ones—as is true for fee-for-service carriers.

At the free health clinic where Emilio volunteers, he has developed an information sheet for patients explaining managed care in simple terms, comparing it with the more familiar fee-for-service structure and including the pros and cons of both. Equipped now with a better understanding of the various structures of health insurance, he is beginning to feel more comfortable in his volunteer work at the free clinic. What it means to be a health insurance professional has taken on a new meaning: it's not just knowing how to complete an insurance form and submitting it—it's also knowing how to build positive relationships with all members of the healthcare team and the patients. Knowing that everyone's job at the clinic is interrelated and that everyone has to work together for the entire system to work efficiently was an important learning experience for Emilio. An appreciation and understanding of the profession is growing as the students continue their lifelong learning experiences in class and in the workplace.

WEBSITES TO EXPLORE

For a live link to the following website, please visit the Evolve® site at http://evolve.elsevier.com/Beik/today/

- To learn more about managed care, visit the websites of the two groups that evaluate MCOs in the United States, the National Committee for Quality Assurance (NCQA) at http://www.ncqa.org/ and the Joint Commission on Accreditation of Healthcare Organizations (JCAHO) at http://www.jcaho.org/

Understanding Medicaid

Chapter Outline

CHAPTER OBJECTIVES

After completion of this chapter, the student should be able to
- Explain what Medicaid is.
- Define the federal government's role in Medicaid.
- Outline how individual states can modify Medicaid coverage.

CHAPTER TERMS

balance billing
budget period
categorically needy
cost avoid(ance)
cost sharing
countable income

disproportionate share hospitals
dual coverage (Medi-Medi)
dual eligibles
federal poverty level (FPL)

CHAPTER OBJECTIVES

- Name the two major groups that qualify for Medicaid and explain both.
- List the services typically covered by Medicaid.
- Explain the various methods for verifying Medicaid eligibility.
- Interpret third-party liability as it relates to Medicaid.
- List common Medicaid billing errors.
- Explain the Medicaid standard remittance advice.
- Discuss fraud and abuse in the Medicaid system.

CHAPTER TERMS

fiscal intermediary (FI) (fiscal agent)
mandated services
Medicaid
Medicaid "simple" claim
medically necessary
medically needy
Medicare hospital insurance (Medicare HI)
Medicare-Medicaid crossover claims
optional services
payer of last resort
pay and chase claims
Program of All-inclusive Care for the Elderly (PACE)
Qualified Disabled and Working Individuals

Qualified Medicare Beneficiaries
reciprocity
remittance advice (RA)
Specified Low-Income Medicare Beneficiaries
spend down
State Children's Health Insurance Program (SCHIP)
supplemental medical insurance (SMI)
supplemental security income (SSI)
Temporary Assistance for Needy Families (TANF)
third-party liability

OPENING SCENARIO

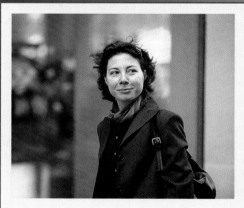

Nela Karnama has been employed as a medical receptionist in a multispecialty medical practice for 9 years. She had heard that there was soon going to be an opening in the Billing Department, which would be a promotion for Nela if she qualified for the position. She had always wanted to specialize in this area, but did not feel qualified, so she enrolled in an evening course at a community college satellite center in a nearby town. Nela thought she knew quite a lot about Medicaid because after her husband was killed in an automobile accident, she and her children became eligible for benefits. After perusing the contents of Chapter 8, it was obvious to her, however, that what she did know about it was limited to the program she and her children were on, and that there was a lot more to learn.

Nela carpooled with Berta Kazinski, a neighbor who also had enrolled in the course. Berta, a nontraditional student, was basically unfamiliar with the program. She recalled that Medicaid had begun paying for part of her mother-in-law's expenses after she had been in a nursing home for several years, but Berta was unaware of the financial implications that led to her mother-in-law's eligibility for this care.

The discussion concerning Medicaid broadened during their commute to the class, and it was obvious that there was more to the Medicaid program than either of the women realized. Using the time study schedule they created in Chapter 2, they laid out their study plans for the next learning phase of their health insurance career.

WHAT IS MEDICAID?

Medicaid is a combination federal and state medical assistance program designed to provide comprehensive and quality medical care for low-income families with special emphasis on children, pregnant women, the elderly, the disabled, and parents with dependent children who have no other way to pay for healthcare. Congress established the Medicaid program under Title XIX of the Social Security Act of 1965. Under the federal Medicaid guidelines, federal and state governments must contribute a specified percentage of total healthcare expenditures. The federal contribution is approximately 50%. The states pay the remaining costs, after which they are relatively free to choose whom to cover and what benefits to provide. There is usually a single state agency in charge of the program in each state, but many states have the program administered by county and city governments.

Although Medicaid benefits vary from state to state, all states have Medicaid programs. As a result, there are essentially 56 different Medicaid programs—one for each state, territory, and the District of Columbia. The individual state programs cover a variety of healthcare services, and each state sets its own guidelines regarding eligibility standards, services, benefits package, payment rates, and program administration within the broader federal guidelines.

What Did You Learn?

1. What is Medicaid?
2. When was the Medicaid program established?
3. Under what major act does the Medicaid program fall?

EVOLUTION OF MEDICAID

Medicaid originally was created to give low-income Americans access to healthcare. Since its inception, Medicaid has evolved from a narrowly defined program available only to individuals eligible for cash assistance (welfare) into a large insurance program with complex eligibility rules. Today, Medicaid is a major social welfare program and is administered by the Centers for Medicare and Medicaid Services (CMS), formerly called the Healthcare Financing Administration (HCFA).

The Medicaid program that was formerly referred to as Aid to Families with Dependent Children is now called **Temporary Assistance for Needy Families (TANF)**. TANF is the federal-state cash assistance program for poor families, typically headed by a single parent. Each state sets its own income eligibility guidelines for TANF, and individuals who are eligible for TANF automatically qualify for Medicaid. Not all states refer to this program as TANF. Many states have coined their own name for this program. Vermont calls it ANFC/RU (Aid to Needy Families with Children/Reach Up); New York calls it simply the Family Assistance (FA) Program; and Kentucky's program is called K-TAP (Kentucky Transitional Assistance Program). For a listing of what all states call their TANF programs, consult Websites to Explore at the end of this chapter.

In 1972, federal law established the **supplemental security income (SSI)** program, which provides federally funded cash assistance to qualifying elderly and disabled poor. Under the SSI program, the Social Security

Administration determines eligibility criteria and sets the cash benefit amounts for SSI. SSI is a cash benefit program controlled by the Social Security Administration; however, it is not related to the Social Security Program.

States may choose to supplement federal SSI payments with state funds. To be eligible for SSI, an individual must be at least 65 years old or blind or disabled and have limited assets (or resources). Income is determined by the standards set forth in the **federal poverty level (FPL)** guidelines (Fig. 8-1). Eligibility for SSI benefits is not based on work record. The income benefits limit is $603 per month (2006 figures). Eligible recipients also qualify for SSI Medicaid assistance for healthcare (for updates, see "Websites to Explore" at the end of this chapter.)

The amount of the SSI payment is the difference between the individual's **countable income** and the Federal Benefit Rate (FBR). Countable income is the amount left over after

1. eliminating all items that are not considered income and
2. applying all appropriate exclusions to the items that are considered income.

During the late 1980s and early 1990s, Congress expanded Medicaid eligibility to include more categories of people—the poor elderly, individuals with disabilities, children, and certain categories of pregnant women. In addition to expanding eligibility parameters, Medicaid programs were broadened as a result of federal mandates. These program expansions include the following:

- Payments to hospitals that serve large numbers of poor, uninsured, or Medicaid recipients
- Coverage of prenatal and delivery services for qualifying pregnant women and their infants who have no other insurance
- Expansion of services to many children in low-income families who do not receive cash assistance (TANF)
- Expansion of Medicaid to fill gaps in Medicare services to the poor elderly or disabled individuals

2006 Federal Poverty Levels (FPL) Chart			
Family Size	100% of FPL	135% of FPL	150% of FPL
1	$9,810	$13,160	$14,595
2	$13,070	$17,561	$19,485
3	$16,330	$21,962	$24,375
4	$19,590	$26,363	$29,265
5	$22,850	$30,764	$34,155
6	$26,110	$35,165	$39,045
7	$29,370	$39,566	$34,935

Fig. 8-1 FPL guidelines.

• Coverage of the full range of federally allowable Medicaid services as medically necessary and appropriate for all children on Medicaid

As a result of these and other federal law changes, the eligibility determination process is more intricate today than in the past. Computer systems designed for a smaller and simpler program now manage information for millions of people in dozens of different eligibility groups.

 HIPAA Tip

Every health insurance professional who files Medicaid claims should be trained in HIPAA policies, procedures, and processes.

What Did You Learn?

1. As it was originally created, what was the only group Medicaid covered?
2. What is TANF?
3. What does SSI provide?
4. What additional group was added to the Medicaid program in 1972?
5. Who administers Medicaid?
6. Why is it difficult to determine Medicaid eligibility in today's healthcare?

STRUCTURE OF MEDICAID

Medicaid is a combination federal and state public assistance program, which pays for certain healthcare costs of individuals who qualify. The program is administered by CMS under the general direction of the Department of Health and Human Services. Eligibility is based on need by meeting certain income and resource limits. The federal government has established broad requirements for eligibility, and the individual states refine eligibility requirements and coverage to the needs of its population.

FEDERAL GOVERNMENT'S ROLE

The federal government establishes broad national guidelines for Medicaid eligibility. Within the federal guidelines, each state establishes its own eligibility standards; determines the type, amount, duration, and scope of services; sets the rate of payment for services; and administers its own program. Under the broadest provisions of the federal statute, individuals, no matter what their financial status, must fall into a designated group before they are eligible for Medicaid. These groups are shown in Fig. 8-2.

CATEGORICALLY NEEDY

Families, pregnant women, and children

• Persons meeting Family Medical criteria (including TANF recipients)
• Children under the age of 1 and pregnant women whose countable income does not exceed 150% of the FPL.
• Children ages 1 – 5 whose countable income does not exceed 133% of the FPL
• Children ages 6 –18 whose countable income does not exceed 100% of the FPL

Aged and Disabled Individuals

• SSI recipients
• Qualified Medicare Beneficiaries (QMBs)

Individuals residing in intermediate or long-term care facilities

• Medicaid beneficiaries
• Dual coverage (Medi-Medi) beneficiaries

MEDICALLY NEEDY

Individuals who do not qualify for Medicaid benefits under the categorically needy programs because of income or resources exceeding the Level of qualifying criteria but are medically indigent.

• Pregnant women
• Children up to age 18 (or age 18 working toward a high school diploma or its equivalent)
• Persons 65 years of age and older
• Persons who are disabled or blind under SSA standards.

Fig. 8-2 Who is eligible for Medicaid.

STATES' OPTIONS

States generally are allowed wide parameters in determining which groups their Medicaid programs cover and the financial criteria for Medicaid eligibility within each particular program. To be eligible for federal funds, however, states are required to provide Medicaid coverage for certain individuals who receive federally assisted income-maintenance payments and for related groups not receiving cash payments. In addition to their Medicaid programs, most states have other "state-only" programs to provide medical assistance for specified poor individuals who do not qualify for Medicaid. Federal funds are *not* provided for state-only programs.

States must cover **categorically needy** individuals, but they have options as to how to define "categorically needy." Categorically needy individuals typically include
• low-income families with children;
• individuals receiving SSI;
• pregnant women, infants, and children with incomes less than a specified percent of the FPL; and
• Qualified Medicare Beneficiaries.

Who qualifies for Medicaid benefits in a particular state varies depending on the options that state has elected to include in the program. States that include the SSI program cover everyone who qualifies for the SSI (aged, blind, and disabled). These states cannot have rules, however, that are more restrictive than the federal government rules for SSI.

In addition to the categorically needy, a state may elect to cover other optional categorical groups, such as

- individuals who have large medical expenses and might qualify for Medicaid categorically, but their income and resources are too high (referred to as **medically needy**) and aged, blind, or disabled individuals;
- members of families with dependent children who have too much income or resources or both to be eligible for cash assistance, but not enough for needed medical care;
- aged and disabled individuals with incomes less than 100% of the FPL; and
- institutionalized individuals with incomes no greater than 300% of the SSI federal benefit rate.

MANDATED SERVICES

Title XIX of the Social Security Act requires that for a state to receive federal matching funds, certain basic services (referred to as **mandated services**) must be offered to the categorically needy population in any state program. These services include

- inpatient and outpatient hospital services;
- physician services;
- medical and surgical dental services;
- nursing facility services for individuals age 21 or older;
- home healthcare for individuals eligible for nursing facility services;
- family planning services and supplies;
- rural health clinic services and any other ambulatory services offered by a rural health clinic that are otherwise covered under the state plan;
- laboratory and x-ray services;
- pediatric and family nurse practitioner services;
- federally qualified health center services and any other ambulatory services offered by a federally qualified health center that are otherwise covered under the state plan;
- nurse-midwife services (to the extent authorized under state law); and
- early and periodic screening, diagnosis, and treatment (EPSDT) services for individuals younger than age 21.

To see a timeline of Medicaid's mandated services, log on to the CMS website, and type "Medicaid mandated services" into the search box at the top of the page.

OPTIONAL SERVICES

There also are federally approved **optional services** for which federal funding is available. They are called optional services because states can provide as many or as few as they choose. Also, individual states can provide these services to their categorically needy population that they do not provide to other groups. These are called optional

services. The most commonly covered optional services under the Medicaid program include

- clinic services,
- nursing facility services for individuals younger than age 21,
- intermediate care facility/mentally retarded services,
- optometrist services and eyeglasses,
- prescribed drugs,
- tuberculosis-related services for tuberculosis-infected individuals,
- prosthetic devices, and
- dental services.

If the state plan includes services in institutions for mental diseases or in intermediate care facilities for the mentally retarded, it must offer certain additional benefits, including

- inpatient psychiatric services for qualifying patients;
- services provided by licensed nonphysician practitioners (e.g., psychologists and social workers);
- case management,
- diagnostic, screening, preventive, and rehabilitative services; and
- clinic services furnished under the direction of a physician.

Individual states also can adopt the medically needy standard. If a state chooses to include the medically needy population, the state plan must provide, as a minimum, the following services:

- Prenatal care and delivery services for pregnant women
- Ambulatory services to individuals younger than age 18 and individuals entitled to institutional services
- Home health services to individuals entitled to nursing facility services

The resource limits for medically needy individuals are higher than the limits for other categories of eligibility. These individuals can **spend down** their assets to the Medicaid eligibility level by deducting incurred medical expenses. A spend down occurs when private or family finances are depleted to the point where the individual/family becomes eligible for Medicaid assistance. Almost any medical bills the applicant or the applicant's family still owes or which were paid in the months for which Medicaid is sought (called the **budget period**) can be used to meet the spend down requirement.

The medically needy spend down process is normally a voluntary process and is frequently done to allow an elderly individual eligibility for Medicaid to help pay for nursing home care that he or she otherwise could not afford. It also is used in certain family situations when an unexpected illness or injury occurs that results in large medical bills the family does not have the funds to pay.

States may provide home and community-based care waiver services to certain individuals who are eligible for Medicaid. The services to be provided to these individuals may include case management, personal care services, respite care services, adult day health services, homemaker/home health aide, habilitation, and other services requested by the state and approved by CMS.

In addition to the assistance Medicaid provides in its federally mandated programs, states have more freedom of choice in the services they may provide for the medically needy category. States also have the option to provide additional services or may cover non–Medicaid eligible individuals for which the federal government will not provide matching funds. There are many different programs in various states, and the rules and regulations vary from program to program and state to state. This can present a confusing situation when one looks at the Medicaid picture as a whole. The health insurance professional must learn the specific guidelines for the programs offered in the state in which he or she is employed to perform his or her job judiciously. The health insurance professional should contact the Medicaid **fiscal intermediary** (a commercial insurer contracted by the Department of Health and Human Services for the purpose of processing and administering claims), in his or her state to obtain a guide as to what programs are available and what each one covers in that state. An alternative resource for this information is listed in Websites to Explore at the end of this chapter.

STATE CHILDREN'S HEALTH INSURANCE PROGRAM

States also can participate in Title XXI of the Social Security Act, which is the **State Children's Health Insurance Program (SCHIP)**. The SCHIP program allows states to expand their Medicaid eligibility guidelines to cover more categories of children. Many states also have programs

---

Imagine This!

Inez Burke, a widow, resides in a nursing home and has complications of diabetes and cellulitis. Six years ago, Inez's husband died, leaving her with a modest savings account. The homestead on which she and her husband raised their family had earlier been divided into parcels for the three children, with the arrangement that Inez would receive life estate in the property. In just a few years, the bills generated as a result of her medical condition depleted her savings account. Realizing that she could no longer live alone, Inez's son arranged for her care at the Sunset Care Center. Because Inez's savings were used up paying her medical bills, Inez qualified for Medicaid. Her monthly Social Security check is applied toward her care at Sunset; other than that, Medicaid pays her room and board plus any medical care she receives from the staff that Medicare does not pay.

---

that assist others not eligible for Medicaid, but who have difficulty paying for medical care. Additionally, most states have programs that provide rehabilitative assistance to the disabled—especially children—and provide medically needy coverage to relatives who care for dependent children. These state programs do not receive matching federal funds, however.

● Stop and Think

Referring back to the Inez Burke scenario in Imagine This!, what Medicaid category does this individual fall into?

Imagine This!

Tyler Strom, a 12-year-old white male, was hospitalized for a serious blood infection resulting from a cat bite, and the hospital bills totaled $8260. Tyler lives with his mother, who is a physical therapist, with a gross monthly income of $4000. Tyler does not meet the SSI definition of a disabled child; his mother is applying to Medicaid for payment of his hospital bills under the Medically Needy Spend Down (for Pregnant Women, Infants and Children) program in their state. Assuming that the medically needy income level for two is $317, to determine eligibility, Medicaid will look at the family's *countable income*, which after allowed deductions, is $2587—$2270 over the $317 limit. Because Tyler's outstanding medical bills total $8260, $2270 of that would be used to "spend down" to the income limit. Medicaid would then pay the remaining $5990 of the charges. Medicaid will not pay the $2270 that was used to spend down to the medically needy income level.

FISCAL INTERMEDIARIES

Medicaid does not, as a rule, process claims. Instead, individual states contract with an organization specializing in administering government healthcare programs, an **FI**, sometimes referred to as a **fiscal agent**. This organization processes all healthcare claims on behalf of the Medicaid program. Some states have more than one FI, one FI for fee-for-service Medicaid claims and a second one for managed care claims. Before an FI is selected by the state, there is a bidding process—similar to when contractors bid for the job of constructing a bridge or building a road. FIs typically contract 1 year at a time and must bid again for subsequent years.

Responsibilities of the FI may differ from state to state; however, more common responsibilities are as follows:

- Process claims
- Provide information for healthcare providers for the particular government program involved
- Generate guidelines for providers to facilitate the claims process
- Answer beneficiary questions about benefits, claims processing, appeals, and the explanation of benefits (**remittance advice [RA]**) document

The health insurance professional should know the name and telephone number of his or her state Medicaid FI and keep it handy, because the FI can offer a wealth of information regarding healthcare claims and administration of the Medicaid program. Additionally, if and when questions arise regarding claims, the FI is there to answer them.

 **HIPAA Tip**

The Medicaid HIPAA Compliant Concept Model (MHCCM)
MHCCM shows how HIPAA affects the Medicaid enterprise and provides practical tools to help a state determine the best course of action for analyzing the HIPAA impact, determine implementation strategies, determine best practices, and validate what a state has accomplished.

Website for MHCCM is at http://www.cms.hhs.gov/medicaid/hipaa/adminsimp/.

What Did You Learn?

1. What is the federal government's role in Medicaid?
2. Explain the state's role in Medicaid.
3. Name the major category of Medicaid eligibles that states must cover under federal mandates.
4. Identify the major categorical group a state might "elect" to cover.
5. Define the term "mandated service."

WHO QUALIFIES FOR MEDICAID COVERAGE?

We already have learned that the Medicaid program is divided into two major groups: the categorically needy and the medically needy. To understand fully who qualifies for inclusion in these two groups, let's examine them more closely.

CATEGORICALLY NEEDY

Individuals in the categorically needy group receive medical assistance because their income falls within the poverty or Family Medical income guidelines or as a result of SSI eligibility. Coverage of the categorically needy is largely mandated by federal law with some limited options. The mandatory groups include

- individuals meeting Family Medical criteria (including TANF recipients),
- SSI recipients,
- pregnant women and children younger than age 1 whose countable income does not exceed 150% of the federal poverty level,
- children age 1 through 5 whose countable income does not exceed 133% of the FPL, and
- children age 6 through 18 whose countable income does not exceed 100% of the FPL.

The categorically needy segment also includes individuals who are believed to be receiving an SSI cash or Family Medical benefit, although are actually ineligible for one because of certain factors. For Family Medical, this would include

- individuals who become ineligible because of increased earnings or an increase in the number of employment hours or because of loss of earned income tax credits,
- individuals ineligible for cash assistance because of requirements that do not apply to medical services, and
- individuals who do not receive cash benefits because of the recovery of an entire grant for overpayment purposes.

For SSI, this would include individuals qualifying for status under the SSI program benefits because they are working but who retain disability.

MEDICALLY NEEDY

The medically needy segment comprises individuals who, although they meet the nonfinancial criteria of one of the categorically needy programs (e.g., age or disability), do not qualify for Medicaid benefits because of excess income or resources or, in the case of pregnant women and children, because they have income that exceeds the FPL guidelines. Most individuals in the medically needy group must pay a share of their medical costs through the spend down process. Coverage of this group is optional under federal law. If a state chooses this option, it must provide coverage for individuals who meet the eligibility standards for one of the following groups:

- Pregnant women
- Children younger than age 18 or age 18 and working toward a high school diploma (or its equivalent)
- Individuals 65 years old and older
- Individuals who are disabled or blind under Social Security Administration standards

Approximately two thirds of the states have medically needy programs. This option allows states to provide Medicaid coverage to individuals who have extensive or costly medical needs and would be eligible for Medicaid if they met the income or resources tests within their category. Depending on how the state structures its program, individuals may qualify categorically or spend down to a certain income or financial level.

PROGRAM OF ALL-INCLUSIVE CARE FOR THE ELDERLY

In addition to mandatory and optional services, there are other program options, such as the **Program of All-inclusive Care for the Elderly (PACE)**. This program provides comprehensive alternative care for noninstitutionalized elderly who otherwise would be in a nursing home. PACE is centered on the belief that it is better for the well-being of elderly with long-term care needs and their families to be served in the community where they live whenever possible. PACE serves individuals who are age 55 or older, certified by their state to need nursing home care, able to live safely in the community at the time of enrollment, and live in a PACE service area. Although all PACE participants must be certified to need nursing home care to enroll in PACE, only a small percentage of PACE participants reside in a nursing home nationally. If a PACE enrollee does need nursing home care, the PACE program pays for it and continues to coordinate his or her care.

What Did You Learn?

1. Name the categorically needy groups that are mandated by federal law.
2. What groups make up the "medically needy" classification?
3. What does the PACE program provide?

PAYMENT FOR MEDICAID SERVICES

Medicaid payments are made directly to the healthcare provider. Providers participating in Medicaid must accept the Medicaid reimbursement as payment in full. Each state is free to determine (within certain federal restrictions) how reimbursements are calculated and the resulting rates for services, with three exceptions:

1. For institutional services, payment may not exceed amounts that would be paid under Medicare payment rates.

2. For **disproportionate share hospitals**, different limits apply. (Disproportionate share hospitals are facilities that receive additional payments to ensure that communities have access to certain high-cost services, such as trauma and emergency care and burn services.)
3. For hospice care.

States may impose nominal deductibles, coinsurance, or copayments on some Medicaid recipients for certain services, such as dental and podiatry care. Emergency services and family planning services must be exempt from such copayments. Certain Medicaid recipients must be excluded from this **cost sharing**, including pregnant women, children younger than age 18, hospital or nursing home patients who are expected to contribute most of their income to institutional care, and categorically needy health maintenance organization enrollees. Cost sharing is a situation in which covered individuals pay a portion of the health costs, such as deductibles, coinsurance, or copayment amounts.

MEDICALLY NECESSARY

As a general rule, Medicaid only pays for services that are determined to be **medically necessary**. For a procedure or service to be considered medically necessary, it typically must be consistent with the diagnosis and in accordance with the standards of good medical practice, performed at the proper level, and provided in the most appropriate setting. If the health insurance professional questions whether a service or procedure is medically necessary, he or she should consult the current Medicaid provider handbook of the state in which he or she is employed or telephone the FI that administers local Medicaid claims. This should be done before the service or procedure is performed to avoid problems with collecting payment from Medicaid or the patient after the fact.

PRESCRIPTION DRUG COVERAGE

Recognizing that prescription drugs are an increasingly important element of comprehensive healthcare, all states have chosen the option of providing prescription drug coverage for their categorically needy populations and most cover some or all of the other groups. Prescription drug coverage is currently a volatile issue, subject to continual modifications. To find out what prescription drugs are covered for the categorically needy group in a particular state, contact the local FI or consult the provider's manual for that state.

Medicaid previously provided drug coverage for more than 6 million Medicare beneficiaries, known as **dual eligibles**. Dual eligibles have Medicare and Medicaid coverage. Beginning January 1, 2006, full benefit dual eligible individuals began receiving drug coverage through the Medicare Prescription Drug Benefit (Part D) of the Medicare Prescription Drug, Improvement, and Modernization Act of 2003, rather than through their state Medicaid programs. Certain drugs are excluded from coverage under the new Medicare Prescription Drug Benefit, however. The Department of Health and Human Services Secretary is responsible for automatically enrolling dual eligible individuals into Part D plans if they do not sign up on their own.

To the extent that state Medicaid programs cover the excluded drugs for Medicaid recipients who are not full benefit dual eligibles, states will be required to cover the excluded drugs for full benefit dual eligibles with federal financial participation. More information on the new Medicare Prescription Drug Plan can be found in Chapter 9.

ACCEPTING MEDICAID PATIENTS

Physicians have the choice of whether or not to accept Medicaid patients. This refers to a patient with Medicaid only or any combination of Medicaid and another insurance company, whether it is a primary or secondary payer. In an emergency, or if it cannot be determined if the patient has Medicaid at the time of treatment, the patient must be informed as soon as possible after identifying Medicaid coverage whether the practice will accept him or her as a Medicaid patient.

Physicians can limit the number of Medicaid patients they accept, as long as there is no discrimination by age, sex, race, or religious preference or national origin, in addition to the limits of their scope of practice. If a practice sees only children, refusing to accept adult patients is not considered discrimination. If a patient has Medicare and Medicaid coverage, however, and the practice does not accept the Medicaid coverage, the health insurance professional must make sure the patient understands this before treatment. The patient then has the opportunity to seek a physician who would accept the patient's Medicaid coverage. If a Medicaid recipient insists on being treated by a nonparticipating healthcare provider (one who does not accept Medicaid), it is recommended that the health insurance professional ask the patient to sign a form verifying his or her understanding that the practice does not accept Medicaid, and he or she will be responsible for paying the deductible and coinsurance amounts.

PARTICIPATING PROVIDERS

The healthcare provider can elect to accept or refuse Medicaid patients; however, many state regulations say if a Medicaid participating provider elects to treat one Medicaid patient, all Medicaid patients must be accepted—the provider cannot single out which ones to

treat. Providers can put a cap, however, on the total number of new patients, including Medicaid patients, that he or she will accept. Additionally, providers must agree to accept what Medicaid pays as payment in full for covered services and are prohibited by law to balance bill Medicaid patients for these services. The healthcare professional should know beforehand whether or not a particular service or procedure is covered by Medicaid. If the patient insists on being treated for a particular noncovered service, it is recommended that he or she sign a waiver that spells out the fact that the service is not covered by Medicaid and that the patient acknowledges responsibility for payment. Some practices even ask the patient to pay for noncovered services in advance.

● Stop and Think

As a general rule, Dr. Vandenberg accepts Medicaid patients in her family practice. After seeing Harold Apple, a patient with a very unpleasant personality, Dr. Vandenberg advised the medical receptionist not to schedule any further follow-up appointments for Mr. Apple. Is Dr. Vandenberg violating any Medicaid principles?

What Did You Learn?

1. Explain the term "cost sharing."
2. What criteria does a procedure or service have to meet to be considered "medically necessary"?
3. Explain the recommended procedure a health insurance professional should follow if a Medicaid recipient insists on being treated in a medical facility that does not accept Medicaid patients.

VERIFYING MEDICAID ELIGIBILITY

Medicaid providers always should ensure that Medicaid will pay for patients' medical care before providing services to determine eligibility for the current date and to discover any limitations to the recipient's coverage. Several methods are available in most states that the health insurance professional can use to verify eligibility, as follows:

• Using the patient's Medicaid identification (ID) card
• Using an automated voice response (AVR) system

- Using electronic data interchange (EDI)
- Using a Point-of-Sale device
- Using a computer software program

MEDICAID IDENTIFICATION CARD

A common method for verifying the patient's Medicaid eligibility is the ID card. This card provides important information regarding eligibility date and type shown on the face of the card. The following steps are suggested for eligibility verification when using the ID card:

- Ensure that the patient's name is on the ID card. (Typically, the patient's birth date and sex also are listed.)
- Unless you know the patient personally, ask to see another form of identification to confirm his or her identity.
- Check the eligibility period. There should be "from" and "through" dates that tell you the time period in which the patient is Medicaid-eligible. Medicaid pays only for dates of service during this eligibility period.
- Look for insurance information. In the example shown in Fig. 8-3, there is a "1" under the "Ins. No." column. The "Insurance Data" block shows details of the patient's insurance coverage.
- Ask the patient if there is any other insurance coverage.
- Photocopy the Medicaid ID card, and enter any new information in the patient's record.

Many states color code the ID cards, which tells the health insurance professional which type of Medicaid program the recipient is enrolled in. Also, the card should be examined closely to see if the patient is in a special program or has special coverage. It is important for the health insurance professional to obtain a provider's guide from the Medicaid FI in his or her state for assistance in interpreting the codes on the Medicaid ID card.

AUTOMATED VOICE RESPONSE SYSTEM

This system involves the use of a touch-tone phone to call an AVR system for eligibility information. For this method of verification, the health insurance professional needs to know the patient's Medicaid ID number or Social Security number and date of birth. The AVR system can provide a variety of eligibility information, including the following:

- Eligibility for specific dates of service
- The type of coverage or special programs in which the patient is enrolled
- If the patient is covered under Medicare Part A and Medicare Part B
- Information known by Medicaid concerning other insurance coverage

If the health insurance professional has access to this type of eligibility verification, he or she should know how to use it correctly and keep current by requesting and reading periodic updates.

ELECTRONIC DATA INTERCHANGE

Providers may obtain Medicaid eligibility information electronically. Online, interactive eligibility verification is available from EDI vendors (sometimes referred to as clearinghouses). Use of an EDI vendor is voluntary to providers. EDI vendors interface directly with the Medicaid recipient database maintained by Electronic Data Services (EDS) for claims processing. The database is updated every day from the state's master eligibility file. This service is available 24 hours a day, 7 days a week, except for periods when it is down for system maintenance. EDI vendors normally charge a fee for their services, and providers might be required to pay a transaction fee to the state's Medicaid FI.

Medicaid Identification Card holds #11 digits

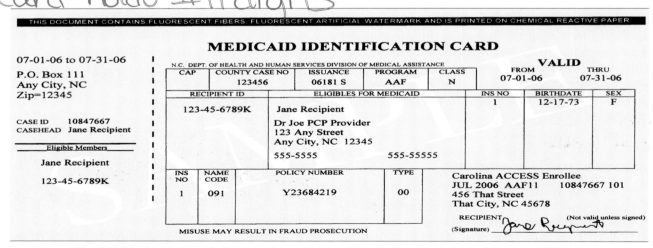

Fig. 8-3 Medicaid ID card. (Source: North Carolina Department of Health and Human Services.)

POINT-OF-SALE DEVICE

With a point-of-sale device, the patient is issued an ID card that is similar in size and design to a credit card. Through the information on the magnetic strip, the provider can swipe the card and can receive an accurate return of eligibility information within a matter of seconds.

COMPUTER SOFTWARE PROGRAM

With this method of eligibility verification, the provider can key the patient's information into a computer software program and in a short time have an accurate return of eligibility information.

BENEFITS OF ELIGIBILITY VERIFICATION SYSTEM

By using one of these eligibility verification system methods, providers can reduce the number of denied claims by verifying recipient eligibility and insurance information before services are provided. Upfront verification using the eligibility verification system results in the submission of more accurate claims and decreases eligibility-related claims denials.

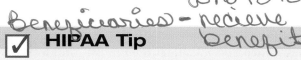

Beneficiaries — who is to recieve benefits

☑ **HIPAA Tip**

Medicaid providers and their vendors who bill electronically need to verify that their systems accept HIPAA-compliant Medicaid transactions.

What Did You Learn?

1. Why is it important for the health insurance professional to verify eligibility?
2. What should the health insurance professional do if a patient insists on receiving non–Medicaid covered services?
3. What are the benefits of the eligibility verification system system?

MEDICARE/MEDICAID RELATIONSHIP

Most elderly or disabled individuals who are very poor are covered under Medicaid and Medicare, commonly referred to as **dual coverage**, dual eligibility, or **Medi-Medi**. These individuals may receive Medicare services for which they are entitled and other services available under that state's Medicaid program. As each state sets up its

Medicaid plan, certain services typically not covered by Medicare (e.g., hearing aids, eyeglasses, and nursing facility care beyond the 100 days covered by Medicare) may be provided to these individuals by the Medicaid program. In addition, the Medicaid program pays all of the cost-sharing portions (deductibles and coinsurance) of Medicare Part A and B for these dually eligible beneficiaries.

deductibles / yearly out of pocket expense before ins

SPECIAL MEDICARE/MEDICAID PROGRAMS

There are other Medicare beneficiaries who are not fully eligible for Medicaid, but who do receive some help through the state's Medicaid program for part or all of the individual's Medicare premiums and cost-sharing expenses. Individuals identified as **Qualified Disabled and Working Individuals**, who lose their Medicare benefits because they returned to work, are allowed to purchase **Medicare hospital insurance (Medicare HI)**. Premiums for such coverage must be paid by the state Medicaid program if the individual qualifies for Qualified Disabled and Working Individuals and his or her income falls below 200% of the FPL. **Supplementary medical insurance (SMI)** coverage also is available to qualifying beneficiaries; however, premiums for SMI coverage are not paid by Medicaid.

Other Medicare beneficiaries who may receive some Medicaid assistance are referred to as **Qualified Medicare Beneficiaries**. These Medicare beneficiaries qualify only if they have incomes below the FPL and resources at or below twice the standard allowed under the SSI program. In this case, the state pays all the Medicare cost-sharing expenses and premiums for Medicare hospital insurance and SMI.

The Medicaid program pays SMI premiums of another classification, known as **Specified Low-Income Medicare Beneficiaries**, which are beneficiaries with resources similar to Qualified Medicare Beneficiaries, but with slightly higher incomes. Medicaid does not pay for the Medicare hospital insurance premium for this group.

In all cases, Medicaid is always the **payer of last resort**, meaning that all other available third-party resources must meet their legal obligation to pay claims before the Medicaid program pays for the care of an individual eligible for Medicaid. If an individual is a Medicare beneficiary, payments for any services covered by Medicare are made by the Medicare program before any payments are made by the Medicaid program. In short, Medicaid pays last.

Co-Insurance — insurance cost sharing 80% self — 20%

MEDICARE AND MEDICAID DIFFERENCES EXPLAINED

People are often confused about the differences between Medicare and Medicaid. Eligibility for Medicare is not tied to individual need. Rather, it is an entitlement program.

Individuals are entitled to it because they or their spouses paid for it through Social Security taxes withheld from their wages. Medicaid is a federal assistance program for low-income, financially needy individuals, set up by the federal government and administered differently in each state. Although an individual may qualify and receive coverage from Medicare and Medicaid, there are separate eligibility requirements for each program, and being eligible for one program does not mean an individual is eligible for the other.

The following lists describe the differences between the two programs:

Medicare
- Provides healthcare insurance for disabled individuals, individuals 65 years old and older, and any age individual with end-stage renal disease
- Must have contributed to Medicare system (deductions from wages) to be eligible
- Pays for primary hospital care and related medically necessary services
- Generally, individuals must be older than 65 to be eligible
- May have a copay provision depending on the services received
- Federally controlled, uniform application across the United States

Medicaid
- Needs-based healthcare program
- Pays for long-term care for qualifying individuals
- Must meet income and financial limitations to be eligible for certain programs
- Must be older than 65, disabled, or blind to qualify for coverage
- Requires mandatory contribution of *all* recipient's income in certain programs
- Individual state-by-state plan options create a different program in each state (generally similar, but may be different in specific application)

Table 8-1 provides a brief summary of the major differences between the two programs.

What Did You Learn?

1. If an individual has dual coverage under Medicaid and Medicare, which claim is filed first?
2. Name two other categories of Medicare beneficiaries who are eligible for partial Medicaid coverage.
3. What are the major differences between Medicaid and Medicare?

MEDICAID CLAIM

The universal CMS-1500 claim is accepted by Medicaid FIs in most states. Some states have their own form, however, that must be used for submitting claims for Medicaid recipients. The health insurance professional must check with the local Medicaid FI to ensure the correct claim form is used. For the exercises in this text and accompanying student workbook, the CMS-1500 form is used.

COMPLETING THE CMS-1500 USING MEDICAID GUIDELINES

Fig. 8-4 provides guidelines on completing the CMS-1500 form for a Medicaid claim. The name and address of the fiscal intermediary is keyed in the upper-right-hand corner. The guidelines used in the form in Fig. 8-4 are generic and may be different from the guidelines used in your state. This example is for a **Medicaid simple claim**—that is, the patient has Medicaid coverage only and no secondary insurance. The health insurance professional must follow the exact guidelines for completing the CMS-1500 form issued by the FI in his or her state.

RECIPROCITY

A simple dictionary definition of reciprocity is the occurrence of a situation in which individuals or entities offer

TABLE 8-1 Medicare and Medicaid: Two Different Programs	
MEDICARE	MEDICAID
Title 18	Title 19
Federal administration	State administration with federal oversight
Work history affects eligibility	Eligibility based on need
Public insurance	Public assistance
For aged, blind, disabled	For aged, blind, disabled, pregnant women, children, and caretaker relatives
Funded by Social Security and Medicare payroll tax deductions	Funded by federal general fund appropriations combined with individual state funds

certain rights to each other in return for the rights being given to them. When one state allows Medicaid beneficiaries from other states (usually states that are adjacent) to be treated in its medical facilities, this exchange of privileges is referred to as **reciprocity**. Health insurance professionals should be aware of which states, if any, offer reciprocity for Medicaid claims in their states.

What Did You Learn?

1. What is a Medicaid "simple" claim?
2. Explain what is meant by "reciprocity"?

Block 1	Enter an "X" in the Medicaid box
Block 1a	Enter the Medicaid recipient's ID number
Block 2	Enter the name of the Medicaid recipient exactly as it appears on the ID card, keying the last name first, followed by the middle name and middle initial (if one is listed).
Block 3	Enter the patient's birth date (using the MM DD YYYY format with spaces), and enter an "X" in the appropriate gender box.
Block 4	This block is left blank.
Block 5	Enter the patient's complete mailing address as indicated on lines 1 and 2 in this block. When keying the telephone number, use spaced rather than dashes and/or parentheses.
Blocks 6 – 9d	These blocks are typically left blank on Medicaid "simple" claims.
Blocks 10a-10c	Key an "X" in the appropriate boxes to indicates whether or not the claim is a result of an auto or other accident or was related to employment. In the case of an auto accident, key the 2-letter state code to indicate the state in which the accident happened.
Block 10d	Usually left blank. Check with your fiscal intermediary for special situations.
Blocks 11–11d	Leave blank.
Blocks 12-13	Leave blank. (Signatures are normally not required on Medicaid claims.)
Blocks 14-16	Leave blank.
Block 17	Enter the full name and credentials of the referring or ordering provider when applicable.
Blocks 17a and b	Enter the unique provider identification number (UPIN) or national provider identifier (NPI) of the individual shown in Block 17. The UPIN can be used until May 22, 2007, and it should appear in Block 17a. Effective May 23, 2007, the NPI must be reported in 17b.
Block 18	If the claim is for in-patient hospital services, enter the admission and discharge dates using the MM DD YYYY format. If the patient is still hospitalized, leave the "To" block blank. If no hospitalization-leave blank.
Block 19	Check the guidelines of your fiscal intermediary.
Block 20	Enter an "X" in the "NO" block. Outside lab facilities must bill Medicaid directly.
Block 21	Enter the patient's diagnosis(es) using ICD-9-CM codes, listing the primary diagnosis first. Note that there is space for up to four codes which should be listed in priority order.
Block 22	If this is a resubmission, enter the applicable Medicaid code.
Block 23	If preauthorization was required, enter this number. (Consult the specific Medicaid guidelines for your state.)
Block 24a	Enter each date of service on a separate line. Enter the month, day, and year in the MMDDYYYY (no spaces) format for each service. Note that Medicaid does not allow "date ranging for consecutive services."
Block 24b	Enter the applicable Place of Service (POS) code.
Block 24c	The block is conditionally required, enter this number. Enter an "X" or an "E" as appropriate for services performed as a result of a medical emergency.

Fig. 8-4 Step-by-step Medicaid claims instructions.

Block 24d	Enter the code number using appropriate 5-digit CPT/HCPCS procedure code and a 2-digit modifier, when applicable. If using an unlisted procedure code (ending in "-99"), a complete description of the procedure must be provided as a separate attachment
Block 24e	Link the procedure code back to the appropriate diagnosis code in Block 21 by indicating the applicable number assigned to the diagnosis (1, 2, 3, or 4).
Block 24f	Enter the amount charged for the service.
Block 24g	Enter the number of days or units for each single visit.
Block 24h	Consult your local Medicaid guidelines. Enter an "E" if the service was performed under the Early and Periodic Screening Diagnosis and Treatment (EPSDT) program. Enter an "F" for Family Planning services.
Block 24i	Enter an "X" if the service was the result of a medical emergency.
Block 24j	Leave blank.
Block 25	Enter the 9-digit Federal tax employer identification number (EIN) assigned to that provider (or group), and check the appropriate box in this field. In the case of an unincorporated practice or a sole practitioner, the provider's Social Security number is typically used.
Block 26	Enter the patient's account number as assigned by the provider's computerized accounting system.
Block 27	Place an "X" in the "YES" box.
Block 28	Enter the total charges for all services listed in column 24f.
Blocks 29-30	Leave blank.
Block 31	Enter the signature of the provider, or his/her representative and initials, and the date the form was signed. The signature may be typed, stamped, or handwritten. Make sure no part of the signature falls outside of the block.
Block 32	Key the name and address of the location where services were provided and enter the Medicaid provider number on the last line of this block. Check for updated changes with your Medicaid FI.
Block 32a	Enter the NPI of the service facility in Block 32.
Block 32b	Enter the appropriate ID qualifier followed by one blank space and then the PIN of the service quality. After May 23, 2007, 32b is not to be reported. Follow the specific guideline of your Medicaid FI.
Block 33	Enter the name, address, zip code, and telephone number of the facility providing services.
Block 33a	Effective May 23, 2007, the NPI of the billing provider or group must be reported here.
Block 33b	Enter the appropriate ID qualifier followed by one blank space and then the PIN of the billing provider or group. Effective May 23, 2007, 33b is not to be reported. Enter the group UPIN, including the 2-digit location identifier, for the performing practitioner/supplier who is a member of a group practice.

Fig. 8-4—cont'd

Imagine This!

Ellen Statler is a single mother of two dependent children living in a small Illinois town along the Mississippi River. Ellen is covered under Illinois Medicaid; however, because the nearest Illinois town where there is a healthcare provider who accepts Medicaid patients is 35 miles away, Ellen travels across the bridge into Iowa and receives care from a family practice clinic there, 2 miles from her home. This arrangement works out much more favorably for Ellen because both of her children have acute asthma, and periodic emergency visits are common.

MEDICAID AND THIRD-PARTY LIABILITY

Third-party liability refers to the legal obligation of third parties to pay all or part of the expenditures for medical assistance furnished under a state plan. Earlier in this chapter, we discussed the fact that the Medicaid program, by law, is intended to be the payer of last resort. Examples of third parties that may be liable to pay for services before Medicaid include
• employment-related health insurance,
• court-ordered health insurance by noncustodial parent,
• workers' compensation,

- long-term care insurance, and
- other state and federal programs (unless specifically excluded by federal statute).

Medicaid pays the bills when due and does not put the burden of collection from a third party on the Medicaid client. Individuals eligible for Medicaid assign their rights to third-party payments to the state Medicaid agency. States are required to take all reasonable measures to ensure that the legal liability of third parties to pay for care and services is met before funds are made available under the state Medicaid plan. Healthcare providers are obligated to inform Medicaid of any known third parties who might have liability. When states have determined that a potentially liable third party exists, the state is required to **cost avoid** or **pay and chase** claims. Cost avoidance is where the healthcare provider bills and collects from liable third parties before sending the claim to Medicaid. Pay and chase is used when the state Medicaid agency goes ahead and pays the medical bills and then attempts to recover these paid funds from liable third parties. States generally are required to cost avoid claims unless they have a waiver approved by CMS that allows them to use the pay and chase method. To learn more about third party liability (TPL), cost avoidance, and collection, refer to Websites to Explore at the end of this chapter.

In the case of third-party liability, certain blocks of the CMS-1500 form are filled out differently (Fig. 8-5). This information is generic, and the health insurance professional must follow the specific Medicaid guidelines in his or her state.

As mentioned previously, in a case in which the patient has dual eligibility for Medicaid and Medicare (Medi-Medi), Medicare is primary. Here, the claim is submitted first to Medicare, who pays their share and then "crosses it over" to Medicaid. More information on **Medicare-Medicaid crossover claims** is given in Chapter 9.

COMMON MEDICAID BILLING ERRORS

The primary goal of the health insurance professional is to create and submit insurance claims in a manner in which the maximum benefits the medical record supports are received in the minimal amount of time. This is a learned process, however, and it takes an experienced individual to avoid making common errors that cause a claim to be delayed or rejected. Fig. 8-6 lists some of these common billing errors.

MEDICAID REMITTANCE ADVICE

Every time a claim is sent to Medicaid, a document is generated explaining how the claim was adjudicated, or

Block 4	Enter the primary policyholder's complete name (last, first, middle initial) as it appears on the ID card.
Block 9	Enter the primary policyholder's complete name (last, first, middle initial) as it appears on the ID card. If it is the same as the patient, key "SAME"
Block 9a	Enter the primary insurer's policy and group numbers as indicated on the ID card.
Block 9b	If the primary policyholder is other than the patient, enter his or her date of birth using the MM DD YYYY format.
Block 9d	Enter the primary policy name.
Block 11	Conditionally required. If the primary payer rejected the claim, enter the rejection code.
Block 11d	"X" the "YES" box.
Block 29	Enter the amount (if any) paid by the primary insurer. If nothing was paid by the primary policy, indicate so using zeroes.
Block 30	If an amount was entered in Block 29, subtract it from Block 28 and enter the balance here.

Fig. 8-5 CMS-1500 guidelines for Medicaid secondary claims.

All claims submitted to Medicaid must pass screening criteria before they can be processed. If one or more of the following conditions are not met the claim will be returned to the provider.

Patient ID (Field 1a) There must always be an 11-digit patient number assigned by Medicaid. If this field is blank, has less than or more than 11 digits, or is invalid, the claim will be returned.

Diagnosis Code (Field 21 and 24-E) There must be a diagnosis code listed in field 21 and/or field 24-E. A claim with a written description without a corresponding diagnosis code is often held until staff is available to code them. If the description is not specific enough to code, the claim will be returned. (**Note:** Diagnosis codes beginning with an E or M are not accepted as a primary diagnosis codes in some states.)

Dates of Service (Field 24-A) There must be a "From" date. If you are billing a date range, both the "From" and "To" date fields must be completed. Future service dates may not be billed.

Place of Service Code (Field 24-B) This must be a two-digit code. If the Place of Service Code is blank, less or more than 2 digits, or an invalid code, the claim will be returned.

Procedure Code (Field 24-D) This must be a 5 or 6 digit code. If the minimum criteria are not met, the claim is returned.

Charges (Field 24-F) There must be a charge for each line billed. (**Note:** Only EPSDT claims will be accepted with a zero line submitted amount.)

Days or Units (Field 24-G) There must be a whole number in this field (No decimals).

Signature (Field 31) There must be a handwritten signature or a computer generated name. The name may not be the provider office name; it needs to be an actual person's name that is responsible for the information submitted on the claim. Initials only are also not accepted.

Billing Date (Field 31) The date billed must be on the claim form in Field 31. If the bill date in Field 31 or the claim received date is prior to the latest date of service on the claim, the claim will be returned.

Total Charge (Field 28) There must be a correct total charge. Claims will be returned for no total charge or for an incorrect total charge. Each claim form must have a total.

Date Received The date received must be no earlier than the latest date of service on the claim. Do not bill for future dates. Claims received prior to the latest date of service on the claim will be returned to the provider.

Fig. 8-6 CMS-1500 common billing errors.

how the payment was determined. In the past, this document was referred to as the explanation of benefits; however, Medicaid now calls it the **remittance advice (RA)**. The RA can be in paper or electronic form (if the medical facility is set up to accept the standard electronic version) and contains information from one or several claims (Fig. 8-7). The RA typically contains several "remark codes" and "reason codes"; the importance of understanding the codes and interpreting this document cannot be stressed enough. Many states generate an RA periodically (e.g., weekly), and the current status of all claims (including adjustments and voids) that have been processed during the past week is indicated. The RA format may differ from state to state;

however, they all furnish basically the same information. It is the health insurance professional's responsibility to interpret and reconcile this document with patient records. All Medicaid claims and RAs should be maintained for 6 years or longer if mandated by state statutes of limitation.

SPECIAL BILLING NOTES

The health insurance professional must keep several things in mind when filing Medicaid claims, as follows.

TIME LIMIT FOR FILING MEDICAID CLAIMS

The time limit for filing Medicaid claims varies from state to state. The health insurance professional should check with the Medicaid FI or carrier in his or her state for the filing deadline. It is good practice, however, to file all claims in a timely manner—typically right after the service has been performed, unless additional services are anticipated within the same month or eligibility period.

COPAYMENTS

Services rendered by some types of healthcare providers (e.g., podiatrists, dentists, chiropractors) often require that the Medicaid recipient make a copayment. If the health insurance professional is employed by one of these types of healthcare providers, he or she should contact the Medicaid FI in his or her state or consult the Medicaid provider manual for information. This information usually is indicated on the Medicaid recipient's ID card. Experienced health insurance professionals suggest that if a copayment is required, it should be collected before services are rendered.

ACCEPTING ASSIGNMENT

As mentioned previously, Medicaid payments are made directly to the healthcare provider. FIs in most states point out, however, that it is still important that assignment is accepted on all Medicaid claims; if Block 27 on the CMS-1500 form is not checked "yes," the claim may be denied. Providers participating in Medicaid must accept the Medicaid reimbursement as payment in full. **Balance billing**, billing the recipient for any amount not paid by Medicaid, is not allowed. Additionally, according to federal law, a provider who accepts Medicaid payment for services furnished to an ill or injured individual has no right to additional payment from a liable third party even if Medicaid has been reimbursed.

PREAUTHORIZATION

Preauthorization is needed for all inpatient hospitalization, unless the hospitalization was due to an emergency.

```
PERF PROV  SERV DATE   POS NOS   PROC   MODS     BILLED    ALLOWED   DEDUCT    COINS       GRP /RC-AMT        PROV  PD

NAME  ALPHA, ALBERT           HIC 699777777A   ACNT 1111111111            ICN 1402065330030   ASG Y  MOA MA01
W88888888  1215 121501  11    1 92547          98.00     27.22     0.00      5.44  CO-42      70.78             21.78
W88888888  1215 121501  11    1 92541          45.00     39.89     0.00      7.98  CO-42       5.11             31.91
PT RESP  13.42                CLAIM TOTALS    143.00     67.11     0.00     13.42             75.89             53.69
                                                                                                              53.69 NET


NAME  BAKER, LEEANN           HIC 699123123A   ACNT 0009                  ICN 1102025001590   ASG Y  MOA MA01 MA18
W88888888  0113 011302  11    1 J9202  GACC   600.00    446.49     0.00     89.30  CO-42     153.51            357.19
                              (J9217)
W88888888  0121 012102  11    1 J9202  CC     600.00    446.49     0.00     89.30  CO-42     153.51            357.19
                                 (J9217)
PT RESP  178.60               CLAIM TOTALS   1200.00    892.98     0.00    178.60            307.02            714.38
                                                                                                             714.38 NET

CLAIM INFORMATION FORWARDED TO:  BCBS OF MINNESOTA    ❹


NAME  CHARLIE, CINDY          HIC 699222222A   ACNT 22222222              ICN 1402008151040   ASG Y  MOA MA01
W88888888  0106 010602  11    1 76091  26      80.00     43.76     0.00      8.75  CO-42      36.24             35.01
W88888888  0106 010602  11    1 G0236  26      50.00      0.00     0.00      0.00  CO-B5      50.00             00.00
REM: M58
PT RESP   8.75                CLAIM TOTALS    130.00     43.76     0.00      8.75             86.24             35.01

ADJS: PREV PD     0.00  INT      0.17   LATE FILING CHARGE     0.00   ❷                                        35.18 NET


NAME  BETA, BOB               HIC 699111111A   ACNT 12345678901234567890 ICN 1402063333010   ASG Y  MOA MA01 MA72
W88888888  0304 030402  11    1 99214         180.00     81.99    47.65      6.87  CO-42      98.01             00.00
W88888888  0304 030402  11    1 82010          30.00      0.00     0.00      0.00  CO-B7      30.00             00.00
W88888888  0304 030402  11    1 J1040          10.00      9.39     0.00      1.88  CO-42      00.61             00.00
PT RESP  56.40                CLAIM TOTALS    220.00     91.38    47.65      8.75            128.62             00.00
                                                                                                              00.00 NET


NAME  BUMAN, JAMES            HIC 699555555A   ACNT 55555555              ICN 1402065200070   ASG Y  MOA MA01
W88888888  0304 030402  11    1 99214          75.00      0.00     0.00      0.00  PR-B7      75.00             00.00
                                                                                  OA-71      20.00
                                                                                  PR-A3     -20.00
PT RESP  55.00                CLAIM TOTALS     75.00      0.00     0.00      0.00             75.00             00.00
                                                                                                              00.00 NET


TOTALS: # OF     BILLED     ALLOWED    DEDUCT      COINS      TOTAL      PROV PD        PROV    ❸   CHECK
        CLAIMS     AMT        AMT       AMT         AMT      RC-AMT       AMT         ADJ AMT        AMT
          5       1768.00    1095.23    47.65      209.52    672.77      803.08       108.50        749.56


PROVIDER ADJ DETAILS:   PLB REASON CODE     FCN              HIC            AMOUNT    ❶
                             CS        1402063333010    699111111A        34.98
                             CS        1402065200070    699555555A        20.00
                             WO        7101347082956                      53.69
                             L6                                           -0.17
```

GLOSSARY: Group, Reason, MOA, Remark and Adjustment Codes:
CO   Contractual Obligation. Amount for which the provider is financially liable. The patient may not be billed for this amount.
PR   Patient Responsibility. Amount that may be billed to a patient or another payee.
OA   Other Adjustment.
A3   Medicare Secondary Payer liability met.
B5   Claim/Service denied/reduced because coverage guidelines were not met or were exceeded.
B7   This provider was not certified for this procedure/service on this date of service.
42   Charges exceed our fee schedule or maximum allowable amount.
71   Primary Payer amount.
M58   Please resubmit the claim with the missing/correct information so that it may be processed.
MA01   If you do not agree with what we approved for these services, you may appeal our decision. To make sure that we are fair to you, we require another individual that did not process your initial claim to conduct the review. However, in order to be eligible for a review, you must write to us within 6 months of the date of this notice, unless you have a good reason for being late.
MA119   Provider level adjustment for late claim filing applies to this claim.
MA18   The claim information is also being forwarded to the patient's supplemental insurer. Send any questions regarding supplemental benefits to them.
MA72   The beneficiary overpaid you for these assigned services. You must issue the beneficiary a refund within 30 days for the difference between his/her payment to you and the total of the amount shown as patient responsibility and as paid to the beneficiary on this notice.
CS   Adjustment
WO   Withholding
L6   Interest

3/25/02

Fig. 8-7 Standard paper remittance (SPR) advice notices, revised format.

In the case of an emergency, most Medicaid FIs require 24-hour notification. Normally, a preadmission/preprocedure review is performed by the provider before the patient is admitted to the hospital and the procedure or service is performed. The areas of required review will not be paid unless the claim denotes review has been performed, the admission is medically necessary, and the setting is appropriate. The Medicaid FI provides a preauthorization number, which should be entered in Block 23 of the CMS-1500 form. The health insurance professional should review and be aware of what procedures and services require a preadmission/preprocedure review and preauthorization. This information usually can be found in the Medicaid provider manual, or the health insurance professional can contact his or her local Medicaid FI.

HIPAA Tip

Paper claim and Prior Authorization Request Form (PA/RF) instructions must be consistent with the Administrative Simplification provisions of the federal Health Insurance Portability and Accountability Act of 1996.

RETENTION, STORAGE, AND DISPOSAL OF RECORDS

The question, "How long should a practice keep medical records?" often generates a challenging discussion. According to HIPAA's proposed privacy regulation, medical records must be maintained for 6 years. According to federal statute, the government can take criminal or civil action up to 7 years. To make it more confusing, the Department of Health and Human Services Privacy Act of 1974 established a new system of records, called the National Provider System. The National Provider System states that "records are retained indefinitely, except in the instance of an individual provider's death, in which case HCFA [now CMS] would retain such records for a 10-year period following the provider's death." In addition, there may be state laws and regulations giving specific time frames for medical record retention. Some practices archive paper records permanently using a photoduplicating process, such as microfilm or microfiche.

Storage of medical records also is important. The healthcare staff needs to be able to find the records they are looking for easily. If dozens of boxes must be searched to find specific medical records, it would cost the practice time and money; it is important that records are stored where they can be located quickly and easily. Computerized records can be stored on electronic media, such as discs, magnetic tape, or CD-ROM. Magnetic storage media

does not guarantee permanency, however. Computer experts suggest using a permanent-type CD-ROM.

When it has been determined that a medical record has met all requirements (state and federal) for disposal, this process should be done according to state statute. Typically, the rule of thumb for paper record disposal is a shredding process. It is unacceptable merely to discard paper records in a trash bin because of security violations. Records kept on magnetic media can be erased or deleted.

What Did You Learn?

1. What is the time limit for filing Medicaid claims?
2. Name the types of providers that might require a copayment.
3. Preauthorization is always needed for what types of Medicaid services?

FRAUD AND ABUSE IN THE MEDICAID SYSTEM

Fraud is an intentional misrepresentation or deception that could result in an unauthorized benefit to an individual or individuals and usually comes in the form of a false statement requesting payment under the Medicaid program. Abuse typically involves payment for items or services in which there was no intent to deceive or misrepresent, but the outcome of poor and inefficient methods results in unnecessary costs to the Medicaid program.

Know 5 of these

WHAT IS MEDICAID FRAUD?

Medicaid fraud occurs when a healthcare provider, such as a physician, dentist, pharmacist, hospital, nursing home, or other healthcare service, engages in one or more of the following practices:

- Billing for medical services not actually performed
- Billing for a more expensive service than was rendered
- Billing separately for several services that should be combined into one billing
- Billing twice for the same medical service
- Dispensing generic drugs and billing for brand name drugs
- Giving or accepting something in return for medical services (kickbacks)
- Bribery
- Providing unnecessary services
- False cost reports
- Billing for ambulance runs when no medical service is provided
- Transporting multiple passengers in an ambulance and billing a run for each passenger

Medicaid fraud and abuse drive up healthcare costs for everyone. The health insurance professional should contact the Attorney General's Medicaid Fraud Control Unit if he or she has evidence of or suspects a healthcare provider (or patient) is committing Medicaid fraud.

PATIENT ABUSE AND NEGLECT

Frequent unexplained injuries or complaints of pain without obvious injury can be indicators of patient abuse and neglect, such as the following:

- Burns or bruises suggesting the use of instruments or cigarettes
- Passive, withdrawn, and emotionless behavior
- Lack of reaction to pain
- Sexually transmitted diseases or injury to the genital area
- Difficulty in sitting or walking
- Fear of being alone with caretakers
- Obvious malnutrition
- Lack of personal cleanliness
- Habitually dressed in torn or dirty clothes
- Obvious fatigue and listlessness
- Begs for food or water
- In need of medical or dental care
- Left unattended for long periods
- Bedsores and skin lesions

Imagine This!

Superior Ambulance Company transports patients from the Coast View Convalescent Home to a nearby medical center. The vehicles are equipped to carry four patients at a time. Shirley Holmes, whose father (a Medicaid recipient) resides at Coast View, received a bill for $800 for an emergency transport. She was with her father at the time of transport and noted that two other residents were occupants of the ambulance at the same time her father was taken to the medical center. Mrs. Holmes discussed the charge with Coast View's administrator, and it was discovered that the ambulance company, rather than splitting the cost of the transport among the three patients who were transported on that run, charged each patient the entire $800 fee.

● Stop and Think

Martin Roble received a prescription for a medication that was to be filled using a generic product. The pharmacist filled the prescription with generic drugs, according to Medicaid rules, but charged Medicaid for the more expensive brand name medication. Would this be considered fraud or abuse?

● Stop and Think

Velma Norton, a health insurance professional working at Klark Rehabilitation Center, noticed that several of the residents wore the same torn clothing every day, and many of them smelled of stale urine. Are these situations indicators of abuse? If so, what should Velma do?

The health insurance professional should learn how to recognize fraud and abuse and do everything possible to prevent it. There is a Medicaid Fraud Control Unit in every state, which is a federally funded state law enforcement entity located in the State Attorney General's office. In addition to investigating fraud committed by healthcare providers, the Medicaid Fraud Control Unit also investigates the abuse, neglect, and exploitation of elderly, ill, and disabled residents of long-term care facilities, such as nursing homes, facilities for the mentally and physically disabled, and assisted living facilities. The investigation of corruption in the administration of the Medicaid program is another important responsibility of the Medicaid Fraud Control Unit. To report fraud or abuse, health insurance professionals may use the state's hotline number or contact the Medicaid Fraud Control Unit nearest them.

Extensive information on Medicaid fraud and abuse can be found on the CMS website. At the CMS home page, click on "Medicaid" under the heading "CMS programs and Information." Under the topic "Medicaid Fraud and Abuse" (on the next screen), click on "Fraud and Abuse for Professionals." Here you will find a related link for state contacts, which will give you information as to how to contact individual state's Medicaid Fraud Control Units.

What Did You Learn?

1. What is the difference between fraud and abuse?
2. What should the health insurance professional do when fraud or abuse is suspected?

SUMMARY CHECK POINTS

☑ Medicaid is a combination federal and state medical assistance program designed to provide medical care for low-income individuals and families, specifically children, pregnant women, the elderly, the disabled, and parents with dependent children.

☑ The federal government establishes broad national guidelines for Medicaid eligibility and contributes approximately 50% of the Medicaid cost to the individual states.

☑ Each state can set its own guidelines regarding Medicaid eligibility standards, services, benefits packages, payment rates, and program administration within the broader federal guidelines. To be eligible for federal funds, however, states are required to provide Medicaid coverage for certain individuals who receive federally assisted income-maintenance payments and for related groups not receiving cash payments. In addition to the federally mandated programs, states can have additional "state-only" programs, but these programs do not receive federal funds.

☑ The two major groups that qualify for Medicaid are the categorically needy and the medically needy. The categorically needy group includes individuals who are eligible for a cash benefit under the SSI program or who meet Family Medical guidelines. Children and pregnant women who have incomes that fall below certain poverty level guidelines also are classified within this group. The medically needy group includes individuals who do not qualify in the categorically needy program (because of excess income or resources), but need help to pay for excessive medical expenses. To qualify for the medically needy group, individuals must spend down their financial assets.

☑ As a general rule, Medicaid pays only for services that are determined to be medically necessary. For a procedure or service to be considered medically necessary, it typically must be consistent with the diagnosis and in accordance with the standards of good medical practice, performed at the proper level, and provided in the most appropriate setting.

☑ Medicaid eligibility can be verified in the following ways:
- Patient's Medicaid ID card
- AVR system, which uses a touch-tone phone process
- EDI, an electronic method that involves online interactive clearinghouses
- Point-of-sale device, in which eligibility information is contained on a magnetic strip similar to a credit card
- Computer software programs, which involves keying patient information into a computer

☑ In insurance terms, a third party is an individual, entity, or a program that, although not directly involved in the implied contract between patient and provider, plays a role in the health insurance claim process—typically paying for a portion of the medical expenses incurred. Medicaid, by law, is the "payer of last resort." Claims must be sent to any third parties involved, and the third parties must meet their legal obligation to pay the claims before Medicaid is billed. Third parties in this case typically would include
- employment-related health insurance,
- court-ordered health insurance by noncustodial parents,
- workers' compensation,
- long-term care insurance, and
- other state and federal programs, such as Medicare

☑ Some of common Medicaid billing errors include
- incorrect patient ID numbers,
- incorrect diagnosis/procedure codes,
- incorrect dates of service format,
- omitting a charge (there must be one for each line of service),
- incorrect billing date, and
- incorrect signature.

☑ Every time a claim is sent to Medicaid, a document is generated explaining how the claim was adjudicated, or how the payment was determined. In the past, this document was referred to as the explanation of benefits; however, Medicaid now calls it the RA. The RA can be in paper or electronic form (if the medical facility is set up to accept the standard electronic version) and contains information from one or several claims. The RA typically contains "remark codes" and "reason codes," which the health insurance professional must be able to understand to interpret and reconcile this document with patient records.

☑ Medicaid fraud occurs when a healthcare provider, such as a physician, dentist, pharmacist, hospital, nursing home, or other healthcare service, deliberately engages in illegal or deceptive practices. Abuse, although not as serious as fraud, also is a growing problem in Medicaid programs. There are countless ways that Medicaid fraud and abuse can occur, and the health insurance professional should learn to recognize fraud perpetrated by the provider and the patient. To report fraud or abuse, the health insurance professional should use the state's hotline number or contact the Medicaid Fraud Control Unit.

CLOSING SCENARIO

When they first began the chapter, Nela and Berta felt as if they were on a ship heading into uncharted waters. Looking over the chapter objectives and terms left them feeling more than slightly apprehensive. There was so much to learn; however, the study plan they laid out before starting Chapter 8 was to "bite off one chunk at a time," which worked well for them in understanding the concepts presented. In addition to what was in the in the chapter, they frequently visited the CMS website for more detailed information. Additionally, they consulted the Medicaid website in their state to become knowledgeable about their individual state's regulations.

Berta, because her mother-in-law was currently in a nursing home, was particularly interested in learning about the "spend down" process, which apparently her mother-in-law went through to become eligible for Medicaid. Nela's interest was in the area of programs for women and children because of her own situation. By now, the women have had enough experience with completing the CMS-1500 claim that they had few problems filling out the blocks for typical Medicaid cases. Understanding the Medicaid remittance advice proved to be more of a challenge, however, and the women admitted that it might take additional experience before they acquired the necessary skill to become efficient. Their instructor assured them that this skill would come with time. It was becoming apparent that a career as a health insurance professional was going to be interesting and rewarding, albeit challenging.

WEBSITES TO EXPLORE

For live links to the following websites, please visit the Evolve® site at http://evolve.elsevier.com/Beik/today/

- To learn about the Medicaid program, visit the website for the Centers of Medicare and Medicaid Services at http://www.cms.hhs.gov/

- To learn about the Medicaid program in your state, log on to http://cms.hhs.gov/medicaid/consumer.asp, and select the applicable state site

- To find out what the TANF program is called in your state, log on to http://www.acf.hhs.gov/programs/ofa/tnfnames.htm

- For state-by-state Medicaid descriptions and plans, research the following website: http://64.82.65.67/medicaid/states.html

- To learn the specific guidelines for the Medicaid programs offered in a particular state, log on to: http://www.cms.hhs.gov/medicaid/consumer.asp, and insert the name of the state in the "select state" box.

- For complete information on the Medicare Prescription Drug, Improvement, and Modernization Act of 2003, log on to http://www.cms.hhs.gov/mmu/default.asp

- The CMS website provides extensive information on third-party liability, cost avoidance, and collection, at http://www.cms.hhs.gov/ThirdPartyLiability

- To learn more about SSI benefits, countable income, and exclusions for the SSI program, log on to www.socialsecurity.gov

- For updates on SSI benefits, log on to www.socialsecurity.gov/pubs/10003.pdf

Chapter 9

Conquering Medicare's Challenges

Chapter Outline

CHAPTER OBJECTIVES

After completion of this chapter, the student should be able to
- Describe the Medicare program and its structure.
- Explain Medicare Parts A, B, C, and D.
- List and discuss Medicare Combination Coverages (Medi-Medi, Medigap, and Medicare Secondary Policy).
- List the advantages and disadvantages of Medicare health maintenance organizations.
- Explain how Medicare determines "medically necessary" services.
- Discuss the purpose of the advance beneficiary notice and determine when it should be used.
- Discuss how to determine correct charges based on the Medicare fee schedule.
- Explain the Medicare "Crossover" Program and how it affects claims submission.
- Define *small providers* and their exemption from filing claims electronically.
- Define the Medicare Summary Notice and discuss what information it contains.
- Explain a Medicare remittance advice and how the health insurance professional uses the information it contains.
- Define electronic remittance advice and explain who can use it and how it works.
- Explain the function and purpose of electronic funds transfer.
- Explain the purpose of quality review studies.
- Define CLIA and explain its function.

CHAPTER TERMS

adjudicated
advanced beneficiary notice (ABN)
allowable charges
beneficiary
benefit period
biologicals
claims adjustment reason codes
Clinical Laboratory Improvement Act (CLIA)
coordination of benefits contractor
coverage requirements
credible coverage
crosswalks
demand bills
denial notice
donut hole
downcoding
dual eligibles
electronic Medicare Summary Notice (MSN)
electronic remittance advice (ERA)
electronic funds transfer (EFT)
end-stage renal disease (ESRD)
Federal Insurance Contribution Act (FICA)
health insurance claim number (HICN)
Health Care Quality Improvement Program

health maintenance organization (HMO) with point-of-service (POS) option
initial claims
lifetime (one-time) release of information form
local coverage decisions (LCDs)
local medical review policies (LMRPs)
mandated Medigap transfer
medically necessary
Medicare
Medicare Beneficiary Protection Program
Medicare gaps
Medicare HMOs
Medicare limiting charge
Medicare managed care plan
Medicare nonparticipating provider (nonPAR)
Medicare participating provider (PAR)
Medicare Part A
Medicare Part A fiscal intermediary (FI)
Medicare Part B
Medicare Part B carrier
Medicare Part B Crossover Program
Medicare Part C (Medicare Advantage Plans)

Medicare Part D
(Prescriptions Drug
Plan)
Medicare Secondary
Payer (MSP)
Medicare Summary
Notice (MSN)
Medicare supplement
policy
Medigap insurance
Medi-Medi
network
noncovered services
open enrollment period
peer review
organization (PRO)
Program of All-inclusive
Care for the Elderly
(PACE)

prospective payment
system (PPS)
provider sponsored
organization (PSO)
quality improvement
organizations
quality review study
remittance remark
codes
resource-based
relative value system
self-referring
standard paper
remittance advice
(SPRA)
trading partner
agreement

OPENING SCENARIO

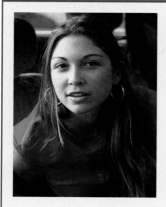

Rita Thomas, a high school dropout, attended an alternative high school to earn her general education diploma (GED). A single mother of a 3-year-old son, Rita lives with her grandmother and works as a waitress in a neighborhood bar and grill. Grandma Nan, as Rita calls her, encourages her granddaughter to enroll in night classes at the local community college. The evening schedule works well because Rita can keep her day job and Grandma Nan is available to babysit for her. Rita signs up for a health insurance course.

"Learn as much as you can about Medicare and then you can explain it all to me," Grandma Nan implores. "It's all so confusing." Encouraged by her grandmother's request, Rita enthusiastically begins her pursuit of "conquering Medicare's challenges." Up to now, Medicare was just a word to Rita without much meaning. She had heard Grandma Nan and her elderly friends discussing it many times, but Rita paid little attention. She was aware, however, that these women did not understand Medicare's whole picture. Now Rita has an opportunity to do something not only for herself, but also for her grandmother who has done so much for her.

MEDICARE PROGRAM

Medicare, a comprehensive federal insurance program, was established by Congress in 1966 to provide individuals age 65 and older financial assistance with medical expenses. In 1972, the Medicare program was expanded to include certain categories of disabled individuals younger than age 65 and individuals of any age who have **end-stage renal disease (ESRD)**, permanent kidney disorders requiring dialysis or transplant (Fig. 9-1). Medicare is administered by the Center for Medicare and Medicaid

Services (CMS), formerly called Healthcare Financing Administration (HCFA). CMS is a division of the Department of Health and Human Services and is based on laws enacted by Congress.

The **Federal Insurance Contributions Act (FICA)** provides for a federal system of old age, survivors, disability, and hospital insurance. The old age, survivors, and disability insurance part is financed by Social Security taxes. The hospital insurance part of Medicare is funded through taxes withheld from employees' wages. In 2006, the individual Medicare contribution rate (amount with-

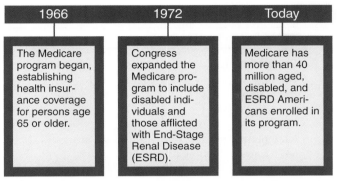

1966	1972	Today
The Medicare program began, establishing health insurance coverage for persons age 65 or older.	Congress expanded the Medicare program to include disabled individuals and those afflicted with End-Stage Renal Disease (ESRD).	Medicare has more than 40 million aged, disabled, and ESRD Americans enrolled in its program.

Fig. 9-1 The Medicare program. (Modified from Centers for Medicare and Medicaid: *World of Medicare*. 2005. Available at http://cms.meridianksi.com/kc/ilc/scorm_course_launch_frm.asp.)

held from wages) was 1.45%. Employers must contribute a matching percentage for a total contribution of 2.9%. All wages are subject to the Medicare tax; there is no wage base limit.

Medicare is not provided free of charge. Medicare requires cost sharing in the form of premiums, deductibles, and coinsurance, all of which are discussed in this chapter.

MEDICARE PROGRAM STRUCTURE

Medicare is composed of four parts:
- **Medicare Part A**—hospital insurance
- **Medicare Part B**—medical (physicians' care) insurance (original Medicare)
- **Medicare Part C**—Medicare Advantage (managed care–type plans, formerly Medicare+Choice)
- **Medicare Part D**—prescription drug program

Medicare Part A

Medicare Part A (hospital insurance) helps pay for services for the following types of healthcare (Table 9-1):
- Inpatient hospital care (including critical access hospitals)
- Inpatient care in a skilled nursing facility (SNF)
- Home healthcare
- Hospice care
- Blood

Medicare Part A does not cover custodial or long-term care.

Coverage requirements under Medicare state that for a service to be covered, it must be considered **medically necessary**—reasonable and necessary for the diagnosis or treatment of an illness or injury or to improve the functioning of a malformed body part.

Noncovered services are situations in which an item or service is not covered under Medicare and include, but are not limited to, the following:
- Program exclusions as designated by CMS
- Medical devices or **biologicals** (drugs or medicinal preparations obtained from animal tissue or other organic

sources) that have not been approved by the Food and Drug Administration
- Items and services that are determined to be investigational in nature

Medicare Part A is free to any individual age 65 or older who is
- eligible to receive monthly Social Security benefits or
- eligible based on wages on which sufficient Medicare payroll taxes were paid.

Medicare Part A also is free to any disabled individual younger than age 65 who has
- received Social Security disability benefits for 24 months as a worker, surviving spouse, or adult child of a retired, disabled, or deceased worker or
- accumulated a sufficient number of Social Security credits to be insured for Medicare and meets the requirements of the Social Security disability program.

A **beneficiary** (an individual who has health insurance through the Medicare or Medicaid program) automatically qualifies for Part A if he or she was a federal employee on January 1, 1983.

Application for Medicare Part A is automatic when an individual applies for Social Security benefits. A husband or wife also may qualify for Part A coverage at age 65, based on the spouse's eligibility for Social Security. If an individual is not eligible for free Part A, he or she may purchase this coverage.

The **Medicare Part A fiscal intermediary (FI)**, a private organization that contracts with Medicare to pay Part A and some Part B bills, determines payment to Part A facilities for covered items and services provided by the facility.

Medicare Part B

Medicare Part B is medical insurance financed by a combination of federal government funds and beneficiary premiums, which helps pay for the following:
- Medically necessary physicians' services
- Outpatient hospital services
- Clinical laboratory services
- Durable medical equipment (DME) (to qualify as DME, it must be ordered by a physician for use in the home and items must be reusable, e.g., walkers, wheelchairs, or hospital beds)
- Blood (received as an outpatient)

| TABLE 9-1 | Medicare Part A Covered Services and Costs |

COVERED SERVICES	WHAT BENEFICIARY PAYS
Hospital Stays Semiprivate rooms, meals, general nursing, and other hospital services and supplies (but not private duty nursing, a television or telephone in the room, or a private room unless medically necessary)	*For each benefit period:* $952 for hospital stay of 1-60 days $238 per day for days 61-90 of hospital stay $476 for each lifetime reserve day* All costs for each day beyond 150 days
SNF Care† Semiprivate rooms, meals, skilled nursing and rehabilitative services, and other services and supplies	*For each benefit period:* Nothing for the first 20 days Up to $119.00 per day for days 21-100 All costs beyond the 100th day in the benefit period
Home Health Care† Intermittent skilled nursing care, physical therapy, occupational therapy, speech language pathology services, home health aide services, DME (e.g., wheelchairs, hospital beds, oxygen, and walkers) and supplies, and other services	*The beneficiary pays:* Nothing for approved home health care services 20% of approved amount for DME (e.g., wheelchairs, hospital beds, oxygen, and walkers)
Hospice Care† Pain and symptom relief and supportive services for the care of a terminal illness Home care is provided. Also covers necessary inpatient care and a variety of services otherwise not covered by Medicare	*The beneficiary pays:* Limited costs for outpatient drugs and inpatient respite care (care given to a hospice patient so that the usual caregiver can rest)
Blood From a hospital or SNF during a covered stay	*The beneficiary pays* For the first 3 pints of blood

*A beneficiary has 60 lifetime reserve days that may only be used once. For each reserve day, Medicare pays all covered costs except for a daily coinsurance.
†The beneficiary must meet certain conditions for Medicare to cover these services.
Benefit period—Starts the day a beneficiary is admitted to a hospital or SNF and ends when the individual has not received hospital inpatient or SNF care for 60 consecutive days.
(From the Centers for Medicare and Medicaid Services.)

If a beneficiary became eligible for Medicare on or after January 1, 2005, Medicare covers a "Welcome to Medicare" one-time physical examination if it is performed within the first 6 months of coverage, if that individual has Part B. Part B also can help pay for many other medical services and supplies that are not covered by Part A and home healthcare if the beneficiary is not enrolled in Medicare Part A. Medicare now covers some preventive healthcare services, such as

- bone mass measurements;
- colorectal cancer screening;
- diabetes services;
- glaucoma testing;
- Pap tests, pelvic examinations, and clinical breast examinations;
- prostate cancer screening;
- screening mammograms; and
- certain vaccinations.

Table 9-2 lists additional services and supplies that Medicare Part B helps pay for and services not covered by Part B.

All Medicare Part B beneficiaries pay for Part B coverage. In 2006, the Part B monthly premium was $88.50. This premium is deducted from the beneficiary's monthly Social Security benefits check.

The health insurance professional should become familiar with Medicare's guidelines to determine if a specific procedure or service is covered. The *Websites to Explore* at the end of this chapter provide several Internet links to follow for additional help and information.

TABLE 9-2	Services and Supplies Medicare Part B Helps Pay for and Services not Covered by Part B
ITEMS MEDICARE PART B HELPS PAY FOR*	**SERVICES NOT COVERED BY MEDICARE PART B†**
Ambulance services	Acupuncture
Certain chiropractic services	Cosmetic surgery
Clinical trials	Custodial care
Diabetic self-management training	Deductibles, coinsurance/copayments
Diabetic supplies (except syringes/insulin)	Dental care/dentures
Diagnostic tests	Eye refractions
DME	Healthcare received outside United States
Emergency department services	Hearing aids/hearing examinations (for the purpose of fitting a hearing aid)
Eyeglasses (limited coverage)	Hearing tests (other than for fitting a hearing aid)
Foot examinations/treatment	Long-term care (custodial care in a nursing home)
Hearing/balance examinations	Orthopedic shoes
Kidney dialysis services	Prescription drugs
Long-term care (skilled care)	Routine foot care
Medical nutrition therapy	Routine eye care and most eyeglasses
Mental health care	Routine physical examinations (Medicare covers a one-time examination for new enrollees)
Practitioner services	Screen tests
Prescription drugs (limited, such as injectable cancer drugs)	Shots/vaccinations (except flu shots)
Prosthetic/orthotic items	Some diabetic supplies
Second surgical opinions	
Smoking cessation counseling	
Surgical dressings	
Telemedicine (in some areas)	
Transplant services	
Travel (limited to specific travel situations outside United States)	
Urgently needed care	

*With certain limitations.
†With certain exceptions.

Similar to a Medicare FI, the **Medicare Part B carrier** determines payment of Part B covered items and services. A Medicare Part B carrier is a private company that contracts with CMS to provide claims processing and payment for Medicare Part B services. The local Medicare carrier also has the ability and authority to designate an item or service as noncovered for its service area or jurisdiction. For a complete list of all noncovered items or services for your state, contact your local Medicare carrier.

ENROLLMENT

Before an individual reaches age 65, he or she must decide whether to enroll in Medicare Part A or Part B or both. If eligible beneficiaries want Medicare coverage to start the month they reach age 65, they should contact their local Social Security office 3 months before their 65th birthday. If they decide not to sign up for Medicare until after their 65th birthday, the Medicare Part B effective date is delayed.

If individuals do not sign up for Medicare Part B when first becoming eligible and later decide to enroll, the monthly premiums are 10% higher than the basic premium for each 12-month period they were eligible to enroll but did not. An eligible beneficiary may delay enrollment without a penalty or a waiting period, however, if the individual was still employed and covered by an employer's group health plan at the time he or she first became eligible for Medicare benefits. Individuals who do not enroll within the 3-month period before becoming age 65 must wait and enroll during the general enrollment period, which is January 1 through March 31 of each year. Medicare Part B coverage becomes effective on July 1 of that year.

PREMIUMS AND COST-SHARING REQUIREMENTS

Medicare Part B (medical insurance) cost-sharing requirements include a monthly premium ($88.50 in 2006). This premium, which is automatically deducted from the beneficiary's monthly Social Security check, is subject to change every year. The second cost-sharing requirement in Medicare Part B is an annual deductible of $124 (2006), after which Medicare pays 80% of **allowable charges**.

Allowable charges are the fees Medicare permits for a particular service or supply. Table 9-3 summarizes the Medicare Part B cost-sharing amounts for various types of services.

A **benefit period** is the duration of time during which a Medicare beneficiary is eligible for Part A benefits for services incurred in a hospital or SNF or both. A benefit period begins the day an individual is admitted to a hospital or SNF. The benefit period ends when the beneficiary has not received care in a hospital or SNF for 60 days in a row. If the beneficiary is readmitted to the hospital or SNF before the 60 days elapse, it is considered to be in the same benefit period. If the beneficiary is admitted to a hospital or SNF after the initial 60-day benefit period has ended, a new benefit period begins. The inpatient hospital deductible must be paid for each benefit period, but there is no limit to the number of benefit periods allowed.

As mentioned previously, Part A is free for individuals who have worked enough quarters to qualify (>40). For 30 to 39 quarters of Social Security work credit, the monthly premium is $216, and for less than 30 quarters of Social Security work credit, the monthly premium is $393. Individuals who enroll after the open enrollment period must pay a 10% premium surcharge for late enrollment.

MEDICARE PART C (MEDICARE ADVANTAGE PLANS)

The Balanced Budget Act of 1997, which went into effect in January 1999, expanded the role of private plans under Medicare+Choice to include preferred provider organizations (PPOs), **provider-sponsored organizations (PSOs)**, private fee-for-service plans, and medical savings accounts (MSAs) coupled with high-deductible insurance plans. The Medicare Prescription Drug, Improvement, and Modernization Act of 2003 renamed the program "Medicare Advantage" and created another option: regional PPOs.

Medicare Advantage plans (formerly Medicare+Choice) are prepaid healthcare plans that offer regular Medicare Parts A and B coverage in addition to *coverage* for other services. Under Medicare Part C, individuals who are eligible for Medicare Parts A and B can choose to get their Medicare benefits through a variety of plans (see previously), with the exception of individuals with ESRD. The primary Medicare Part C plans include the following:

- *Medicare managed care plans,* such as health maintenance organizations (HMOs), PSOs, PPOs, and other certified public or private coordinated care plans that meet the standards under the Medicare law.
- *Medicare private, unrestricted fee-for-service plans* that allow beneficiaries to select certain private providers.

TABLE 9-3	Medicare Part B Covered Services and Costs	
COVERED SERVICES	**WHAT BENEFICIARY PAYS**	
Medical Expenses	$124 deductible (pay once per year)	
Physician services; inpatient and outpatient medical and surgical services and supplies; physical, occupational, and speech therapy; diagnostic tests; and DME	20% of approved amount after the deductible except in the outpatient setting	
	50% for most outpatient mental health	
	20% for all outpatient physical, occupational, and speech-language services	
Clinical Laboratory Service	Nothing for approved services	
Blood tests, urinalysis		
Home Health Care	Nothing for approved services	
Intermittent skilled care, home health aide services, DME and supplies, and other services	20% of approved amount for DME	
Outpatient Hospital Services	Coinsurance or fixed copayment amount, which may vary according to service	
Services for the diagnosis or treatment of an illness or injury		
Blood	For the first 3 pints plus 20% of approved amount for additional pints (after the deductible)	
As an outpatient, or as part of a Part B covered service		

Note: Actual amounts the beneficiary must pay for coinsurance are higher if the provider does not accept assignment.
(From the Centers for Medicare and Medicaid Services.)

These providers must accept the plan's payment terms and conditions.

• *MSA plans* that allow beneficiaries to enroll in a plan with a high deductible. After the deductible is met, the MSA plan pays providers. Money remaining in the MSA can be used to pay for future medical care, including some services not usually covered by Medicare Part A and Part B, such as dentures.

Medicare Part C coverage not only includes Part A and Part B coverage, but also pays for services not covered under the original Medicare plan, such as

• preventive care,
• prescription drugs,
• eyeglasses,
• dental care, and
• hearing aids

For a Medicare beneficiary to qualify for one of these Medicare Advantage options, he or she must be eligible for Medicare Parts A and B and live in the service area of the plan. Generally, an individual is not eligible to elect a Medicare Advantage plan if he or she has been diagnosed with ESRD. There are exceptions to this eligibility rule, however, such as individuals who are already members of a Medicare Advantage plan when they develop ESRD and individuals who received a kidney transplant and no longer require a regular course of dialysis treatments.

MEDICARE PART D (MEDICARE PRESCRIPTION DRUG BENEFIT PLAN)

The Medicare Prescription Drug Improvement and Modernization Act of 2003, signed into law in December 2003, introduced significant changes to the Medicare program. Included in the Act is the new Medicare Part D coverage for prescription drugs. On January 1, 2006, this revised Medicare plan went into effect.

The main change in this plan is that all Medicare beneficiaries are asked to choose a prescription drug plan to help offset the increasing cost of prescription drugs. If they enroll in Medicare Part D, they pay an additional premium (which can be deducted from their monthly Social Security check). Premiums range from $2 to $100, depending on the plan, with a national average of approximately $35. Individual plans offer varying benefits; however, each must offer no less than the basic Medicare coverage referred to as "credible coverage." Under Medicare's basic benefits, each year, Medicare beneficiaries pay up to $250 in prescription drug costs out of their own pocket (deductible). For the next $2000 in drug costs, Medicare pays 75% ($1500), and the Medicare beneficiary pays 25% ($500). After that, the Medicare beneficiary is responsible for all prescription drug expenses until a total of $3600 is spent out-of-pocket. (This period of noncoverage is referred to as the "donut hole.") After yearly prescription drug expenditures reach this limit, Medicare pays 95% of the

beneficiary's prescription drug costs. Medicare beneficiaries still must pay a 5% copayment.

Individuals qualifying for Medicare and Medicaid benefits (**dual eligibles**, sometimes referred to as **Medi-Medi**) who receive the full Medicaid benefits package lose their prescription drug coverage under Medicaid, but can enroll in the Medicare Part D Prescription Drug Benefit Plan. Medicare pays the $250 Part D deductible for all dual eligibles and their monthly premiums, if they enroll in an average or low-cost Part D plan. These subsidies eliminate the gap in coverage for dual eligibles that Medicare beneficiaries who do not qualify for Medicare and Medicaid face. Dual eligibles are responsible, however, for small copays ranging from $1 to $5. Dual eligibles residing in nursing homes or other institutions are exempt from copays because they already are contributing all but a small portion of their income to the cost of their nursing home care.

Although the new law shifts drug coverage for dual eligibles from Medicaid to Medicare, there is no provision for providing full financial assistance to states. States are required to pay for most of the cost of providing the Medicare Part D prescription drug benefit to dual eligibles through payments to the federal government. Under the new bill, states are not allowed to use federal Medicaid matching funds to supplement prescription drug coverage for dual eligibles under Part D plans. A state can choose, however, to use state-only funds to offset the cost of the prescription drug benefit.

Medicare Part D basic plan includes the following guidelines for all Medicare beneficiaries:

• An average of $35 per month premium, which is in addition to the monthly Medicare Part B premium
• $250 annual deductible (for 2006)
• 25% coinsurance up to $2250 per year in out-of-pocket expenses
• No coverage for $2251 through $5100 in out-of-pocket expenses (the donut hole)
• "Catastrophic coverage" from $5100 with 5% copayment (for 2006)

Many plans offer more comprehensive coverage.

PROGRAM OF ALL-INCLUSIVE CARE FOR THE ELDERLY

The **Program of All-inclusive Care for the Elderly (PACE)** provides community-based acute and long-term care services. A multidisciplinary team composed of a physician, nurse, therapists (physical, occupational, or recreational), dietitian, social worker, home care coordinator, and transportation supervisor completes an initial and semiannual assessment of each participant with a documented plan of treatment. Most services are provided at a licensed day activity center. Participants must accept the PACE organization and its contractors as their only service provider for all Medicaid and Medicare services. PACE is available only in areas where a PACE organization is under contract to deliver services.

To be eligible for the PACE program, an individual must meet the following criteria:

- Age 55 or older
- Meet the nursing facility medical need criteria
- Live in a area serviced by a PACE organization
- Be safely served in the community according to the PACE organization

To be eligible for PACE Medicaid, the following criteria must be met:

- Be eligible for supplemental security income benefits
- Have been eligible for Medicaid as a result of protective coverage mandated by federal law
- Be eligible for Medicaid benefits if institutionalized

What Did You Learn?

1. What are Medicare's two *primary* parts?
2. Name four common services Medicare B does not cover.
3. What are Medicare's cost-sharing requirements?
4. What type of service does Medicare Advantage cover that fee-for-service Medicare does not?
5. List the eligibility requirements for PACE.

MEDICARE COMBINATION COVERAGES

Because Medicare does not cover some services, and there are deductibles and copayments that patients must pay out-of-pocket for most services, beneficiaries often have added health insurance coverage to help with the gaps in Medicare's coverage. This extra coverage can be one of the following:

- Medicare/Medicaid dual eligibility
- Medicare supplement policies
- Medicare Secondary Payer (MSP)

The following sections explain each of these supplemental types of healthcare coverage.

MEDICARE/MEDICAID DUAL ELIGIBILITY

Dual eligibility, as stated earlier, refers to individuals who qualify for benefits under the Medicare and Medicaid programs. Most dual eligibles are low-income elderly and individuals younger than 65 with disabilities. Medicare does not pay for all health services, just basic physician and hospital care. In addition, Medicare beneficiaries have to meet a yearly deductible and pay a monthly premium and a 20% copayment (cost sharing) for all covered services. Dual eligibles rely on Medicaid to pay Medicare premiums and cost-sharing expenses and to pay for the needed benefits Medicare does not cover, such as long-term care.

MEDICARE SUPPLEMENT POLICIES

The traditional Medicare program provides valuable coverage of healthcare needs, but it leaves uninsured areas with which elderly and disabled Americans need additional help. To ensure that they are adequately protected, many seniors purchase a **Medicare supplement policy**. A Medicare supplement policy is a health insurance plan sold by private insurance companies to help pay for healthcare expenses not covered by Medicare and Medicare's deductibles and coinsurance. An individual may qualify for supplemental insurance through an employer-sponsored retirement plan or, more commonly, through a Medigap plan.

Medigap Insurance

Sometimes Medicare supplement policies are referred to as **Medigap insurance**. Medigap insurance is designed specifically to supplement Medicare benefits and is regulated by federal and state law. A Medigap policy must be clearly identified as Medicare supplemental insurance, and it must provide specific benefits that help fill the gaps in Medicare coverage. Other kinds of insurance may help with out-of-pocket healthcare costs, but they do not qualify as Medigap plans.

There are 12 standard Medicare supplement plans called "A" through "L." Each plan has a different set of benefits. Plan "A" is the basic plan, and it has the least amount of benefits. Plan "J" is the most comprehensive. Table 9-4 shows Medigap plans A through L and what each covers.

When an individual buys a Medicare supplement policy, he or she pays a premium to the private insurance company. This premium is above and beyond the Medicare Part B premium. If the individual has a Medicare Advantage plan, it is not necessary to have a Medicare supplement policy because these plans typically include much of the same coverages as Medigap. *Note:* Since the new Medicare D plan became effective in January of 2006, insurance companies are no longer allowed to sell Medicare supplement policies H, I, and J, which include prescription drug coverage.

Standard Medigap Policies. The 12 standard Medigap policies were developed by the National Association of Insurance Commissioners and incorporated into state and federal law. The plans cover specific expenses not covered or not fully covered by Medicare. Insurance companies are not permitted to change the combination of benefits or the letter designations of any of the plans.

All states must allow the sale of plan A, and all Medigap insurers must make plan A available if they are going to sell any Medigap plans in their state. Although not required to offer any of the other plans, most insurers do offer several of these alternate plans to pick from; some offer all 12. Insurers can decide which of the optional plans they will sell as long as the state in which the plans are sold approves.

TABLE 9-4 Twelve Standard Medicare Supplemental Plans

BASIC BENEFITS	PLAN A	PLAN B	PLAN C	PLAN D	PLAN E	PLAN F	PLAN G	PLAN H	PLAN I	PLAN J	PLAN K	PLAN L
Part A Hospital												
Day 61-90 Coinsurance	X	X	X	X	X	X	X	X	X	X	X	X
Day 91-150 Coinsurance	X	X	X	X	X	X	X	X	X	X		
365 more days – 100%	X	X	X	X	X	X	X	X	X	X		
Part B Coinsurance or Copay	X	X	X	X	X	X	X	X	X	X	50%*	75%*
Parts A & B Blood	X	X	X	X	X	X	X	X	X	X	50%	75%
ADDITIONAL BENEFITS	A	B	C	D	E	F	G	H	I	J	K	L
Skilled Nursing Facility Coinsurance Day 21-100			X	X	X	X	X	X	X	X	50%	75%
Part A Deductible		X	X	X	X	X	X	X	X	X	50%	75%
Part B Deductible			X			X				X		
Part B Excess						100%	80%		100%	100%		
Foreign Travel Emergency			X	X	X	X	X	X	X	X		
At-Home Recovery				X			X		X	X		
Preventive Medical Care					X					X		
Out-of-pocket annual limit											$4000	$2000

*Plan K and L pay 100% of Part B coinsurance for preventive services.
(Source: Iowa Medicare Supplemental Premium Comparison Guide, Iowa Insurance Division, 2006.)

Although insurers must offer the same coverage in each plan, they do not have to charge the same premium rates; it is strongly suggested that individuals shop around and compare prices before purchasing a Medigap policy.

Where the Gaps Are. Box 9-1 describes the **Medicare gaps** in various types of care.

What Medigap Plans Cover. Medigap policies pay most, if not all, of the Medicare coinsurance amounts and may provide coverage for Medicare's deductibles. Some standard plans pay for services not covered by Medicare, such as at-home recovery, preventive screening, and emergency medical care while traveling outside the United States. Coverage also is provided in some plans for healthcare provider charges in excess of Medicare's approved amount and for some care in the home.

Eligibility. If an individual enrolls in Medicare Part B when he or she turns 65, federal law forbids insurance companies from denying eligibility for Medigap policies for 6 months. This 6-month period is called the **open enrollment period**. If the individual did not enroll in Medicare Part B when turning 65, he or she can sign up for it later during the yearly general enrollment period—January to March. The individual has a 6-month open enrollment period for Medigap policies beginning July 1 of that year. Individuals who were covered by a group health insurance plan when they turned 65 have a 6-month open enrollment period for Medigap policies beginning

Box 9-1

Medicare Gaps by Care Type

During a hospital stay, Medicare Part A does not pay
- yearly deductible;
- coinsurance amount for each day of hospitalization more than 60 days and up to 90 days for any one benefit period;
- coinsurance amount for each day of hospitalization more than 90 days and up to 150 days, for any one benefit period past a 150-day hospitalization;
- anything past a 150-day hospitalization;
- the cost of 3 pints of blood, unless replaced; or
- medical expenses during foreign travel.

During a stay in a skilled nursing facility, Medicare Part A does not pay
- coinsurance amount for each day in the facility more than 20 days and up to 100 days for any one benefit period or
- anything for a stay of more than 100 days.

For home healthcare, Medicare Part A does not pay
- 20% of the approved cost of DME or approved nonskilled care or
- anything for nonmedical personal care services.

For physicians, clinics, laboratories, therapies, medical supplies, and equipment, Medicare Part B does not pay
- yearly deductible,
- 20% of the Medicare-approved amount,
- 15% above the Medicare-approved amount if provider does not accept assignment,
- preventive or routine examinations and testing, except for the "Welcome to Medicare" exam if received within the first 6 months of eligibility,
- treatment that is not considered medically necessary,
- prescription medication that can be self-administered,
- general dental work,
- routine eye and hearing examinations, or
- glasses or hearing aids.

the date their Part B coverage begins, regardless of when they sign up for it.

Medicare Secondary Payer

MSP is the term used when Medicare is not responsible for paying first because the beneficiary is covered under another insurance policy. The MSP program, enacted in 1980, was created to preserve Medicare funds and to ensure that funds would be available for future generations. Since the program's beginning, a series of federal laws has changed the coordination of benefits provision between Medicare and other insurance carriers. These federal laws take precedence over individual state law and private insurance contracts. For certain categories of individuals, Medicare is the secondary payer regardless of state law or plan provisions. Medicare most likely would be the secondary payer in any of the following situations:

- Workers' compensation (injury or illness that occurred at work)
- Working aged (age >65 years) who are covered by a group health plan through their own or their spouse's current employment
- Disabled individuals age 64 and younger who are covered by a large group health plan (>100 employees) through their own or a family member's current employment
- Medicare beneficiaries with permanent kidney failure covered under a group health plan
- Individuals with black lung disease covered under the Federal Black Lung Program.
- Veterans Administration benefits
- Federal Research Grant Program

It is often the responsibility of the health insurance professional to determine, in cases where the Medicare beneficiary has other insurance coverage, to which third-party payer the CMS-1500 claim is submitted first. Many medical practices use a structured form, such as a MSP questionnaire, to simplify this process. An example MSP questionnaire is shown in Fig. 9-2.

Medicare Secondary Payer Questionnaire

Patient Name: _____   Date: _____

HICN: _____

Medicare law requires that we determine if your medical services might be covered by another insurer. In order to assist us in the correct billing of these services, please answer the following questions:

1. Is your injury/illness due to:
    A. Work-related accident/condition?
        ☐ No
        ☐ Yes, name and address of worker's compensation plan: _____
        _____
        _____
        Policy or ID#: _____
        Accident date: _____

    B. A condition covered under the Federal Black Lung Program?
        ☐ No
        ☐ Yes

    C. An automobile accident?
        ☐ No
        ☐ Yes, name and address of auto insurance: _____
        _____
        _____
        Name of insured: _____
        Policy or ID#: _____
        Accident date: _____ Accident location: _____

    D. An accident other than an automobile accident?
        ☐ No
        ☐ Yes, name and address of no-fault insurer: _____
        _____
        _____
        Name of insured: _____
        Policy or ID#: _____
        Accident date: _____ Accident location: _____

    E. The fault of another party?
        ☐ No
        ☐ Yes, name and address of no-fault insurer: _____
        _____
        _____
        Name of insured: _____
        Policy or ID#: _____
        Accident date: _____ Accident location: _____

DMERC Region D Supplier Manual   *(Rev. 1/2001) Exhibit 1*

Fig. 9-2 MSP questionnaire. (Source: U. S. Department of Health & Human Services, Centers for Medicare & Medicaid Services.)

Medicare Secondary Payer Questionnaire (cont'd)

2. Are you eligible for coverage under the Veterans' Administration?
    ☐ No
    ☐ Yes

3. Are you employed?
    ☐ No. Date of retirement:
    ☐ Yes, employer name and address: _____
    _____

    Do you have employer group health plan coverage?
    ☐ No
    ☐ Yes, insurer name and address: _____
    _____

    Policy #: _____
    Group #: _____

4. Is your spouse employed?
    ☐ No. Date of retirement, if applicable:
    ☐ Yes, spouse's name: _____
    Employer name and address: _____

    Are you covered under your spouse's employer group health plan?
    ☐ No
    ☐ Yes, insurer name and address: _____
    _____

    Policy #: _____
    Group #: _____

5. Are you a dependent covered under a parent's/guardian's employer group health plan?
    ☐ No
    ☐ Yes, employer name and address: _____
    _____

    Insurer name and address: _____
    _____

    Name of insured: _____
    Policy #: _____
    Group #: _____

Thank you for your cooperation in ensuring that your medical services will be billed to the proper insurer(s).

Exhibit 1 (Rev. 1/2001)   *DMERC Region D Supplier Manual*

Fig. 9-2—cont'd

In 2001, the CMS created a separate entity called the **coordination of benefits contractor**. This individual assumes responsibility for nearly all initial MSP development activities formerly performed by Medicare intermediaries and carriers. The main job of the coordination of benefits contractor is to ensure that the information on Medicare's eligibility database regarding other health insurance primary to Medicare is up to date and accurate. The coordination of benefits contractor also handles MSP-related inquiries other than those related to specific claims or recoveries.

The goal of these MSP information-gathering activities is to identify MSP situations quickly, ensuring correct primary and secondary payments by the responsible party. Healthcare providers and other suppliers benefit from this activity because the total payments received for services provided to Medicare beneficiaries are greater when Medicare is a secondary payer to a group health plan than when Medicare is the primary payer. Table 9-5 illustrates the role of the coordination of benefits contractor in various processes.

MEDICARE AND MANAGED CARE

Medicare-eligible individuals have a choice of whether they receive Medicare benefits through traditional Medicare or through a managed care plan. A **Medicare managed care plan** is an HMO or PPO that uses Medicare to pay for part of its services for eligible beneficiaries. Medicare managed care plans fill the gaps in basic Medicare similar to Medigap policies; however, Medicare managed care plans and Medigap policies function differently. Medigap policies work along with Medicare to pay for medical expenses. Medical claims are sent to Medicare and then to a Medigap insurer, and each pays a portion of the approved charges. Medicare managed care plans provide all basic Medicare benefits, plus some additional coverages (depending on the plan) to fill the gaps Medicare does not pay. The extent of coverage beyond Medicare, the size of premiums and copayments, and decisions about paying for treatment all are controlled by the managed care plan itself, not by Medicare.

The basic premise of managed care is that the patient/enrollee agrees to receive care only from an approved list of physicians, hospitals, and other providers—called a **network**—in exchange for reduced overall healthcare costs. There are several types of Medicare managed care plans. Some have tight restrictions concerning members visiting specialists or seeing providers outside the network. Others give members more freedom to choose when they see providers and which providers they may consult for treatment.

Medicare Health Maintenance Organizations

Similar to the structure of the HMOs we learned about in Chapter 7, **Medicare HMOs** maintain a network of physicians and other healthcare providers. The HMO member/enrollee must receive care only from the providers in the network except in emergencies. If a member sees a provider outside the network, the HMO usually pays nothing toward the bill. Because an HMO plan member has technically withdrawn from traditional Medicare by opting to join the managed care organization, Medicare also pays nothing. The result in this case: the plan member must pay the entire bill out-of-pocket.

The HMO is the least expensive and most restrictive Medicare managed care plan; it has four main restrictions:
- Care from network providers only
- All care coordinated through primary care physician
- Prior HMO approval of certain services

TABLE 9-5	Role of the Coordination of Benefits Contractor	
PROCESS	**DESCRIPTION**
First claim development	When a Medicare intermediary or carrier receives the first claim for a Medicare beneficiary, the claim is processed, and a questionnaire is sent to the provider to collect information on the existence of other insurance that may be primary to Medicare
Secondary claim development	When a claim is submitted with an EOB attached from an insurer other than Medicare, a questionnaire is sent to the beneficiary to collect information on the existence of other insurance that may be primary to Medicare
Trauma code development	When a diagnosis appears on a claim that indicates a traumatic accident, injury, or illness, which might form the basis of MSP, a questionnaire is sent to the beneficiary to collect information on the existence of other insurance that may be primary to Medicare
Self-report development	A self-report covers the full spectrum of MSP situations. Any source that contacts the coordination of benefits contractor initiates this type of development process to address these inquiries and to ensure that the information provided is accurate
CFR 411.25	This process confirms MSP information received from a third-party payer

• Limited rights to appeal the plan's decisions (typically limited to appeals outside the HMO or to Medicare).

Health Maintenance Organization with Point-of-Service Option

One type of HMO has a significant modification that makes it more popular, albeit more costly, than the standard HMO plan. This plan offers what is referred to as an **HMO with point-of-service (POS) option**. A member is allowed to see providers who are not in the HMO network and receive services from specialists without first going through a primary care physician. This method is called **self-referring**. When a member does go outside the network or sees a specialist directly, however, the plan pays a smaller portion of the bill than if the member had followed regular HMO procedures. The member pays a higher premium for this plan than for a standard HMO plan and a higher copayment each time the option is used.

Preferred Provider Organization

A PPO works much the same as an HMO with POS option. If a member receives a service from a PPO's network of providers, the cost to the member is lower than if the member sees a provider outside the network. In contrast to an HMO with POS option, a member does not have to go through a primary care physician for referrals to specialists. PPO patients usually are allowed to self-refer to specialists. PPOs tend to be more expensive than standard HMOs, charging a monthly premium and a higher copayment for non-network services. For many individuals, this extra flexibility in selecting the provider of their choice is an important reassurance to them, however, and worth the extra money.

Provider Sponsored Organization

A **PSO** is a group of medical providers—physicians, clinics, and hospitals—that skips the insurance company middleman and contracts directly with patients. As with an HMO, members pay a premium and a copayment each time a service is rendered. Some PSOs in urban areas are large conglomerations of physicians and hospitals that offer a wide choice of providers. Some PSOs are small networks of providers that contract through a particular employer or other large organization or that serve a rural area where no HMO is available.

Advantages and Disadvantages of Medicare Health Maintenance Organizations

As with most areas of healthcare insurance, there are advantages and disadvantages of enrolling in a Medicare HMO.

Advantages.
• HMOs often do not health screen; enrollment may not be denied because of health status.
• HMOs may cover services that traditional Medicare does not cover, such as routine physical examinations, eyeglasses, hearing aids, prescriptions, and dental coverage.
• Enrollees do not need Medigap insurance.
• Paperwork is limited or nonexistent, in contrast to traditional Medicare coverage.
• Enrollees do not have to pay the Medicare deductibles and coinsurance.

Disadvantages.
• Choice of healthcare providers and medical facilities is limited.
• Members/enrollees are covered only for healthcare services received through the HMO except in emergency and urgent care situations.
• Prior approval usually is needed from a primary care physician for a specialist's services, surgical procedures, medical equipment, and other healthcare services.
• Enrollees who travel out of the HMO's service area do not receive coverage except in emergency and urgent care situations.
• If an enrollee decides to switch from the HMO to the traditional Medicare plan, coverage does not begin until the first day of the month after the disenrollment request.

WHY THIS INFORMATION IS IMPORTANT TO THE HEALTH INSURANCE PROFESSIONAL

As a health insurance professional, you will be doing more than sitting at a desk entering data into a computer or at a typewriter filling in the blocks of CMS-1500 forms. In your job, you no doubt will become a liaison between many third-party payers and the entire healthcare team. Additionally, you must be able to answer patients' questions about Medicare accurately. The Medicare program and all its various parts and choices can be very confusing to people, especially the elderly. Although it is important that the health insurance professional learn all the intricacies of the Medicare program from the provider standpoint, he or she also must become an expert from the beneficiaries' perspective. Just the fact alone that the fee-for-service (called *original* or traditional Medicare) plan covers 80% of *allowed charges* is enough to create confusion. When you present an elderly patient with an advanced beneficiary notice (ABN) or begin discussing Medicare's lifetime release of information form you must be prepared to answer questions in layman's language.

Clara Thornton visited her family practice provider for a yearly wellness examination 8 months after becoming eligible for Medicare. When she received the MSN from Medicare, she noticed that Medicare did not pay for the service. Disturbed, she called her daughter, saying, "Medicare is supposed to pay for a Welcome to Medicare exam. Why didn't they pay this?" Together they read through the beneficiary booklet "Medicare & You" that Medicare had sent to Clara when she enrolled. Only then did she learn that Medicare pays for a one-time physical examination, but it must be within 6 months of becoming eligible for Part B.

What Did You Learn?

1. What categories of people make up the "dual eligible" classification?
2. How does Medicaid assist Medicare beneficiaries?
3. List two types of Medicare supplement policies.
4. What do most Medigap plans cover?
5. Name four payers that typically would be primary to Medicare.

PREPARING FOR THE MEDICARE PATIENT

When a Medicare beneficiary comes to the office for an appointment, the procedure for handling the encounter is basically the same as with non-Medicare patients with a few exceptions.

MEDICARE'S LIFETIME RELEASE OF INFORMATION FORM

The medical facility should maintain a current release of information for every patient. Among other things, this allows the health insurance professional to complete and submit the insurance form legally. Typically, a release of information is valid only for 1 year; however, with Medicare, a **lifetime (one-time) release of information form** may be signed by the beneficiary, eliminating the necessity of annual updates. Fig. 9-3 is an example of a lifetime release of information.

DETERMINING MEDICAL NECESSITY

Before Medicare pays for a service or procedure, it must be determined if it is medically necessary. To meet

Medicare's definition of medical necessity, the service or procedure must meet the following criteria:
- Consistent with the symptoms or diagnosis of the illness or injury being treated
- Necessary and consistent with generally accepted professional medical standards
- Not furnished primarily for the convenience of the patient or physician
- Furnished at the most appropriate level that can be provided safely to the patient

CMS has the power under the Social Security Act to determine if the method of treating a patient in a particular case is reasonable and necessary on a case-by-case basis. Even if a service is reasonable and necessary, coverage may be limited if the service is provided more frequently than allowed under a national coverage policy, a local medical policy, or a clinically accepted standard of practice.

Imagine This!

Arlene Sorensen had been told by her gynecologist when she was younger that it was important to receive a Pap smear every year. After she became eligible for Medicare, she told her family practice provider that she wanted to continue this practice. The first Pap smear was covered by Medicare; however, a subsequent Pap smear a year later was not. When she questioned her physician, he referred her to the health insurance professional, who informed Mrs. Sorensen that Medicare only considers Pap smears "medically necessary" every 2 years, unless the patient is considered high risk.

Claims for services that are not medically necessary are denied, but not getting paid is not the only risk. If Medicare or other payers determine that services were medically unnecessary *after* payment already has been made, it is treated as an *overpayment*, and the beneficiary is asked to refund the money, with interest. If a pattern of such claims is evident, and the provider knows or should have known that the services were not medically necessary, the provider may face large monetary penalties, exclusion from the Medicare program, and possibly criminal prosecution.

One of the most common reasons for denial of Medicare claims is that the provider did not know the services provided were not medically necessary. Lack of knowledge is not a defense, however, because a general notice to the medical community from CMS or a carrier (including a Medicare report or special bulletin) that a certain service is not covered is considered sufficient notice. If a provider was on Medicare's mailing list as of the publication date, CMS considers it sufficient evidence to establish that the

---

LIFETIME AUTHORIZATION AND REQUEST FOR MEDICAL INFORMATION

I hereby release Charles H. Shaw M.D., P.A. DBA Gainesville Orthopaedic Group to release my records to the physician individual I direct verbally or in writing.

RELEASE OF MEDICAL INFORMATION
I, the below named patient, hereby authorize Charles H. Shaw, M.D./D. Troy Trimble, D.O. Gainesville Orthopaedic Group to release to my referring physician and/or family physician and any third party payer (such as an insurance company or government agency, e.g. Blue Cross or Medicare) any medical information and records concerning my treatment when requested or by such third party payer or other entity for use in connection with making or determining claim payment for such treatment and/or diagnosis.

ASSIGNMENT OF BENEFITS AND GUARANTEE OF PAYMENT
I, the below named patient/subscriber, hereby absolutely assign payments directly to Charles H. Shaw, M.D./D. Troy Trimble, D.O. Gainesville Orthopaedic Group and any group and/or individual surgical and/or major medical benefits herein specified and otherwise payable to me for their services as described.

Medicare/Medicaid: I certify that the information given me in applying for payment under title XVIIIVXIX of the Social Security Administration or its intermediaries or carriers any information needed for this or a related Medicare claim. I request that payment of authorized benefits be made on my behalf. I assign the benefits payable for physician's services to Charles H. Shaw, M.D./D. Troy Trimble, D.O. Gainesville Orthopaedic Group.

I/We hereby guarantee payment of all charges incurred for the below named patient from the date of the first treatment until discharged from care by Charles H. Shaw/D. Troy Trimble, D.O. Gainesville Orthopaedic Group. I/We agree that should the amount of insurance benefit to be insufficient to cover the expenses. I/We will be responsible for the entire amount due for services rendered. I/We understand that statements are due when received unless other arrangements have been made with Charles H. Shaw, M.D./D. Troy Trimble, D.O. DBA Gainesville Orthopaedic Group. I/We understand that if there is no response or payment from the insurance company within 60 days of billing, I/We will be responsible for the balance due on account.

_____   _____
Subscriber (insured person) Signature   Date

_____   ☐ Checking this box indicates a digital signature.
Subscriber Printed Name

_____   _____
Patient Signature (if different from the subscriber)   Date

_____
Patient Printed Name

Fig. 9-3 CMS lifetime (one-time) release authorization for Medicare beneficiaries.

provider received the notice. Courts have concluded that it is reasonable to expect providers to comply with the published policies or regulations they receive, and no other evidence of knowledge may be necessary. This is one reason why it is important for the health insurance professional to attend periodic educational seminars, read all Medicare/Medicaid-related publications, and make every conceivable effort to keep up with these changes. Something else to be aware of is that if a provider fails to read Medicare's publications, but delegates that responsibility to others, the physician or the professional corporation still may be held liable for what the physician should have known.

Health insurance professionals can protect the physicians they work for by obtaining up-to-date information on services covered by Medicare from several sources.

Imagine This!

Shelly Jennings, a health insurance professional employed by Medical Specialties, Inc., asked all Medicare patients receiving a "screening" colonoscopy to sign an ABN because when she first started working at the facility, Medicare did not cover this procedure unless there were symptoms indicating a problem. After several patients complained, Medicare made an inquiry. Shelly's excuse was that she did not have time to read all the publications Medicare sent or attend periodic educational seminars and did not realize that Medicare now paid for a colonoscopy screening every 10 years, unless the patient is considered high risk.

CMS publishes a periodical called *The CMS Quarterly Provider Update*. These quarterly updates include all changes to Medicare instructions that affect physicians, provide a single source for national Medicare provider information, and give physicians advance notice on upcoming instructions and regulations. (See Websites to Explore.)

LOCAL MEDICAL REVIEW POLICIES

Local Medical Review Policies (LMRPs) outline general provisions for acceptance or rejection of Medicare claims. CMS maintains an official list describing approximately 600 covered items, services, and procedures in its *Coverage Issues Manual*. If a service or procedure is not on that list, the local Medicare carrier uses locally acceptable standards of practice, called LMRPs to determine coverage.

LMRPs were developed by insurance carriers that serve as Medicare intermediaries. Effective January 2001, CMS required that all intermediaries for Medicare establish a process that must be open to the public for the development of their LMRPs.

LOCAL COVERAGE DECISIONS

In December 2003, CMS began the 2-year transition of LMRPs to **local coverage decisions (LCDs)**. In contrast to LMRPs, LCDs are pure medical-necessity documents. LCDs focus exclusively on whether a service is reasonable and necessary according to the ICD-9-CM code for that particular CPT procedure code. Everything else is separate.[1]

This is an important transition because it changes the process for deciding whether Medicare will pay for a particular service considering the patient's diagnosis. By December 2005, all Medicare FIs and carriers must complete the shift from LMRPs to LCDs. Although they both are issued by Medicare FIs and carriers, LMRPs and LCDs are different. LMRPs are comprehensive documents, which list the tests and procedures that are considered medically necessary and are covered by Medicare for a specific diagnosis; this is accomplished by pairing the ICD-9 and CPT codes that trigger Medicare reimbursement. LMRPs contain more than just medical-necessity information. For example, there are

1. frequency limits (e.g., only one mammogram is covered each year);
2. statutory exclusions (Medicare does not cover preventive care except for certain initial screenings, e.g., colonoscopies);
3. national coverage decisions (e.g., Medicare does not pay for removal of benign keratosis unless there is a medical, noncosmetic reason, such as interference with vision); and

4. various other rules (e.g., Medicare will not pay for a complex procedure for a certain diagnosis unless other measures are taken first).

ADVANCED BENEFICIARY NOTICE

In addition to ascertaining that a valid release of information form is on file for a Medicare patient, the health insurance professional should ensure that the service requested is eligible for Medicare coverage. Medicare pays only for services that it considers medically necessary.

The health insurance professional must have the essential current publication on hand to consult if a question arises as to whether or not a particular service is included on the Medicare-eligible list. If, after checking the coverage rules, the health insurance professional believes that it is likely that Medicare *would not* pay for a test or procedure the provider orders, the patient should be asked to sign an **ABN**. The ABN is a form that Medicare requires all healthcare providers to use when Medicare does not pay for a service. This form ensures that beneficiaries have a choice about their healthcare in the event that Medicare does not pay. Fig. 9-4 is an example of a typical ABN.

When patients are asked to sign an ABN, they have two options:
• They may choose to receive the test or procedure, agree to be responsible for payment, and sign the ABN.
• They may choose not to receive the test or procedure, refuse to be responsible for payment, and sign the ABN.

When patients are given an ABN, the health insurance professional should be able to answer questions about financial responsibility and payment options so that patients can make informed decisions about their healthcare. If the patient refuses to sign the ABN and still demands the service, it should be made clear that he or she will be held personally and fully responsible for payment. In such cases, some practices ask for payment for the service in advance.

Supplemental insurance policies may pay for some services not paid for by Medicare, depending on the particular coverage. If the patient thinks that his or her secondary insurance may pay for the service not covered by Medicare, the health insurance professional can bill Medicare for a **denial notice**, an explanation that an LCD does not cover a certain item or service. After it has been established that Medicare will not pay the claim, the secondary insurer can be billed.

---

[1]Article reprinted from "Report on Medicare Compliance," January 29, 2004.

● Stop and Think

Gladys Larson calls the office to schedule an appointment to "have Dr. Clifford remove all these ugly spots on my chest." Looking through her health record, you notice the physician's reference to "benign keratosis." How do you determine if an ABN is needed?

Patient's Name: Medicare # (HICN):

ADVANCE BENEFICIARY NOTICE (ABN)

NOTE: You need to make a choice about receiving these health care items or services.

We expect that Medicare will not pay for the item(s) or service(s) that are described below. Medicare does not pay for all of your health care costs. Medicare only pays for covered items and services when Medicare rules are met. The fact that Medicare may not pay for a particular item or service does not mean that you should not receive it. There may be a good reason your doctor recommended it. Right now, in your case, **Medicare probably will not pay for –**

Items or Services:
Because:

The purpose of this form is to help you make an informed choice about whether or not you want to receive these items or services, knowing that you might have to pay for them yourself. Before you make a decision about your options, you should **read this entire notice carefully.**

- Ask us to explain, if you don't understand why Medicare probably won't pay.
- Ask us how much these items or services will cost you (**Estimated Cost: $_____**), in case you have to pay for them yourself or through other insurance.

PLEASE CHOOSE **ONE** OPTION. CHECK **ONE** BOX. **SIGN & DATE** YOUR CHOICE.

☐ **Option 1. YES.** **I want to receive these items or services.**

I understand that Medicare will not decide whether to pay unless I receive these items or services. Please submit my claim to Medicare. I understand that you may bill me for items or services and that I may have to pay the bill while Medicare is making its decision. If Medicare does pay, you will refund to me any payments I made to you that are due to me. If Medicare denies payment, I agree to be personally and fully responsible for payment. That is, I will pay personally, either out of pocket or through any other insurance that I have. I understand I can appeal Medicare's decision.

☐ **Option 2. NO.** **I have decided not to receive these items or services.**

I will not receive these items or services. I understand that you will not be able to submit a claim to Medicare and that I will not be able to appeal your opinion that Medicare won't pay.

_____   _____
Date   **Signature of patient or person acting on patient's behalf**

NOTE: Your health information will be kept confidential. Any information that we collect about you on this form will be kept confidential in our offices. If a claim is submitted to Medicare, your health information on this form may be shared with Medicare. Your health information which Medicare sees will be kept confidential by Medicare.

OMB Approval No. 0938-0566   Form No. CMS-R-131-G   (June 2002)

Fig. 9-4 Example of ABN.

HEALTH INSURANCE CLAIM NUMBER AND IDENTIFICATION CARD

The Medicare beneficiary's **health insurance claim number (HICN)** is in the format of nine numeric characters, usually the beneficiary's Social Security number, followed by one alpha character. It also might be a 6-digit or 9-digit number with one or two letter prefixes or suffixes. This type of coding allows the health insurance professional to look at the patient's identification (ID) card and immediately determine what the coverage is. When the status of a beneficiary changes, it is possible for the prefix or suffix of his or her claim number to change. Fig. 9-5 shows an example of a Medicare ID card. Table 9-6 lists alpha codes for HICNs and what they stand for. Patients belonging to a Medicare Advantage do not have the traditional ID card, but instead use the ID card of the plan in which they are enrolled.

What Did You Learn?

1. What are the criteria for meeting Medicare's "medically necessary" guidelines?
2. What are LMRPs?
3. When should an ABN be used?
4. How is the HICN structured?

MEDICARE BILLING

Billing for services rendered to Medicare beneficiaries is slightly different than that of non-Medicare patients. The health insurance professional must divert from the regular physician's fee schedule and use Medicare's special fee schedule. The fees contained in this schedule for the service performed by the physician are dictated by a complex formula worked out by the federal government and printed periodically in the Medicare Physician Fee Schedule.

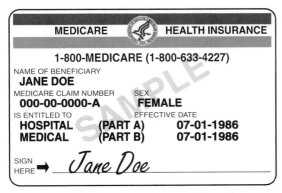

Fig. 9-5 Sample Medicare ID card.

TABLE 9-6	Traditional Medicare HICN Alpha Code Types
A	Wage Earner (Retirement)
B	Wife
B1	Husband
B2	Young Wife
C1-C9	Child (Includes Disabled or Student)
D	Aged Widow
D1	Widower
D6	Surviving Divorced Wife Benefits
E	Widowed Mother
E1	Surviving Divorced Mother
E4	Widowed Father
E5	Surviving Divorced Father
F1	Father
F2	Mother
F3	Stepfather
F4	Stepmother
F5	Adopting Father
F6	Adopting Mother
G	Claimant of Lump-Sum Death Benefits
HA	Wage Earner (Disability)
HB	Wife of Disabled Wage Earner
HB1	Husband of Disabled Wage Earner
HC	Child of Disabled Wage Earner
M	Uninsured—Premium Health Insurance Benefits (HIB) (Part A)
M1	Uninsured—Qualified for but refused HIB (Part A)
T	Uninsured—Entitled to HIB (Part A) under deemed or renal provisions
W	Disabled Widow
W1	Disabled Widower
W6	Disabled Surviving Divorced Wife

PHYSICIAN FEE SCHEDULE

Healthcare providers must use the Medicare fee schedule when billing Medicare for beneficiary services. CMS publishes an updated Medicare Physician Fee Schedule every year. In the last decade, the Medicare fee schedule was changed from fee-for-service to a **resource-based relative value system**. This means that each of the payment values is found within a range of payments. Table 9-7 is a portion of a sample page from the 2006 Medicare Physician Fee Schedule.

Payment for each service in the fee schedule is based on three factors:

1. A nationally uniform relative value for the specific service. This relative value is based on calculations for each service based on components of work, practice overhead, and professional liability and is referred to as a relative value unit.
2. A geographically specific modifier that considers variation in different areas of the United States. Each different area of the United States has its own

TABLE 9-7		2006 Medicare Fee Schedule					
PROC	S	PAR	NON-PAR	LIMITING CHARGE	GLB	INTR	P/T
97001	A	61.40	58.33	67.08	XXX	0.00	7
97002	A	37.66	35.78	41.15	XXX	0.00	7
*97002	A	30.75	29.21	33.59	XXX	0.00	7
97003	A	75.76	71.97	82.77	XXX	0.00	7
*97003	A	59.97	56.97	65.52	XXX	0.00	7
97004	A	45.22	42.96	49.40	XXX	0.00	7

*These amounts apply when service is performed in a facility setting.
Credit line: (Data from U. S. Department of Health and Human Services, Centers for Medicare & Medicaid Services.)

geographic practice cost indices for each of the relative value factors of work, practice overhead, and professional liability.

3. A nationally uniform conversion factor that is updated annually.

MEDICARE PARTICIPATING AND NONPARTICIPATING PROVIDERS

In its simplest explanation, a **Medicare participating provider (PAR)** or supplier is one who has signed a contract with Medicare; a **Medicare nonparticipating (nonPAR) provider** or supplier has not. Medicare PARs agree to accept Medicare's allowed amount as payment in full. Medicare typically pays 80% of the *allowed* fee for medically necessary procedures and services after the annual deductible has been met. **Medicare nonPARs** and suppliers may choose whether to accept Medicare's approved amount as payment on a case-by-case basis. If they do not accept the approved amount, the beneficiary pays the full billed amount. The "full billed" amount cannot exceed **Medicare's limiting charge**, however, which is 115% of Medicare's allowed amount.

Medicare PARs agree to accept Medicare fee schedule amounts as full payment for Medicare services. Medicare pays 80% of the fee schedule amount for a physician's service, and the beneficiary is responsible for 20% of the fee schedule amount. Medicare PARs benefit from the following advantages:

• Their Medicare fee schedule is 5% higher than that of nonPARs.
• They are provided with toll-free lines if they submit claims electronically.
• Their names are listed in the Medicare Participating Physician/Supplier Directory, which is furnished to senior citizen groups.

NonPARs not accepting assignments are advised they can charge beneficiaries no more than 115% of Medicare allowance. All Medicare providers, regardless of whether or not they accept assignment, must submit Medicare claims for the patient.

DETERMINING WHAT FEE TO CHARGE

It is important that the health insurance professional knows how to interpret the Medicare fee schedule so that he or she can determine the correct fee to charge the patient. Using the example fee schedule shown in Table 9-7 and choosing CPT code 97001 (a physical therapy evaluation), the amount Medicare allows a PAR to charge the patient is the amount shown in column 3 under the heading "PAR," or $61.40. A Medicare nonPAR accepting assignment can charge the amount in the next column under the heading "NON-PAR," or $58.33. The limiting charge for providers *not accepting* assignment is the amount in the next column under the heading "LIMITING," or $67.08—15% more than the nonPAR amount.

What Did You Learn?

1. Who uses Medicare's "limiting charge"?
2. List three advantages of becoming a Medicare PAR.
3. How does a health insurance professional determine what fee to charge for a Medicare-eligible service?

COMPLETING THE CMS-1500 FORM FOR MEDICARE CLAIMS

To ensure accurate and quick claim processing, the following guidelines should be followed for paper claims:
• Do not staple, clip, or tape anything to the CMS-1500 claim form.
• Place all necessary documentation in the envelope with the CMS-1500 claim form.
• Include the patient's name and Medicare number on each piece of documentation submitted.
• Use dark ink.
• Use only uppercase (CAPITAL) letters.

- Use 10 or 12 pitch (pica) characters and standard dot-matrix fonts.
- Do not mix character fonts on the same form.
- Do not use italics or script.
- Avoid using old or worn print bands or ribbons.
- Do not use dollar signs, decimals, or punctuation.
- Enter all information on the same horizontal plane within the designated field.
- Do not print, hand-write, or stamp any extraneous data on the form.
- Ensure data are in the appropriate fields and do not overlap into other fields.
- Remove pin-fed edges at side perforations.
- Use only an original red-ink-on-white-paper CMS-1500 claim form.

Submission of paper claims that do not meet the carrier's requirements may delay payments.

The process of completing the CMS-1500 form for Medicare claims is similar to that of a commercial claim with a few exceptions. Table 9-8 provides complete Medicare claims filing instructions, which are effectively the same as those provided on the NUCC website.

 HIPAA Tip

The determining factor for the correct place of service (POS) for Medicare beneficiaries is determined by the status of the patient. When a patient is registered as an inpatient (POS 21) or outpatient (POS 22), one of these POS codes must be used to bill Medicare.

TABLE 9-8   CMS-1500 Claim Form Instructions for Medicare

Throughout these instructions, the following formats are used to report dates:

MM|DD|YY or MM|DD|CCYY—indicates that a space must be reported between month, day, and year. This space is delineated by a dotted vertical line on the CMS-1500 claim form.

MMDDYY or MMDDCCYY—indicates that no space must be reported between month, day, and year. The date must be reported as one continuous number.

Block 1	Show the type of health insurance coverage applicable to this claim by checking the appropriate box, e.g., if a Medicare claim is being filed, check the Medicare box
Block 1a	Enter the patient's Medicare HICN whether Medicare is the primary or secondary payer (do not include spaces or hyphens)
Block 2	Enter the patient's last name, first name, and middle initial, if any, *exactly* as shown on the patient's Medicare card
Block 3	Enter the patient's 8-digit birth date (MM|DD|CCYY) and sex
Block 4	When the insured and the patient are the same, enter the word "SAME." If the patient has insurance primary to Medicare, through the patient's or spouse's employment or any other source, list the name of the insured here. If Medicare is primary, leave blank
Block 5	On the first line, enter the patient's street address; the second line, the city and 2-letter state code; the third line, the Zip Code and phone number
Block 6	Check the appropriate box for the patient's relationship to the insured when Block 4 is completed. If Medicare is the primary insurance, leave this block blank
Block 7	Complete this block only when Blocks 4 and 11 are completed. Enter the insured's address and telephone number. When the address is the same as the patient's, enter the word "SAME"
Block 8	Check the appropriate box for the patient's marital status and whether employed or a student
Block 9	Enter the last name, first name, and middle initial of the enrollee in a Medigap policy, if it is different from that shown in Block 2. Otherwise, enter the word "SAME." If no Medigap benefits are assigned, leave blank. This field may be used in the future for supplemental insurance plans.*
Block 9a	Enter the policy or group number of the Medigap insured preceded by MEDIGAP, MG, or MGAP. Block 9d must be completed if you enter a policy or group number in Block 9a
Block 9b	Enter the Medigap insured's 8-digit birth date (MMDDCCYY) and sex
Block 9c	Leave blank if a Medigap PayerID is entered in Block 9d. Otherwise, enter the claims processing address of the Medigap insurer. Use an abbreviated street address, 2-letter postal code, and Zip Code copied from the Medigap insured's Medigap ID card. *For example:* 1257 Anywhere Street, Baltimore, MD 21204 is shown as "1257 Anywhere St MD 21204."

TABLE 9-8	**CMS-1500 Claim Form Instructions for Medicare—cont'd**
Block 9d	Enter the 9-digit (alpha-numeric and up to 9-digit) PAYERID number of the Medigap insurer. If no PAYERID number exists, enter the Medigap insurance program or plan name. If you are PAR facility and the beneficiary wants Medicare payment data forwarded to a Medigap insurer under a mandated Medigap transfer, all of the information in Blocks 9, 9a, 9b, and 9d must be complete and accurate. Otherwise, the Medicare carrier cannot forward the claim information to the Medigap insurer
Blocks 10a-10c	Check "YES" or "NO" to indicate whether employment, auto liability, or other accident involvement applies to one or more of the services described in Block 24. For auto accidents, enter the 2-letter state code in which the accident occurred. Any Block checked "YES" indicates there may be other insurance primary to Medicare. If any items in this block are checked "YES," identify primary insurance information in Block 11
Block 10d	**Use this Block exclusively for Medicaid (MCD) information**. If the patient is entitled to Medicaid, enter the patient's Medicaid number preceded by MCD. *This Medicare carrier does not use this field*
Block 11	This block must be completed on Medicare claims. By doing so, the provider acknowledges having made a good faith effort to determine whether Medicare is the primary or secondary payer. If there is insurance primary to Medicare for the service date on the claim, enter the insured's policy or group number and proceed to Blocks 11a-11c. Note: Enter the appropriate information in Block 11c if insurance primary to Medicare is indicated in Block 11. If there is no insurance primary to Medicare, enter the word "NONE," and proceed to Block 12.† If the insured reports a terminating event with regard to insurance that had been primary to Medicare (e.g., insured retired), enter the word "NONE," and proceed to Block 12. Circumstances under which Medicare payment may be secondary to other insurance include: Group Health Plan Coverage, Working Aged, Disability (Large Group Health Plan), End Stage Renal Disease, No Fault and/or Other Liability, Work-Related Illness/Injury, Workers' Compensation, Black Lung; and Veterans Benefits. If Medicare is secondary, enter the insured's policy or group number within the confines of the box, or if there is no insurance primary to Medicare, enter the word "NONE"
Block 11a	Enter the insured's 8-digit birth date (MM|DD|CCYY) and sex if different from that in Block 3. *If entered as a 6-digit date, use hyphens or other punctuation, called "delimiters." If entered as an 8-digit date, do not use delimiters. This item is mandatory if a policy or group number is submitted in Block 11 and is different from the date in Block 3*
Block 11b	Enter employer's name, if applicable. If there is a change in the insured's insurance status, e.g., retired, enter either a 6-digit (MM|DD|YY) or 8-digit (MM|DD|CCYY) retirement date preceded by the word "RETIRED." *Please add employer's address and phone number to attached copy of EOB. This item is mandatory if a policy or group number is submitted in Block 11*
Block 11c	Enter the 9-digit PAYERID number of the primary insurer. If no PAYERID number exists, enter the complete primary payer's program or plan name. If the primary payer's EOB does not contain the claims processing address, record the primary payer's claims processing address directly on the EOB. Include the telephone number of the primary payer. **This item is mandatory if a policy or group number appears in Block 11**
Block 11d	Leave blank. Not required by Medicare
Block 12	The patient or authorized representative must sign and enter a 6-digit date (MM|DD|YY), 8-digit date (MM|DD|CCYY), or an alphanumeric date (e.g., January 1, 1998) unless a signature is on file.‡ *If entered as a 6-digit date, use delimiters. If entered as an 8-digit date, do not use delimiters.* "Signature on file" indicators (SOF) should be on the signature line, immediately following the word "signed." If the signature is not in the correct area, the information may be missed, and the claim could be denied
Block 13	A signature in this block authorizes payment of mandated Medigap benefits to the PAR if required Medigap information is included in Block 9 and its subdivisions. The patient or his or her authorized representative signs this item, or the signature must be on file as a separate Medigap authorization. The Medigap assignment on file in the PAR of service/supplier's office must be insurer specific. It may state that the authorization applies to all occasions of service until it is revoked. "Signature on file" indicators (SOF) should be on the signature line, immediately following the word "signed." If the signature is not in the correct area, the information may be missed, and the claim would not be crossed over to the Medigap insurance company. Block 13 is mandatory when the provider is PAR, and Medigap information is submitted in Blocks 9-9d

TABLE 9-8	CMS-1500 Claim Form Instructions for Medicare—cont'd
Block 14	Enter either a 6-digit (MM|DD|YY) or 8-digit (MM|DD|CCYY) date of current illness, injury, or pregnancy.
Block 15	Leave blank. Not required by Medicare
Block 16	If the patient is employed and is unable to work in current occupation, enter 6-digit (MM|DD|YY) or 8-digit (MM|DD|CCYY) date when patient is unable to work. An entry in this field may indicate employment-related insurance coverage. Refer back to Blocks 10a and 11c. *Block 16 is mandatory if Blocks 10a and 11c are completed*
Block 17	Enter the name of the referring or ordering physician if the service or item was ordered or referred by a physician. **Referring physician**—a physician who requests an item or service for the beneficiary for which payment may be made under the Medicare program. **Ordering physician**—a physician or, when appropriate, a non-physician practitioner, who orders non-physician services for the patient. Examples of services that might be ordered include diagnostic laboratory tests, clinical laboratory tests, pharmaceutical services, durable medical equipment, and services incident to that physician's or non-physician practitioner's service.
Blocks 17a and b	An entry in Block 17a and/or 17b is required when a service listed on the form was ordered or referred by a physician. When a claim involves multiple referring and/or ordering physicians, a separate CMS-1500 form must be used for each referring/ordering physician. The provider's unique provider identification number (UPIN) can be used until May 22, 2007. The UPIN should appear in Block 17a. Effective May 23, 2007, the UPIN in 17a is *not* to be reported. Instead, the NPI must be reported in 17b when a service was ordered or referred by a physician.
Block 18	Enter a 6-digit (MM|DD|YY) or 8-digit (MM|DD|CCYY) date when a medical service is furnished as a result of, or subsequent to, a related hospitalization.
Block 19	Enter either a 6-digit or 8-digit date when the patient was last seen and the UPIN (NPI when it becomes effective) of his/her attending physician when an independent physical or occupational therapist submits claims or a physician providing routine foot care submits claims.
Block 20	Complete this block when billing for diagnostic tests subject to purchase price limitations. Enter the purchase price under charges if the "yes" block is checked. A "yes" check indicates that an entity other than the one billing for the service performed the diagnostic test. A "no" check indicates that "no purchased tests are included on the claim." When "yes" is checked, Block 32 must be completed.
Block 21	Enter the patient's diagnosis/condition. All providers must use an ICD-9-CM code number and code to the highest level of specificity. *Enter four codes in priority order (primary, secondary condition).*
Block 22	Leave blank. Not required by Medicare
Block 23	Enter the Quality Improvement Organization (QIO) prior authorization number for procedures requiring QIO prior approval or the Investigational Device Exemption (IDE) number when an investigational device is used in an FDA-approved clinical trial. Enter the 10-digit Clinical Laboratory Improvement Act (CLIA) certification number for laboratory services billed by an entity performing CLIA covered procedures. When a physician provides services to a beneficiary residing in a SNF and the services were rendered to a SNF beneficiary outside of the SNF, the physician shall enter the Medicare facility provider number of the SNF in item 23. NOTE: Item 23 can contain only one condition. Any additional conditions should be reported on a separate CMS-1500 form.
Block 24a	Enter a 6-digit or 8-digit (MMDDCCYY) date for each procedure, service, or supply. When "from" and "to" dates are shown for a series of identical services, enter the number of days or units in column G. This is a required field. Claim will be returned as unprocessable if a date of service extends more than one day and a valid "to" date is not present.
Block 24b	Enter the appropriate place of service code for each item used or service performed. This is a required field. NOTE: When a service is rendered to a hospital inpatient, use the "inpatient hospital" code.
Block 24c	Medicare providers are not required to complete this item.

TABLE 9-8	CMS-1500 Claim Form Instructions for Medicare—cont'd
Block 24d	Enter the procedures, services, or supplies using the appropriate 5-digit CPT or CMS Healthcare Common Procedure Coding System (HCPCS) code. When applicable, show HCPCS code modifiers. When reporting an "unlisted procedure code" or a "not otherwise classified" (NOC) code, include a narrative description in item 19 if a coherent description can be given within the confines of that box. Otherwise, an attachment should be submitted with the claim. This is a required field.
Block 24e	Enter the diagnosis code reference number as shown in item 21 to relate the date of service and the procedures performed to the primary diagnosis. Enter only one reference number per line item. When multiple services are performed, enter the primary reference number for each service, either a 1, or a 2, or a 3, or 4. This is a required field. If a situation arises where two or more diagnoses are required for a procedure code (e.g., pap smears), the provider shall reference only one of the diagnoses in item 21.
Block 24f	Enter the charge for each listed service.
Block 24g	Enter the number of days or units. This field is most commonly used for multiple visits, units of supplies, anesthesia minutes, or oxygen volume. If only one service is performed, enter the number 1.
Block 24h	Leave blank. Not required by Medicare
Block 24i	Enter the ID qualifier 1C in the shaded portion for Medicare claims
Block 24j	Prior to May 23, 2007, enter the rendering provider's PIN in the shaded portion. After May 23, 2007, enter the rendering provider's NPI number in the lower portion. In the case of a service provided incident to the service of a physician or non-physician practitioner, when the person who ordered the service is not supervising, enter the PIN of the supervisor in the shaded portion.
Block 25	Enter the provider of service or supplier Federal Tax ID (Employer Identification Number) or Social Security Number. The participating provider of service or supplier Federal Tax ID number is required for a mandated Medigap transfer.
Block 26	Enter the patient's account number assigned by the provider's accounting system. This field is optional to assist the provider in patient identification.
Block 27	Check the appropriate block to indicate whether the provider accepts assignment of Medicare benefits. If Medigap is indicated in item 9 and Medigap payment authorization is given in item 13, the provider of service or supplier shall also be a Medicare participating provider of service or supplier and accept assignment of Medicare benefits for all covered charges for all patients.
Block 28	Enter total of all charges in item 24f.
Block 29	Enter the total amount the patient paid on the covered services only. Leave blank if no payment has been made.
Block 30	Leave blank. Not required by Medicare.
Block 31	Enter the provider's signature or his/her representative, and either the 6- or 8-digit date, or alpha-numeric date (e.g., January 1, 1998) the form was signed. Computer generated signature are acceptable.
Block 32	Medicare requires the name, address, and zip code of the facility regardless of where services were performed and does not allow "SAME."
Block 32a	Enter the NPI of the service facility in Block 32a.
Block 32b	Enter the appropriate ID qualifier followed by one blank space and then the PIN of the service facility. After May 23, 2007, 32b is not to be reported. Note: Providers of service (namely physicians) must identify the supplier's PIN when billing for purchased diagnostic tests.
Block 33	Enter the provider's billing name, address, zip code, and telephone number.
Block 33a	Effective May 23, 2007, the NPI of the billing provider or group must be reported here.
Block 33b	Enter the appropriate ID qualifier followed by one blank space and then the PIN of the billing provider or group. Effective May 23, 2007, and later, 33b is not to be reported. Enter the group UPIN, including the 2-digit location identifier, for the performing practitioner/supplier who is a member of a group practice.

TABLE 9-8	CMS-1500 Claim Form Instructions for Medicare—cont'd

Note: Only PARs are to complete Block 9 and its subdivisions and only when the beneficiary wishes to assign his or her benefits under a Medigap policy to the participating physician or supplier. PARs must enter information required in Block 9 and its subdivisions if requested by the patient. PARs sign an agreement with Medicare to accept assignment of benefits for all Medicare patients. A claim for which a beneficiary elects to assign his or her benefits under a Medigap policy to a participating physician/supplier is called a mandated Medigap transfer. Do not list other supplemental coverage in Block 9 and its subdivisions at the time a Medicare claim is filed. Other supplemental claims are forwarded automatically to the private insurer if the private insurer contracts with the carrier to send Medicare claim information electronically. If there is no such contract, the beneficiary must file his or her own supplemental claim.

†*Note:* For a paper claim to be considered for Medicare Secondary Payer benefits, a copy of the primary payer's EOB notice must be attached to the claim form. *If a policy or group number is entered, an EOB MUST be attached.*

‡*Note:* In lieu of signing the claim, the patient may sign a release of information statement to be retained in the provider's file. If the patient is physically or mentally unable to sign, a representative may sign on the patient's behalf. In this case, the statement's signature line must indicate the patient's name followed by "by," the representative 's name, address, relationship to the patient, and the reason the patient cannot sign. The authorization is effective indefinitely unless the patient or the patient's representative revokes this arrangement. The patient's signature authorizes release of medical information necessary to process the claim. It also authorizes payment of benefits to the provider of service or supplier, when the provider of service or supplier accepts assignment on the claim. When an illiterate or physically handicapped enrollee signs by mark, a witness must enter his or her name and address next to the mark.

§*Note:* When the ordering physician is also the performing physician (as often is the case with in-office clinical laboratory tests), the performing physician's name and assigned UPIN must appear in Blocks 17 and 17a. All physicians who order or refer Medicare beneficiaries or services must obtain a UPIN even though they may never bill Medicare directly. A physician who has not been assigned a UPIN must contact the Medicare carrier. When a physician extender or other limited licensed practitioner refers a patient for consultative service, the name and UPIN of the physician supervising the limited licensed practitioner must appear in Blocks 17 and 17a. When a patient is referred to a physician who also orders and performs a diagnostic service, a separate claim form is required for the diagnostic service. Enter the original ordering/referring physician's name and UPIN in Blocks 17 and 17a of the first claim form. Enter the ordering (performing) physician's name and UPIN in Blocks 17 and 17a of the second claim form.

Surrogate UPINs: If the ordering/referring physician has not been assigned a UPIN, a surrogate UPIN must be used in Block 17a. The surrogate UPIN used depends on the circumstances and is used only until the physician is assigned a UPIN. Enter the physician's name in Block 17 and the surrogate UPIN in Block 17a. All surrogate UPINs, with the exception of retired physicians (RET000), are temporary and may be used only until a UPIN is assigned.

From the CMS (http://www.cms.hhs.gov/transmittals/downloads/R735CP.pdf).

COMPLETING A MEDIGAP CLAIM

Completion of Blocks 9 through 9d is conditional for insurance information related to Medigap. Only PARs are required to complete Block 9 and its subdivisions and only when the patient wishes to assign his or her benefits under a Medigap policy to the PAR. PARs of service and suppliers must enter information required in Block 9 and its subdivisions if requested by the beneficiary. (PARs sign an agreement with Medicare to accept assignment of Medicare benefits for *all* Medicare patients. NonPARs can accept assignment on a case-by-case basis.)

A claim for which a beneficiary elects to assign his or her benefits under a Medigap policy to a PAR is called a **mandated Medigap transfer**. If a PAR and the patient want Medicare payment data forwarded to a Medigap insurer under a mandated Medigap transfer, all of the information in Blocks 9, 9a, 9b, and 9d must be complete and accurate. Otherwise, Medicare cannot forward the claim information to the Medigap insurer.

If the health insurance professional wishes to use the statement "Signature on File" in Block 13 in lieu of the patient's actual signature, a statement must be signed and dated by the patient and maintained in the practice's records (Fig. 9-6). Table 9-9 contains instructions for completion of blocks that are affected by Medigap policies.

MEDICARE SECONDARY POLICY

When Medicare is the secondary payer, the claim must be submitted first to the primary insurer. The primary insurer processes the claim in accordance with the coverage provisions in the contract. If, after processing the claim, the primary insurer does not pay in full for the services, the claim may be submitted to Medicare electronically or via a paper claim for consideration of secondary benefits. It is the provider's responsibility to obtain primary insurance information from the beneficiary and bill

(Name of Beneficiary) (Health Insurance Claim Number) (Medigap Policy Number)

I request that payment of authorized Medigap benefits be made either to me or on my behalf to the provider of service and (or) supplier for any services furnished to me by that the provider of service and (or) supplier. I authorize any holder of Medicare information about me to release to (Name of Medigap Insurer) any information needed to determine these benefits payable for related services.

_____
(Signature) (Date)

Fig. 9-6 Example of "signature on file" statement.

TABLE 9-9	Modifications to the CMS-1500 Form for a Medigap Claim
Block 9	Enter the last name, first name, and middle initial of the Medigap enrollee, if it is different from that shown in Block 2. Otherwise, enter the word "SAME"
Block 9a	Enter the policy and/or group number of the Medigap insured preceded by MEDIGAP, MG, or MGAP. *Note:* Block 9d must be completed if a policy and/or group number is in Block 9a
Block 9b	Enter the Medigap enrollee's birth date (MMDDCCYY) and sex
Block 9c	Disregard "employer's name or school name," which is printed on the form. Enter the claims processing address for the Medigap insurer. Use an abbreviated street address, 2-letter state postal code, and Zip Code copied from the Medigap insured's Medigap ID card. For example: 1257 Anywhere Street, Baltimore, MD 21204, is shown as "1257 Anywhere St MD 21204." *Note:* If a carrier-assigned unique identifier of a Medigap insurer appears in Block 9d, Block 9c may be left blank
Block 9d	Enter the name of the Medigap insured's insurance company or the Medigap insurer's unique identifier provided by the local Medicare carrier. If you are a participating provider of service or supplier, and the beneficiary wants Medicare payment data forwarded to a Medigap insurer under a mandated Medigap transfer, all of the information in Block 9 and its subdivisions must be complete and correct. Otherwise, the claim information cannot be forwarded to the Medigap insurer
Block 12	All Medicare/Medigap claims must have Block 12 completed. Failure to include an appropriate signature and 6-digit date or a "signature on file" statement results in claim rejection. A Medigap authorization signature in Block 13 does not satisfy the Block 12 signature requirement
Block 13	Completion of this block is conditional for Medigap. The signature in Block 13 authorizes payment of mandated Medigap benefits to the PAR of service or supplier if required Medigap information is included in Block 9 and its subdivisions. The patient or his or her authorized representative signs this block, or the signature must be on file as a separate Medigap authorization. The Medigap assignment on file in the participating physician or supplier's office must be list the name of the specific Medigap insurer. It may state that the authorization applies to all occasions of service until it is revoked

Medicare appropriately. Claim filing extensions are not granted because of incorrect insurance information.

Insurance Primary to Medicare

Circumstances under which Medicare payment may be secondary to other insurance include the following:
• Group health plan coverage: working aged, disability (large group health plan), and ESRD
• No fault or other liability
• Work-related illness/injury: workers' compensation, black lung, and veterans benefits
For a paper claim to be considered for MSP benefits, a copy of the primary payer's explanation of benefits (EOB) notice must be forwarded along with the claim form.

● Stop and Think

Franklin Elmore is a new patient in your office. When he filled out the patient information form, he indicated that he was born February 26, 1939, and is employed full-time at Alamo Distributing Company. Under the insurance section, Mr. Elmore lists Medicare as his primary insurer and group coverage with Amax Quality Assurance through his employer as his secondary insurance. Is Mr. Elmore's information form correct? Which insurer should receive the CMS-1500 claim first?

Completing Medicare Secondary Policy Claims

When Medicare is the secondary payer, the health insurance professional must include a copy of the primary insurer's EOB with the claim. The EOB should include the following information:
• Name and address of the primary insurer
• Name of subscriber and policy number
• Name of the provider of services
• Itemized charges for all procedure codes reported
• Detailed explanation of any denials or payment codes
• Date of service

A detailed explanation of any primary insurer's denial or payment codes must be submitted with the claim to Medicare. If the denial/payment code descriptions or any of the above-listed information is not included with the claim, it may result in a delay in processing or denial of the claim. If the beneficiary is covered by more than one insurer primary to Medicare (e.g., a working aged beneficiary who was in an automobile accident), the EOB statement from plans must be submitted with the claim.

To submit MSP claims electronically, the health insurance professional should refer to the American National Standards Institute (ANSI) ASC X12N Implementation Guide or the National Standard Format Specifications for reporting requirements.

When submitting a paper claim to Medicare as the secondary payer, the following instructions apply:
• The CMS-1500 form must indicate the name and policy number of the beneficiary's primary insurance in Blocks 11 through 11c.
• Providers, whether they are PAR or nonPAR, must submit a claim to Medicare if a beneficiary provides a copy of the primary EOB.
• The claim must be submitted to Medicare for secondary payment consideration with a copy of the EOB. If the beneficiary is not cooperative in supplying the EOB, the beneficiary may be billed for the amount Medicare would pay as the secondary payer.
• Providers must bill the primary insurer and Medicare the same charge for rendered services. If the primary insurer is billed $50.00 for an office visit and they pay $35.00, do not bill Medicare the remaining $15.00.

Medicare also must be billed for the $50.00 charge, and a copy of the primary insurer's EOB must be attached to the completed claim form.

It was stated previously that when submitting paper or electronic claims for Medicare, Block 11 must be completed. By completing this block, the physician/supplier acknowledges having made a good faith effort to determine whether Medicare is the primary or secondary payer. A claim without this information would be returned.

When there is insurance primary to Medicare, as in the MSP situation, the health insurance professional should enter the insured's policy or group number in Block 11 and proceed to Blocks 11a through 11c. (When there is no insurance primary to Medicare, enter the word "NONE" in Block 11 and proceed to Block 12.) Completion of Blocks 11b and 11c is conditional for insurance information primary to Medicare. Table 9-10 gives instructions for how Blocks 11a through 11d should be completed for MSP claims.

Medicare Secondary Policy Conditional Payment

Medicare may make a conditional payment if they have knowledge that another insurer is primary to Medicare, but the primary payer does not made prompt payment (within 120 days) or has denied the claim for a reason Medicare considers acceptable. (This conditional payment is applicable, however, only for black lung, workers' compensation, and accidents). From a reimbursement standpoint, a claim paid conditionally pays the same as if there were no insurance other than Medicare.

MEDICARE PART B CROSSOVER PROGRAM

The **Medicare Part B Crossover program** is a fee-per-claim service that Medicare Part B offers to private insurers and retirement plans. Medicare Part B and a supplemental insurer enter into a formal contract called a **trading partner agreement** for the electronic data interchange of claim information. Trading partners are Medigap insurers, supplemental retirement plans, or other healthcare payers.

TABLE 9-10	Modifications to the CMS-1500 for Medicare Secondary Payer Claims
Block 11a	Enter the insured's birth date (MMDDCCYY) and sex, if different from Block 3
Block 11b	Enter the employer's name, if applicable. If there is a change in the insured's insurance status, such as retired, enter the 6-digit retirement date (MMDDYY) preceded by the word "RETIRED"
Block 11c	Enter the *complete* insurance plan or program name (e.g., Blue Shield of [State]). If the primary payer's EOB does not contain the claims processing address, record the primary payer's claims processing address directly on the EOB
Block 11d	Can be left blank. Not required by Medicare

The crossover process, in contrast to Medigap, does not require input from the provider. After a trading agreement is signed, the insurer sends an eligibility file to Medicare, and Medicare sends corresponding claim information back to the healthcare payer. The eligibility file contains the beneficiary's name, Medicare HICN, and policy effective dates. Medicare matches the trading partner's HICN against its own Medicare files. Any resulting claims are automatically sent to the payer for additional payment considerations. This process results in a significant number of claims sent to each supplemental payer.

Some private insurers may choose to be Medigap and Crossover participants. When private insurance companies send a list of their insureds to Medicare, any resulting claims are handled as Crossover claims. If a Medicare beneficiary's file does not show a private insurer, but a claim from a PAR shows Medigap information, Medicare forwards the information to the supplemental payer.

The Health Insurance Portability and Accountability Act (HIPAA) has made Medicare Crossover systems easier to develop and maintain. Examples of benefits through HIPAA are as follows:

- The uniform provider number eliminates the need for **crosswalks** (the process of matching one set of data elements or category of codes to their equivalents within a new set of elements or codes) between the Medicare and Medicaid provider numbering systems.
- With a uniform insurer/payer number, crossover systems are able to forward claims to Medicare carriers if the claim is billed to the state Medicaid agency because the claims can be forwarded easily between payers. In addition, if the beneficiary has a Medicare supplemental policy, the state Medicaid agency can forward the Medicare adjudicated invoice directly to the supplemental insurer, simply by using the uniform payer ID number.
- The transaction sets allow the state Medicaid agency to have all required data on claims crossed over from the carrier or intermediary. Eligibility verification between the Medicaid agency and the carrier or intermediary can be accomplished online through the use of the eligibility inquiry and response transactions. These transactions also can be used to verify Medicare supplemental insurance.
- Because all payers use the same remittance transactions and coding, providers may be able to use a single program to post the payments to their accounts receivable systems. Direct deposit of provider payments also is beneficial because the cost of printing and mailing checks is eliminated.

MEDICARE/MEDICAID CROSSOVER CLAIMS

Modifications must be made on the CMS-1500 form for dual-eligible beneficiaries. The claim is sent to Medicare first, who determines their liability portion of the charges. Then the claim is automatically *crossed over* to Medicaid

directly from the Medicare carrier. The following blocks are affected:

Block 1—The Medicare and Medicaid boxes should be checked.

Block 10d—Enter the abbreviation MCD followed by the beneficiary's Medicaid ID number.

Block 27—PARs and nonPARS should place an "X" in the "YES" box because assignment must be accepted on Medicare/Medicaid crossover claims.

Filing Medicare Claims Electronically

The Administrative Simplification Compliance Act (ASCA) requires that all **initial claims** for reimbursement under Medicare be submitted electronically as of October 16, 2003. Initial claims are as follows:

- Claims submitted to a Medicare fee-for-service carrier or FI for the first time, including resubmitted previously rejected claims.
- Claims with paper attachments.
- **Demand bills**. Under Medicare rules, a beneficiary, on receiving notification of noncoverage, has the right to request that a FI review that determination. Such a request is known as a demand bill (Fig. 9-7). Before using a demand bill, the beneficiary must sign an ABN and agree to pay for the services in full if Medicare coverage is denied. It is up to the medical facility to ensure that this request is filed.
- Claims for which Medicare is the secondary payer and there is only one primary payer.
- Nonpayment claims.

 HIPAA Tip

With the implementation of HIPAA, it is possible to submit an electronic claim and submit a separate paper attachment for that claim. When an electronic claim is filed, an attachment control number is assigned. The paper attachment is sent with a cover page containing the attachment control number.

Initial claims do not include:
- adjustments,
- previously submitted claims, or
- appeal requests.

This requirement does not apply to claims submitted by
- beneficiaries,
- providers that furnish services only outside the United States, or
- managed care plans or health plans other than Medicare.

DEPARTMENT OF HEALTH AND HUMAN SERVICES
CENTERS FOR MEDICARE & MEDICAID SERVICES

MEDICARE RECONSIDERATION REQUEST FORM

1. Beneficiary's Name:_____

2. Medicare Number:_____

3. Description of Item or Service in Question: _____

4. Date the Service or Item was Received: _____

5. I do not agree with the determination of my claim. MY REASONS ARE:

_____

_____

_____

6. Date of the redetermination notice_____
(If you received your redetermination more than 180 days ago, include your reason for not making this request earlier.)

_____

_____

_____

7. Additional Information Medicare Should Consider:_____

_____

_____

_____

8. Requester's Name:_____

9. Requester's Relationship to the Beneficiary: _____

10. Requester's Address: _____

_____

11. Requester's Telephone Number: _____

12. Requester's Signature:_____

13. Date Signed: _____

14. ❑ I have evidence to submit. (Attach such evidence to this form.)
❑ I do not have evidence to submit.

15. Name of the Medicare Contractor that Made the Redetermination:_____

NOTICE: Anyone who misrepresents or falsifies essential information requested by this form may upon conviction be subject to fine or imprisonment under Federal Law.

Form CMS-20033 (05/05) EF (05/2005)

Fig. 9-7 Sample demand bill.

HIPAA Tip

As of October 16, 2003, electronically submitted claims must comply with the appropriate claim standards adopted for national use under HIPAA or with standards supported under the Medicare HIPAA contingency plan during the period that plan is in effect.

 **HIPAA Tip**

HIPAA defines a clearinghouse as an entity that translates data to or from a standard format for electronic transmission. HIPAA requires that clearinghouses submit claims electronically effective October 16, 2003, without exception

Exceptions

The guidelines that were issued by CMS that went into effect January 20, 2004, state that, "In some cases, it has been determined that due to limitations in the claims transaction formats adopted for national use under HIPAA, it would not be reasonable or possible to submit certain claims to Medicare electronically. Providers are to self-assess to determine if they meet these exceptions." There are limited exceptions to the government mandate that all Medicare claims be filed electronically. Earlier, we talked about the *small provider* exception. To meet this "small provider" exception, the provider must be defined as either

a provider of services (as that term is defined in section 1861(u) of the Social Security Act) with fewer than 25 full-time equivalent (FTE) employees or

a physician, practitioner, facility, or supplier that is not otherwise a provider under section 1861(u) with fewer than 10 FTE employees.

To simplify implementation, Medicare considers all providers falling into either of the aforementioned two categories, and that are required to bill a Medicare intermediary, to be small and qualify for the exception to the rule. These regulations do not modify preexisting laws or employer policies defining full-time employment.

Although small providers who meet the exception ruling are exempt from the mandatory electronic claim requirement, they are encouraged to file Medicare claims electronically, if possible. The small provider exception does not apply to healthcare claim clearinghouses that are agents for small providers.

● Stop and Think

You are employed by a two-physician practice. In addition to you, the health insurance professional, there is a medical receptionist, two medical assistants, and a registered nurse. You have just completed transferring all patient accounts over to a computerized patient accounting system. Are you now required to submit all Medicare claims electronically?

The CMS website furnishes a list of other claim types that are considered to meet the exemption criteria (see Websites to Explore).

DEADLINE FOR FILING MEDICARE CLAIMS

Medicare's fiscal year begins October 1 and ends September 30. Claims typically must be filed no later than the end of the calendar year (December 31) following the fiscal year in which services were provided. Assigned claims can take longer (27 months, depending on the date the service was performed) if the provider has good reason for delaying claims submission. If not, a 10% reimbursement penalty is assessed to the claim. The health insurance professional always should file claims in a timely manner if for no other reason out of courtesy to the patient and financial benefit to the provider.

What Did You Learn?

1. What blocks on the CMS-1500 form are typically affected by Medigap claims?
2. What is the significance of a signature in Block 13 on a Medigap claim?
3. Name three circumstances under which Medicare may be the secondary insurer.
4. What must accompany a Medicare secondary payer paper claim?
5. What blocks on the CMS-1500 form are typically affected by MSP claims?

MEDICARE SUMMARY NOTICE

When a Medicare claim is filed, the beneficiary receives a document called the **Medicare Summary Notice (MSN)**. The MSN (Fig. 9-8) replaced the Explanation of Medicare Benefits form in 2001. The MSN form is an easy-to-read monthly statement that lists Part A and Part B claims information, including the patient's deductible status. The health insurance professional should make it clear to the patient that the MSN is not a bill, and he or she

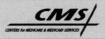

Medicare Summary Notice

Page 1 of 2

July 1, 2004

BENEFICIARY NAME
STREET ADDRESS
CITY, STATE   ZIP CODE

CUSTOMER SERVICE INFORMATION

Your Medicare Number: 111-11-1111A

If you have questions, write or call:
Medicare
555 Medicare Blvd., Suite 200
Medicare Building
Medicare, US XXXXX-XXXX

BE INFORMED: Beware of telemarketers offering free or discounted medicare items or services.

Local: (XXX) XXX-XXXX
Toll-free: 1-800-XXX-XXXX
TTY for Hearing Impaired: 1-800-XXX-XXXX

This is a summary of claims processed from 05/10/2004 through 06/10/2004.

PART B MEDICAL INSURANCE – ASSIGNED CLAIMS

Dates of Service	Services Provided	Amount Charged	Medicare Approved	Medicare Paid Provider	You May Be Billed	See Notes Section
Claim Number: 12435-84956-84556						a
Paul Jones, M.D., 123 West Street, Jacksonville, FL 33231-0024						
Referred by: Scott Wilson, M.D.						
04/19/04	1 Influenza immunization (90724)	$5.00	$3.88	$3.88	$0.00	b
04/19/04	1 Admin. flu vac (G0008)	5.00	3.43	3.43	0.00	b
	Claim Total	**$10.00**	**$7.31**	**$7.31**	**$0.00**	
Claim Number: 12435-84956-84557						a
ABC Ambulance, P.O. Box 2149, Jacksonville, FL 33231						
04/25/04	1 Ambulance, base rate (A0020)	$289.00	$249.78	$199.82	$49.96	
04/25/04	1 Ambulance, per mile (A0021)	21.00	16.96	13.57	3.39	
	Claim Total	**$310.00**	**$266.74**	**$213.39**	**$53.35**	

PART B MEDICAL INSURANCE – UNASSIGNED CLAIMS

Dates of Service	Services Provided	Amount Charged	Medicare Approved	Medicare Paid You	You May Be Billed	See Notes Section
Claim Number: 12435-84956-84558						a
William Newman, M.D., 362 North Street Jacksonville, FL 33231-0024						
03/10/04	1 Office/Outpatient Visit, ES (99213)	$47.00	$33.93	$27.15	$39.02	c

THIS IS NOT A BILL – Keep this notice for your records.

Fig. 9-8 Example of Medicare Summary Notice Part B. (Source: U. S. Department of Health & Human Services, Centers for Medicare & Medicaid Services.)

should **not** send any money to the provider or supplier until a statement is received.

Medicare began testing a new service in 2004—the **Electronic Medicare Summary Notice (electronic MSN)**. The electronic MSN allows beneficiaries to look at their MSN on the World Wide Web and print copies from their home computers. The electronic MSN does not replace the paper MSN, which is still mailed each month when a claim is processed, but it is a quick and convenient way for beneficiaries to track their claims.

INFORMATION CONTAINED ON THE MEDICARE SUMMARY NOTICE

The MSN gives a breakdown of Medicare claims billed on the patient's behalf and processed by the FI or carrier. In addition to listing the services received along with the name of the provider, the MSN lists
• the total amount billed by providers,
• Medicare's approved payment amount for services,
• amount paid to the beneficiary or his or her provider,
• costs the beneficiary is responsible for, and
• deductible information.
If there is a supplemental insurance policy or Medigap, these insurers also may need a copy of the MSN to process their share of the bill.

The health insurance professional should know how to read the MSN so that he or she can answer any questions beneficiaries might have. Detailed instructions on how to read the MSN can be found on the CMS website.

MEDICARE REMITTANCE ADVICE

When a claim has gone through the processing stage, Medicare notifies the provider as to how the claim was **adjudicated** (how the decision was made as to the payment). This notification is referred to as a remittance advice (RA). The RA is notification Medicare sends to the provider and includes a list of all claims paid and claims rejected or denied during a particular payment period. A paper RA is generated for all providers whether they file paper or electronic claims. The only exception is when the provider has been approved to receive the RA electronically.

Each RA contains a list of claims that Medicare has cleared for payment since the last RA was generated. Also included in the RA are any claims that have moved to a "deny status" since the last RA was sent. RAs are generated in a weekly cycle. Each claim listed on the RA contains detailed processing information. A reimbursement amount, **Claim Adjustment Reason Codes**, and **Remittance Remark Codes** are included for each claim. Claim adjustment reason codes and remittance remark codes are used in the **electronic remittance advice (ERA)** and the **standard paper remittance advice (SPRA)** to relay information relevant to the adjudication of Medicare Part B claims. Reason codes detail the reason why an adjustment was

made to a healthcare claim payment by the payer, and remark codes represent nonfinancial information crucial to understanding the adjudication of the claim.

Standard Paper Remittance Advice

The SPRA is the product of standardization by CMS of the provider payment notification. The form was created to (1) provide a document that is uniform in content and format and (2) ease the transition to the electronic remittance format. The SPRA displays the same reason codes, remark codes, messages, and other data as the ERA for Medicare Part A providers.

Fig. 9-9 shows the SPRA along with a list of the various fields depicted on the SPRA and their definitions. One claim is listed in each block of the remittance and is separated from other claims with a line. The claims on the remittance are organized in alphabetical order, by beneficiary name within each type of claim (i.e., Inpatient, Part A). At the end of each type of claim, there is a subtotal of the information included on the remittance. At the end of the remittance is a total summation.

Electronic Remittance Advice

An ERA is one of several different types of electronic formats that is generated rather than a paper document. Information contained in an ERA furnishes the same information as that contained on the SPRA. An ERA allows automatic posting of claims payment information directly into the facility's practice management system. ERAs eliminate the need for manual posting of Medicare payment information, which saves the provider time and money. Automatic ERA information transfer also eliminates errors made by manual posting of information from the SPRA to the ledger accounts.

Who Can Receive Electronic Remittance? Any provider or supplier enrolled in the Medicare program who submits claims electronically may receive ERAs. It is not required that a provider be Medicare PAR to receive ERAs. Additionally, providers may allow a billing agent (billing service or clearinghouse) to receive ERAs on their behalf.

How Does It Work? The provider receives a paper Medicare check and SPRA just as before. The Medicare check number appears on paper and electronic versions of the RA. Production of paper remittance notices may be discontinued at the discretion of the provider or CMS or both after a reasonable phase-in period.

Steps for Enrolling in Electronic Remittance. Receiving ERAs is not automatic. The provider must go through an enrollment process, which typically includes several steps, as follows:

Standard Paper Remittance (SPR) Advice Notices - Revised Format

The Centers for Medicare & Medicaid Services (CMS) has revised the format of the Standard Paper Remittance (SPR) Advice Notices to correspond with the changes made to the X12 835 as a result of HIPAA. These changes are effective with SPRs printed on and after **April 1, 2002**. Following is a summary of the SPR changes and an example of the revised SPR highlighting these changes.

SPR Changes:

* The "TOTAL PD TO BENE" and "TOTAL MSP" amount fields used in computing provider payment will now be reported as reason code adjustments, rather than in separate fields at the provider summary level. Please refer to Reference❶ in the attached example.
* The "OFFSET DETAILS" section has been replaced with the "PLB REASON CODE". Please refer to Reference ❶ in the attached example. Some of the offset codes have been replaced and some new offset codes were added. The following is a crosswalk of the codes used in Medicare processing:

Current ADJ/ Offset Reason Code	New Code	Description	Comments
AP	AP	Acceleration of Benefits	Advance Payments
RF	B2	Rebate	Refund, HPSA
RI	CS	Adjustment	Used for multiple reasons
BF	FB	Forwarding Balance	
AJ, J1	J1	Adjustment	Nonreimbursable
IN	L6	Interest	Interest applied on the claim.
OF	WO	Withholding	Offset as a result of a previous overpayment
LF	50	Late Filing Reduction	

* Any adjustment to the submitted charge and/or units will continue to be reported next to the claim line with the appropriate group, reason and remark codes explaining the adjustment. Every provider level adjustment will now be reported in the provider level adjustment section of the SPR as well. Please refer to Reference ❶ in the attached example.
* The "TOTAL PD TO BENE" has been deleted from the provider summary level. The "PD TO BENE" has also been deleted from the claim level field. Amounts paid to the beneficiary will now be reported as a "CS" adjustment reason code in the "PLB REASON CODE" section. Please refer to Reference ❶ in the attached example.
* The "TOTAL INT" has been deleted from the provider summary level but the "INT" remains on the claim level field. Please refer to Reference ❷ in the attached example. Interest amounts will also be reported as a "L6" adjustment reason code in the "PLB REASON CODE" section. Please refer to Reference ❶ in the attached example. The interest amount reported in this section will be displayed as a negative amount if the amount has been included in the "NET" field at the claim level.
* A new claim level field, "LATE FILING CHARGE" has been added for the reporting of late filing reductions. Please refer to Reference ❷ in the attached example. This amount will be reported in the "PLB REASON CODE" section with a "50" adjustment reason code.
* The "TOTAL PREV PD" has been deleted from the provider summary level. This amount will now be reported only in the claim level field "PREV PD". Please refer to Reference ❷ in the attached example.
* The "TOTAL OFFSET" field at the provider summary level has been renamed as "TOTAL PROV ADJ AMT". Please refer to Reference ❸ in the attached example.
* Only the first crossover carrier name will be reported on the SPR, even if COB information is sent to more than one payer. Please refer to Reference ❹ in the attached example.

Note for MSP Claims: The amount of the payment for an MSP claim will not be reflected on the remittance under "NET". This amount is the amount of payment from the primary payer, plus the amount allowed from Medicare. To determine the amount that Medicare paid as their portion, you must deduct the amount in the "PROV ADJ DETAILS" for that claim from the "NET" in the claim detail. In the example shown, the NET was $20.00. The ADJ detail for that claim was also $20.00. The difference is $0, so Medicare did not pay anything on this particular claim. See Reference ❶ and ❺.

Fig. 9-9 Example of Standard Paper Remittance Advice (SPRA). (Source: U. S. Department of Health & Human Services, Centers for Medicare & Medicaid Services.)

Standard Paper Remittance (SPR) Advice Notices - Revised Format (continued)

EXAMPLE OF REVISED SPR

```
PERF PROV  SERV DATE  POS NOS  PROC  MODS    BILLED   ALLOWED   DEDUCT    COINS     GRP /RC-AMT    PROV PD

NAME  ALPHA, ALBERT         HIC 699777777A  ACNT 1111111111     ICN 1402065330030  ASG Y  MOA MA01
W88888888 1215 121501 11   1 92547           98.00    27.22     0.00      5.44  CO-42    70.78       21.78
W88888888 1215 121501 11   1 92541           45.00    39.89     0.00      7.98  CO-42     5.11       31.91
PT RESP   13.42                CLAIM TOTALS  143.00    67.11     0.00     13.42           75.89       53.69
                                                                                                53.69 NET


NAME  BAKER, LEEANN         HIC 699123123A  ACNT 0009           ICN 1102025001590  ASG Y  MOA MA01 MA18
W88888888 0113 011302 11   1 J9202 GACC     600.00   446.49     0.00     89.30  CO-42   153.51      357.19
          (J9217)
W88888888 0121 012102 11   1 J9202 CC       600.00   446.49     0.00     89.30  CO-42   153.51      357.19
          (J9217)
PT RESP  178.60                CLAIM TOTALS 1200.00   892.98     0.00    178.60          307.02      714.38
                                                                                               714.38 NET

CLAIM INFORMATION FORWARDED TO:  BCBS OF MINNESOTA   ❹


NAME  CHARLIE, CINDY        HIC 699222222A  ACNT 22222222       ICN 1402008151040  ASG Y  MOA MA01
W88888888 0106 010602 11   1 76091  26       80.00    43.76     0.00      8.75  CO-42    36.24       35.01
W88888888 0106 010602 11   1 G0236  26       50.00     0.00     0.00      0.00  CO-B5    50.00       00.00
REM: M58
PT RESP    8.75                CLAIM TOTALS  130.00    43.76     0.00      8.75  ❷        86.24       35.01
ADJS: PREV PD    0.00 INT      0.17 LATE FILING CHARGE    0.00                                  35.18 NET


NAME  BETA, BOB             HIC 699111111A  ACNT 12345678901234567890 ICN 1402063333010  ASG Y  MOA MA01 MA72
W88888888 0304 030402 11   1 99214          180.00    81.99    47.65      6.87  CO-42    98.01       27.47
W88888888 0304 030402 11   1 82010           30.00     0.00     0.00      0.00  CO-B7    30.00       00.00
W88888888 0304 030402 11   1 J1040           10.00     9.39     0.00      1.88  CO-42    00.61        7.51
PT RESP   56.40                CLAIM TOTALS  220.00    91.38    47.65      8.75          128.62       34.98
                                                                                                34.98 NET


NAME  BUMAN, JAMES          HIC 699555555A  ACNT 55555555       ICN 1402065200070  ASG Y  MOA MA01
W88888888 0304 030402 11   1 99214           75.00     0.00     0.00      0.00  PR-B7    75.00       20.00
                                                                               OA-71    20.00
                                                                               PR-A3   -20.00
PT RESP   55.00                CLAIM TOTALS   75.00     0.00     0.00      0.00           75.00       20.00  ❺
                                                                                                20.00 NET


TOTALS: # OF      BILLED     ALLOWED    DEDUCT     COINS      TOTAL     PROV PD       PROV  ❸    CHECK
        CLAIMS    AMT        AMT        AMT        AMT        RC-AMT    AMT           ADJ AMT     AMT
        5         1768.00    1095.23    47.65      209.52     672.77    858.06        108.50     749.56


PROVIDER ADJ DETAILS:  PLB REASON CODE    FCN              HIC            AMOUNT   ❶
                       CS                 1402063333010    699111111A      34.98
                       CS                 1402065200070    699555555A      20.00
                       WO                 7101347082956                    53.69
                       L6                                                  -0.17
```

GLOSSARY: Group, Reason, MOA, Remark and Adjustment Codes:

CO	Contractual Obligation. Amount for which the provider is financially liable. The patient may not be billed for this amount.
PR	Patient Responsibility. Amount that may be billed to a patient or another payee.
OA	Other Adjustment.
A3	Medicare Secondary Payer liability met.
B5	Claim/Service denied/reduced because coverage guidelines were not met or were exceeded.
B7	This provider was not certified for this procedure/service on this date of service.
42	Charges exceed our fee schedule or maximum allowable amount.
71	Primary Payer amount.
M58	Please resubmit the claim with the missing/correct information so that it may be processed.
MA01	If you do not agree with what we approved for these services, you may appeal our decision. To make sure that we are fair to you, we require another individual that did not process your initial claim to conduct the review. However, in order to be eligible for a review, you must write to us within 6 months of the date of this notice, unless you have a good reason for being late.
MA119	Provider level adjustment for late claim filing applies to this claim.
MA18	The claim information is also being forwarded to the patient's supplemental insurer. Send any questions regarding supplemental benefits to them.
MA72	The beneficiary overpaid you for these assigned services. You must issue the beneficiary a refund within 30 days for the difference between his/her payment to you and the total of the amount shown as patient responsibility and as paid to the beneficiary on this notice.
CS	Adjustment
WO	Withholding
L6	Interest

Fig. 9-9—cont'd SPRA.

Step 1. Providers must contact their software vendor to determine if ERA capability is available for the facility's practice management system. Special programming usually is required to extract the information from the electronic remittance file and automatically post this information to the patient accounts. (An example of an ERA is shown in Fig. 9-10.)

Step 2. The provider must complete an ERA enrollment form (Fig. 9-11).

ELECTRONIC FUNDS TRANSFER

Payments from Medicare may be automatically deposited to a provider's designated bank account using **electronic funds transfer** (EFT). Each EFT transaction is assigned a unique number, which functions the same way as a Medicare check number. The EFT number appears on the RA (paper or electronic) in the same field/location as the Medicare check number. EFT is available to all providers who bill Medicare. Providers must request an EFT enrollment form from their Medicare carrier. A request for EFT authorization form is shown in Fig. 9-12.

What Did You Learn?

1. What is an MSN?
2. Explain the difference between the MSN and the Medicare RA.
3. Who is eligible to receive an ERA?
4. What is an EFT?

MEDICARE AUDITS AND APPEALS

AUDITS

Medicare audits fall into two broad categories: prepayment audits, which, as the name suggests, review claims before Medicare pays the provider, and postpayment audits, which analyze claims after Medicare reimbursement. Some medical facilities believe they can avoid audits because they choose to report lower level Evaluation and Management Medicare codes on the claims; this is referred to as **downcoding**. Many audits target physicians' offices that practice downcoding because this type of practice "raises a red flag" to auditors. Downcoding on a claim is discouraged when the reason for doing so is simply that documentation in the health record does not meet the carriers' guidelines. If a particular code accurately describes the service or procedure performed, a provider should not voluntarily lower the code simply because he or she fears a documentation deficiency.

Stop and Think

You are having lunch with your friend Nellie Shumway, who works for a family practice clinic across the courtyard from your building. Over lunch one day, Nellie confides, "In our office, we code all new Medicare patient visits at Level 1 (99201). It's so much easier, and we don't have to worry about Medicare auditing our records." What, if anything, might you tell your friend?

If a carrier believes that a provider has a universal billing problem, the carrier may place that provider on prepayment review, which requires the provider to submit documentation for every claim before Medicare allows reimbursement. Prepayment review is a tremendous burden on the medical facility because it can no longer submit electronic claims. If the prepayment review involves documentation of hospital visits, the physician must obtain the records from the facility for each visit before submitting the claim; this delays reimbursement and creates administrative problems.

Postpayment audits are most commonly triggered by statistical irregularities. A postpayment audit can result if a provider uses a certain code much more frequently or less frequently than other providers of the same specialty in the same area. Patient complaints also can trigger audits and reviews.

APPEALS

Medicare regulations allow providers and beneficiaries who are dissatisfied with Medicare's determination to request that the determination be reconsidered. Through the appeals process, Medicare seeks to ensure that the correct payment is made or a clear and adequate explanation is given supporting nonpayment.

A physician or supplier providing items and services payable under Medicare Part B may appeal an initial determination if

• he or she accepted assignment;
• he or she did not accept assignment on a claim that was denied on the basis as being not reasonable and necessary;
• the beneficiary did not know or could not have been expected to know that the service would not be covered, requiring the provider/supplier to refund the beneficiary any payment received for the services; or
• he or she did not accept assignment, but is acting as the authorized representative of the beneficiary, and indicates this in the appeal (attaching a copy of the beneficiary's MSN indicates the provider/supplier is authorized to act on the beneficiary's behalf).

Provider Name   Provider #:

Address   Page #:   1 of 2

City State Zip   Date: 08/27/03

                                                                Check/EFT #:

```
************************************************************************************
*                                                                                  *
*     Effective Monday, September 15, 2003, the phone numbers to contact Noridian  *
*     Administrative Services' Phone Appeals and Provider Enrollment teams will be *
*     changing. The Phone Appeals number will be 1-800-279-5331 and the Provider   *
*     Enrollment number will be 1-888-608-8816.                                    *
*                                                                                  *
************************************************************************************
```

PERF PROV	SERV DATE	POS NOS	PROC	MODS	BILLED	ALLOWED	DEDUCT	COINS	GRP/RC-AMT	PROV PD
NAME		HIC	ACNT				ICN 1703219015000		ASG Y MOA	MAO1 MA18
	0701 070103 11	1 99213		180.00	44.16	0.00	8.83 CO-42	135.84	35.33	
PT RESP 8.83		CLAIM TOTALS	180.00	44.16	0.00	8.83	135.84	35.33	
CLAIM INFORMATION FORWARDED TO: BCMNX/BC/BC MINNESOTA									35.33 NET	

NAME		HIC	ACNT				ICN 1803171001050		ASG Y MOA	MAO1
	0402 040203 11	1 76091		150.00	0.00	0.00	0.00 CO-50	150.00	0.00	
REM: M25										
PT RESP 0.00		CLAIM TOTALS	150.00	0.00	0.00	0.00	150.00	0.00	
									0.00 NET	

NAME		HIC	ACNT				ICN 0102247015010		ASG Y MOA	MAO1 N154
	0510 051002 11	1 99213		150.00	45.79	0.00	9.16 CO-42	104.21	36.63	
PT RESP 9.16		CLAIM TOTALS	150.00	45.79	0.00	9.16	104.21	36.63	
ADJS: PREV PD 0.00 INT 0.02 LATE FILING CHARGE 0.00									36.65 NET	

TOTALS:	# OF CLAIMS	BILLED AMT	ALLOWED AMT	DEDUCT AMT	COINS AMT	TOTAL RC-AMT	PROV PD AMT	PROV ADJ AMT	CHECK AMT

PROVIDER ADJ DETAILS: PLB REASON CODE   FCN   HIC   AMOUNT
                          WO   7102352195000   35.33

SUMMARY OF NON-ASSIGNED CLAIMS

PERF PROV	SERV DATE	POS NOS	PROC	MODS	BILLED	ALLOWED	DEDUCT	COINS	GRP/RC-AMT	PROV PD
NAME		HIC	ACNT				ICN 1703219015010		ASG N MOA	MA28
	0704 070403 11	1 99214		200.00	69.11	0.00	13.82 PR-42	10.37	0.00	
								CO-45	120.52	
								PR-100	55.29	
PT RESP 79.48		CLAIM TOTALS	200.00	69.11	0.00	13.82	186.18	0.00	
									0.00 NET	

Glossary: Group, Reason, MOA, Remark and Adjustment Codes

CO   Contractual Obligation. Amount for which the provider is financially liable. The patient may not be billed for this amount.

PR   Patient Responsibility. Amount that may be billed to a patient or another payer.

100   Payment made to patient/insured/responsible party.

42   Charges exceed our fee schedule or maximum allowable amount.

45   Charges exceed your contracted/legislated fee arrangement.

MAO1   If you do not agree with what we approved for these services, you may appeal our decision. To make sure that we are fair to you, we require another individual that did not process your initial claim to conduct the review. However, in order to be eligible for a review, you must write to us within 120 days of the date of this notice, unless you have a good reason for being late. An institutional provider, e.g., hospital, SNF, HHA or a hospice may appeal only if the claim involves a reasonable and necessary denial, a SNF non-certified bed denial, or a home health denial because the patient was not homebound or was not in need of intermittent skilled nursing services, or a hospice care denial because the patient was not terminally ill, and either the patient or the provider is liable under Section 1879 of the Social Security Act, and the patient chooses not to appeal. If your carrier issues telephone review decisions, a professional provider should phone the carrier's office for a telephone review if the criteria for a telephone review are met.

MA18   The claim information is also being forwarded to the patient's supplemental insurer. Send any questions regarding supplemental benefits to them.

Fig. 9-10 ERA. (Source: U. S. Department of Health & Human Services, Centers for Medicare & Medicaid Services.)

Submitter Name: _____   Submitter ID: _____

Contact Person: _____   Phone Number: _____

Remittance Format and version:

ANSI X12 835, version 4010 A1 _____   ANSI X12 835, version 3030 _____

National Standard Format, version 1.04 _____   ANSI X12 835, version 3051,3B.00 _____

National Standard Format, version 2.0 _____   ANSI X12 835, version 3051,4B.00 _____

National Standard Format, version 2.01 _____   ANSI X12 835, version 4010 _____

In compliance with the Health Insurance Portability and Accountability Act (HIPAA), effective October 16, 2003 the only remittance format and version that NHIC will provide is ANSI X12 835, version 4010A1. If your practice management accommodates a remittance module, we recommend that you work with your vendor to install the 4010A1 version.

Provider Numbers:
Please list all provider numbers to receive remittance. If billing with a group provider number, list only the group number. Please attach a separate sheet if necessary. The provider must sign the form to be activated.

Provider ID (9) characters   **Printed Provider Name**   **Provider Signature**

_____   _____   _____

_____   _____   _____

A billing service or clearinghouse may accept remittance files on behalf of a provider(s), but the billing service or clearinghouse is prohibited from viewing, storing, modifying or reporting the data for its own use. The billing service or clearinghouse's signature on this form signifies their agreement with this requirement.

Billing Service/Clearinghouse Representative (if applicable)

Please fax or mail this form to the NHIC office that processes your Medicare Part B claims:

Fig. 9-11 ERA enrollment form.

Claims submitted with incomplete or invalid information are not given appeal rights and are returned as unprocessable. The provider has two options for correcting the claim, as follows:
- Submit an entirely new claim (electronic or paper) with complete, valid information
- Submit corrections in writing

Table 9-11 lists the types of appeal actions available to Medicare beneficiaries and providers.

Telephone Review Requests

Providers or suppliers may request a review by telephone, if the appeal request is not complex. If an appeal from a provider or supplier is complex, or if significant documentation is needed to adjudicate the appeal request, a written review must be filed within the timely filing period. Examples of review request clarifications or problems that can be handled over the telephone include the following:
- The diagnosis was not linked properly on the original claim.

- The number of services or units is incorrect or missing.
- The anesthesia time is missing.
- The date of service is incorrect (except for changes to the year).
- The CPT code is incorrect, and changing it would not create an overpayment.
- The services are incorrectly denied as duplicate charges.
- A modifier is being added or corrected (except for returned unprocessable claim, or RUC, rejections).
- The place of service is incorrect.

Written Part B Determination

For Part B appeals, Medicare regulations state that any party who is dissatisfied with the initial determination may request the carrier review such determination. Effective January 1, 2003, a request for review must be filed within 4 months after the date of the notice of the initial determination. Medicare cannot accept an appeal for which no initial determination has been made. The request for review not only must identify the initial determination

AUTHORIZATION AGREEMENT FOR ELECTRONIC FUNDS TRANSFER (EFT)

Reason for Submission:
❑ New EFT Authorization
❑ Revision to Current Authorization *(i.e. account or bank changes)*
❑ EFT Termination Request

Chain Home Office:
❑ Check here if EFT payment is being made to the Home Office of Chain Organization
(Attach letter Authorizing EFT payment to Chain Home Office)

Physician/Provider/Supplier Information

Physician's Name _____

Provider/Supplier Legal Business Name _____

_____

Chain Organization Name _____

Home Office Legal Business Name *(if different from Chain Organization Name)* _____

_____

Tax ID Number: *(Designate SSN ❑ or EIN ❑)* ___ ___ ___ ___ ___ ___ ___ ___ ___

Doing Business As Name_____

Medicare Identification Number *(OSCAR, UPIN, or NSC only)* _____

Depository Information (Financial Institution)

Depository Name _____

Account Holder's Name _____

Street Address _____

City _____ State _____ Zip Code _____

Depository Telephone Number_____

Depository Contact Person _____

Depository Routing Transit Number *(nine digit)* ___ ___ ___ ___ ___ ___ ___ ___ ___

Depositor Account Number _____

Type of Account *(check one)* ❑ Checking Account ❑ Savings Account

Please include a voided check, preprinted deposit slip, or confirmation of account information on bank letterhead with this agreement for verification of your account number.

Authorization

I hereby authorize the Medicare contractor, _____, hereinafter called the COMPANY, to initiate credit entries, and in accordance with 31 CFR part 210.6(f) initiate adjustments for any credit entries made in error to the account indicated above. I hereby authorize the financial institution/bank named above, hereinafter called the DEPOSITORY, to credit and/or debit the same to such account.

If payment is being made to an account controlled by a Chain Home Office, the Provider of Services hereby acknowledges that payment to the Chain Office under these circumstances is still considered payment to the Provider, and the Provider authorizes the forwarding of Medicare payments to the Chain Home Office.

If the account is drawn in the Physician's or Individual Practitioner's Name, or the Legal Business Name of the Provider/Supplier, the said Physician/Provider/Supplier certifies that he/she has sole control of the account referenced above, and certifies that all arrangements between the DEPOSITORY and the said Physician/Provider/Supplier are in accordance with all applicable Medicare regulations and instructions.

FORM CMS-588 (09/03)

Fig. 9-12 Authorization agreement for EFT. (Source: U. S. Department of Health & Human Services, Centers for Medicare & Medicaid Services.)

This authorization agreement is effective as of the signature date below and is to remain in full force and effect until the COMPANY has received written notification from me of its termination in such time and such manner as to afford the COMPANY and the DEPOSITORY a reasonable opportunity to act on it. The COMPANY will continue to send the direct deposit to the DEPOSITORY indicated above until notified by me that I wish to change the DEPOSITORY receiving the direct deposit. If my DEPOSITORY information changes, I agree to submit to the COMPANY an updated EFT Authorization Agreement.

Signature Line

Authorized/Delegated Official Name *(Print)* _____

Authorized/Delegated Official Title _____

Authorized/Delegated Official Signature_____Date_____

PRIVACY ACT ADVISORY STATEMENT

Sections 1842, 1862(b) and 1874 of title XVIII of the Social Security Act authorize the collection of this information. The purpose of collecting this information is to authorize electronic funds transfers.

The information collected will be entered into system No. 09-70-0501, titled "Carrier Medicare Claims Records," and No. 09-70-0503, titled "Intermediary Medicare Claims Records" published in the Federal Register Privacy Act Issuances, 1991 Comp. Vol. 1, pages 419 and 424, or as updated and republished. Disclosures of information from this system can be found in this notice.

Furnishing information is voluntary, but without it we will not be able to process your electronic funds transfer.

You should be aware that P.L. 100-503, the Computer Matching and Privacy Protection Act of 1988, permits the government, under certain circumstances, to verify the information you provide by way of computer matches.

According to the Paperwork Reduction Act of 1995, no persons are required to respond to a collection of information unless it displays a valid OMB control number. The valid OMB control number for this information collection is 0938-0626. The time required to complete this information collection is estimated to average 2 hours per response, including the time to review instructions, search existing data resources, gather the data needed, and complete and review the information collection. If you have any comments concerning the accuracy of the time estimate(s) or suggestions for improving this form, please write to: CMS, Attn: PRA Reports Clearance Officer, 7500 Security Boulevard, Baltimore, Maryland 21244-1850.

FORM CMS-588 (09/03)

Fig. 9-12—cont'd

TABLE 9-11	Types of Appeal Actions	
TYPE OF APPEAL	**CRITERIA NECESSARY**	**TIME LIMITS**
Telephone review	May be requested by providers, beneficiaries, or their representative. Allowed only for assigned claims, unless beneficiary is present at the time of the request and gives Medicare the authorization to proceed with review. Providers may be limited in the number of reviews made per call (See "Telephone Review Requests" section below).	*Before January 1, 2003:* Must be requested within 6 months of date of initial determination *January 1, 2003 and after:* Must be requested within 4 months of initial determination
Written review	Requests must be made in writing and must be signed.	*Before January 1, 2003:* Must be requested within 6 months of date of initial determination *January 1, 2003 and after:* Must be requested within 4 months of initial determination
Fair hearing	Requested if provider is dissatisfied with the review determination. Amount in controversy must be at least $110.00. May request the hearing be held in person, by telephone, or on-the-record. If you request hearing on-the-record, a decision is made based on information currently on file. If you request an in-person or telephone hearing, it is scheduled.	Must be filed within 6 months after the date of the review determination
Administrative law judge	Filed if provider is dissatisfied with determination made by the hearing officer. Amount in controversy must be at least $500.00. May request a hearing before an Administrative Law Judge (ALJ) of the Social Security Administration (SSA).	Must be made in writing and filed within 60 days of the date of the carrier's fair hearing decision of record
Judicial review	Requested if provider is still dissatisfied with the determination of the Administrative Law Judge. Amount in controversy must be at least $1090.00.	No time limits.

with which the party is dissatisfied, but also must meet the requirements for the contents of an appeal request as follows:
• A request for a review may be filed on HCFA-1964, Request for Review of Part B Medicare Claim.
• A request for a review may be a signed written statement from the provider or supplier expressing disagreement with the initial determination or indicating that the review or a re-examination should be made.
• A request for a review may be filed on the provider's or supplier's letterhead or on a Physician/Supplier Inquiry Form (this form may be requested by calling your carrier.)

The review request must include the following information:
• Beneficiary name
• Medicare HICN
• Name and address of provider/supplier of item/service
• Date of initial determination

• Date of service for which the initial determination was issued (dates must be reported in a manner that comports with the Medicare claims filing instructions; ranges of dates are acceptable only if a range of dates is properly reportable on the Medicare claim form)
• The item, if any, and service that is at issue in the appeal

The provider RA should accompany the review request along with any pertinent data that provide additional information (information not submitted with the initial claim). It is not necessary to send another CMS-1500 form. Any corrected information should be included with the written request.

Providers and suppliers are responsible for submitting documentation, if any, that supports the reason for the appeal. This documentation may be supplied with the appeal request or at the request of the carrier. Failure to submit documentation in a timely manner may result in processing delays. A sample request for review form is shown in Fig. 9-13.

REQUEST FOR REVIEW OF PART B MEDICARE CLAIM
Medical Insurance Benefits – Social Security Act

NOTICE – Anyone who misrepresents or falsifies essential information requested by this form may upon conviction be subject to fine and imprisonment under Federal Law.

1. Carrier's Name and Address	2. Name of Patient
	3. Health Insurance Claim Number

4. I do not agree with the determination you made on my claim as described on my Explanation of Medicare Benefits dated:

5. MY REASONS ARE: (Attach a copy of the Explanation of Medicare Benefits, or describe the service, date of service, and physician's name. NOTE: If the date on the Explanation of Medicare Benefits mentioned in Item 4 is more than six months ago, include your reason for not making this request earlier.)

6. Describe illness or injury:

7. ☐ I have additional evidence to submit. (Attach such evidence to this form.)
   ☐ I do not have additional evidence.

COMPLETE ALL OF THE INFORMATION REQUESTED. SIGN AND RETURN THE FIRST COPY AND ANY ATTACHMENTS TO THE CARRIER NAMED ABOVE. IF YOU NEED HELP, TAKE THIS AND YOUR NOTICE FROM THE CARRIER TO A SOCIAL SECURITY OFFICE, OR TO THE CARRIER. KEEP THE DUPLICATE COPY OF THIS FORM FOR YOUR RECORDS.

8. SIGNATURE OF *EITHER* THE CLAIMANT *OR* HIS REPRESENTATIVE

Claimant	Representative	
Address	Address	
City, State and ZIP Code	City, State and ZIP Code	
Telephone Number	Date	Telephone Number	Date

Form CMS-1964 (9/91)

Carrier's Copy

Fig. 9-13 Request for review of Medicare Part B claim. (Source: U. S. Department of Health & Human Services, Centers for Medicare & Medicaid Services.)

What Did You Learn?

1. Name the two categories into which Medicare audits fall.
2. List two things that might prompt a Medicare audit.
3. Under what circumstances might a provider initiate an appeal?
4. Name four types of claim errors that can be handled via a telephone review.

QUALITY REVIEW STUDIES

Regulations define a **quality review study** as "an assessment, conducted by or for a **peer review organization [PRO]**, of a patient care problem for the purpose of improving patient care through peer analysis, intervention, resolution of the problem, and follow-up."[2] Quality review studies typically follow a set of related structured activities designed to achieve measurable improvement in processes and outcomes of care. Improvements are achieved through interventions that target healthcare providers, practitioners, plans, or beneficiaries.

QUALITY IMPROVEMENT ORGANIZATIONS

Medicare **quality improvement organizations** work with consumers, physicians, hospitals, and other caregivers to refine care delivery systems to ensure patients receive the right care at the right time, particularly among underserved populations. The program also safeguards the integrity of the Medicare trust fund by ensuring payment is made only for medically necessary services and investigates beneficiary complaints about quality of care. Under the direction of CMS, the program consists of a national network of 53 quality improvement organizations responsible for each state, territory, and the District of Columbia.

 HIPAA Tip

Covered entities may disclose protected health information about non-Medicare patients without their permission when the information involves Quality Improvement Organizations quality-related activities under its contract. (Under HIPAA, a "covered entity" is a health plan, healthcare clearinghouse, or healthcare provider who transmits information in electronic form.)

MEDICARE BENEFICIARY PROTECTION PROGRAM

Medicare quality improvement organizations, such as the **Medicare Beneficiary Protection Program**, help protect the safety and health of Medicare beneficiaries through numerous activities, such as
• responding to beneficiary complaints,
• Hospital Issued Notice of Noncoverage (HINN) and Notice of Discharge and Medicare Appeal Rights (NODMAR) reviews, and
• physician review of medical records.

Beneficiary Complaints

If a Medicare beneficiary or representative has a concern about the quality of care, especially if the beneficiary believes that the care was inadequate or inappropriate, the beneficiary may contact one of the Medicare beneficiary protection programs and initiate a complaint. More information about Medicare beneficiary rights is available on the Medicare website.

Hospital Issued Notice of Noncoverage and Notice of Discharge and Medicare Appeal Rights Reviews

When a hospital issues a HINN, or a managed care organization issues a NODMAR, a beneficiary or representative may request an immediate review. The purpose of the review is to ensure that the HINN or NODMAR is correct, and that beneficiaries are not discharged prematurely from care.

PEER REVIEW ORGANIZATIONS

PRO review is governed by Titles XI and XVIII of the Social Security Act and by regulations contained in various sections of the Social Security Act. Each state has its own PRO, and although each is unique, there are certain guidelines they must all follow in relation to the review of items or services provided to Medicare beneficiaries to determine the following:
• Whether services provided or proposed to be provided are reasonable and medically necessary for the diagnosis and treatment of illness or injury, or to improve functioning of a malformed body member, or (with respect to pneumococcal vaccine and mammograms) for prevention of an illness, or (in the case of hospice care) for the relief of symptoms or effects of and management of terminal illness.
• Whether the services furnished or proposed to be furnished on an inpatient basis could be performed effectively on an outpatient basis or in an inpatient healthcare facility of a different type.

[2]http://www.cms.hhs.gov/manuals/19_pro/pr16.asp#_1_2.

- The medical necessity, reasonableness, and appropriateness of inpatient hospital care for which additional payment is sought under the outlier provisions of the **prospective payment system (PPS)**. PPS is a method of reimbursement in which Medicare payment is made based on a predetermined, fixed amount. The payment amount for a particular service is derived based on the classification system of that service (e.g., DRGs for inpatient hospital services).
- Whether a hospital has misrepresented admission or discharge information or has taken an action that results in the unnecessary admission of an individual entitled to benefits under Part A, unnecessary multiple admissions of an individual, or other inappropriate medical or other practices with respect to beneficiaries, or billing for services furnished to beneficiaries.
- The validity of diagnostic and procedural information supplied by the provider to the intermediary for payment purposes.
- The completeness and adequacy of hospital care provided.
- Whether the quality of services meets professionally recognized standards of healthcare.

PHYSICIAN REVIEW OF MEDICAL RECORDS

Physician reviewers conduct medical record review to determine if the care received was medically necessary and appropriate. Reviews may include utilization, coding, or quality of care issues. The reviewer is generally from the same specialty as the physician who provided the care. This peer review is an important component of the quality-of-care oversight provided by Medicare quality improvement organizations and external quality review organizations.

HEALTHCARE QUALITY IMPROVEMENT PROGRAM

The **Health Care Quality Improvement Program** was created to improve health outcomes of all Medicare beneficiaries regardless of personal characteristics (e.g., socioeconomic status, health status, ethnic group), physical location (urban or rural), or setting (e.g., physicians' offices, Medicare Advantage organizations, hospitals, nursing homes). The PRO's Statement of Work sets forth specific quality indicators for national health improvement priorities, which reflect the current state of PRO program experience, measurement systems, and data sources. These quality indicators neither address the entire spectrum of healthcare nor reflect fully the unique circumstances of each state. CMS requires state PROs to conduct the following:

- For Medicare beneficiaries in a specific state, implement quality improvement projects on a standardized set of quality indicators in each of the following six clinical topics:

- Acute myocardial infarction
- Pneumonia
- Diabetes
- Breast cancer
- Stroke, transient ischemic attack, or atrial fibrillation
- Congestive heart failure
- Initiate local projects within the specific state in the following three areas:
  - Quality improvement projects in alternate settings
  - Projects designed to reduce the disparity of care received by members of disadvantaged groups and all other beneficiaries in the PRO's state
  - Projects in response to local interests and needs
- For Medicare Advantage organizations in a specific state, offer technical assistance services, and encourage the organizations to collaborate with healthcare facilities in any or all of their health improvement projects. This specifically includes the diabetes and influenza immunization projects that the Medicare Advantage organizations are required to conduct under their Quality Improvement System for Managed Care regulations.

PAYMENT ERROR PREVENTION PROGRAM

The Office of Inspector General Audit Opinion Financial Statement found that a considerable amount of improper payments were made for inpatient services under the PPS. To reduce this payment error rate, the PRO must initiate a program of payment error prevention projects. CMS defines the payment error rate as the number of dollars found to be paid in error out of the total of all dollars paid for inpatient PPS services. CMS implements a surveillance system to provide state-specific estimates of the payment error rate. These estimates are used as performance indicators on which to evaluate performance.

CLINICAL LABORATORY IMPROVEMENT AMENDMENT

Congress established the **Clinical Laboratory Improvement Amendments (CLIA)** program in 1988 to regulate quality standards for all laboratory testing done on humans to ensure the safety, accuracy, reliability, and timeliness of patient test results regardless of where the test was performed. CMS assumes primary responsibility for financial management operations of the CLIA program. Although all clinical laboratories must be properly certified to receive Medicare or Medicaid payments, CLIA has no direct Medicare or Medicaid program responsibilities.

To enroll in the CLIA program, laboratories (including laboratories located in physician offices) first must register by completing an application, paying a fee, being surveyed if applicable, and becoming certified. CLIA fees are structured depending on the type of certificate requested by the laboratory based on the complexity of the tests it performs. After all these preliminary measures are taken, the laboratory is issued an 11-digit CLIA certificate number. This information is significant to the health insurance professional because the 11-digit CLIA certificate number must appear in Block 23 of the CMS-1500 form for Medicare claims when laboratory services have been performed in a physician office laboratory.

What Did You Learn?

1. Define a "quality review study."
2. How does the Medicare Beneficiary Protection Program aid beneficiaries?
3. What is the purpose of PROs?
4. Where on the CMS-1500 form should the CLIA number be entered?

SUMMARY CHECK POINTS

☑ Medicare is a comprehensive federal insurance program established by Congress in 1966 to provide limited healthcare to people age 65, certain categories of disabled individuals younger than age 65, and individuals of any age who have ESRD. Medicare is administered by CMS.

☑ *Medicare Part A* (hospital insurance) helps pay for *medically necessary* services for the following types of healthcare:
  • Inpatient hospital care
  • Inpatient care in SNF
  • Home healthcare
  • Hospice care

☑ *Medicare Part B* is medical insurance financed by a combination of federal government funds and beneficiary premiums, which helps pay for
  • medically necessary physicians' services,
  • outpatient hospital services,
  • DME, and
  • some other services/supplies not covered by Part A

☑ *Medicare Part C* (Medicare Advantage, formerly Medicare+Choice) is a managed healthcare structure that offers regular Part A and Part B Medicare coverage and other services. Primary Medicare Part C plans include
  • Medicare managed care plans;
  • Medicare private, unrestricted fee-for-service plans; and
  • MSA plans.

☑ Medicare Part C not only includes Part A and Part B coverage, but also pays for services not covered under the original Medicare plan, such as
  • preventive care,
  • prescription drugs,
  • eyeglasses,
  • dental care, and
  • hearing aids.

☑ As of January 2006, *Medicare Part D* (Prescription Drug Plan) will pay a portion of prescription drug expenses and cost sharing for qualifying individuals.

☑ *Medi-Medi* refers to individuals who qualify for benefits under the Medicare and Medicaid Programs, sometimes referred to as *dual eligibles*. Most individuals who qualify for Medi-Medi are low-income elderly and individuals younger than 65 with disabilities.

☑ *Medigap* is a Medicare supplement insurance policy sold by private insurance companies to fill "gaps" in the original (fee-for-service) Medicare plan coverage. There are 12 standardized plans labeled Plan A through Plan L. Medigap policies work only with the original Medicare plan.

☑ *MSP* is the term used when Medicare is not responsible for payment healthcare charges first when the beneficiary is covered under another insurance policy. Medicare may be the secondary payer in any of the following situations:
  • Workers' compensation
  • Working aged (people age >65 years who are covered by a group health plan through their own or their spouse's current employment)
  • Disabled individuals age 64 and younger who are covered by a large group health plan (>100 employees) through their own or a family member's current employment
  • Medicare beneficiaries with ESRD who are covered under a group health plan
  • Individuals covered under the Federal Black Lung Program
  • Individuals receiving Veterans Administration benefits
  • Individuals who are covered under a Federal Research Grant Program

☑ Advantages of Medicare HMOs include the following:
  • HMOs often do not health screen; enrollment may not be denied because of health status.
  • HMOs may cover services that traditional Medicare does not cover, such as routine physical examinations, eyeglasses, hearing aids, prescriptions, and dental coverage.
  • Enrollees do not need Medigap insurance.

☑ There is limited or no paperwork to deal with, contrary to traditional Medicare coverage.
• Enrollees do not have to pay the Medicare deductibles and coinsurance.

☑ Disadvantages of Medicare HMOs include the following:
• Choice of healthcare providers and medical facilities is limited.
• Members/enrollees are covered only for healthcare services received through the HMO except in emergency and urgent care situations.
• Prior approval usually is needed from a primary care physician for a specialist's services, surgical procedures, medical equipment, and other healthcare services.
• Enrollees who travel out of the HMO's service area do not receive coverage except in emergency and urgent care situations.
• If an enrollee decides to switch from the HMO to the traditional Medicare plan, coverage does not begin until the first day of the month after the disenrollment request.

☑ For a service or procedure to be determined *medically necessary* under Medicare guidelines, the service or procedure must meet the following criteria:
• Consistent with the symptoms or diagnosis of the illness or injury being treated
• Necessary and consistent with generally accepted professional medical standards
• Not furnished primarily for the convenience of the patient or physician
• Furnished at the most appropriate level that can be provided safely to the patient

☑ The ABN is a form that Medicare requires all healthcare providers to use when Medicare does not pay for a service to ensure that beneficiaries have a choice about their healthcare in the event that Medicare does not pay. When patients are asked to sign an ABN, they have two options:
• To receive the test or procedure, agree to be responsible for payment, and sign the ABN
• Not to receive the test or procedure, refuse to be responsible for payment, and sign the ABN

☑ The health insurance professional must use the Medicare fee schedule to determine the amount Medicare allows PARs and nonPARs accepting assignment to charge a patient for a particular service or procedure. Medicare PARs use the amount shown under the heading "PAR." A Medicare nonPAR can charge the amount in the next column under the heading "NON-PAR." The limiting charge for providers *not accepting* assignment is the amount under the heading "LIMITING," which is 15% more than the nonPAR amount.

☑ The Medicare Crossover Program is a service that Medicare Part B offers to private insurers and retirement plans, such as Medigap insurers, supplemental retirement plans, or other healthcare payers wherein the insurer sends an eligibility file to Medicare, and Medicare sends corresponding claim information back to the healthcare payer. The eligibility file contains the beneficiary's name, Medicare HICN, and policy effective dates. Medicare matches the trading partner's HICN against its own Medicare files. Any resulting claims are automatically sent to the payer for additional payment considerations.

☑ A *small provider* is defined as follows:
• A provider of services (as that term is defined in section 1861(u) of the Social Security Act) with fewer than 25 FTE employees
• A physician, practitioner, facility or supplier that is not otherwise a provider under section 1861 (u) with fewer than 10 FTE employees

☑ MSN is a document sent to the Medicare beneficiary after a provider files a claim for Part A and Part B services in the original Medicare plan. It explains what the provider billed for, the Medicare-approved amount, how much Medicare paid, and what the beneficiary must pay (sometimes called an Explanation of Medicare Benefits).

☑ A Medicare RA is the document Medicare sends to the provider of services that explains how claims were adjudicated. The RA contains detailed processing information, including claims adjustment reason codes that tell why an adjustment was made to the claim payment and remittance remark codes, which represent nonfinancial information. The health insurance professional must be able to decipher these codes to understand why the payment is less than that shown on the claim.

☑ Any Medicare provider (PAR and nonPAR) who submits electronic claims can receive an ERA. Additionally, providers may allow a billing agent (billing service, clearinghouse) to receive ERAs on their behalf. The provider receives a paper Medicare check and SPRA just as before. The check number appears on paper and electronic versions of the RA.

☑ Medicare payments can be automatically deposited to a provider's designated bank account using EFT.

With EFT, each transaction is assigned a unique number, which functions the same way as a Medicare check number. EFT is instantaneous, which allows funds to become immediately available for practice or other expenses.

☑ Quality review studies are performed to
- improve the processes and outcomes of patient care,

- safeguard the integrity of the Medicare trust fund by ensuring payments are made only for medically necessary services, and
- investigate beneficiary complaints.

☑ CLIA was established to set quality standards for all laboratory testing to ensure the safety, accuracy, reliability, and timeliness of patient test results regardless of where the test was performed.

CLOSING SCENARIO

Rita felt relieved yet satisfied after completing the chapter on Medicare. As she had anticipated at the beginning, there was a lot to learn. Each evening after class, Grandma Nan had waited up for Rita, and they talked about what the lesson had been about that day. Grandma Nan's interest inspired Rita to listen closely, take detailed notes, and ask questions when she did not understand a particular concept. Soon, Rita found herself caught up in Medicare's challenges.

Rita became a big help to Grandma Nan and her elderly friends. When one of them brought over a Medicare Summary Notice, Rita went through it with them, explaining each detail line by line. She also was able to explain to them the concept of "medically necessary" and the fact that Medicare pays only 80% of "covered" charges—not *all* services and supplies. The light of understanding in their eyes was the only reward Rita needed, and she decided then and there that she wanted to work in a medical facility specializing in the treatment of elderly patients. Rita believed that she could establish a similar rapport with elderly patients as she had with Grandma Nan and her friends.

WEBSITES TO EXPLORE

For live links to the following websites, please visit the Evolve® site at http://evolve.elsevier.com/Beik/today/

- For extensive information on Medicare, log on to http://www.medicare.gov/

- National Medicare Coverage Policies are found on the following website: http://cms.hhs.gov/

- For more information about CMS log on to http://www.cms.hhs.gov/home/aboutcms.asp

- To peruse an issue of *The CMS Quarterly Provider Update*, log on to www.cms.hhs.gov/providerupdate

- LMRPs can be found on the following link: http://www.lmrp.net

- The *Medicare Coverage Issues Manual* is searchable on the following: http://cms.hhs.gov/

- For information on how to submit MSP claims electronically, log on to the following website: http://www.ansi.org/ for the American National Standards Institute (ANSI) ASC X12N Implementation Guide

- Or for the National Standard Format (NSF) Specifications log on to http://www.hipaanet.com/hisb_nsf.htm

- For instructions on how to read the beneficiary MSN, log on to the following website: http://www.medicare.gov/Basics/SummaryNotice_HowToRead.asp

- Information on filing complaints for Medicare beneficiaries is available at www.medicare.gov/Publications/Pubs/pdf/10050.pdf

- For more information on CLIA, log on to the CMS website at http://www.cms.hhs.gov/ and click on CLIA in the left-hand column

Chapter 10

Military Carriers: TRICARE and CHAMPVA

CHAPTER OBJECTIVES

After completion of this chapter, the student should be able to

- Describe TRICARE's role in military insurance.
- List and explain TRICARE's three choices for healthcare.
- Distinguish eligibility criteria among the three TRICARE plans.
- Define a nonavailability statement and advise when it must be used.
- Compare TRICARE participating providers and nonparticipating providers as they relate to claims processing.
- Explain CHAMPVA's role in military insurance.
- List the criteria necessary for CHAMPVA eligibility.
- Discuss the CHAMPVA-Medicare connection.
- List the important steps for filing military claims.
- Explain how to use the Internet to find addresses for military claims submission.
- State the deadlines for filing military claims.
- Discuss what the Department of Defense has done to implement HIPAA's privacy rules.

CHAPTER TERMS

beneficiaries
catastrophic cap (cat cap)
CHAMPUS Maximum Allowable Charge
CHAMPVA for Life (CFL)
Civilian Health and Medical Program of the Department of Veterans Affairs (CHAMPVA)
Civilian Health and Medical Program of the Uniformed Services (CHAMPUS)
claims processor
covered charges
Defense Enrollment Eligibility Reporting System (DEERS)
lead agent
Military Health System
military treatment facility (MTF)

nonavailability statement (NAS)
other health insurance (OHI)
primary care manager (PCM)
remote assignment
reserve components (RCs)
sponsor
TRICARE
TRICARE Extra
TRICARE-for-Life (TFL)
TRICARE Management Activity
TRICARE Prime
TRICARE Prime Remote
TRICARE Standard
TRICARE Standard Supplemental Insurance
TRICARE's allowable charge
XPress Claim

OPENING SCENARIO

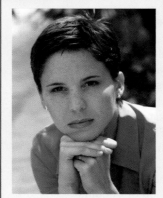

Sally Curtis is looking forward to the chapter on military insurers. She comes from a long line of military people. Both her parents are in the Army Reserves, her uncle is currently a Marine stationed in Iraq, her maternal grandfather was a Green Beret, and her great-grandfather was stationed in England during World War II. Until now, Sally was not even aware that the military had their own insurance. During a family discussion, a lot of questions were raised about TRICARE and CHAMPVA that Sally could not answer.

Sally's Aunt Betty said she was aware that there were three plans available to spouses and dependents of active service members, but she didn't know which was the best plan for her. The health insurance professional where Aunt Betty received her healthcare was little help because she didn't know much about military insurance either, and Aunt Betty wonders if her claims were handled properly. "She calls it CHAMPUS," Aunt Betty said, "not TRICARE. What's the difference?" Sally promised her family members that she would be able to give them the answers they were looking for after she had completed Chapter 10.

MILITARY HEALTH PROGRAMS

The federal government has provided healthcare for the military from the earliest years of U.S. history. In 1884, Congress requested that Army medical officers and surgeons should attend to the families of the officers and soldiers free of charge whenever possible. During World War II, Congress authorized the creation of the Emergency Maternal and Infant Care Program (EMIC), which provided maternity care and care of infants up to 1 year of age for wives and children of service members. During the Korean War in 1956, the Dependents Medical Care Act became law.

The 1966 amendments to this law initiated what later became the **Civilian Health and Medical Program of the Uniformed Services (CHAMPUS)**, a military healthcare program that existed for more than 30 years until it was replaced with TRICARE in 1998.

TRICARE

TRICARE developed from the CHAMPUS Reform Initiative, which began in 1988. It was a demonstration program for CHAMPUS-eligible individuals in California and Hawaii. TRICARE is a regionally based managed healthcare program for active duty and retired members of the uniformed services, their families, and survivors. **TRICARE Standard** has basically the same benefits and cost-sharing structure as the original CHAMPUS program.

TRICARE brings together the healthcare resources of the Army, Navy, and Air Force and supplements them with networks of civilian healthcare professionals to provide them with better access to healthcare and high-quality service while maintaining the capability to support military operations. TRICARE's main objectives are *accessibility* and *affordability*, which serve as ways to
- improve overall access to healthcare for beneficiaries;
- provide faster, more convenient access to civilian healthcare;
- create a more efficient way to receive healthcare;
- offer enhanced healthcare services, including preventive care;
- provide choices for healthcare; and
- control escalating healthcare costs.

TRICARE is administered on a regional basis. There are 11 regions encompassing the 50 United States, the Virgin Islands and Puerto Rico, Canada, Latin America, and Europe as denoted on the map pictured in Figure 10-1. Each region is managed by a **lead agent** or director. A lead agent is a military officer who is at the head of a TRICARE region and represents all of the military medical services in that region, dealing with the TRICARE support contractor. The lead agent/director, along with assistance from the **military treatment facility (MTF)** commanders, is responsible for the development and execution of an integrated plan for the delivery of healthcare within that region.

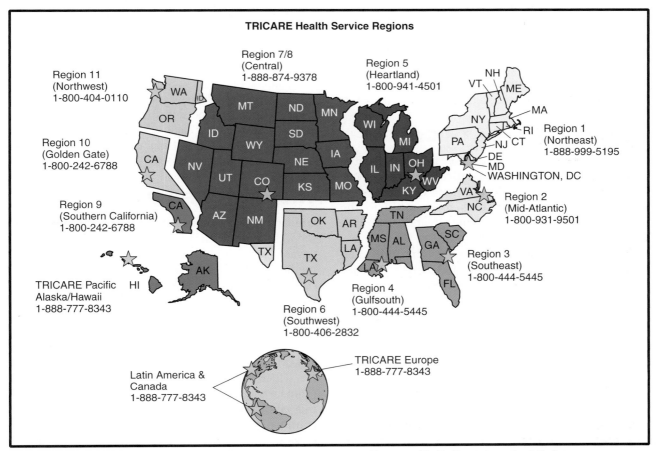

Fig. 10-1 TRICARE healthcare service regional map. (Source: U. S. Department of Defense, TRICARE Management Activity.)

Military Health System is the name for the total health-care system of the U.S. uniformed services. The Military Health System includes MTFs and various programs in the civilian healthcare market, such as TRICARE. An MTF is a clinic or hospital operated by the Department of Defense located on a military base that provides care to military personnel, their dependents, and military retirees and their dependents. The Military Health System provides healthcare to roughly 9 million beneficiaries, including active duty military personnel and their dependents, retired military personnel and their dependents, and survivors of military personnel.

The Department of Defense established the **TRICARE Management Activity**, which began operations in 1998, to oversee the TRICARE managed healthcare program. TRICARE Management Activity has headquarters in the Washington, DC, area and in Aurora, Colorado, the location of the former TRICARE Support Office. The main purpose of TRICARE Management Activity is to enhance the performance of TRICARE worldwide. One of the initial tasks of TRICARE Management Activity was to conduct a survey of approximately 10,000 beneficiaries, which gathered information about beneficiary information needs, preferred sources, and information-seeking strategies. Results of this survey will be used to develop a new national compilation of beneficiary education products and services.

There are three basic plans under TRICARE—TRICARE Standard, TRICARE Extra, and TRICARE Prime. To use TRICARE Extra or TRICARE Prime, the individual receiving care must live in an area where these options are available, and civilian provider network has been established to support these plans.

WHO IS ELIGIBLE FOR TRICARE

Similar to Medicaid and Medicare, TRICARE-eligible individuals are referred to as **beneficiaries**. The service member, whether in active duty, retired, or deceased, is called the **sponsor**. The sponsor's relationship to the beneficiary (spouse, child, parent) creates eligibility under TRICARE.

After eligibility has been established, the individual must be listed in the Department of Defense's **Defense Enrollment Eligibility Reporting System (DEERS)**. DEERS is a computerized data bank that lists all active and retired military service members. Active and retired service members are listed automatically, but it is the sponsor's responsibility to list dependents and report any changes to family members' status (e.g., marriage, divorce, birth of a child, adoption) or changes in mailing addresses. TRICARE contractors (TRICARE's term for fiscal intermediaries) check DEERS before processing claims to ensure patients are eligible for TRICARE benefits.

Categories of individuals eligible for TRICARE include
• active duty military members and their dependent family members,

• military retirees and their eligible family members, and
• survivors of all uniformed service members who are not eligible for Medicare.

Box 10-1 provides a more detailed list of TRICARE eligible categories.

Imagine This!

Alan Workman is a Marine serving on active duty in Iraq. He has a wife and two children (ages 2 and 7) at home in the United States. In this scenario, TRICARE considers Alan the sponsor, and his wife and two children are the beneficiaries.

WHO IS NOT ELIGIBLE FOR TRICARE

Categories of individuals *not* eligible for TRICARE benefits include the following:
• Most individuals who are 65 years old and eligible for Medicare (except active duty family members) are not TRICARE-eligible. Individuals younger than age 65 who are Medicare-eligible because of a disability or end-stage renal disease may retain TRICARE eligibility until age 65, but must be enrolled in Medicare Part B.
• Parents and parents-in-law of active duty service members or uniformed services retirees, or of deceased active duty members or retirees, are not TRICARE-eligible. They may be able to receive treatment in military medical facilities if space permits, however.
• Individuals who are eligible for benefits under the Civilian Health and Medical Program of the Department of Veterans Affairs (CHAMPVA) are not TRICARE-eligible.

WHAT TRICARE PAYS

Similar to most insurers, TRICARE pays for only their *allowed* services, supplies, and procedures, which they refer to as **covered charges**. TRICARE's covered charges include medical and psychological services and supplies that are considered appropriate care and are generally accepted by qualified professionals to be reasonable and adequate for the diagnosis and treatment of illness, injury, pregnancy, and mental disorders or well-child care.

TRICARE's allowable charge, also known as the **CHAMPUS Maximum Allowable Charge**, is the amount on which TRICARE figures a beneficiary's cost share (coinsurance) for covered charges. TRICARE calculates this allowable charge by looking at all professional (noninstitutional) providers' fees for the same or similar services nationwide over the past year, with adjustments for specific localities. If the health insurance professional does not know what the allowable charge is for a particular

Box 10-1

Detailed List of TRICARE-Eligible Categories

1. *Active duty service members* themselves are enrolled automatically in TRICARE Prime and may use the local military and civilian provider network (if one is in place) with proper authorization. Their healthcare remains the top priority of the military healthcare system, and they would be the first to be allowed to sign up with PCMs at MTFs.

2. *Eligible family members of active duty service personnel* include spouses and unmarried children who are young enough (in most cases, <21 years old or <23 years old if in school full-time) to retain their eligibility. These children (including stepchildren who are adopted by the sponsor) are covered by TRICARE, even if the spouse gets divorced or remarried. Stepchildren *do not* have to be adopted by the sponsor to be covered by TRICARE while the sponsor and the mother or father of the stepchildren remain married. In the case of divorce, a stepchild who was *not* adopted by the sponsor loses eligibility on the date the divorce decree is final.

3. *Military retirees and their eligible family members* have the same conditions for eligibility as above (these eligibility conditions for children are the same throughout all categories of eligibility).

4. *Spouses and unmarried children of reservists* who are ordered to active duty for more than 30 consecutive days or reservists who die during active duty. (Coverage is in force only during the reservist's active duty tour; they can use TRICARE Extra and TRICARE Standard, but they cannot enroll in TRICARE Prime unless the reservist's active duty period lasts at least 180 days).

5. *Surviving spouses who have not remarried and unmarried children* of active or retired service members who have died.

6. *Surviving spouses who have not remarried and unmarried children of reservists*, if the reservists are injured or aggravate an injury, illness, or disease during—or on the way to—active duty training for a period of 30 days or less or a period of inactive duty training and die as a result of the specific injury, illness, or disease.

7. *Some unremarried former spouses* of active or retired service members, who meet certain length-of-marriage rules and other requirements.

8. *Unmarried children of military sponsors*, who are age 21 and older (to age 23, if the child is a full-time student), and who are severely disabled and the disability existed before the child's 21st birthday (or before the 23rd birthday, if the child is a full-time student).

9. *Dependent wards placed in the custody of a service member or former member* by a court or by a recognized adoption agency for at least 12 months. TRICARE eligibility is effective July 1, 1994, if the child is placed by a court. A child placed by a recognized adoption agency is eligible effective on the date the child is placed by the agency, or on October 5, 1994, whichever date is later.

10. *Certain family members of active duty service members* who were court-martialed and separated for spouse or child abuse or were administratively discharged as a result of such an offense. The victims of the abuse within the family are eligible for treatment of illnesses and injuries related to the abuse for 1 year from the date of the sponsor's separation from the service. Cost-sharing would be the same as for other active duty families.

11. *Certain abused spouses, former spouses, or dependent children* of service members who were retirement-eligible, but who lost that eligibility as a result of abuse of the spouse or child. This benefit is effective for medically necessary services and supplies provided under TRICARE Standard on or after October 23, 1992. It is not limited to 1 year of eligibility (as is the category described immediately above), and it is not limited to illnesses and injuries resulting from the abuse.

12. *Illegitimate children* of current or retired service members or their spouses may be eligible for TRICARE benefits under certain circumstances. Check with your nearest health benefits adviser, healthcare finder, or TRICARE service center.

13. *Spouses and children of North Atlantic Treaty Organization (NATO) nation representatives*, under certain circumstances (outpatient care only).

14. *Certain former active duty members and their families* may be eligible for limited periods of TRICARE benefits under the Transitional Assistance Management Program. Check with your health benefits adviser or your military personnel office for details.

service or supply, he or she can telephone the regional claims processor for this information or consult the TRICARE handbook. It is advisable to keep a current copy of the TRICARE handbook on file for information regarding TRICARE billing and claims submission guidelines.

✓ **HIPAA Tip**

TRICARE/CHAMPVA beneficiaries and providers of care benefit from HIPAA in the following ways:
- Improves uniformity and efficiency of communication among providers
- Increases protection of patients' private, personal health information
- Makes transferring enrollment between plans easier

What Did You Learn?

1. List TRICARE's two main healthcare objectives.
2. What category of individuals are TRICARE sponsors?
3. Name the three categories of individuals eligible for TRICARE benefits.

TRICARE'S THREE CHOICES FOR HEALTHCARE

As mentioned earlier, TRICARE typically (depending on the geographic area) offers eligible beneficiaries three different healthcare plans to choose from.

TRICARE Standard

TRICARE Standard is a fee-for-service option that has basically the same benefits as the original CHAMPUS program. Under this plan, eligible enrollees can see the authorized provider of their choice. In some locations, TRICARE Standard may be the only option available.

Eligibility Anyone who is CHAMPUS-eligible may use TRICARE Standard. (Active duty personnel are not CHAMPUS-eligible and are automatically enrolled in TRICARE Prime.) Family members of military service personnel in the Army Reserves and National Guard, called **reserve components (RCs)**, are eligible for TRICARE Standard only if the RC is ordered to active duty for more than 30 consecutive days or if the orders are for an indefinite period. The RC is entitled to TRICARE Prime benefits as soon as he or she goes into active duty.

Advantages
- Broadest choice of providers
- Widely available
- No enrollment fee
- Eligible members also may use TRICARE Extra

Disadvantages
- No **primary care manager (PCM)**
- Patient pays deductible and copayment
- Patient pays up to 15% over and above allowable charge for nonparticipating providers (nonPARs)
- Beneficiaries may have to do their own paperwork and file their own claims if provider is nonPAR

Summary
- Greatest flexibility in choosing healthcare providers
- Most convenient when away from home
- Potentially most expensive of all options
- Enrollment not required
- Allow for space-available care in military hospitals, but at low priority

TRICARE Extra

TRICARE Extra is a preferred provider option (PPO). The enrollee chooses a physician, hospital, or other medical provider listed in the TRICARE Provider Directory. With TRICARE Extra, there are no enrollment criteria to meet, and enrollees do not pay an annual fee. There is, however, an annual deductible and cost sharing for outpatient care. In the TRICARE Extra program, when an enrollee receives care from a TRICARE Extra network provider, he or she gets a discount on cost sharing, and patients do not have to file their own claims. TRICARE Extra may be used on a case-by-case basis just by choosing a provider within the network. TRICARE Extra is not available overseas or to active duty service members.

TRICARE Standard, Extra, and Prime have an annual **catastrophic cap (cat cap)**, which is a maximum cost limit placed on out-of-pocket expenses for covered medical bills. The limit that a family of an active duty member will have to pay in any given year is $1000. For all others (other than Active Duty Families), using TRICARE Standard or Extra, there is a $3000 cat cap per fiscal year (October 1st- September 30th) that is applied to out-of-pocket expenses for TRICARE-covered benefits (2006 figures). For more details on the cat cap, the health insurance professional should check with the nearest TRICARE Service Center (TSC). Also, see the list of websites at the end of this chapter.

Eligibility Anyone who is CHAMPUS-eligible may use TRICARE Extra. (Active duty personnel are not CHAMPUS-eligible and are automatically enrolled in TRICARE Prime.)

Advantages

- Copayment 5% less than TRICARE Standard
- No balance billing
- No enrollment fee
- No deductible when using retail pharmacy network
- Patient not responsible for filing forms
- Enrollees also may use TRICARE Standard

Disadvantages

- No PCM
- Provider choice is limited
- Patient must pay deductible and cost share
- Nonavailability statement *may* be required for civilian inpatient care for areas surrounding MTFs
- Not available everywhere

Summary

- Patients can choose any provider in the TRICARE Extra network
- Less expensive than TRICARE Standard
- Enrollment not required
- Eligible for space-available care in MTF, but at low priority

TRICARE Prime

TRICARE Prime is a health maintenance organization (HMO)–type managed care option in which MTFs are the principal source of healthcare. When eligible beneficiaries enroll in TRICARE Prime, they are assigned to a PCM, which is a healthcare provider or a team of healthcare providers that the enrollee must see first for all routine medical care, similar to a primary care provider or gatekeeper in civilian managed care plans. The PCM

- provides or coordinates all healthcare,
- maintains patient health records, and
- arranges referrals to specialists if necessary (to be covered, specialty care must be arranged and approved by the PCM).

Similar to most managed healthcare plans, TRICARE Prime emphasizes preventive healthcare, including health risk assessments, screening tests (e.g., cholesterol, hypertension, mammogram, Pap and prostate screening), advice on nutrition, and smoking cessation classes designed to guide the enrollee to a healthy lifestyle. Retired military beneficiaries and their eligible family members also can enroll in TRICARE Prime. There is an annual enrollment fee for retired military beneficiaries, whereas active duty family members pay no enrollment fee.

When active duty service members are automatically enrolled in TRICARE Prime, they are assigned to a PCM, generally at an MTF. For all other eligible individuals, including family members, enrollment in TRICARE Prime is voluntary and can be done any time of the year. None of the three TRICARE options—Standard, Extra, or Prime—has preexisting condition limitations.

If the beneficiary lives in an area where TRICARE Prime is offered, he or she can call the regional TRICARE contractor and ask for an enrollment packet by mail. Enrollment must be in writing; enrollment by telephone is not an option. Healthcare usually is provided at an MTF, but civilian clinics may be used in some cases.

The Point-of-Service option under TRICARE Prime allows enrollees the freedom to seek and receive non-emergency healthcare services from any TRICARE authorized civilian provider, in or out of the network, without requesting a referral from their PCM.

Eligibility There is no enrollment fee for TRICARE Prime, but there is a registration process. Besides active service members' automatic enrollment, the following categories of individuals may enroll in TRICARE prime:

- Dependent family members and survivors of active duty personnel
- Retirees and their family members and survivors younger than age 65
- RCs and their family members called to active duty for 179 days or more

RCs and their family members may enroll in TRICARE Prime or may be eligible for TRICARE Prime Remote. Enrollment forms must be completed, and MTFs or TRICARE Prime network providers must be used.

TRICARE Prime Remote provides healthcare coverage through civilian networks or TRICARE-authorized providers for uniformed service members and their families who are on **remote assignment**, which is 50 miles or more from an MTF. TRICARE Prime Remote for Active Duty Family Members (TPRADFM) is the TRICARE Prime Remote plan for family members with similar benefits and program requirements. TRICARE Prime Remote/TPRADFM is offered in the 50 United States only, and both programs require enrollment.

The cat cap on most medical expenses (other than active duty enrollees) for TRICARE Prime managed care plan is $3000 per 12-month enrollment period. This means that for 1 year (beginning with the date of enrollment), TRICARE Prime enrollees pay a maximum of $3000 for enrollment fees, inpatient and outpatient cost shares, and copayments for professional services and supplies. After the $3000 maximum is reached, enrollees pay nothing more for care received through the TRICARE Prime network of providers until a new enrollment period begins (2006 figures).

Advantages

- No enrollment fee for active duty service members and their families
- Pay only a small fee per visit to civilian providers (no fee for active duty members)
- No balance billing
- Guaranteed appointments (access standards)
- PCM supervises and coordinates care
- Away-from-home emergency coverage
- Point-of-Service option

Disadvantages
- Enrollment fee for retirees and their families
- Provider choice limited to providers belonging to network
- Specialty care by referral only
- Not available outside the 50 United States

Summary
- Guaranteed access to timely medical care
- Priority for care at military hospitals and clinics
- PCM provides and coordinates healthcare delivery
- Lowest cost for treatment among three options
- Requires enrollment for 1 year
- Retirees pay enrollment fee
- Very expensive to receive care outside TRICARE Prime (Point-of-Service option)
- Not available everywhere

It can be a challenge to decide which TRICARE option—Prime, Extra, or Standard—to choose (Fig. 10-2). As stated, active duty personnel are automatically enrolled in TRICARE Prime and pay no fees. Active duty family members pay no enrollment fees, but they have to choose a TRICARE option, and they must apply for enrollment if they choose TRICARE Prime.

Nonavailability Statement

As discussed previously, military personnel and their TRICARE-eligible dependents typically receive healthcare at an MTF. If treatment is not available at an MTF, the individual must sometimes obtain a **nonavailability statement (NAS)** (Figs. 10-3 and 10-4) indicating that care is not available from the MTF. An NAS is certification from the MTF that says it cannot provide the specific healthcare the beneficiary needs at that facility. The statements must be entered electronically in the Department of Defense's DEERS computer files by the MTF.

As of December 2002, individuals covered by TRICARE Standard no longer need approval from their MTF to seek inpatient care at civilian hospitals. A requirement still exists, however, for TRICARE Standard beneficiaries to get an NAS before seeking *nonemergency inpatient mental healthcare* services. This requirement applies only to beneficiaries who use TRICARE Standard or Extra, who are not Medicare eligible, and who have no other health insurance that is primary to TRICARE. Preauthorization for TRICARE beneficiary inpatient mental healthcare is not needed when Medicare is the primary payer.

With this change in policy, beneficiaries have the freedom to choose an MTF or a civilian facility without this extra paperwork. Nevertheless, TRICARE beneficiaries are urged to consider the Military Health System as their first choice for healthcare (Table 10-1).

OTHER HEALTH INSURANCE

If a TRICARE-eligible beneficiary has other healthcare coverage besides TRICARE Standard, Extra, or Prime through an employer, an association, or a private insurer,

TRICARE's Three Options

Topic	TRICARE Prime	TRICARE Extra	TRICARE Standard
Definition	TRICARE Prime is a managed care option similar to a health maintenance organization (HMO).	TRICARE Extra is similar to a preferred provider organization (PPO) where the beneficiary selects from a network of providers.	TRICARE Standard has the same benefits and cost shares as the former CHAMPUS.
Cost vs. Choice	Least out-of-pocket costs with some restrictions on freedom-of-choice.	Copayment 5% less than TRICARE Standard and no deductible when using the retail network pharmacy.	Highest out-of-pocket costs with the greatest degree of freedom to choose health care providers.

Fig. 10-2 TRICARE's three options. (Source: U. S. Department of Defense, TRICARE Management Activity.)

ENCLOSURE 1   DD 1251 (SAMPLE)

UNIFORMED SERVICES MEDICAL TREATMENT FACILITY NONAVAILABILITY STATEMENT (NAS)	REPORT CONTROL SYMBOL

Privacy Act Statement

AUTHORITY: 44 USC 3101, 41 CFR 101 et seq., 10 USC 1066 and 1079, and EO 9397, November 1943 (SSN).

PRINCIPAL PURPOSE: To evaluate eligibility for civilian health benefits authorized by 10 USC, Chapter 55, and to issue payment upon establishment of eligibility and determination that the medical care received is authorized by law. The information is subject to verification with the appropriate Uniformed Service.

ROUTINE USE: CHAMPUS and its contractors use the information to control and process medical claims for payment; for control and approval of medical treatments and interface with providers of medical care; to control and accomplish reviews of utilization; for review of claims related to possible third party liability cases and initiation of recovery actions; and for referral to Peer Review Committees or similar professional review organizations to control and review providers' medical care.

DISCLOSURE: Voluntary; however, failure to provide information will result in denial of, or delay in payment of, the claim.

1. NAS NUMBER *(Facility) (Yr-Julian) (Seq. No.)*	2. PRIMARY REASON FOR ISSUANCE *(X one)*

	a. PROPER FACILITIES ARE TEMPORARILY NOT AVAILABLE IN A SAFE OR TIMELY MANNER
3. MAJOR DIAGNOSTIC CATEGORY FOR WHICH NAS IS ISSUED *(Use code from reverse)*	b. PROFESSIONAL CAPABILITY IS TEMPORARILY NOT AVAILABLE IN A SAFE OR TIMELY MANNER
	c. PROPER FACILITIES OR PROFESSIONAL CAPABILITY ARE PERMANENTLY NOT AVAILABLE AT THIS FACILITY
	d. IT WOULD BE MEDICALLY INAPPROPRIATE TO REQUIRE THE BENEFICIARY TO USE THE MPT *(Explain in Remarks)*

4. PATIENT DATA

a. NAME *(Last, First, Middle Initial)*	b. DATE OF BIRTH *(YYMMDD)*	c. SEX

d. ADDRESS *(Street, City, State, and ZIP Code)*	e. PATIENT CATEGORY *(X one)*	f. OTHER NON CHAMPUS HEALTH INSURANCE *(X one)*
	(1) Dependent of Active Duty	
	(2) Dependent of Retiree	(1) Yes, but only CHAMPUS Supplemental
	(3) Retiree	
	(4) Survivor	(2) Yes *(List in Remarks)*
	(5) Former Spouse	(3) No

5. SPONSOR DATA *(if you marked 4e(3) Retiree above, print "Same" in 5a.)*

a. NAME *(Last, First, Middle Initial)*	b. SPONSOR'S OR RETIREE'S SOCIAL SECURITY NO.

6. ISSUING OFFICIAL DATA

a. NAME *(Last, First, Middle Initial)*	b. TITLE	
c. SIGNATURE	d. PAY GRADE	e. DATE ISSUED *(YYMMDD)*

7. REMARKS *(Indicate block number to which the answer applies.)*

DD Form 1251, JUL 91	*Outside the United States and Puerto Rico, previous editions may be used until exhausted* *Inside the United States and Puerto Rico, previous editions are obsolete*

Fig. 10-3 Sample NAS for inpatient care. (Source: U. S. Department of Defense, TRICARE Management Activity.)

Application For Nonavailability Statement	Date:

TO: Health Benefits Advisor, Managed Care Division, DeWitt Army Community Hospital, Fort Belvoir 22060-5901

A Nonavailability Statement (DD Form 1251) is required when nonemergency inpatient care and certain outpatient care is to be provided to dependents of active duty personnel residing with, or apart from sponsor retirees and their dependents and dependents of deceased/former spouses residing within a ZIP Code Catchment area of this hospital. The following is required to evaluate a request for issuance of DD Form 1251:

Patient Name (Last, First, MI):		Status (wife, son, etc.)

Home Address (street, city, state, ZIP):		Home Telephone:
		Work Telephone:

Date of Birth:	Sponsor's Name:	Rank:

Sponsor's Category: (active duty, retired, deceased, former spouse, if active duty his/her unit/organization and BRANCH OF SERVICE (Army, Navy, Marines, Air Force or other)

Other Primary Health Insurance (yes or no) If you have private health insurance that pays first for the cost of medical services, you do not need a nonavailability statement from the local MTF.

All retroactive requests for nonavailability statements require summary of hospitalization or history and physical examination. If maternity care, name of hospital where delivery will take place, date of first civilian prenatal visit and delivery date. All other requests require name of civilian hospital and date of hospitalization. MEDICARE, ACTIVE DUTY, DEPENDENT PARENTS AND PARENTS-IN-LAW ARE NOT ELIGIBLE FOR CHAMPUS.

Reason for Request

Submit

Fig. 10-4 Application form for an NAS. (Source: U. S. Department of Defense, TRICARE Management Activity.)

☑ HIPAA Tip

HIPAA privacy applies to individually identifiable health information, including paper, electronic, or oral communications. This includes information that identifies the patient and relates to his or her past, present, or future health condition.

Imagine This!

In February 2003, Kim Sun Hwa, a TRICARE Standard enrollee, sought care for a serious cardiac condition at the MTF near the town where she lived. The MTF did not have the facilities to perform the needed quadruple bypass surgery and referred her to Genesis Cardiac and Rehabilitation Center 150 miles away. The MTF filed a nonavailability statement with DEERS; however, the health insurance professional at Genesis advised Kim that an NAS was no longer necessary for beneficiaries enrolled in TRICARE Standard. After the surgery, Kim experienced post-surgical depression and returned to Genesis for outpatient psychotherapy. Because she did not need an NAS from the MTF for her surgery, Kim assumed she would not need an NAS for the treatment of her mental health condition; however, without it, TRICARE refused the second claim.

or if a student in the family has a healthcare plan obtained through his or her school, TRICARE considers this **other health insurance (OHI)**. It also may be called double coverage or coordination of benefits. OHI does not include TRICARE supplemental insurance or Medicaid.

TABLE 10-1 TRICARE Comparison Chart (2006)

	TRICARE PRIME	TRICARE EXTRA	TRICARE STANDARD
Active Duty Family Members			
Annual deductible	None	$150/individual or $300/family for E-5 and above; $50/$100 for E-4 and below	$150/individual or $300/family for E-5 and above; $50/$100 for E-4 and below
Annual enrollment fee	None	None	None
Civilian outpatient visit	No cost	15% of negotiated fee	20% of allowed charges for covered service
Civilian inpatient admission	No cost	Greater of $25 or $14.35/day	Greater of $25 or $14.35/day
Civilian inpatient mental health	No cost	Greater of $20/day or $25/admission	Greater of $20/day or $25/admission
Civilian inpatient skilled nursing facility care	$0 per diem charge per admission. No separate cost share for separately billed professional charges	$11/day ($25 minimum) charge per admission	$11/day ($25 minimum) charge per admission
Retirees, Their Family Members, and Others			
Annual deductible	None	$150/individual or $300/family	$150/individual or $300/family
Annual enrollment fee	$230/individual or $460/family	None	None
Civilian cost shares	—	20% of negotiated fee	25% of allowed charges for covered service
Outpatient	$12	—	—
Emergency care	$30	—	—
Mental health visit	$25; $17 for group visit	—	—
Civilian inpatient cost share	Greater of $11/day or $25/admission; no separate co-payment for separately billed professional charges	Lesser of $250/day or 25% of negotiated charges plus 20% of negotiated professional fees	Lesser of $535/day or 25% of billed charges plus 25% of allowed professional fees
Civilian inpatient skilled nursing facility care	$11/day ($25 minimum) charge per admission	$250 per diem cost share or 20% cost share of total charges (whichever is less), institutional services, plus 20% cost share of separately billed professional charges	25% cost share of allowed charges for institutional services, plus 25% cost share of allowable for separately billed professional charges.
Civilian inpatient behavioral health	$40/day; no charge for separately billed professional charges	20% of total charge plus 20% of the allowable charge for separately billed professional services	High Volume Hospitals—25% hospital specific per diem, plus 25% of the allowable charge for separately billed professional services; Low Volume Hospitals—$175/day or 25% of the billed charges (whichever is lower) plus 25% of the allowable charge for separately billed services

TRICARE STANDARD SUPPLEMENTAL INSURANCE

TRICARE Standard Supplemental Insurance policies, similar to Medicare supplemental insurance policies, are health benefit plans that are designed specifically to supplement TRICARE Standard benefits. These plans are frequently available from military associations or other private organizations and firms. They generally pay most or all of whatever is left after TRICARE Standard has paid its share of the cost of covered healthcare services and supplies. Such policies are not specifically for retirees and may be useful for other TRICARE-eligible families as well.

TRICARE-FOR-LIFE

TRICARE-for-Life (TFL) is a comprehensive health benefits program established by the National Defense Authorization Act. This program is available to uniformed services retirees, their spouses, and their survivors who are age 65 or older, are Medicare-eligible, are enrolled in Medicare Part A, and have purchased Medicare Part B coverage. TFL has no monthly premium cost and is a permanent healthcare benefit for all uniformed service branches.

Who Is Eligible for TRICARE-for-Life

The following individuals are eligible for TFL:
- All Medicare-eligible military retirees, regardless of age (retirees are individuals who had more than 20 years of active duty service)
- Spouses and survivors, regardless of age, who are eligible for Medicare Part A and who are enrolled in Medicare Part B
- Certain qualifying former spouses
- Reservists, including guardsman, drawing reserve retired pay, their spouses, and other eligible family members become eligible for TFL when they turn 65
- Medal of Honor winners who left the service before retirement plus their spouses and survivors

In addition to the qualifying members of the uniformed service branches listed, individuals belonging to or employed by Public Health Service groups and the National Oceanic and Atmospheric Administration may enroll in TFL if they meet the eligibility criteria.

How TRICARE-for-Life Works to Supplement Medicare

TFL functions much the same as Medicare supplemental insurance; TFL enrollees do not need a Medicare supplement policy. For individuals who are eligible for Medicare TFL and Medicare, the following applies:
- Eligible individuals pay no premium to be enrolled in TFL.
- Medicare automatically crosses claims over to TRICARE.
- TRICARE pays Medicare deductibles and coinsurance or copayment amounts up to 115% of Medicare-allowable charges.

For procedures *not covered* by Medicare (e.g., chiropractic care), beneficiaries are responsible for TRICARE deductibles and copayment amounts. When the annual out-of-pocket limit has been reached, TRICARE pays 100% of TRICARE-allowed charges for the remainder of the year. When a claim is submitted for a Medicare/TFL beneficiary, TRICARE pays last. Medicare/TFL beneficiaries have the same coverage for prescription drugs as that provided under Medicare Prescription Drug Coverage (Part D) (Table 10-2).

Imagine This!

Benjamin Hudson, a dual-eligible enrollee under TRICARE and Medicare, visited Dr. Alton Simmons, an ophthalmologist, for vision problems. Benjamin subsequently opted to receive laser surgery to correct his myopia. When he received a statement for the entire fee, he telephoned the health insurance professional in Dr. Simmons' office stating that because he had Medicare and TRICARE coverage, one or the other should pay. Under the impression that an error had been made, Benjamin insisted that the claim be resubmitted; however, the health insurance professional informed him that because laser surgery was a noncovered expense under Medicare, TRICARE would not pay it either. Mr. Hudson refused to pay the bill on the grounds that the health insurance professional should have informed him that this was a noncovered service before the procedure. Dr. Simmons ultimately adjusted the charge off Benjamin's account.

TABLE 10-2	TRICARE-for-Life: What Healthcare Services Are Covered, and Who Pays?		
	MEDICARE PAYS[a]	TRICARE PAYS[b]	BENEFICIARY PAYS[c]
Inpatient Services (Medicare Part A) *Inpatient Hospitalization (Medical-Surgical) and hospital-based psychiatric care*			
Days 1-60	100% (after $952 deductible)[d]	$952 deductible	Nothing for Medicare-covered services
Days 61-90	All but $238/day[d]	$238/day[d]	Nothing for Medicare-covered services
Days 91-150[e]	All but $476/day[d]	$476/day[d]	Nothing for Medicare-covered services[e]
Days 151+	Not covered	The DRG-allowed[g] amount minus patient's co-payment/ cost share	$250/day or 20% of the institutional charges (whichever is less) if care is delivered in a TRICARE network hospital[h]; $535/day or 25% of billed charges for institutional charges (whichever is less), plus 25% of allowable for professional charges if care is delivered in a non-network hospital
Inpatient Mental Health (Psychiatric Facility) Inpatient mental healthcare requires preauthorization; care for >30 days requires a waiver for secondary TRICARE coverage; if authorized, TRICARE pays cost share or deductible; *a new benefit period[g] must begin before Medicare covers additional days*			
Days 1-60	100% (after $952 deductible)[d]	$952 deductible	Nothing for services payable by Medicare and TRICARE
Days 61-90	All but $238/day[d]	$238/day[d]	Nothing for services payable by Medicare and TRICARE
Days 91-150	All but $476/day[d]	$476/day[d]	Nothing for services payable by Medicare and TRICARE
Days 151+	Not covered	80% if network hospital[h]; 75% if non-network hospital	20% of institutional charges plus 20% of professional charges for services received in a network hospital.[h] For services received in a non-network hospital, see TRICARE Reimbursement Manual Ch. 2, Addendum A, page 10 on the TRICARE Web site at www.tricare.osd.mil/tricaremanuals/
Skilled Nursing Facility A beneficiary must be admitted to an inpatient hospital during a benefit period for at least 3 days before receiving Medicare authorization to receive this benefit			

TABLE 10-2	TRICARE-for-Life: What Healthcare Services Are Covered, and Who Pays?—cont'd

	MEDICARE PAYS[a]	TRICARE PAYS[b]	BENEFICIARY PAYS[c]
Days 1-20	100%	Remaining beneficiary liability (if any)	Nothing for services payable by Medicare and TRICARE
Days 20-100	All but $119/day[d]	$119/day	Nothing for services payable by Medicare and TRICARE
Days 101+	Not covered	80% if network hospital[h]	20% of TRICARE allowable charges if care delivered in a network hospital; 25% of TRICARE allowable charges if care delivered in a non-network hospital
Hospice Care	95%	Remaining beneficiary liability 5%	Nothing for services payable by Medicare and TRICARE
Outpatient Services (Medicare Part B)			
Physician's Visit (Outside MTF)	80%	20%	Nothing for services payable by Medicare and TRICARE
Emergency Department Visit	80%	20%	Nothing for services payable by Medicare and TRICARE
Mental Health Visit	50%	50%	Nothing for services payable by Medicare and TRICARE
Laboratory Services	100%	Remaining beneficiary liability (if any)	Nothing for services payable by Medicare and TRICARE
Radiology (X-Rays)	80%	20%	Nothing for services payable by Medicare and TRICARE
Home Health Care	100% for approved services	Remaining beneficiary liability (if any)	Nothing for services payable by Medicare and TRICARE
Durable Medical Equipment	80%	20%	Nothing for services payable by Medicare and TRICARE
Outpatient Hospital Services	80%	20%	Nothing for Medicare-covered services
Blood	80%	Not covered	20% Medicare cost-share

[a]All percentages paid by Medicare are for the Medicare-approved amounts for services received from Medicare providers who accept Medicare assignment.

[b]TRICARE pays the difference between Medicare's paid amount and Medicare's limiting charge (up to 115% of the allowable amount) for nonPAR claims.

[c]TRICARE has a $3000 per fiscal year (October 1-September 30) catastrophic cap (maximum out-of-pocket expense).

[d]Medicare amount that changes every calendar year.

[e]Lifetime reserve days (91-150) are 60 additional days that Medicare will pay for minus $406/day (in 2002) deductible, when the beneficiary is in a hospital for >90 consecutive days. These 60 reserve days can be used only once.

[f]A benefit period begins when a beneficiary is admitted to a hospital or skilled nursing facility and continues until the beneficiary has been out of the facility for at least 60 consecutive days.

[g]A reimbursement system using Diagnosis Related Groups (DRGs) that assigns payment levels to each DRG based on the average cost of treating all patients in a given DRG.

[h]A network hospital is one that has a contractual agreement with TRICARE.

VERIFYING ELIGIBILITY

When a patient comes to the office for an appointment and informs the health insurance professional that he or she is eligible for benefits under one of the military's healthcare programs, it should be verified immediately. Box 10-2 lists some suggestions for verification. Figure 10-5 shows sample ID cards.

TRICARE PARTICIPATING PROVIDERS

Healthcare providers who participate in TRICARE (participating providers [PAR]), also referred to as *accepting assignment,* agree to accept the TRICARE allowable charge (including the cost share and deductible, if any) as payment in full for the healthcare services provided and cannot balance bill. Individual providers who do not accept assignment on all claims (nonPARs) can participate in TRICARE on a case-by-case basis. PARs and nonPARs who accept assignment must file the claim for the patient, and TRICARE sends the payment (if any) directly to the provider. Hospitals that participate in Medicare, by law, also must participate in TRICARE Standard for inpatient care. For outpatient care, hospitals may choose whether or not participate.

TRICARE CLAIMS PROCESSING

The facility that handles TRICARE claims for healthcare received within a particular state or region is called a **claims processor**. In some regions, they are called TRICARE contractors or fiscal intermediaries. All claims processors (fiscal intermediaries) have toll-free phone numbers to handle questions that a health insurance professional might have regarding TRICARE claims. The health insurance professional should have the latest TRICARE handbook on file or log onto the TRICARE website for an electronic version of the handbook. In addition to the handbook, a file should be kept that has an up-to-date list of telephone numbers and addresses to facilitate claims processing.

Submitting Paper Claims

Providers submitting paper claims should use the standard CMS-1500 claim form. Patients who file their own claims must use Form 2692 (CHAMPUS Claim Patient Request for Medical Payment), which can be downloaded from the TRICARE website. If the patient files his or her own claim, the provider's detailed itemized statement and an NAS (if necessary) must be attached. Completed claims are sent to the TRICARE claims processor in the region in which the enrollee resides. For information on where to file paper claims, the TRICARE website (http://www.tricare.osd.mil/) lists the names and addresses of claims processors by region. At the TRICARE home page, click on "site map," choose "claims," and select the region of choice to access the chart of pertinent information.

Who Submits Claims

If the patient is enrolled in TRICARE Prime and goes to a Prime provider, the provider submits the claims. After the claims are submitted, the beneficiary and provider receive an explanation of benefits (EOB) from the claims processor showing the services performed and the adjudication.

Sample Military ID

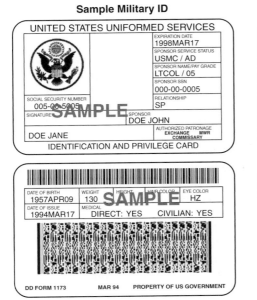

Sample TRICARE Prime ID

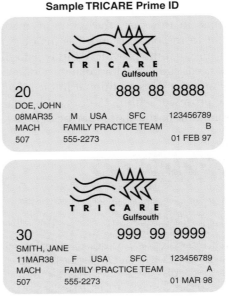

Fig. 10-5 Examples of military ID cards. (Source: U. S. Department of Defense, TRICARE Management Activity.)

Box 10-2

Suggestions for Verifying Eligibility

- Ask to see a Uniformed Services ID card or a family member's Uniformed Services ID card. Anyone 10 years old or older should have a personal ID card.
- Check the back of the card for TRICARE/CHAMPUS eligibility and the expiration date.
- Prime enrollees must show their Uniformed Services ID card and their TRICARE Prime ID card. The Prime ID card does not specify the beneficiary's period of eligibility, so the health insurance professional needs to verify the current eligibility status by calling the beneficiary services hotline. Failure to verify eligibility may result in claim denial.
- The Prime sponsor's Social Security number is included in the 11-digit number on the Prime ID card. Verify the Prime sponsor's Social Security number with the patient. It should match the final nine digits of the number given on the TRICARE Prime ID card.
- If you are the patient's PCM, you also should verify that you are the PCM listed on the Prime card and note the effective date of the coverage.
- In most cases, active duty personnel must seek nonemergency healthcare from their host MTF. Under certain circumstances, such as nonavailability of needed services at the MTF, active duty personnel may obtain Prime benefits from civilian providers under the Supplemental Healthcare Program. Because active duty personnel are not issued Prime ID cards, they must show their green (active duty) ID cards to verify eligibility.
- Make a copy of the front and back of all ID cards for your records.

Patients using TRICARE Standard are usually responsible for submitting their own claims to the appropriate *claims processor*. If the patient has access to the Internet, these forms can be downloaded from the TRICARE website. They are in Portable Document Format (PDF). PDF is a universal file format that preserves the fonts, images, graphics, and layout of any source document, regardless of the application and platform used to create it. PDF files are compact and complete and can be shared, viewed, and printed by anyone with free Adobe Reader software. It may be necessary first to *download* the Adobe Reader software. Instructions for downloading and installing the software are available at the download site.

In the case of nonPARs, TRICARE Standard patients must file their own claims. In this case, the reimbursement check would be sent to the patient, and it is his or her responsibility to ensure that the provider's bill is paid. If the claims processor needs additional information, whoever filed the claim is contacted. This additional information must be sent to the processor within 35 days of the date of the letter or phone call, or the claim may be denied.

● Stop and Think

Ruth Carson is a 36-year-old teacher and a TRICARE Standard beneficiary. On March 30, she visits her family physician, Dr. Bennett, for a routine yearly examination. As Dr. Bennett's health insurance professional, you must advise Ruth that Dr. Bennett does not accept assignment on TRICARE claims and that Ruth will have to file her own claim. Ruth asks you how to file the claim. What are your instructions?

Electronic Claims Submission

As with other third-party payers, TRICARE claims can be filed electronically, and providers are encouraged to do so. The numerous advantages to electronic claims filing include the following:
- Saves time by sending claims directly into the TRICARE processing system
- Saves money with no-cost or low-cost claims filing options
- Improves cash flow with faster payment turnaround
- Expedites claim confirmation—usually the next day with batch processing
- Reduces postage costs and mailing time
- Reduces paper handling
- Provides a better audit trail (the electronic media claims response reports shows which claims were accepted for processing and which were denied)

Front-end electronic media claims edits claims and provides feedback more quickly when there are claim problems, allowing correction and resubmission in hours or days instead of weeks, as is common with paper claims. Software also is available to electronic media claims submitters that allows online claims status inquiry and DEERS eligibility inquiry. Some TRICARE regions allow required documentation for claim support to be faxed.

XPressClaim is a secure, streamlined World Wide Web–based system that allows providers to submit TRICARE claims electronically and, in most cases, receive instant results. XPressClaim is the fastest way available to get TRICARE claims processed, and it is free. Filing a TRICARE claim with XPressClaim is relatively straightforward. If the provider is already a member of *myTRICARE claims for Providers,* all the health insurance professional has to do is sign on and click the XPressClaim tab on the top left. To submit the claim, the health insurance professional

1. selects the location where the patient received care, the physician who provided it, and the patient who received it;
2. enters the services and charges for claim;
3. clicks "Submit;" and
4. makes any necessary online corrections.

In most cases, providers receive immediate claim results. Figure 10-6 illustrates the process that TRICARE paper claims undergo.

Deadline for Submitting Claims

TRICARE claims should be submitted within 30 days from the date services were rendered or as soon as possible after the care is rendered. No payment is made for incomplete claims or claims submitted *more than 1 year* after services are rendered for PARs and nonPARs. In addition, PARs are required to participate in Medicare (accept assignment) and submit claims on behalf of TRICARE beneficiaries and Medicare beneficiaries. It is important

for TRICARE providers to adhere to specific guidelines in claims preparation to ensure smooth and timely processing and payment of claims.

The sooner the TRICARE contractor gets the claim forms and other papers, the sooner the claim is paid. As mentioned, the contractor must receive claims within 1 year of the date the service was received or, in the case of inpatient care, within 1 year of the date of an inpatient's discharge. If the claim covers several different medical services or supplies that were provided at different times, the aforementioned 1-year deadline applies to each item on the claim. When a claim is submitted on time, but the claims contractor returns it for more information, the claim must be resubmitted, along with the requested information, so that it is received by the contractor no later than 1 year after the medical services or supplies were provided, or 90 days from the date the claim was returned, whichever is later.

TRICARE EXPLANATION OF BENEFITS

If there are no problems with the claim, the contractor should send whoever filed the claim a written notice, known as an EOB, in about 1 month.

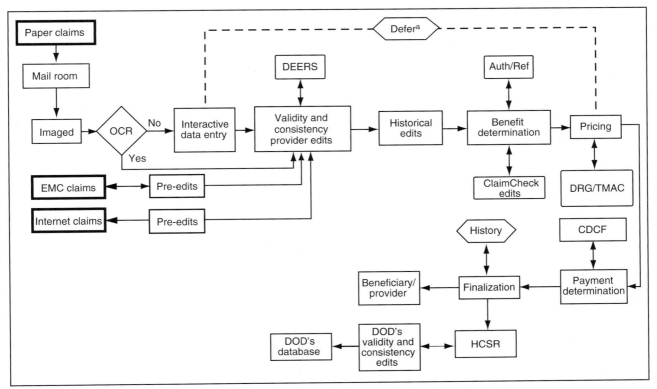

Source: GAO.
Fig. 10-6 TRICARE claims flow chart.* (Source: U. S. Department of Defense, TRICARE Management Activity.) *At any point between Interactive Data Entry and Pricing, processing can be deferred, and the claim can loop back to obtain additional information, usually requiring manual intervention.

TRICARE Explanation of Benefits

TRICARE EXPLANATION OF BENEFITS

This is a statement of the action taken on your TRICARE Claim.
Keep this notice for your records.

PGBA or WPS
TRICARE Claims Administrator for Your Region

1*

2*

3*

4*

5*

Date of Notice:	August 02, 2000
Sponsor SSN:	000-00-0000
Sponsor Name:	NAME OF SPONSOR
Beneficiary Name:	NAME OF BENEFICIARY

7*   Benefits were payable to:

6*

PATIENT, PARENT/GUARDIAN
ADDRESS
CITY STATE ZIP CODE

PROVIDER OF MEDICAL CARE
ADDRESS
CITY STATE ZIP CODE

8*

Claim Number: 919533693-00-00

Services Provided By Date of Services	Services Provided	Amount Billed	TRICARE Approved	See Remarks
9*	10*	11*	12*	13*

PROVIDER OF MEDICAL CARE

Date		Services	Code	Amount Billed	TRICARE Approved	See Remarks
07/08/2000	1	Office/outpatient visit, est	(99213)	$ 45.00	$ 38.92	1
07/08/2000	1	Comprehen metabolic panel	(88054)	20.00	19.33	1
07/08/2000	1	Automated hemogram	(85025)	12.00	12.00	1
Totals:				**$ 77.00**	**$ 70.25**	

Claim Summary	Beneficiary Liability Summary	Benefit Period Summary
	15*	16*

Amount billed:	77.00	Deductible	0.00	**Fiscal Year Beginning:** October 01, 1999
TRICARE Approved:	70.25	Copayment:	0.00	Individual Family
Non-Covered: 14*	6.75	Cost Share	17.56	Deductible: 150.00 150.00
Paid by Beneficiary:	0.00			Catastrophic Cap:
Other Insurance:	0.00			**Enrollment Year Beginning:**
Paid to Provider:	52.69			December 01, 1999
Paid to Beneficiary:	0.00			Individual Family
Check Number:		POS Deductible:		300.00 600.00
		Prime Cap:		856.32

Remarks 17*

1 – CHARGES ARE MORE THAN ALLOWABLE AMOUNT

1-888-XXX-XXXX 18*

THIS IS NOT A BILL
If you have questions regarding this notice, please call or write us at the telephone number/address listed above

1. PGBA or WPS processes all TRICARE claims depending on the region where you live.

2. Prime Contractor: The name and logo of the company that provides managed care support for the region where you live will appear here.

3. Date of Notice: PGBA or WPS prepared your TRICARE Explanation of Benefits (TEOB) on this date.

4. Sponsor SSN/Sponsor Name: Your claim is processed using the Social Security Number of the military service member (active duty, retired or deceased) who is your TRICARE sponsor.

5. Beneficiary Name: The patient who received medical care and for whom this claim was filed.

Fig. 10-7 Example of TRICARE EOB. (Source: U. S. Department of Defense, TRICARE Management Activity.)

TRICARE Explanation of Benefits

6. Mail To Name and Address: We mail the TRICARE Explanation of Benefits (TEOB) directly to the patient (or patient's parent or guardian) at the address given on the claim. (HINT: Be sure your doctor has updated your records with your current address.)

7. Benefits Were Payable To: This field will appear only if your doctor accepts assignment. This means the doctor accepts the TRICARE Maximum Allowable Charge (TMAC) as payment in full for the services you received.

8. Claim Number: Each claim is assigned a unique number. This helps PGBA or WPS keep track of the claim as it is processed. It also helps them find the claim quickly whenever you call or write us with questions or concerns.

9. Service Provided By/Date of Services: This section lists who provided your medical care, the number of services and the procedure codes, as well as the date you received the care.

10. Services Provided: This section describes the medical services you received and how many services are itemized on your claim. It also lists the specific procedure codes that doctors, hospitals and labs use to identify the specific medical services you received.

11. Amount Billed: Your doctor, hospital or lab charged this fee for the medical services you received.

12. TRICARE Approved: This is the amount TRICARE approves for the services you received.

13. See Remarks: If you see a code or a number here, look at the Remarks section (17) for more information about your claim.

14. Claim Summary: A detailed explanation of the action taken by PGBA or WPS taken on your claim is given here. You will find the following totals: amount billed, amount approved by TRICARE, non-covered amount, amount (if any) that you have already paid to the provider, amount your primary health insurance paid (if TRICARE is your secondary insurance), benefits we have paid to the provider, and benefits paid to the beneficiary by PGBA or WPS. A Check Number will appear here only if a check accompanies your TEOB.

15. Beneficiary Liability Summary: You may be responsible for a portion of the fee your doctor has charged. If so, you'll see that amount itemized here. It will include any charges that we have applied to your annual deductible and any cost-share or copayment you must pay.

16. Benefit Period Summary: This section shows how much of the individual and family annual deductible and maximum out-of-pocket expense you have met to date. If you are a TRICARE Standard or Extra beneficiary, PGBA or WPS calculates your annual deductible and maximum out-of-pocket expense by fiscal year. See the Fiscal Year Beginning date in this section for the first date of the fiscal year. If you are a TRICARE Prime beneficiary, we calculate your maximum out-of-pocket expense by enrollment and fiscal year. See Enrollment Year Beginning date in this section for the first date of your enrollment year. (Note: the Enrollment Year Beginning will appear on your TEOB only if you are enrolled in TRICARE Prime.)

17. Remarks Explanations of the codes or numbers listed in See Remarks will appear here.

18. Toll-Free Telephone Number: Questions about your TRICARE Explanation of Benefits? Please call PGBA or WPS at this toll-free number. Their customer service representatives will assist you.

Fig. 10-7—cont'd

The EOB shows the following (Fig. 10-7):
• What the provider billed
• The TRICARE allowable charge at the time of care
• How much of the patient's annual deductible has been met
• How much the patient has paid toward the annual cost cap
• The patient's cost share for the care
• How much TRICARE paid
• Any reasons for denying services on a claim

What Did You Learn?

1. What types of third-party coverage does TRICARE consider OHI?
2. When a beneficiary has TRICARE and Medicare, which pays first?
3. Define a dual-eligible beneficiary under TRICARE.
4. Under what circumstances do beneficiaries have to submit their own claims?
5. List six items of information contained on a TRICARE EOB.

CHAMPVA

The **Civilian Health and Medical Program of the Department of Veterans Affairs (CHAMPVA)** is a healthcare benefits program for dependents of veterans who

1. have been rated by the Department of Veterans Affairs (VA) as having a total and permanent service-connected disability;
2. are survivors of veterans who died from VA-rated service-connected conditions or who, at the time of death, were rated permanently and totally disabled from a VA-rated service-connected condition; and
3. survivors of individuals who died in the line of duty that was not due to misconduct and who are not otherwise entitled to TRICARE benefits.

Under CHAMPVA, the VA shares the cost of covered healthcare services and supplies with eligible beneficiaries. CHAMPVA is managed by the VA's Health Administration

Center in Denver, Colorado. There is no cost to CHAMPVA beneficiaries when they receive healthcare treatment at a VA facility.

HIPAA Tip

TRICARE and military treatment facilities are required to give health information about any individual to the Department of Health and Human Services for use in an investigation of a complaint.

ELIGIBILITY

The precise eligibility criteria of individuals who are entitled to CHAMPVA benefits are as follows:

- *The spouse or dependent child* of a veteran who has been rated by a VA regional office as having a permanent and total service-connected condition/disability
- *The surviving spouse or dependent child* of a veteran who died as a result of a VA-rated service-connected condition or who, at the time of death, was rated permanently and totally disabled from a service-connected condition
- *The surviving spouse or dependent child* of a person who died in the line of duty and the death was not due to misconduct

CHAMPVA eligibility can be lost if certain demographic changes occur, such as a widow remarrying, divorcing the sponsor, or becoming eligible for Medicare or TRICARE. Dependent children lose their eligibility on reaching age 18 years. This age is extended to 23 years if they are attending an accredited college full-time (a minimum of 12 credit hours). CHAMPVA recipients should report any changes in status to CHAMPVA immediately.

Imagine This!

Scott Talbott was an Army corporal stationed in Haiti in 2004 during their civil war. One evening, Scott and two other enlisted men went to a local bar. After an evening of drinking, they got into a brawl with a group of civilian townsmen. During the altercation, Scott sustained a knife wound to the chest and subsequently died of his injuries. Jenny Talbott, his widow, was informed that she and her three children were not eligible for CHAMPVA benefits because Scott's death was due to "misconduct." Jenny appealed but lost.

● Stop and Think

Harold and Patsy Yates were divorced 12 years ago. Harold, a double amputee Vietnam veteran, was rated by the regional VA office as having a permanent and total service-connected disability. Harold and Patsy are CHAMPVA-eligible; however, Patsy plans to remarry. How, if at all, will this affect her eligibility?

● Stop and Think

Suppose that Harold Yates had been killed in Vietnam, rather than disabled, and he and Patsy were married at the time of his death, which makes her eligible for CHAMPVA benefits. In this scenario, if Patsy remarries, how would this affect her eligibility?

CHAMPVA BENEFITS

In general, CHAMPVA covers most healthcare services and supplies that are medically and psychologically necessary. Prescription medications are free; however, over-the-counter medications are not covered. CHAMPVA benefits do not normally include dental or most eye care. Exceptions are limited to services directly related to treatment of certain medical conditions of the eyes or mouth. CHAMPVA-eligibles may see any provider of their choice as long as the provider is properly licensed.

On confirmation of eligibility, applicants receive program materials that specifically address covered and noncovered services and supplies. Preauthorization is required for certain types of services, as follows:

- Dental care (other than the exceptions mentioned previously)
- Durable medical equipment with a total purchase price or total rental price of more than $300
- Hospice services
- Mental health/substance abuse services
- Organ and bone marrow transplants

Failure to acquire preauthorization results in denial of the claim. Preauthorization for visits to specialists or diagnostic tests is unnecessary.

WHAT CHAMPVA PAYS

CHAMPVA pays the allowable amount of covered services generally equivalent to the TRICARE and Medicare rates for same or similar services. In 2006, CHAMPVA had an outpatient deductible of $50 per person up to $100 per family per year and a cost share (coinsurance) of 25% up to the cat cap. If the patient has OHI, CHAMPVA pays the lesser of 75% of the allowable amount after the $50 calendar year deductible is met or the remainder of the charges. The beneficiary normally has no cost share. CHAMPVA also covers any medical expenses incurred overseas.

It is advised that the health insurance professional collect the 25% of the charges at the time services are rendered, unless the patient has a supplemental policy or OHI. If the beneficiary has OHI, such as group health insurance, the OHI is primary to CHAMPVA and must be billed first. After the OHI has paid, the EOB should be filed with the CHAMPVA claim.

The cat cap for CHAMPVA is $3000 per year. The cat cap time period begins on January 1 of each year and runs through December 31. When the beneficiary has met his or her cat cap, cost sharing for covered services for the remaining calendar year is waived, and CHAMPVA pays 100% of the *allowable* amount.

CHAMPVA offers a more cost effective prescription drug benefit than Medicare Part D, and has no monthly premium. Under CHAMPVA, the prescription plan is considered "credible coverage," and beneficiaries typically do not have to sign up for a Medicare Part D prescription drug plan. If CHAMPVA beneficiaries get their maintenance medications through the CHAMPVA Meds by Mail program and do not routinely use a local pharmacy, they will continue to have those prescriptions provided cost free and delivered directly to their home.

If there is any question whether or not a particular service is payable under CHAMPVA guidelines, the health insurance professional should consult the CHAMPVA handbook or contact the VA Health Administration Center using their toll free phone line or e-mail at HAC.INQ@MED.VA (Table 10-3).

TABLE 10-3 CHAMPVA Costs/Patient Summary (2006)

BENEFITS	DEDUCTIBLE?	BENEFICIARY PAYS	CHAMPVA PAYS
Ambulatory surgery facility services	No	25% of CHAMPVA allowable	75% of CHAMPVA allowable
Professional services	Yes	25% of CHAMPVA allowable after deductible	75% of CHAMPVA allowable
Durable medical equipment: non-VA source	Yes	25% CHAMPVA allowable after deductible	75% of CHAMPVA allowable
Inpatient services: DRG based	No	Lesser of (1) per day amount × number of inpatient days, (2) 25% of billed amount, or (3) DRG rate	CHAMPVA allowable less beneficiary cost share
Inpatient Services: non-DRG based	No	25% of CHAMPVA allowable	75% of CHAMPVA allowable
Mental health: high volume/residential treatment center (RTC)	No	25% of CHAMPVA allowable	75% of CHAMPVA allowable
Mental health: low volume	No	Lesser of (1) per day amount × number of inpatient days or (2) 25% of billed amount	CHAMPVA allowable less beneficiary cost share
Outpatient services (i.e., physician visits, laboratory/radiology, home health, skilled nursing visits, ambulance)	Yes	25% of CHAMPVA allowable after deductible	75% of CHAMPVA allowable
Pharmacy services	Yes	25% of CHAMPVA allowable after deductible	75% of CHAMPVA allowable
VA source (durable medical equipment, Meds by Mail, CHAMPVA In-house Treatment Initiative)	No	Nothing	100% of VA cost

TABLE 10-3 CHAMPVA Costs/Patient Summary (2006)—cont'd

SERVICE	MEDICARE PAYS	CHAMPVA PAYS (AFTER $100 DEDUCTIBLE MET)	BENEFICIARY PAYS (AFTER $50 DEDUCTIBLE MET)
Part B-Outpatient			
Outpatient medical care to include:	80% of Medicare allowable amount	In most cases, the CHAMPVA allowable covers the Medicare copay and a portion of the beneficiary's Medicare outpatient deductible	In most cases, $0
Office visits (physician)			
Durable medical equipment			
Cancer screenings			
Mammograms			
PAP smears			
Immunizations (including flu shots)			
Diabetes supplies (e.g., test strips, monitors)			
Diabetes self-management training			
Bone mass measurements			
Clinical laboratory	100% of Medicare allowable	CHAMPVA allowable less Medicare's payment	$0*
Mental health visit	50% of Medicare allowable	CHAMPVA allowable less Medicare's payment	In most cases, $0
Hospice	100% of Medicare allowable	CHAMPVA allowable less Medicare's payment	$0*
Outpatient medications	All but $5 per prescription		
Respite care	95% of Medicare allowable		
Pharmacy	$0 (with a few exceptions)	Retail, 75% of allowable amount; Meds by Mail, 100%	Retail, 25% of CHAMPVA allowable amount; by mail: $0

*Where Medicare has paid 100% of the allowable representing payment in full, in most cases, there will be no out-of-pocket expense for beneficiary.

● Stop and Think

Elaine Porter is employed by Harper Products, Inc. She has single coverage under her employer's group healthcare plan. Elaine's husband, a helicopter pilot, was killed when his Chinook helicopter was shot down by an air-to-ground missile during Desert Storm. Because Elaine also is covered under CHAMPVA, which payer in this case would be primary?

CHAMPVA-TRICARE CONNECTION

CHAMPVA and TRICARE are federal programs; however, an individual who is eligible for TRICARE is not eligible for CHAMPVA. Although similar, TRICARE should not be confused with CHAMPVA. TRICARE provides coverage to the families of active duty service members, families of service members who died while on active duty, and retirees and their families, whether or not the veteran is disabled. CHAMPVA provides benefits to eligible family members of veterans who have been declared 100% permanently disabled from service-connected conditions, survivors of veterans who died from service-connected conditions, and survivors of service members who died in the line of duty who are not otherwise entitled to TRICARE benefits.

CHAMPVA-MEDICARE CONNECTION

CHAMPVA and Medicare are federal programs; however, CHAMPVA is the last payer after all other third-party payers have met their obligations except for Medicaid and CHAMPVA supplemental insurance. Another exception to third-party payer priority is when a CHAMPVA-eligible beneficiary resides or travels overseas. When this is the case, if all eligibility criteria are met, CHAMPVA is the primary payer (unless there is OHI) until the individual returns to the United States.

When a beneficiary is eligible for healthcare benefits under Medicare and CHAMPVA, Medicare is the primary payer. For healthcare services covered under both plans, there are often no out-of-pocket expenses for covered services. It is important for the beneficiary to be aware that if he or she has Medicare and CHAMPVA, Medicare's rules and procedures must be followed for covered services. Failure to do so means the service would not be covered under CHAMPVA. If Medicare determines that the service is not medically necessary or appropriate, CHAMPVA also would deny coverage. If the beneficiary or the provider disagrees with the Medicare decision, an appeal should be made with Medicare, rather than with CHAMPVA.

CHAMPVA AND HEALTH MAINTENANCE ORGANIZATION COVERAGE

If a CHAMPVA-eligible beneficiary has an HMO plan, CHAMPVA would pay any copayments under the HMO. When medical services are available through the HMO, and the patient chooses to seek care outside the HMO (e.g., from a physician who is not associated with the HMO or does not follow the rules and procedures of the HMO to obtain the care), CHAMPVA would not pay for that medical care. When submitting the OHI Certification (Form 10-7959c), the patient or health insurance professional should include a copy of the HMO copayment information or schedule of benefits.

CHAMPVA PROVIDERS

Healthcare providers may elect to participate in CHAMPVA simply by agreeing to see the beneficiary and submitting a claim to CHAMPVA on the beneficiary's behalf. Providers who accept CHAMPVA patients also must accept the CHAMPVA allowable rate as payment in full and cannot balance bill. Providers may choose not to participate; and in this case, patients typically pay the entire bill and submit

their own claims to CHAMPVA for personal reimbursement of the allowable amount. Even in the case of nonPARs, providers must accept the allowable rate and cannot balance bill. Under the CHAMPVA program, however, the patient is responsible for paying the CHAMPVA cost share and any charges for noncovered services.

CHAMPVA FOR LIFE

The **CHAMPVA for Life (CFL)** program became effective October 1, 2001. This relatively new benefit is designed for spouses or dependents of veterans who are age 65 or older. They must be family members of veterans and meet one of the following conditions:
- The veteran has a permanent and total service-connected disability.
- The veteran died of a service-connected condition.
- The veteran was totally disabled from a service-connected condition at the time of death.
- The spouses and dependents must have Medicare coverage.

Similar to TFL, CFL pays benefits for covered medical services to eligible beneficiaries who are 65 or older and enrolled in Medicare Parts A and B. The CFL benefit is payable after Medicare pays their share. If the beneficiary has a Medigap-type insurance policy, CHAMPVA becomes third in line for payment. If a beneficiary is eligible for TFL, he or she is *not* eligible for CHAMPVA because TFL is for military retirees and their dependents. CFL combined with Medicare gives the beneficiary extensive coverage that covers most healthcare needs. There are exceptions, however. If a particular procedure is *not* covered by Medicare, it probably would not be covered by CHAMPVA (e.g., eye glasses, dental care). CHAMPVA would not pay Medicare Part B premiums, but it does pay Medicare's first-day hospital deductible. CFL beneficiaries cannot use a VA medical center.

FILING CHAMPVA CLAIMS

As with TRICARE, providers accepting assignment for CHAMPVA claims must submit the claim for the beneficiary. Beneficiaries who receive treatment from nonPARs usually are required to submit their own claims. All CHAMPVA claims, whether electronic or paper, should be sent to the following address:

VA Health Administration Center
CHAMPVA
PO Box 65024
Denver, CO 80206-9024

As stated earlier, if the beneficiary has OHI, claims should be sent to the OHI first. The EOB from the OHI should be attached to the claim and submitted to CHAMPVA. By law, CHAMPVA is always secondary payer except to Medicaid and CHAMPVA supplemental policies.

CHAMPVA CLAIMS FILING DEADLINES

CHAMPVA claims follow the same filing deadline specifications as TRICARE with the exception that all CHAMPVA claims are sent to the VA Health Administration Center in Denver, Colorado. A TRICARE contractor can grant exemptions from the filing deadlines under certain circumstances. Box 10-3 lists circumstances that qualify for a time filing exemption.

● Stop and Think

Maria Delgado received care from her family physician, Imari Deili, on July 1, 2003. Anne Jenkins, Dr. Deili's health insurance professional, neglected to file a claim until Ms. Delgado telephoned inquiring about a series of statements she received. Anne completed the claim and mailed it to the TRICARE contractor on June 30, 2004. She then told Ms. Delgado that the claim would be paid by TRICARE because it would be postmarked within the 1-year time limit. Is Anne correct?

What Did You Learn?

1. What categories of individuals qualify for CHAMPVA benefits?
2. List five types of services for which CHAMPVA requires preauthorization.
3. If a Medicare/CHAMPVA-eligible beneficiary resides or travels overseas, which payer is primary?
4. On what factor does CHAMPVA base their allowable amount?
5. Where does the health insurance professional send CHAMPVA claims?
6. What is the deadline for filing CHAMPVA claims?

INSTRUCTIONS FOR COMPLETING TRICARE/CHAMPVA CLAIM FORMS

All professional charges must be submitted on a CMS-1500 claim form according to TRICARE guidelines. Guidelines are provided in Table 10-4. It is important to remember when completing the claim that the "sponsor" is the member or was active duty military. The sponsor's dependent (spouse

Box 10-3

Circumstances for Exemptions to the Claims Deadline Date

1. If CHAMPUS headquarters or a CHAMPUS/TRICARE contractor made a mistake that resulted in a claim being improperly denied for lack of timely filing.
2. If mental incompetency of the patient (or of a guardian or sponsor, in the case of a minor child) resulted in a claim not being filed in a timely manner. The incompetency may include an inability to communicate, even if the inability is the result of a physical disability. It must be documented by a physician.
3. If the provider agreed to participate in CHAMPUS (also known as accepting assignment) on the claim, and to bill CHAMPUS/TRICARE directly, but failed to do so.
4. If delays by other health insurance plans (health plans that must pay first, before a claim for the care may be filed with CHAMPUS/TRICARE) in making their payment determinations cause the person or organization filing the claim to miss the deadline. Delays must not be the fault of the CHAMPUS/TRICARE-eligible patient.
5. If billings are made directly by participating providers, and they request an exception to the deadline.
6. If a patient is found to have been CHAMPUS/TRICARE-eligible after the care was received, but claims were not filed with the contractor in time to meet the deadline because of the delay in determining eligibility. Individuals who want to request an exception to the claim-filing deadline may submit a request to the CHAMPUS/TRICARE contractor for the state or region in which the medical services or supplies were provided. Such requests must include a complete explanation of the circumstances of the late filing, together with all available documentation supporting the request, along with the claim denied for late filing.

TABLE 10-4	**Instructions for Filing TRICARE/CHAMPVA Paper Claims**
Block 1	Required. Place an "X" in the CHAMPUS box for TRICARE claims; place an "X" in the CHAMPVA for CHAMPVA claims.
Block 1a	Required. Enter the sponsor's Social Security number (not the beneficiary's) unless they are one and the same. If the beneficiary is a NATO beneficiary, enter "NATO" here.
Block 2	Required. Enter the patient's last name, first name, and middle initial (if any) *exactly* as shown on the TRICARE or CHAMPVA ID card.
Block 3	Required. Enter the patient's 8-digit birth date (MM DD YYYY) as shown on the ID card, and place an "X" in the appropriate box indicating sex.
Block 4	Required. Enter the sponsor's last name, first name, and middle initial, or if the sponsor and the patient are one and the same, enter the word "SAME."
Block 5	Required. Enter the complete address of the patient's place of residence at the time of service and the telephone number. Do not use PO Box numbers. For rural addresses, indicate the box number and rural route or 911E number.
Block 6	Required. If the beneficiary is the sponsor, indicate "SELF" or provide the relationship to the sponsor. If "other" is checked, indicate how the beneficiary is related to the sponsor (e.g., former spouse). *Note:* Parents, parents-in-law, stepparents, and any grandchildren who are not adopted are *not* eligible for TRICARE despite the fact that they may have a military ID card. Be sure to check the *back* of the dependent beneficiary's ID card to ensure it indicates authorization for civilian/TRICARE benefits.
Block 7	Required. Enter the address of the active duty sponsor's duty station or the retiree's mailing address. If the address if the same as the beneficiary's, enter "SAME." If the sponsor resides overseas, enter the APO/FPO address.
Block 8	Required. Check the appropriate box for the patient's marital status and whether employed or a student.
Block 9	Enter the name of the insured if different from that shown in Block 2. If the beneficiary is covered by a spouse's insurance, Blocks 11a-d should be used to show other health insurance held by the beneficiary.
Note: Block 11d should be completed before determining the need for completing Blocks 9a-d. If Block 11d is checked "yes," Blocks 9a-d must be completed before claims processing as follows:	
Block 9a	Provide the policy number/group number of the insured's policy.
Block 9b	Enter the other insured's date of birth and check the appropriate box for sex.
Block 9c	Enter the name of the employer or name of the school.
Block 9d	Enter the name of the insurance plan or the program name where the individual has OHI coverage. If the other coverage is truly supplemental to TRICARE (Medicaid or a plan specifically stating it is supplemental to TRICARE), enter the name and the word "SUPPLEMENTAL" in this block.
Blocks 10a-c	Required. Check "YES" or "NO" to indicate whether employment, auto liability, or other accident involvement applies to one or more of the services described in Block 24. Provide information concerning potential third-party liability. The claims processor will send a DD form 2527, "Statement of Personal Injury—Possible Third Party Liability," to the beneficiary if the diagnosis code(s) fall within the 800-999 range.
Block 10d	Required. Use this block to indicate that other health insurance is attached.
Block 11	Conditionally required. If the beneficiary has OHI, enter the policy/group number here. Indicate if the beneficiary is covered by Medicare. (Blocks 9a-d should be used to report other primary coverage held by family members that includes coverage of the beneficiary).
Block 11a	Conditionally required. If the beneficiary has OHI, enter the date of birth and sex if different from Block 3.
Block 11b	Conditionally required. Enter the employer or school name, if applicable.
Block 11c	Conditionally required. Enter the OHI plan or program name. If the beneficiary is covered by a supplemental policy (Medicaid or a policy specifically stating it is supplemental to TRICARE), indicate "SUPPLEMENTAL".
Block 11d	Required. Indicate if there is or is not another health benefit plan that is primary to TRICARE. The beneficiary may be covered under a plan held by a spouse, a parent, or some other person. If this block is checked "yes," Blocks 9a-d must be completed.
Block 12	Required. "SIGNATURE ON FILE" or "SOF" can be used here if the beneficiary's signature is on file in the provider's office (and on a document that includes a release of information statement). If not on file, the beneficiary must sign and date Block 12. If the patient is under 18 years old, either parent should sign the claim unless the services are confidential. If the patient is over 18 years old, but cannot sign the claim, the person who signs must be the legal guardian or, in the absence of a legal guardian, a spouse or parent of the patient. The signer should write the beneficiary's name in Block 12, followed by the word, "by" and his/her own signature. A statement must be attached giving the signer's full name, address, relationship to the beneficiary, and the reason the signer is unable to sign. Also, documentation must be attached showing the signer's appointment as legal guardian or power of attorney.

TABLE 10-4	Instructions for Filing TRICARE/CHAMPVA Paper Claims—cont'd
Block 13	Leave blank for TRICARE and CHAMPVA claims. Claims checks are forwarded to PAR and nonPAR accepting assignment. On nonPAR claims, benefit checks are mailed to the patient.
Block 14	Conditionally required. Enter the 8-digit (MM DD YYYY) date of current illness, injury, or pregnancy, if it is documented in the health record.
Block 15	Conditionally required. If it is documented in the health record that the patient has had same or similar condition previously, enter that date here.
Block 16	Conditionally required. If the patient is employed and unable to work in his or her current occupation, enter the 8-digit (MM DD YYYY) date when patient was unable to work. (*Note:* An entry in this field may indicate employment-related insurance coverage).
Block 17	Required. Enter the name and address of the entity that referred the patient to the provider of services identified on the claim. This is required for all charges for a consultation or the claims processor will have to pay the claim at the rate for the lowest category of office visit. If the beneficiary was referred from an MFT, enter the name of the MTF and attach a copy of the military referral form (DD 2161 or SF 513).
Block 17a and 17b	Enter the unique provider identification number (UPIN) or national provider identifier (NPI) of the individual shown in Block 17. The UPIN can be used until May 22, 2007, and it should appear in Block 17a. Effective May 23, 2007, the NPI must be reported in 17b.
Block 18	Conditionally required. If the patient was hospitalized as an inpatient, enter the "FROM" and "TO" dates here.
Block 19	Not required. Leave blank.
Block 20	Conditionally required. Indicate whether laboratory work was performed outside of the provider's office, and if so, enter the total amount charged by the laboratory for work being reported on the claim.
Block 21	Required. Enter the patient's diagnosis/condition using an ICD-9-CM code number (s).
Block 22	Not required. Leave blank.
Block 23	Conditionally required. Enter the prior authorization number if the services require preauthorization/preadmission review.
Block 24a	Required. Enter the month, day, and year for each procedure/service or supply using the MM DD YYYY format. If "from" and "to" dates are shown here for a series of identical services, enter the total number of units in Block 24g.
Block 24b	Required. Enter the appropriate 2-digit numeric place of service (POS) code. See Table 10-5 for the list of applicable codes.
Block 24c	This block is conditionally required. Enter an "X" or an "E" as appropriate for services performed as a result of a medical emergency.
Block 24d	Required. Enter the appropriate CPT code for each service. If using one of the "not elsewhere classified" codes, you must supply a narrative description of the service/supply.
Block 24e	Required. Enter the appropriate diagnosis reference code as shown in Block 21 to relate to each service/procedure. If multiple services/procedures were performed, enter the diagnosis code reference number for each service/procedure.
Block 24f	Required. Enter the charge for each listed service. Please include the cents with dollar amounts. *For example, $24.00 should be entered as 24 00 rather than $24. Dashes or lines should not be used in this item.*
Block 24g	Required. Provide the days or units for each line item. This block should be used for multiple visits for identical services, number of miles, units of supplies, or oxygen volume. If anesthesia, provide the beginning and end time of administration, time in minutes, or 15-minute units.
Block 24h	Not required. Leave blank.
Block 24i	Conditionally required. Enter the appropriate ID qualifier. Contact your local TRICARE/CHAMPVA FI for this information.
Block 24j	Prior to May 23, 2007, enter the provider's PIN in the shaded portion. After May 23, 2007, enter the provider's NPI number in the lower, unshaded portion. In the case of a service-provided incident to the service of a physician or non-physician practitioner, when the person who ordered the service is not supervising, enter the PIN of the supervisor in the shaded portion.
Block 25	Required. Enter the 9-digit Federal tax ID (employer identification number) assigned to that provider (or group), and check the appropriate box. In the case of an unincorporated practice or a sole practitioner, the provider's social security number is typically used.
Block 26	Conditionally required. Enter the patient's account number assigned by the provider of service's or supplier's accounting system.

Government claim

TABLE 10-4	Instructions for Filing TRICARE/CHAMPVA Paper Claims—cont'd
Block 27	Required. PARs and nonPARs accepting assignment should check this box "Yes." Failure to complete this box or if the "X" is outside the box means assignment was not accepted. To accept assignment under TRICARE guidelines means that the provider will accept the TRICARE-determined allowed amount as payment in full for services. If a provider does not accept assignment, payment and the EOB go to the beneficiary *only*. The provider would not be given any information on the claim other than receipt. On claims where assignment is not accepted, the provider may collect only up to 115% of the TRICARE-determined allowed amount for the services.
Block 28	Required. Enter total charges for the services (i.e., total of all charges in Block 24f).
Block 29	Required. Enter the amount received by the provider or supplier from OHI. If no payment was made by the primary payer, an EOB should be attached to the claim indicating why the primary payer made no payment. If the primary payer is Medicare or an HMO, an EOB should be attached whether payment was made or not. Any payment received from the beneficiary should not be included in this box.
Block 30	Not required. Leave blank.
Block 31	Required. This block must contain the signature of the provider and date or that of his or her authorized representative. If someone other than the provider of services signs on the provider's behalf, there should be a notarized statement on file with the claims processor indicating the provider's permission to accept someone else's signature. This "representative" should sign his or her name and title so as not to be confused with the actual provider.
Block 32a	Enter the NPI of the service facility in Block 32.
Block 32b	Enter the appropriate ID qualifier followed by one blank space and then the PIN of the service facility. After May 23, 2007, 32b is not to be reported. Follow the specific guidelines of your Medicaid FI.
Block 33	Enter the name, complete address, and telephone number (including area code) where the provider's office is physically located.
Block 33a	Effective May 23, 2007, The NPI of the billing provider must be reported here.
Block 33b	Enter the approriate ID qualifier followed by one blank space and then the PIN of the billing provider or group. Effective May 23, 2007, 33b is not to be reported. Enter the group UPIN, including the 2-digit location identifier, for the performing practitioner or supplier who is a member of a group practice.

or child) is the "patient" or "beneficiary," as these terms are often used interchangeably. The instructions in Table 10-4 are generic and may not be exactly the same as required by the claims processor in each area. The health insurance professional should obtain complete, detailed, and up-to-date claims completion guidelines from the TRICARE claims processor in his or her area to ensure the CMS-1500 forms are completed correctly to expedite reimbursement.

CLAIMS FILING SUMMARY

The following are some important points to consider when filing claims:
- Claims should be submitted as soon as services are rendered to expedite the claims process.
- Claims filing deadline is 1 year from the date of service or 1 year from the date of discharge for inpatient hospitalization.
- Copies should be kept of all information submitted to the TRICARE claims processor or CHAMPVA.
- It is not beneficial to hold multiple claims over a period of time and submit them all at once. If numerous claims are submitted, and there is a problem with one, it could delay the processing of all claims.

CHAMPVA EXPLANATION OF BENEFITS

On completion of the processing of a CHAMPVA claim, an EOB form is sent to the beneficiary and to the provider, if the claim was filed by the provider. The EOB is a summary of the action taken on the claim and contains the following information (Fig. 10-8):
- Provider name
- Date of service
- Description of service
- Amount billed by the provider
- CHAMPVA-allowed amount
- Amount not covered
- Amount paid by OHI
- Amount applied to the beneficiary's annual deductible requirement
- Beneficiary and family deductible accrual
- CHAMPVA payment
- Annual cat cap accrual
- Remarks

CLAIMS APPEALS AND RECONSIDERATIONS

In the event a provider or beneficiary disagrees with the manner in which a claim was processed and considers it

TABLE 10-5 POS/TOS Codes

PLACE-OF-SERVICE CODES (FOR USE IN BLOCK 24B OF CMS-1500 FORM)	
11	Office
12	Home
21	Inpatient
22	Outpatient, hospital
23	Emergency department—hospital
24	Ambulatory surgical center
25	Birthing center
26	Military treatment facility
31	Skilled nursing facility
33	Custodial care facility
34	Hospice
41	Ambulance, land
42	Ambulance, air or water
51	Inpatient psychiatric facility
52	Psychiatric facility (partial hospitalization)
53	Community mental health center
54	Intermediate care facility (mentally handicapped)
55	Residential substance abuse treatment facility
56	Psychiatric residential treatment facility
61	Comprehensive outpatient rehabilitation facility
71	State or local public health clinic
72	Rural health clinic
81	Independent laboratory
99	Other, unlisted facility

necessary to file a claims appeal or have the processing of a claim reconsidered, such an appeal must be filed within 90 days of the receipt of the EOB. The EOB contains the pertinent information on the procedures for filing an appeal. All appeals must be in submitted in writing. On receipt of the written appeal, all claims for the entire course of treatment are reviewed. Health insurance professionals should contact the claims processor in their region or the CHAMPVA office in Denver for details on how to submit an appeal.

Imagine This!

Dr. Serjio Manya, a psychiatrist, provided psychiatric treatment to Samuel Fortune, a Gulf War veteran, for clinical depression. Samuel, who was determined to be CHAMPVA-eligible after his diagnosis, subsequently was admitted to the Trenton Mental Healthcare Facility because of a suicide attempt, where he remained for 15 months. Because Dr. Manya was nonPAR and Samuel's mental condition rendered him incompetent, the claim was not filed within the time limit. Because Samuel's illness was documented by Dr. Manya, however, Samuel was able to get a filing extension and ultimately received CHAMPVA benefits.

What Did You Learn?

1. In which block on the claim form should the "sponsor's" name appear?
2. List at least five items of information shown on the CHAMPVA EOB.
3. What is the deadline for filing a CHAMPVA appeal?

HIPAA AND MILITARY INSURERS

All military medical facilities have implemented the privacy rules of the Health Insurance Portability and Accountability Act (HIPAA) of 1996. The Military Health System always has had privacy standards in place to limit unauthorized access and disclosure of personal health information. The new HIPAA rules heighten awareness, raise the level of oversight, and provide a standard set of guidelines to protect the privacy of all patients.

 HIPAA Tip

HIPAA requires all employees, contractors, and volunteers of healthcare provider organizations, healthcare insurers, and healthcare clearinghouses, including those associated with TRICARE and CHAMPVA, who come in contact with Protected Health Information to be trained annually in the areas of privacy and security.

In preparation to become HIPAA compliant by the required date, the Department of Defense mailed approximately 5 million MTF notices of privacy practices—one to each beneficiary enrolled in DEERS. Each MTF has an assigned, trained privacy officer available to respond to any questions or concerns that beneficiaries may have regarding the new privacy rules. The privacy officers also serve as patient advocates ensuring that personal health information maintained by the MTF remains protected yet accessible to beneficiaries and their providers. A copy of the notice to privacy practice is available on the TRICARE website for sponsors and family members to download; copies also are available for distribution at each Department of Defense MTF.

What Did You Learn?

1. What steps did CHAMPVA take to become HIPAA compliant?
2. What is the role of the privacy officer?

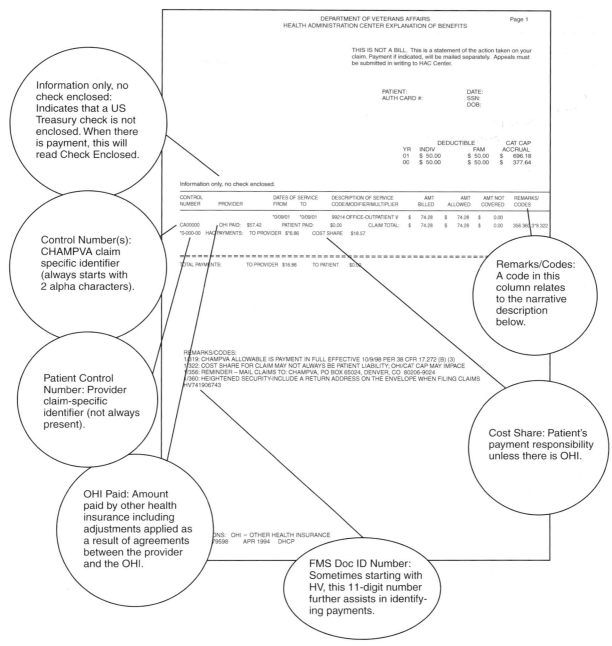

Fig. 10-8 Sample CHAMPVA EOB. (Source: U. S. Department of Veterans Affairs, Health Administration Center.)

SUMMARY CHECK POINTS

☑ Through its main objectives of accessibility and affordability, TRICARE brings together the healthcare resources of the Army, Navy, and Air Force and supplements them with networks of civilian healthcare professionals to provide better access to healthcare and high-quality service, while maintaining the capability to support military operations.

☑ TRICARE's three choices for healthcare are as follows:
- *TRICARE Standard:* The standard fee-for-service (indemnity) option, formerly called CHAMPUS. This program provides greater personal choice in the selection of healthcare providers, although it requires higher individual out-of-pocket costs than a managed care plan.

☑ • *TRICARE Extra:* A preferred provider option through which, rather than an annual fee, a yearly deductible is charged. Healthcare is delivered through a network of civilian healthcare providers who accept payments from TRIACARE and provide services at negotiated, discounted rates.

• *TRICARE Prime:* A HMO-type plan in which enrollees receive healthcare through a Military Treatment Facility PCM or a supporting network of civilian providers.

☑ Eligibility under TRICARE's three plans is as follows:

• *TRICARE Standard eligibles* include spouses and dependents of active service members, military retirees and their eligible family members, and survivors of all uniformed services who are not eligible for Medicare. Dependents of military service members in the Army and National Guard Reserves, known as RCs, also are eligible for TRICARE Standard, if the RC is ordered to active duty for more than 30 consecutive days, or if the orders are for an indefinite period. All TRICARE eligibles must be listed in DEERS.

• *TRICARE Extra eligibles* include any individual who is eligible for TRICARE Standard.

• *TRICARE Prime eligibles* include retired military beneficiaries and their eligible family members. Active military members are automatically enrolled in TRICARE Prime.

☑ An NAS is a document of certification from the MTF that says it cannot provide the specific healthcare the beneficiary needs. The statements must be entered electronically in the Defense Department's DEERS computer files by the MTF. An NAS is no longer needed for TRICARE Standard beneficiaries except for nonemergency mental health services.

☑ TRICARE PARs agree to accept the TRICARE allowable charge on all claims as payment in full for the healthcare services provided and not balance bill. NonPARs can participate in TRICARE on a case-by-case basis. PARs and nonPARs who accept assignment must file the claim for the patient, and TRICARE sends the payment (if any) directly to the provider.

☑ CHAMPVA is a healthcare benefits program for qualifying dependents and survivors of veterans. Under CHAMPVA, VA shares the cost of covered healthcare services and supplies with eligible beneficiaries. CHAMPVA is managed by the VA's Health Administration Center in Denver, Colorado.

☑ Individuals who are entitled to CHAMPVA benefits include

• *the spouse or dependent child* of a veteran who has been rated by a VA regional office as having a permanent and total service-connected condition/disability;

• *the surviving spouse or dependent child* of a veteran who died as a result of a VA-rated service-connected condition or who, at the time of death, was rated permanently and totally disabled from a service-connected condition; and

• *the surviving spouse or dependent child* of a person who died in the line of duty, and the death was not due to misconduct.

☑ A qualifying beneficiary can be eligible for healthcare benefits under Medicare and CHAMPVA. For healthcare services covered under both plans, there are often no out-of-pocket expenses for covered services. The beneficiary should know that if he or she has Medicare and CHAMPVA, Medicare's rules and procedures must be followed for covered services. If the beneficiary fails to do so, the service will not be covered under CHAMPVA. Also, if Medicare finds the service is not medically necessary or appropriate, CHAMPVA will not provide coverage either. Medicare is primary to CHAMPVA.

☑ Providers filing claims should
• use the standard CMS-1500 claim form,
• follow the TRICARE guidelines for completing the form,
• ensure the information is complete and accurate,
• affix the required signature format,
• date the claim form,
• make and keep a copy of all paper claims, and
• send completed claims (electronic or paper) to the TRICARE claims processor in the region in which the enrollee resides.

☑ Patients who file their own claims
• must use Form 2692 (CHAMPUS Claim Patient Request for Medical Payment) and
• attach the provider's detailed itemized statement and an NAS (if necessary).

☑ All CHAMPVA claims, whether electronic or paper, should be sent to VA Health Administration Center, CHAMPVA, PO Box 65024, Denver, CO 80206-9024.

☑ For information regarding where to file paper claims, the TRICARE website lists the names and addresses of claims processors by region. At the TRICARE home page, click on "site map," choose "claims," and select the region of choice to access the chart of pertinent information.

☑ The deadline for submitting all military claims is 1 year from the date of service. If the service was rendered on August 30, 2003, the claim must be in the hands of the claims processor by the end of the working day on August 30, 2004. For inpatient hospital claims, the deadline is 1 year from the date of discharge.

☑ In preparation to become HIPAA compliant, the Department of Defense mailed notices of privacy practices to all MTFs and to every beneficiary enrolled in DEERS. In addition, each MTF has an assigned, trained privacy officer available to respond to any questions or concerns that beneficiaries may have regarding the new privacy rules. A copy of the notice of privacy practices also is available on the TRICARE website for sponsors and family members to download; copies also are available for distribution at each Department of Defense MTF.

CLOSING SCENARIO

After completing the chapter on military carriers, Sally thinks she is ready to answer her Aunt Betty's questions. She agrees with her aunt that the various plans available under TRICARE can be confusing, and it may be difficult to decide which plan best suits a military spouse's or dependent's needs. First, Sally explained that CHAMPUS was the former name, and it was now called TRICARE (*TRI* because it offers three plans). Additionally, Sally outlined the three plans along with the advantages and disadvantages of each. She gave her aunt several Internet websites from which to get further details regarding TRICARE and suggested that she sit down with the health insurance professional at the medical clinic to resolve some of the confusion over claims.

Sally also discovered that her grandfather was eligible to receive his prescription medicine by mail through the VA. This would be a tremendous cost savings for him because he was on seven different medications. It gave Sally a good feeling to know that she was able to help her family. Now, she looked forward to helping others through her career as a health insurance professional.

WEBSITES TO EXPLORE

For live links to the following websites, please visit the Evolve® site at http://evolve.elsevier.com/Beik/today/

- To find the nearest uniformed services personnel office, log on to http://www.dmdc.osd.mil/rsl/

- For detailed information on TRICARE, log on to their information-filled website at http://www.tricare.osd.mil/hipaa/

- To view the TRICARE handbook, log on to http://www.tricare.osd.mil/tricarehandbook/

- For details regarding the cat cap in a particular area, log on to the website at http://www.tricare.osd.mil/tricareservicecenters/default.cfm

- To view the CHAMPVA handbook, log on to http://www.va.gov/hac/forbeneficiaries/champva/handbook.asp

- Additional information on HIPAA, TRICARE, and the new privacy standards is available on the TRICARE website at http://www.tricare.osd.mil/hipaa

- To report fraud, waste, or abuse in federal programs, log on to www.gao.gov/fraudnet/fraudnet.htm

Chapter 11

Miscellaneous Carriers: Workers' Compensation and Disability Insurance

Chapter Outline

CHAPTER OBJECTIVES

After completion of this chapter, the student should be able to
- Explain the purpose of workers' compensation.
- Discuss workers' compensation eligibility requirements, exemptions, and benefits.
- Understand the reporting requirements of workers' compensation claims.
- Describe how disability is determined in workers' compensation cases.
- Explain the purpose of disability income insurance.
- Differentiate between Social Security Disability Insurance and supplemental security income.
- Summarize the Centers for Disease Control and Prevention's Disability and Health Team Activities.
- Explain the Ticket to Work Program.
- Discuss the process for filing Social Security Disability Insurance and supplemental security income claims.
- List the health insurance professional's responsibilities that can facilitate disability claims processing.

CHAPTER TERMS

activities of daily living
Americans with
    Disabilities Act (ADA)
benefit cap
Black Lung Benefits Act
casual employee
coming and going rule
Disability and Health
    Team
disability income
    insurance
earned income
egregious
employment network
Federal Employment
    Compensation Act
    (FECA)
Federal Employment
    Liability Act
financial means test
instrumental activities
    of daily living
interstate commerce
job deconditioning
Longshore and Harbor
    Workers'
    Compensation Act
long-term disability

Merchant Marine Act
    (Jones Act)
modified own-
    occupation policy
no-fault insurance
ombudsman
own-occupation policy
permanent and
    stationary
permanent partial
    disability
permanent total disability
progress or
    supplemental report
protected health
    information
short-term disability
Social Security Disability
    Insurance (SSDI)
supplemental security
    income (SSI)
temporarily disabled
temporary partial
    disability
temporary total disability
Ticket to Work Program
vocational rehabilitation
workers' compensation

OPENING SCENARIO

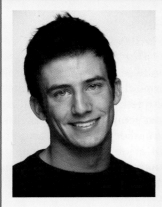

The terms "workers' compensation" and "disability insurance" were familiar to Jim Lightfoot. His father had been a construction worker on a high-rise apartment building and had fallen to his death 6 years earlier. Even though Jim was young at the time, he remembers the monthly benefit checks his mother received, which were so vital in helping pay living expenses for the family. Now, Jim was anxious to learn as much as he could about the various types of disability listed in the chapter outline.

Tammy Hansen, a classmate, didn't share Jim's enthusiasm for the subject at first, but her uncle was an insurance salesman. The day before Jim and Tammy were to begin the chapter on workers' compensation and disability insurance, Uncle Niles stopped by her house, and Tammy overhead her father and uncle discussing disability income insurance. "I can't afford to have disability insurance," her father stated, to which her uncle replied: "With your growing family, you can't afford not to!" The tone of her uncle's voice made Tammy sit up and listen. Why, she wondered, did her uncle believe that disability income insurance was important? Perhaps this chapter might be more informative and interesting than she first thought.

WORKERS' COMPENSATION

Workers' compensation is a type of insurance regulated by state laws that pays medical expenses and partial loss of wages for workers who are injured on the job or become ill as a result of job-related circumstances. If death results, benefits are payable to the surviving spouse and dependents as defined by law. Most U.S. workers are covered by the

Workers' Compensation Law. The employer, not the employee, pays the premiums. Each state sets up its own workers' compensation laws and regulations; however, they are basically the same from state to state.

HISTORY

Workers' compensation began in Germany in the 1800s when it was determined that something needed to be done to take care of injured workers to limit their physical and financial suffering from injuries or illnesses resulting from their jobs. Workers' compensation became common in the United States in the 1930s and 1940s, and it exists today in all 50 states and territories.

When workers' compensation was first proposed, U.S. companies were hesitant to accept full responsibility for paying the premiums. Their argument was that on top of the premium expense, they still could be financially liable in a worker-initiated lawsuit. A compromise was reached between businesses and workers: Companies would pay the premiums for the insurance that protected workers, and the workers would give up the right to sue the employer for damages resulting from a job-related illness or injury. This principle continues essentially intact to this day. Workers' compensation is not considered a "benefit"; rather, it is a legally mandated right of the worker.

Companies that meet specific state requirements must provide workers' compensation for all employees. There are fines and sometimes other penalties for businesses that do not provide coverage as required by law. Workers' compensation can be purchased from several possible sources—private insurance companies, state funds, insurance pools, and self-insurance programs.

State statutes establish the framework and set up the laws for most workers' compensation insurance. As we learned earlier, these laws provide benefits not only for workers, but also dependents of workers who are killed or die because of job-related accidents or illnesses. Many state laws also protect employers and their fellow workers by limiting the amount an injured employee can recover from an employer and by eliminating the liability of coworkers in most accidents.

FEDERAL LEGISLATION AND WORKERS' COMPENSATION

Besides the workers' compensation programs offered at the state level, there are several categories of federal programs for workers who do not fall under the umbrella of covered employees under state laws.

The **Federal Employment Compensation Act (FECA)** provides workers' compensation for nonmilitary federal employees. Many of its provisions are similar to state workers' compensation laws; however, awards are limited to disability or death incurred while in the performance of the employee's duties, but not caused willfully by the employee or by intoxication or other illegal acts. The act covers medical expenses resulting from the disability and can require the employee to undergo job retraining. Under this act, a disabled employee receives two thirds of his or her normal monthly salary during the disability period and may receive more for permanent physical injuries or if he or she has dependents. The act provides compensation for survivors of employees who are killed while on the job or die from a job-related illness or condition. The Federal Employment Compensation Act is administered by the Office of Workers' Compensation Programs.

The **Federal Employment Liability Act,** although not a workers' compensation statute, states that companies in which railroads are engaged in **interstate commerce** (trade that involves more than one state) are liable for injuries to their employees if they have been negligent.

The **Merchant Marine Act (Jones Act)** provides seamen (individuals involved in transporting goods by water between U.S. ports) with the same protection from employer negligence that Federal Employment Liability Act provides railroad workers.

Congress enacted the **Longshore and Harbor Workers' Compensation Act** to provide workers' compensation to specified employees of private maritime employers. The Office of Workers' Compensation Programs administers the act.

The **Black Lung Benefits Act** provides compensation for miners with *black lung* (pneumoconiosis). This act requires liable mine operators to award disability payments and establishes a fund administered by the Secretary of Labor providing disability payments to miners where the mine operator is unknown or unable to pay. The Office of Workers' Compensation Programs regulates the administration of the act.

ELIGIBILITY

In the United States, any employee who injures himself or herself on the job or develops an employment-related illness that prevents the employee from working is likely to be eligible to collect workers' compensation benefits. The same applies to the spouse and dependents of a family member who dies because of a job-related accident or illness. If the disability is permanent or the employee has dependents, benefits include a specific percentage (often two thirds) of regular wages or salary.

As with many rules and regulations, there are exceptions. Benefits are awarded only for disability or death occurring while the employee was in the process of performing lawful duties. If any horseplay, drunken stumbling, or illegal drugs are involved, workers' compensation usually does not pay. The same applies for self-inflicted injuries and for injuries incurred while a worker is off the job, committing a crime, or violating company policy.

Exemptions

Not all business organizations are required to purchase workers' compensation insurance for their employees. Exemption criteria vary, however, from state to state. The following list presents various exemption classifications (keep in mind, however, that these classifications are not nationwide but vary from state to state):

- Employers with a minimum number of full-time employees (fewer than three and up to five, depending on the state)
- Executive officers
- Individuals who are business partners (coverage is optional)
- Sole proprietors (most states allow optional coverage)
- "Casual" employees. (A **casual employee** is one who is not entitled to paid holiday or sick leave, has no expectation of ongoing employment, and for whom each engagement with the employer constitutes a separate contract of employment. Casual employees often receive a higher rate of pay to compensate for a lack of job security and benefits.)
- Volunteers
- Part-time domestic employees, agricultural workers, and emergency relief workers. (These categories of employees are typically excluded, but employees can obtain workers' compensation and employers' liability insurance coverage by agreement between their employer and an insurance carrier.)

Benefits

Workers' compensation insurance is **no-fault insurance**. Benefits are paid to the injured (or ill) worker regardless of who is to blame for the accident or injury barring the exceptions mentioned previously. There are four major benefit components to workers' compensation:

1. *Medical expense*—pays the expenses involved for hospitalization, physicians' visits, and any necessary medical treatment
2. *Disability pay*—can be temporary or permanent if it is determined that the worker will never fully recover
3. *Vocational rehabilitation*—if the injury or illness results in the worker being unable to perform the usual duties of his or her occupation, retraining may be necessary for the worker to enter into a new trade or business; also, physical therapy may be needed
4. *Death benefits*—paid to surviving dependents

Because workers' compensation imposes strict liability without inquiry into fault, an employer could be penalized if the cause of injury or illness was **egregious**, meaning the employer was conspicuously negligent, such as violating federal or state safety standards, failing to correct known defects, or other such careless conduct.

Most state workers' compensation laws exclude coverage for injuries sustained while an employee is commuting to and from work. This is referred to as the **coming and going rule**. There are exceptions to this rule, however, such as in the case where the scope of the employee's duties includes travel or where the employee is running an errand for the employer during the commute. Inquiry as to whether the coming and going rule applies to a particular situation should be made before simply ruling out the possibility of coverage for an accident that occurred during a worker's commute to or from work. If an employee is injured during a lunch period, it is usually considered outside the scope of the employment relationship.

● Stop and Think

Carol Brown, bookkeeper at the Memorial Health Clinic, drops off the bank deposit each evening on her way home from work. One evening, as she is in the process of making the deposit, she slams her hand in the depository door, sustaining a laceration to her middle and index finger. Several weeks later, as Carol is on her way to the bank to make the daily deposit, she stops at a convenience store for a cup of coffee and a donut. In her haste, she spills the coffee, sustaining second-degree burns to her torso. Does either of these scenarios represent a legitimate workers' compensation claim?

☑ HIPAA Tip

HIPAA requirements do not apply to certain types of benefit plans known as *excepted benefits*, which include coverage only for accidents (including accidental death or dismemberment) or certain categories of disability income insurance.

Denial of Benefits and Appeals

Employees who believe they have been wrongly denied workers' compensation benefits can appeal or resort to litigation. Some states have an **ombudsman**, who is an individual responsible for investigating and resolving workers' complaints against the employer or insurance company that is denying the benefits.

Most work injuries result in granted benefits because it is usually obvious when an injury is work-related. In these cases, if the claim were filed in a timely manner and according to a company's work rules, benefits would be awarded. There are a variety of situations, however, that may justify an employer or the insurer contesting a claim for workers' compensation benefits. It may be believed that an injury or resulting disability does not meet one or more of the legal requirements for entitlement to benefits. In these cases, a notice that the claim has been denied, containing reasons for the denial, must be issued promptly to the worker by the employer or by the employer's workers' compensation insurance company.

Imagine This!

Louise Carson has been a teacher at Harrison Junior High School for 10 years. At her yearly physical examination, her healthcare provider informs her that she is dangerously hypertensive. Louise attributes her hypertension to stress from her teaching responsibilities plus increasing pressure from her supervisor to maintain better discipline in the classroom. Louise's blood pressure does not respond to conventional antihypertensive medication, so her physician suggests a 6-week leave of absence from her job. Louise files a workers' compensation claim with the Harrison City School District; however, the claim is denied. The reason for denial, TEL-Abbot, Harrison's insurer informs her, is that high stress is a normal part of the teaching profession.

Stop and Think

Benjamin Abbott, owner of Abbott Manufacturing, holds an annual Christmas party every year in the company cafeteria. Attendance to the party is optional, but Mr. Abbot uses this occasion to hand out the employee Christmas bonuses. Night shift foreman Ken Carter sustains a back injury while doing the limbo at the party. Abbott's insurer denies the claim stating that even though, technically, the injury occurred at work, it was not during regular work hours, and the employee was not engaged in his usual work duties. Can Ken appeal this decision?

The appeal process differs from state to state. In many states, if the employee disagrees with the decision to deny the claim, he or she may appeal, but it must be done within a specific time, depending on state statutes. The appeal process can be started by contacting the appropriate state agency or by hiring an attorney. If all attempts at appeal do not reverse the decision, and the denial becomes final, the worker is responsible for payment of all medical bills. If the individual has other health insurance, a claim can be submitted to that insurer. Most health insurance companies ask that a copy of the workers' compensation claim denial be included with the claim.

Time Limits

Each state has rules established under which an employee is required to file a claim within a certain time limit. Usually, traumatic claims must be brought within a time frame that runs from the date of the accident, date of last medical treatment, or date of the last payment of benefits. In cases where a job-related disease does not manifest immediately (i.e., lung cancer, toxic disease, or mesothelioma [a type of lung disease caused by asbestos exposure]), the time limit may extend from the date of the last exposure, date of the first symptoms of the disease, or date the diagnosis was determined. The time limits for filing claims and issuing appeals are established by individual state statutes and vary from state to state; it is important that the health insurance professional becomes familiar with the workers' compensation regulations in the state in which he or she is employed.

WORKERS' COMPENSATION CLAIMS PROCESS

The workers' compensation claims process can be long and arduous. Various steps must be followed, and report forms must be completed. This process can be facilitated, however, if the individual steps are adhered to carefully and the forms are completed correctly and in a timely manner. The following sections discuss the steps for successful workers' compensation claim processing.

First Report of Injury

Employees who are injured, suspect they have been injured, or have contracted a disease they believe is related to their job should take immediate steps to protect their rights and to ensure that their claim is processed properly. Failure to seek timely medical treatment within the workers' compensation network may cause a delay in claim processing and perhaps denial of benefits. Injured workers should be transported to a medical treatment facility without delay in the case of an emergency. For nonemergency situations, the employee should take the following steps:

- Notify a supervisor of the incident immediately, and provide the names of witnesses, if any.
- Complete the initial accident report or necessary paperwork. It does not matter whether the injury is severe or minor; it *must* be documented. The employer should supply the necessary forms (Fig. 11-1).
- The employer should report the incident to their workers' compensation carrier.
- The injured or ill worker should be sent to a medical facility for treatment or diagnosis, if not already done.

WORKERS COMPENSATION - FIRST REPORT OF INJURY OR ILLNESS

Employer(Name & Address with Zip Code)	Carrier/Administrator Claim Number	Report Purpose Code
	Jurisdiction	Jurisdiction Claim Number

Insured Report Number

SIC Code	Employer Fein	Employer's Location Address(If different)	Location #:
			Phone #

CARRIER/CLAIMS ADMINISTRATOR

Carrier(Name, Address & Phone No)	Policy Period To	Claims Administrator(Name, Address & Phone Number)
	Check if Appropriate ☐ Self Insurance	

Carrier Fein	Policy/Self-Insured Number	Administration Fein

Agent Name & Code Number

EMPLOYEE / WAGE

Name (Last, First, Middle)	Birth Date	Social Security Number	Hire Date	State of Hire

Address (include Zip Code)	Sex	Marital Status	Occupation/Job Title
			Employment Status
			NCCI Class Code
Phone	# Dependants		

Rate Per ☐ Day ☐ Month ☐ Week ☐ Other:	# Days Worked/Week	Full Pay for Day of Injury? ☐ Yes ☐ No Did Salary Continue? ☐ Yes ☐ No

OCCURANCE/TREATMENT

Time Employee Began Work	Date of Injury/Illness	Time of Occurrence AM PM	Late Work Date	Date Employer Notified	Date Disability Began

Contact Number/Phone Number	Type of Injury/Illness	Part of Body Affected

Did Injury/Illness Exposure Occur on Employer's Premises? Yes ☐ No ☐	Type of Injury/Illness Code	Part of Body Affected Code

Department or Location Where Accident or Illness Exposure Occurred	All Equipment, Materials, or Chemicals Employee was using when Accident or Illness Exposure Occurred
Specific Activity the Employee was Engaged in When the Accident or Illness Exposure Occurred	Work Process The Employee was engaged in When Accident or Illness Exposure Occurred

How Injury or Illness/Abnormal Health Condition Occurred. Describe the Sequence of Events and Include Any Objects or substances that Directly Injured the Employee or Made the Employee ILL	Cause of Injury Code

Date Return(ed) To Work	If Fatal, Give Date of Death	Were Safeguards or Safety Equipment Provided? ☐ Yes ☐ No Were They Used ☐ Yes ☐ No

Physician/Health Care Provider(Name & Address)	Hospital(Name & Address)	Initial Treatment

Witness (Name & Phone #)

Date Administrator Notified	Date Prepared	Preparer's Name & Title	Phone Number

Fig. 11-1 Sample workers' compensation first report of injury form.

Employer's Instructions
DO NOT ENTER DATA IN SHADED FIELDS

Preferred Formats for Date and Time: Dates should be entered as MM/DD/YYYY, and times as HH:MM a (am) / p (pm)

SIC Code: This is the code which represents the nature of the employer's business which is contained in the Standard Industrial Classification Manual published by the Federal Office of Management and Budget.

Carrier: The licensed business entity issuing a contract of insurance and assuming financial responsibility on behalf of the employer of the claimant.

Claims Administrator: Enter the name of the carrier, third party administrator, state fund, or self-insured responsible for administering the claim.

Agent Name & Code Number: Enter the name of your insurance agent and his/her code number if known. This information can be found on your insurance policy.

Employee/Wage Section: When filling in Social Security Number, do **NOT** include dashes.

Occupation/Job Title: This is the primary occupation of the claimant at the time of the accident or exposure.

Employment Status: Indicate the employee's work status. The valid choices are:

Apprenticeship Full-Time	Apprenticeship Part-Time	Disabled	Full-Time
Not Employed	On Strike	Part-Time	Piece Worker
Retired	Seasonal	Unknown	Volunteer

Date Disability Began: The first day on which the claimant originally lost time from work due to the occupation injury or disease or otherwise deigned by statute.

Contact Name/Phone Number: Enter the name of the individual at the employer's premises to be contacted for additional information.

Type of Injury/Illness: Briefly describe the nature of the injury or illness, (e.g. Lacerations to the forearm).

Part of Body Affected: Indicate the part of body affected by the injury/illness, (e.g. Right forearm, lower back). Part of Body Affected Code does not allow multiple body parts to be selected. Please choose the most dominant body part affected from the list.

Department or Location Where Accident or Illness Exposure Occurred: (e.g. Maintenance Dept or Client's Office at (address). If the accident or illness exposure did not occur on the employer's premises, enter address or location. Be specific.

All Equipment, Material or Chemicals Employee Was Using When Accident or Illness Exposure Occurred: (e.g. Acetylene cutting torch, metal plate) List of all the equipment, materials, and/or chemicals the employee was using, applying, handlings or operating when the injury or illness occurred. Be specific, for example: decorator's scaffolding, electric sander, paintbrush, and paint. Enter "NA" for not applicable if no equipment, materials, or chemicals were being used. NOTE: The items listed do not have to be directly involved in the employee's injury or illness.

Specific Activity the Employee Was Engaged In When the Accident or Illness Exposure Occurred: (e.g. Cutting metal plate for flooring). Describe the specific activity the employee was engaged in when the accident or illness exposure occurred, such as sanding ceiling woodwork in preparation for painting.

Work Process the Employee Was Engaged In When Accident or Illness Exposure Occurred:
Describe the work process the employee was engaged in when the accident or illness exposure occurred, such as building maintenance. Enter "NA" for not applicable if employee was not engaged in a work process (e.g. walking along a hallway).

How Injury or Illness/Abnormal Health Condition Occurred. Describe the Sequence of Events And Include Any Objects Or Substances That Directly Injured The Employee Or Made The Employee Ill:
(Worker stepped back to inspect work and slipped on some scrap metal. As worker fell, worker brushed against the hot metal.) Describe how the injury or illness/abnormal health condition occurred. Include the sequence of events and name any objects of substance that directly injured the employee or made the employee ill. For example: Worker stepped to the edge of the scaffolding to inspect work, lost balance and fell six feet to the floor. The worker's right wrist was broken in the fall.

Date Return(ed) To Work: Enter the date following the most recent disability period on which the employee returned to work.

Fig. 11-1—cont'd

Some states have a time limit for this initial reporting process—ranging from 24 to 72 hours. Other states' laws consider a workers' compensation claim filed as soon as an employee verbally informs the supervisor that he or she has been injured or is ill. Larger organizations often retain their own company-elected medical practitioner for workers' compensation claims. If there is no specific physician indicated, workers are normally allowed to see their own physician.

Physician's Role

Physicians have two distinct roles in the workers' compensation process:

1. To diagnose and treat work-related injuries and illnesses
2. To provide claims administrators opinions in response to specific medical and legal questions about work-related injuries or illnesses, including:
   - Was the injury or illness caused by the employee's work?
   - Is the condition **permanent and stationary**, meaning has the employee reached a state of maximal medical improvement?
   - If an employee is permanent and stationary, has the injury caused permanent disability that limits the ability to compete in the open labor market?
   - Can the employee return to his or her usual and customary work assignment? If not, does he or she need some type of accommodations because of work restrictions, or does the employee need to be retrained for a new job?
   - Will the employee who has attained permanent and stationary status require access to future medical treatment for the condition?

Usually, a single physician fills both roles in workers' compensation cases; however, an independent medical evaluator commonly addresses the specific medical and legal questions. When the injured or ill employee visits the medical facility, the attending physician should
- obtain a complete history of the condition, including preexisting conditions or disability;
- obtain a thorough work history, including any exposures as they pertain to the chief complaint;
- perform a physical examination, focusing on the system or systems involved;
- consider restrictions (e.g., no typing for >1 hour) before taking the patient off work to prevent **job deconditioning** (where the patient psychologically or physically or both loses his or her ability to perform normal job duties at the previous level of expertise as a result of being absent from work);
- make a diagnostic evaluation; and

- complete all paperwork promptly because the patient may have no source of income if the paperwork is delayed (Fig. 11-2).

Determining Disability

When the injured or ill worker visits the healthcare facility for treatment, the provider completes an attending physician statement (as discussed in the previous section), which should indicate any physical or mental impairments resulting from the incident. The classification of workers' compensation disability cases, mandated by federal law, is as follows:
- *Medical treatment only*—this category comprises minor injuries or illnesses that are resolved relatively quickly, resulting in a minimal loss of work time with no residual limitations. Compensation is made for medical expenses rendered that are necessary to cure and relieve the effects of the injury or illness.
- *Temporary disability*—benefits in this category are paid so long as the physician's opinion concurs with that claim of status. Temporary disability includes two subcategories:
  - *Temporary total disability*—where the worker's ability to perform his or her job responsibilities is totally lost, but on a temporary basis.
  - *Temporary partial disability*—involves an injury or illness that impairs an employee's ability to work for a limited time. The impairment is such that the individual is able to perform limited employment duties and is expected to recover fully.
- *Permanent disability*—the ill or injured employee's condition is such that it is impossible to return to work. Compensation is awarded to the worker for the loss of value of his or her skills in the open labor market. As with temporary disability, permanent disability has two classifications:
  - *Permanent partial disability*—prevents the individual from performing one or more occupational functions, but does not impair his or her capability of performing less demanding employment.
  - *Permanent total disability*—where the employee's ability to work at any occupation is totally and permanently lost.

● Stop and Think

George Meade makes his living as a concert pianist. To relax between concerts, George takes up woodworking and inadvertently severs his right index finger, preventing him from performing. What classification would George's disability fall into?

Health Care Provider Report
See Instructions on Reverse Side
(WHEN COMPLETED RETURN TO REQUESTER)

H C 0 1

DO NOT USE THIS SPACE

Please PRINT or TYPE your responses.
Enter dates in MM/DD/YYYY format.

SOCIAL SECURITY NUMBER | DATE OF INJURY

EMPLOYEE | EMPLOYER

INSURER/SELF-INSURER/TPA | INSURER CLAIM NUMBER

INSURER ADDRESS

CITY | STATE | ZIP CODE

REQUESTER must specify all items to be completed by health care provider. ☐ Items: _____ ☐ MMI (#9) ☐ PPD (#10)

HEALTH CARE PROVIDER TO COMPLETE ITEMS REQUESTED ABOVE

1. Date of first examination for this injury by this office: _____ (date)
2. Diagnosis (include all ICD-9-CM codes):

3. History of injury or disease given by employee:

4. In your opinion (as substantiated by the history and physical examination) was the injury or disease caused, aggravated or accelerated by the employee's alleged employment activity or environment? ☐ No ☐ Yes

5. Is there evidence of pre-existing or other conditions that affect this disability? ☐ No ☐ Yes   If yes, describe:

6. Is further treatment of this injury or referral to another doctor planned? ☐ No ☐ Yes   If yes, describe:

7. Has surgery been performed? ☐ No ☐ Yes   If yes, date and describe: _____ (date)

8. Attach the most recent Report of Work Ability. Date of report: _____ (date)
9. **Has the employee reached maximum medical improvement?** ☐ No ☐ Yes   Date reached: _____
   (If yes, complete item #10) (See definition on back)
10. **Has the employee sustained any permanent partial disability from the injury?** ☐ No ☐ Yes ☐ Too early to determine
    The permanent partial disability is ____ % of the whole body. This rating is based on Minn. Rules:

| 5223. | % | 5223. | % |
| 5223. | % | 5223. | % |

NAME (Type or Print) | SIGNATURE | DEGREE

ADDRESS | STATE | LICENSE #/REGISTRATION #

CITY | STATE | ZIP CODE | AREA CODE | TELEPHONE # | DATE SIGNED

MN HC01 (7/01)

Fig. 11-2 Sample healthcare provider report.

NOTICE TO EMPLOYEE: SERVICE OF THIS REPORT OF MAXIMUM MEDICAL IMPROVEMENT (SEE DEFINITION IN INSTRUCTIONS FOR ITEM 9) MAY HAVE AN IMPACT ON YOUR TEMPORARY TOTAL DISABILITY WAGE LOSS BENEFITS. IF THE INSURER PROPOSES TO STOP YOUR BENEFITS, A NOTICE OF INTENTION TO DISCONTINUE BENEFITS SHOULD BE SENT TO YOU. IF YOU HAVE ANY QUESTIONS CONCERNING YOUR BENEFITS OR MAXIMUM MEDICAL IMPROVEMENT, YOU MAY CALL THE CLAIM REPRESENTATIVE OR THE DEPARTMENT OF LABOR AND INDUSTRY, WORKERS' COMPENSATION DIVISION.

INSTRUCTIONS TO THE INSURER AND HEALTH CARE PROVIDER

Within ten (10) calendar days of receipt of a request for information on the Health Care Provider Report from an employer, insurer, or the commissioner, a health care provider must respond on the report form or in a narrative report that contains the same information. (Minn. Rules 5221.0410, subp. 2)

A. **The employer, insurer, or Commissioner may request required medical information on the Health Care Provider Report form.**

- The requester must complete the general information identifying the employee, employer, and insurer.

- The requester must specify all items to be answered by the health care provider.

- For those injuries that are required to be reported to the Division, the self-insured employer or insurer must file reports with the Division. (M.S. § 176.231, subd. 1 and Minn. Rules 5221.0410, subp. 5 and subp. 8)

- The self-insured employer or insurer must serve the report of maximum medical improvement (MMI) on the employee. (M.S. § 176.101, subd. 1(j) and Minn. Rules 5221.0410, subp. 3)

B. **Instructions to the Health Care Provider for completing the Health Care Provider Report:**

- Items 1 - 5: Fill in all information as required.

- Item 6: Indicate if further treatment or referral is planned. Describe the treatment plan (e.g., continue medication, refer to physical therapy, refer to a specialist, perform surgery).

- Item 7: State if surgery has been performed. If yes, fill in the date performed and describe the procedure.

- Item 8: Attach the most recent Report of Work Ability. (Minn. Rules 5221.0410, subp. 6)

- Item 9: Indicate if the employee has reached MMI. If yes, fill in the date MMI was reached. At MMI, permanent partial disability (PPD) must be reported (item 10). (M.S. § 176.011, subd. 25 and Minn. Rules 5221.0410, subp. 3)

  MAXIMUM MEDICAL IMPROVEMENT means "The date after which no further significant recovery from or significant lasting improvement to a personal injury can reasonably be anticipated, based upon reasonable medical probability, irrespective and regardless of subjective complaints of pain."

- Item 10: The health care provider must render an opinion of PPD when ascertainable, but no later than the date of MMI. (M.S. § 176.011, subd. 25 and Minn. Rules 5221.0410, subp. 4)

  Indicate if the employee sustained PPD from this injury. Check one of the three boxes (too early to determine, no, yes). If yes, specify any applicable category of the PPD schedule in effect for the employee's date of injury. Report any zero ratings.

- Identify the health care provider completing the report by name, professional degree, license or registration number, address, and phone number.

- The health care provider must sign and date the report.

This material can be made available in different forms, such as large print, Braille or on a tape.

ANY PERSON WHO, WITH INTENT TO DEFRAUD, RECEIVES WORKERS' COMPENSATION BENEFITS TO WHICH THE PERSON IS NOT ENTITLED BY KNOWINGLY MISREPRESENTING, MISSTATING, OR FAILING TO DISCLOSE ANY MATERIAL FACT IS GUILTY OF THEFT AND SHALL BE SENTENCED PURSUANT TO SECTION 609.52, SUBDIVISION 3.

Fig. 11-2—cont'd

Vocational Rehabilitation

When employees cannot return to their previous job because of a workers' compensation injury or illness, they often are entitled to **vocational rehabilitation** services if it is reasonable to assume that these individuals can be trained for some alternative type of employment. The goal of vocational rehabilitation is to return the injured worker to some sort of suitable, gainful employment that he or she can reasonably achieve and that offers an opportunity to restore the injured worker to maximum self-support as soon as practical and as near as possible to what it was before the incident.

Waiting Periods

Workers' compensation benefits normally do not begin immediately. Table 11-1 shows a list of waiting periods for several states. Most states allow for retroactive compensation when disability continues for a certain period from the date of injury or illness.

Imagine This!

Frank Turner sustains a serious cut to his right hand while operating a band saw at work. Frank's injury qualifies him for workers' compensation benefits, which start 1 week after the incident occurred. Larry Boggs, a coworker in the millroom with Frank, becomes ill the same week. Thinking he was just suffering from a minor cold, Larry does not file for workers' compensation; however, 2 weeks later, his cold is no better. Larry returns to his physician who determines he has pneumonia. Larry subsequently is hospitalized for 1 week, during which time further tests reveal that Larry's condition is caused by breathing minute particles of sawdust. When Larry is discharged from the hospital, he files a workers' compensation claim. The claim is approved, but Larry's benefits do not begin until 4 weeks after his illness began.

Claim Forms

In contrast to most major third-party payer claims, there is no universal form to use when filing a workers'

compensation claim. Some states (e.g., Iowa) allow workers' compensation claims to be submitted on the CMS-1500 form. Private insurance carriers typically have their own forms. The health insurance professional should determine if it is cceptable to submit a workers' compensation claim on the CMS-1500 form; if not, the health insurance professional should ask the patient to request the required form from his or her employer or insurer.

Normally, multiple copies of all workers' compensation reports are essential for proper distribution as follows:

1. Original form to the insurance carrier
2. One copy to the appropriate state agency
3. One copy to the patient's employer
4. One copy to be retained in the healthcare provider's files

When special claim forms are to be used, instructions usually are provided—often on the back side of the form. If instructions do not come with the form, the health insurance professional should ask the patient to obtain detailed guidelines from the employer or insurer.

Because there are literally thousands of different forms used for workers' compensation claims in the United States, to avoid confusion, instructions for completing the standard CMS-1500 claim form are used in this chapter. These instructions are generic, and the health insurance professional should obtain exact guidelines from the employer, the insurer, or the particular state the claim occurs in to prevent delays or rejections.

Before completing the blocks, the health insurance professional should determine the name and address of the insurer to whom the claim will be sent. This informa-

TABLE 11-1	Partial List of States Showing Waiting Periods
STATE	WAITING PERIOD
Alabama	21 days
Alaska	>28 days
California	14 days (also retroactive if person is hospitalized)
Colorado	>2 weeks
Connecticut	7 days
Delaware (no waiting period in the case of amputation of an extremity, or a part thereof, or when the injury results in hospitalization of the employee)	7 days, including date of injury
District of Columbia	>14 days
Hawaii (temporary total disability only)	None
Illinois (temporary total disability only)	>14 days
Iowa (temporary total disability only)	>14 days
Maryland	>14 days
Minnesota (temporary total disability only)	10 days
Missouri	>14 days
New Hampshire	>14 days
Oklahoma	None
Oregon (temporary total disability only)	14 days (inpatient in hospital receive compensation from date of incapacity)

tion should appear in the in the upper right-hand corner of the claim form. Table 11-2 provides step-by-step instructions for completing the CMS-1500 form for a workers' compensation claim.

Progress Reports

Keeping the employer and insurance carrier apprised of the patient's treatment plan, progress, and status is a priority

TABLE 11-2	Step-by-Step Guidelines for Workers' Compensation Claims
Block 1	"Other" should be checked for workers' compensation claims unless the claim is for patients who are receiving Black Lung benefits.
Block 1a	Enter the claim number if one has been assigned (check your state's requirements for this block if no claim number has been assigned, or use the patient's Social Security number).
Block 2	Use the same guidelines as with all other carriers.
Block 3	Indicate the patient's 8-digit birthdate and sex.
Block 4	The *employer's name* is entered here as the "insured."
Block 5	Use the same guidelines as with all other carriers.
Block 6	Check "other."
Block 7	Enter the address of the insuring company/corporation.
Block 8	Check "employed." Consult your local state guidelines as to whether or not it is necessary to indicate marital status.
Block 9	For most claims, leave blank. If there is a question as to whether or not the injury/illness falls under workers' compensation, enter the applicable information for the patient's other insurance.
Blocks 9a-d	Leave blank.
Block 10a	Check "yes" to indicate that the injury occurred while the patient was on the job.
Blocks 10b-c	Check "no".
Block 10d	Leave blank.
Blocks 11-11c	Leave blank.
Block 11d	Normally, this is left blank; however, if the workers' compensation case is pending, check with your local state agency's guidelines as to whether or not this box would be checked "yes".
Blocks 12-13	No signature is required.
Block 14	Enter the date that the injury occurred or the date on which the illness first was noticed by the patient (this date must coincide with the employer's First Report of Injury and the provider's First Report of Treatment).
Block 15	If a date is documented in the patient's record, indicate it in this block; otherwise, leave blank.
Block 16	Enter the first full day patient was unable to perform his or her job duties to the first day the patient is back to work (this should be documented in the provider's First Report of Treatment).
Blocks 17-17b	Enter the unique identification number (UPIN) or national provider identifier (NPI) of the individual shown in Block 17. The UPIN can be used until May 22, 2007, and it should appear in Block 17a. Effective May 23, 2007, the NPI must be reported in 17b.
Block 18	Use the same guidelines as with all other carriers.
Block 19	Leave blank.
Block 20	Use the same guidelines as with all other carriers.
Block 21	Use the same guidelines as with all other carriers.
Blocks 22-23	Leave blank.
Blocks 24a-j	Use the same guidelines as with all other carriers or consult the appropriate state agency's guidelines.
Block 25	Use the same guidelines as with all other carriers.
Block 26	Use the same guidelines as with all other carriers.
Block 27	Leave blank; not applicable because all workers' compensation payments go to the provider.
Block 28	Use the same guidelines as with all other carriers.
Block 29-30	Leave blank.
Block 31	Use the same guidelines as with all other carriers.
Block 32	Key the name and address of the location where services were provided.
Block 32a	Enter the NPI of the service facility in Block 32.
Block 32b	Enter the appropriate ID qualifier followed by one blank space and then the PIN of the service facility. After May 23, 2007, 32b is not to be reported. Follow the specific guidelines of your Medicaid FI.
Block 33	Enter the name, address, zip code, and telephone number of the billing provider.
Block 33a	Effective May 23, 2007, the NPI of the billing provider or group must be reported here.
Block 33b	Enter the appropriate ID qualifier followed by one blank space and then the PIN of the billing provider or group. Effective May 23, 2007, and later, 33b is not to be reported. Enter the group UPIN, including the 2-digit location identifier, for the performing practitioner/supplier who is a member of a group practice. (Refer to specific carrier guidelines.)

in workers' compensation cases. The health insurance professional should be well versed in the particulars of workers' compensation reporting so that written communications meet all accepted legal standards. After the initial visit to the physician has occurred, and the attending physician report has been filed, unless the employee has returned to work full-time, periodic reports have to be filed. These are referred to as **progress or supplemental reports** (Fig. 11-3). Often, there are no special printed forms for progress reports, and copies of clinical notes from the patient's health record or a letter from the attending physician giving a detailed account of the patient's progress are acceptable. When the patient's disability ends, and he or she is able to return to work, the physician submits a final report.

SPECIAL BILLING NOTES

Most states have a fee schedule that providers must use when billing a workers' compensation claim, and as long as a workers' compensation claim is pending, the provider cannot bill the patient. Additionally, balance billing is not allowed on workers' compensation claims. If the claim has been denied, and all efforts for appeal have been exhausted, the health insurance professional should issue a letter of reply immediately, after which direct billing to the patient or the patient's private insurance company for the services rendered is allowed. The workers' compensation fee schedule does not apply to denied claims; instead, the provider's usual and customary fees apply. Workers' compensation claims are handled differently in each state, and the health insurance professional must follow the guidelines set forth by the law in his or her state.

Imagine This!

Sandra Cotter was injured at work when a filing cabinet fell on her foot. The human relations officer advised Sandra to see her own physician because the company did not have a specific workers' compensation physician. Sandra was treated at the Heartland Medical Clinic, which billed her health insurer, Blue Cross and Blue Shield. Blue Cross and Blue Shield refused payment, so Heartland billed Sandra. Sandra refused to pay the bill, stating that it was a workers' compensation case. Heartland argued that they had not received a call from Sandra's employer authorizing treatment. Still, Sandra refused to pay. After sending Sandra statements for 6 months, Heartland sent her a certified letter stating they were refusing all future medical treatment at the clinic. Sandra filed a complaint with the State Workers' Comp Board, and the case eventually was resolved; however, Heartland still refused to see Sandra for subsequent visits.

HIPAA AND WORKERS' COMPENSATION

The Health Insurance Portability and Accountability Act (HIPAA) Privacy Rule does not apply to workers' compensation insurers, workers' compensation administrative agencies, or employers. The Privacy Rule recognizes the legitimate need for insurers and other entities involved in the workers' compensation system to have access to an injured worker's **protected health information** as authorized by state or other law. Workers' compensation patients may or may not be required to sign a release of information form for a claim form to be filed. Additionally, employers and claims adjusters retain the right of access to workers' compensation files. If the health insurance professional encounters a workers' compensation case for an established patient who already has a health record in that office, a separate record should be created and kept separate from that individual's regular health record. Some medical offices color code or flag workers' compensation records or file them in a separate area to avoid confusion. The health insurance professional should check the regulations in his or her state regarding protected health information regulations.

WORKERS' COMPENSATION FRAUD

As with any type of insurance, fraud occurs in workers' compensation cases. Most states require workers' compensation insurers, self-insured employers, and third-party administrators to report fraud to the State Insurance Commissioner's office or to the local District Attorney's Office or both. Anyone can report workers' compensation fraud, however. When fraud is suspected, a report should be made within a reasonable time, usually within 30 days from the time the person reporting knows or reasonably believes he or she knows the identity of a person or entity that has committed workers' compensation fraud or has knowledge that such fraud has been committed. This often can be accomplished by a telephone call to the either of the above-named offices.

What Did You Learn?

1. How did workers' compensation originate?
2. Who is eligible for workers' compensation benefits?
3. List four exemption classifications.
4. What is "no-fault" insurance?
5. What does an ombudsman do?

Plan Progress Report

Please PRINT OR TYPE your responses
All dates must be entered in MM/DD/YYYY

PR01

DO NOT USE THIS SPACE

1. DATE OF THIS REPORT

2. SOCIAL SECURITY NUMBER | 3. DATE OF INJURY

4. EMPLOYEE NAME

5. EMPLOYEE ADDRESS

CITY   STATE   ZIP CODE | 6. EMPLOYEE PHONE NUMBER | 7. DATE OF BIRTH

8. EMPLOYER | 9. EMPLOYER CONTACT PERSON | 10. PHONE #

11. EMPLOYER ADDRESS | CITY   STATE   ZIP CODE

12. INSURER CLAIM NUMBER | 17. QRC NAME

13. INSURER/SELF-INSURER/TPA | 18. QRC FIRM

14. INSURER ADDRESS | 19. ADDRESS

CITY   STATE   ZIP CODE | CITY   STATE   ZIP CODE

15. CLAIM REPRESENTATIVE | 16. PHONE NUMBER | 20. QRC # | 21. QRC FIRM # | 22. PHONE NUMBER

23. Is the employee released to return to work?   ☐ Yes, with restrictions   ☐ Yes, without restrictions   ☐ No

Health Care Provider Report Date

24. Current work status: ☐ Not Working   ☐ Part Time   ☐ Full Time   ☐ Seasonal Layoff

If working, is this a temporary job?   ☐ Yes   ☐ No

25. Is the plan still current?   ☐ Yes   ☐ No

26. Of the _____ services outlined in the plan, _____ services have been accomplished. **(Attach most recent narrative report)**

| QRC | Registered Rehab Vendor | Other Rehab Provider Costs | Other Costs Necessary to Complete Plan | Estimated Total Cost |

27. Costs to Date ☐ + ☐ + ☐ + ☐ = ☐

28. Plan Duration from plan filing date (in days) | Duration to Date | Expected Additional Duration to Plan Completion | Estimated Total Duration

☐ + ☐ = ☐

Fig. 11-3 Sample plan progress report. (Source: Minnesota Department of Labor and Industry.)

PRIVATE AND EMPLOYER-SPONSORED DISABILITY INCOME INSURANCE

Most people think about insurance coverage as it relates to health, life, home, or auto, but the most crucial aspect of personal and family finances is **earned income—** income from employment. If an illness or injury occurred and this income stopped, most people would quickly find it difficult or impossible to maintain a home and provide for their family. **Disability income insurance** replaces a *portion* of earned income when an individual is unable to perform the requirements of his or her job because of injury or illness (that is not work-related).

Imagine This!

Paul Graham, a self-employed auto mechanic, purchased private disability income insurance from Excel Coverage Experts. When he became disabled because of a shoulder injury, his monthly disability benefits paid his house and car payments. Stanley Morgan, Paul's neighbor, fell from a ladder while fixing his roof, resulting in multiple fractures in both legs. Stanley did not have disability income insurance. Stanley was disabled for 6 months, during which time the bank foreclosed on his house because he could not pay the mortgage.

Disability insurance can be purchased privately through a commercial insurance company, or it is sometimes furnished by the employer. There are two major types of disability coverage:

1. **Short-term disability**, which provides an income for the early part of a disability—typically 2 weeks up to 2 years
2. **Long-term disability**, which helps replace income for a longer time—up to 5 years or until the disabled person turns 65.

DEFINING DISABILITY

Disability is commonly defined one of two ways:

1. An individual is unable to perform in the occupation or job that he or she was doing before the disability occurred. (This definition of disability is covered in what is referred to as **own-occupation policies**. A variation is the **modified own-occupation policy**, which covers workers for their own occupation as long as they are not gainfully employed elsewhere.)
2. An individual is unable to perform *any* occupation for which he or she is suited by education and experience.

The distinction between these two definitions can be crucial. If a surgeon loses a hand, he or she may not be able to perform surgery. In the case of an *own-occupation policy*, the surgeon would be able to recover, even though he or she was able to work as a physician in a nonsurgical field. With the inability to perform *any occupation*, there would be no recovery, even if the surgeon could work as a tour guide.

Short-Term Disability

Short-term disability pays a percentage of an individual's wages or salary if and when he or she becomes **temporarily disabled,** meaning that the person is not able to work for a short time because of sickness or injury (excluding job-related illnesses or injuries). A typical short-term disability policy pays one half to two thirds percent for a specific number of weeks, depending on the policy. Most short-term disability policies have a **benefit cap**, meaning there is a maximum benefit amount paid per month.

A worker generally begins receiving money from a short-term disability policy within 1 to 14 days after becoming sick or disabled. The actual time elapsed before payments begin depends on the stipulations in the policy. Often, if the individual sustains an injury, benefits begin immediately. An illness usually takes longer because there needs to be enough time to show that the illness is severe enough to be disabling. If the disability insurance is furnished by the employer, there may be additional restrictions as to when the short-term disability benefits begin. The employer may require all sick days to be used up before the employee begins receiving disability payments. Typically, if the condition worsens over time, the individual would receive disability pay retroactive to the first sick day.

Long-Term Disability

As with short-term disability, a **long-term disability** insurance policy protects an individual from the loss of ability to earn an income because of an illness or injury that is not work-related. It pays a monthly amount to help cover expenses when an individual is unable to perform his or her job or function in a chosen occupation or profession.

There are two major types of individual long-term disability insurance: no cancelable and guaranteed renewable. In the case of no cancelable or guaranteed renewable policies, the insurer cannot cancel or refuse to renew the policy as long as the required premiums are paid on time. The key difference between the two major types of policies is that under a no cancelable contract, the individual has the extra security that premiums can never be raised above those shown in the policy as long as the required premiums are paid. With a guaranteed renewable policy, the premiums can be raised, but only if the change affects an entire class of policyholders. For this reason, initial premiums for guaranteed renewable policies can be less expensive than no cancelable policies.

DISABILITY CLAIMS PROCESS

As with workers' compensation, there are several steps to the disability claims process. There are certain responsibilities to which the employee and the employer must attend to allow this process to work efficiently and effectively.

Employee's Responsibilities

First, the worker must notify the proper party that he or she intends to file a disability claim. To do this, the individual first needs to submit a claim request. If disability insurance is provided through the employer, a claim form may be obtained from the company's human resources department. Some insurers allow telephone submission of claims. In this case, the human resources department should provide a toll-free number and specific instructions for calling in the claim. In the case of an individual or private disability policy, a claim form may be obtained from the insurance company where the policy was purchased. The claim request should include everything needed to process the claim, including

1. information the employee provides (Fig. 11-4),
2. information the employer provides (Fig. 11-5),
3. the attending physician statement (Fig. 11-6), and
4. an authorization release form that enables the insurer to gather additional information as it becomes necessary (Fig. 11-7).

Employer's Responsibilities

If the disability insurance is provided by the employer, a statement that helps identify the benefits available should accompany the claim. The employer also must provide detailed information as to the type of coverage, policy number, division/class number, and division/class description.

Attending Physician's Statement

It is important that the injured or ill worker be examined by a physician as soon as possible after the disability has occurred and within the time limit allowed by the insurer. The physician must determine that the individual is disabled as defined by the policy. To accomplish this, an attending physician's statement must be completed, which typically includes such information as
• the diagnosis,
• the first day the individual was unable to work,
• whether or not the illness or injury was work-related,
• the nature of the treatment or suggested treatment, and
• restrictions and limitations.

✓ HIPAA Tip

HIPAA mandates that, if an employer provides insurance to its employees and their dependents, *all* employees and dependents must be covered regardless of medical condition.

Health Insurance Professional's Role

Frequently, disability claim handling gets tied up in time-consuming tasks, such as document processing, record keeping, written correspondence, telephone inquiries, photocopying, and sending faxes. The process involves a lot of human interaction, which complicates the process, especially if all phases are not properly documented and monitored. Everyone involved can become quickly frustrated and impatient. It is the health insurance professional's responsibility to see that everything possible is done to facilitate the claims process for the benefit of the medical practice and the disabled patient. This can be accomplished by seeing to it that claim forms and statements are completed correctly and submitted promptly, and all necessary documentation is included.

The health insurance professional's role also might be to educate the patient regarding disability benefits. With disability insurance, the insurer does not reimburse the patient strictly according to the fees charged for medical services rendered by the attending physician. Disability insurance benefits are paid to compensate for loss of income from wages. Periodic payments (typically monthly) are made directly to the patient to use for expenses as he or she sees fit. It is hoped that the patient has a separate health insurance policy to pay the cost of needed healthcare.

What Did You Learn?

1. What do disability income insurance benefits pay?
2. What items should a typical claim request include?
3. List five things the attending physician's statement should address.
4. What is the health insurance professional's role in the disability claims process?

FEDERAL DISABILITY PROGRAMS

Federal disability programs provide services such as cash support, healthcare coverage, and direct supportive services to eligible individuals with disabilities. These programs

EMPLOYEE'S CLAIM FOR COMPENSATION

ANSWER ALL QUESTIONS FULLY - PRINT OR TYPE CLEARLY

IMPORTANT: Your Social Security Number Must Be Entered:

IMPORTANTE: El Numero de su Seguro Social Debe Ser Indicado:

WCB Case No. (If known)_____ Carrier Case No.(if known)_____

A.
Injured person
	1. Name..
	       First Name Middle Name Last Name
	2.MailingAddress..
	       Number and Street (includeApartment No.) City State Zip Code.
	3. Sex ☐Male ☐Female Date of Birth.............................Telephone No. ( )...............
	4. Do you speak English? ☐Yes ☐No If no, what language do you speak?...............
	5. Name of union and local number, if member...
	6. State what your regular work/occupation was...
	7. Wages or average earnings per day, including overtime, board, rent and other allowances............
	8. Were you paid full wages for the day of injury? ☐Yes ☐No
	9. Your work week at time of injury was: ☐Five day ☐Six day ☐Seven day ☐Other.............

B. Employer(s)	1. Employer..Telephone No. ( )............... 2. Employer's Address.. 3. Were you employed by any other employer or employers at the time of your injury/illness? ☐Yes ☐No 4. If yes, did you lose time from work at this other employment as a result of your injury/illness? ☐Yes ☐No
C. Place/Time	1. Address where injury occurred..County..................... 2. Date of Injury........................at................o'clock, ☐ AM ☐ PM
D. The Injury	1. How did injury/illness occur?... ....
E. Nature and Extent of Injury/ Illness	1. State fully the nature of your injury/illness, including all parts of body injured............... .... 2. Date you stopped work because of this injury/illness?.......................... 3. Have you returned to work? ☐Yes ☐No If yes, on what date?................. 4. Does injury/illness keep you from work? ☐Yes ☐No 5. Have you done any work during period of disability? ☐Yes ☐No 6. Have you received any wages since your injury/illness? ☐Yes ☐No

F.
Medical Benefits
	1. Did you receive or are you now receiving medical care? ☐Yes ☐No
	2. Are you now in need of medical care? ☐Yes ☐No
	3. Name of attending doctor...
	    Doctor's address..
	4. If you were in a hospital, give the dates hospitalized........................
	    Name of hospital...
	    Hospital's Address...

G. Comp. Payments	1. Have you received or are you now receiving workers' compensation payments for the injury reported above? ☐Yes ☐No 2. Do you claim further workers' compensation payments? ☐Yes ☐No
H. Notice	1. Have you given your employer (or supervisor) notice of injury? ☐Yes ☐No 2. If yes, notice was given ☐orally ☐in writing, on.............................. to ....

ANY PERSON WHO KNOWINGLY AND WITH INTENT TO DEFRAUD PRESENTS, CAUSES TO BE PRESENTED, OR PREPARES WITH KNOWLEDGE OR BELIEF THAT IT WILL BE PRESENTED TO, OR BY AN INSURER, OR SELF INSURER, ANY INFORMATION CONTAINING ANY FALSE MATERIAL STATEMENT OR CONCEALS ANY MATERIAL FACT SHALL BE GUILTY OF A CRIME AND SUBJECT TO SUBSTANTIAL FINES AND IMPRISONMENT.

Signed by...Dated...
          (Claimant)

C-3 (2-04)

Fig. 11-4 Employee's statement form.

typically are limited to individuals younger than age 65. There are nine major federal disability programs that include sizable proportions of individuals age 50 to 64, as follows:

1. Social Security Disability Insurance (SSDI)
2. Supplemental security income (SSI)
3. Medicare
4. Medicaid

EMPLOYER'S REPORT OF NON-WORK-RELATED ACCIDENT/OCCUPATIONAL DISEASE

Send this notice directly to the Chair, Workers' Compensation Board at the address shown on the reverse side within ten (10) days after an accident occurs. ANSWER ALL QUESTIONS FULLY. A copy should also be provided to or retained by your workers' compensation insurance carrier.

Any employer who fails to timely file Form C-2, as required by Section 110 of the Workers' Compensation Law, is subject to a fine of not more than $1,000. In addition, the Board or Chair may impose a penalty of up to $2,500.

TYPEWRITER PREPARATION IS STRONGLY RECOMMENDED - INCLUDE ZIP CODE IN ALL ADDRESSES-EMPLOYEE'S S.S.NO. MUST BE ENTERED BELOW ↓

WCB CASE NO.(If Known)	CARRIER CASE NO.	CARRIER CODE NO.	WC POLICY NO.	DATE OF ACCIDENT	EMPLOYEE'S S.S. NO.

1.(a) EMPLOYER'S NAME | (b) EMPLOYER'S MAILING ADDRESS | (c) OSHA CASE/FILE NO.

(d) LOCATION (If Different From Mailing Address) | (e) NATURE OF BUSINESS (Principal Products, Services, etc.) | (f) NY UI EMPLOYER REG. NO. | (g) FEIN - if UI Emp. Reg. No. Unknown

2.(a) INSURANCE CARRIER | (b) CARRIER'S ADDRESS

3.(a) INJURED EMPLOYEE (First, M.I., Last) | (b) ADDRESS (Includes No. & Street, City, State, Zip & Apt. No.)

ACCIDENT

4. (a) ADDRESS WHERE ACCIDENT OCCURRED | (b) COUNTY | (c) WAS ACCIDENT ON EMPLOYER'S PREMISES? ☐ Yes ☐ No

5. HOUR EMP. BEGAN WORK h h : m m ☐ AM ☐ PM | 6. TIME OF ACCIDENT h h : m m ☐ AM ☐ PM | 7. DEPT. WHERE REGULARLY EMPLOYED | 8.(a) DATE STOPPED WORK BECAUSE OF THIS INJURY/ILLNESS | (b) WAS EMPLOYEE PAID IN FULL FOR DAY? ☐ Yes ☐ No

INJURED PERSON

9. SEX ☐ Male ☐ Female | 10. DATE OF BIRTH | 11. OCCUPATION (Specific job title at which employed) | 12. DATE HIRED

13.(a) AVERAGE EARNINGS PER WEEK? $ .0 0 | (b) TOTAL EARNINGS PAID DURING 52 WEEKS PRIOR TO DATE OF ACCIDENT (Include bonuses, overtime, value of lodging, etc.) $ .0 0 | 14. (a) EMPLOYEE IS: ☐ Full Time ☐ Part Time | (b) INJURED EMPLOYEE'S WORK WEEK (Check days usually worked.) Mon ☐ Tue ☐ Wed ☐ Thu ☐ Fri ☐ Sat ☐ Sun ☐

NATURE OF INJURY

15. NATURE OF INJURY AND PART(S) OF BODY AFFECTED | 16. (a) DID YOU PROVIDE MEDICAL CARE? ☐ Yes ☐ No | (b) IF YES, WHEN?

17. WAS EMPLOYEE TREATED IN AN EMERGENCY ROOM? ☐ Yes ☐ No | 18. WAS EMPLOYEE HOSPITALIZED OVERNIGHT AS AN IN-PATIENT? ☐ Yes ☐ No

19. (a) NAME AND ADDRESS OF DOCTOR | (b) NAME AND ADDRESS OF HOSPITAL

20. (a) HAS EMPLOYEE RETURNED TO WORK? ☐ Yes ☐ No | (b) IF YES, GIVE DATE: | (c) AT WHAT WEEKLY WAGE? $, .0 0

NOTE: FORM C-11 MUST BE FILED EACH TIME THERE IS A CHANGE IN EMPLOYMENT STATUS

CAUSE OF ACCIDENT

21. WHAT WAS EMPLOYEE DOING WHEN INJURED? (Please be specific. Identify tools, equipment or material the employee was using.)

22. HOW DID THE ACCIDENT OR EXPOSURE OCCUR? (Please describe fully the events that resulted in injury or occupational disease. Tell what happened and how it happened. Please use separate sheet if necessary.)

23. OBJECT OR SUBSTANCE THAT DIRECTLY INJURED EMPLOYEE. e.g., the machine employee struck against or which struck him/her, the vapor or poison inhaled or swallowed, the chemical that irritated his/her skin. In cases of strains, the thing (s)he was lifting, pulling, etc.

FATAL CASES

24. (a) DATE OF DEATH | (b) NAME AND ADDRESS OF NEAREST RELATIVE | (c) RELATIONSHIP

PREPARATION

DATE EMPLOYER/SUPERVISOR FIRST KNEW OF INJURY | DATE OF THIS REPORT | IF FORM IS SUBMITTED BY EMPLOYER, COMPLETE A & B BELOW. IF FORM IS SUBMITTED BY THIRD PARTY, COMPLETE A,B,C & D BELOW.

A. EMPLOYEE PREPARING FORM OR SUPPLYING INFORMATION TO THIRD PARTY | B. TITLE | TELEPHONE NUMBER & EXTENSION

C. IF REPORT PREPARED BY THIRD PARTY, COMPANY NAME AND ADDRESS

D. THIRD PARTY CONTACT NAME | TELEPHONE NUMBER & EXTENSION

Fig. 11-5 Sample employer's statement form.

Health Care Provider Report
See Instructions on Reverse Side
(WHEN COMPLETED RETURN TO REQUESTER)

Please PRINT or TYPE your responses.
Enter dates in MM/DD/YYYY format.

SOCIAL SECURITY NUMBER	DATE OF INJURY	
EMPLOYEE	EMPLOYER	
INSURER/SELF-INSURER/TPA	INSURER CLAIM NUMBER	
INSURER ADDRESS		
CITY	STATE ZIP CODE	

REQUESTER must specify all items to be completed by health care provider. ☐ Items: _____ ☐ MMI (#9) ☐ PPD (#10)

HEALTH CARE PROVIDER TO COMPLETE ITEMS REQUESTED ABOVE

1. Date of first examination for this injury by this office: _____ (date)

2. Diagnosis (include all ICD-9-CM codes):

3. History of injury or disease given by employee:

4. In your opinion (as substantiated by the history and physical examination) was the injury or disease caused, aggravated or accelerated by the employee's alleged employment activity or environment?   ☐ No ☐ Yes

5. Is there evidence of pre-existing or other conditions that affect this disability?   ☐ No ☐ Yes   If yes, describe:

6. Is further treatment of this injury or referral to another doctor planned?   ☐ No ☐ Yes   If yes, describe:

7. Has surgery been performed?   ☐ No ☐ Yes   If yes, date and describe: _____ (date)

8. Attach the most recent Report of Work Ability. Date of report: _____ (date)

9. **Has the employee reached maximum medical improvement?**   ☐ No ☐ Yes   Date reached: _____
   (If yes, complete item #10) (See definition on back)

10. **Has the employee sustained any permanent partial disability from the injury?** ☐ No ☐ Yes ☐ Too early to determine
    The permanent partial disability is _____ % of the whole body. This rating is based on Minn. Rules:

5223.	%	5223.	%
5223.	%	5223.	%

NAME (Type or Print)	SIGNATURE		DEGREE
ADDRESS	STATE	LICENSE #/REGISTRATION #	
CITY STATE ZIP CODE	AREA CODE TELEPHONE #	DATE SIGNED	

MN HC01 (7/01)

Fig. 11-6 Attending physician statement form.

CLAIMANT'S AUTHORIZATION TO DISCLOSE HEALTH INFORMATION
(Pursuant to HIPAA)

INSTRUCTIONS

To the Claimant: The Health Insurance Portability and Accountability Act of 1996 (HIPAA) set standards for guaranteeing the privacy of individually identifiable health information and the confidentiality of patient medical records. By completing and signing this form, you authorize your health care provider to file medical reports with the parties that you choose (such as the Workers' Compensation Board, your employer's insurance carrier, your attorney or representative, etc.) by checking the appropriate boxes below.

You have the right to refuse to sign this Authorization. If you sign, you have the right to revoke this Authorization at any time by mailing a request to revoke to the health care provider. You have the right to receive a copy of this Authorization.

IMPORTANT: Failure to execute this authorization may interfere with your ability to obtain workers' compensation benefits.

CLAIMANT'S NAME	CLAIMANT'S SOCIAL SECURITY NUMBER	CLAIMANT'S DATE OF BIRTH
LIST ALL WCB CASE NUMBER(S) AND CORRESPONDING DATE(S) OF ACCIDENT FOR WHICH YOU ARE GRANTING AUTHORIZATION		

I, _____, hereby authorize my treating health provider,
Claimant's Name

_____, to disclose the following described health information:
Health Provider's Name

_____

_____

_____

This information can be disclosed to the following parties: *(check all that apply; give names and addresses, if known)*

☐ New York State Workers' Compensation Board

☐ My current/former employer _____

☐ Workers' compensation insurance carrier(s) _____

☐ Third-party administrator _____

☐ My attorney/licensed representative _____

☐ The Uninsured Employer's Fund (this fund is responsible for paying the medical bills and lost wage benefits when an employer is uninsured.)

☐ Special Funds Conservation Committee (for cases under Section 25-a or 15-8 of the Workers' Compensation Law)

Section 25-a: If your claim is being reopened after being previously closed, the Special Fund for Reopened Cases may be responsible for paying your medical bills and lost wage benefits.

Section 15-8: If you had a medical condition that existed prior to this injury, the Special Fund for Second Injuries may be responsible for reimbursing your employer's insurance carrier after a period of time has elapsed.

Redisclosure: I understand that once the above-referenced health care provider discloses health information based on this Authorization, that health information is no longer protected by HIPAA and the Privacy Rule.
Expiration Date: This Authorization expires upon the final closing of the workers' compensation claim(s) for which it is executed.

I have had the opportunity to review and understand the content of this Authorization. By signing this Authorization, I confirm that it accurately reflects my wishes.

_____   _____   _____
Printed Name of Claimant or Legal Representative   Signature of Claimant or Legal Representative   Date

If Authorization signed by a legal representative on behalf of claimant, state relationship to claimant_____and
basis for authority (e.g. claimant is a minor; patient is deceased and representative is the claimant in a workers' compensation proceeding or represents the estate) _____

TO THE HEALTH PROVIDER: Keep the original of this Authorization on file. A copy must be given to the patient/claimant upon request.

Fig. 11-7 Authorization release form.

5. Workers' compensation
6. Black Lung
7. Department of Veterans Affairs (VA) Disability Compensation Program
8. VA Pension Programs
9. VA Health Services Program

An individual may receive benefits from more than one program if he or she meets all the eligibility requirements. Specific eligibility requirements typically vary, depending on the purpose of the program, and eligibility requirements may change over time, as the result of amendments to the law, new regulations, or court decisions that affect eligibility criteria.

Disability under the federal programs generally is defined as significant difficulty with or the inability to perform certain day-to-day functions as a result of a health condition or impairment. For adults age 18 through 64, these functions often involve working or keeping house. For individuals age 65 and older, the functions may involve the inability to carry out routine daily tasks. Some commonly used factors federal programs look at in assessing disability are as follows:

- Sensory impairments—difficulty with or the inability to see, hear, or speak
- Cognitive/mental impairments—the presence of or resulting disabilities from cognitive/mental impairments (e.g., Alzheimer's disease, mental illness, mental retardation)
- Functioning of specific body systems—capacity of specific body systems (e.g., climbing stairs, walking 3 blocks, lifting 10 lb)
- **Activities of daily living/instrumental activities of daily living**—difficulty with or the inability to perform without the help of another person or a device the activities of daily living, which typically include bathing, dressing, eating, toileting, getting in or out of a bed or chair, and walking, or the instrumental activities of daily living, which generally include using the telephone, shopping, preparing meals, keeping house, doing laundry, doing yard work, managing personal finances, and managing medications
- Working—inability to work; limitations in the amount or kind of work; or ability to work only occasionally, irregularly, or part-time.

AMERICANS WITH DISABILITIES ACT

The intent of the **Americans with Disabilities Act (ADA)** of 1990 is to protect the civil rights of individuals with disabilities. Equal opportunity provisions pertain to employment, public accommodation, transportation, state and local government services, and telecommunications. Disability is present for purposes of the ADA if an individual meets one of the following three criteria:

1. There is a physical or mental impairment that substantially limits one or more of the major life activities.

2. There is a record of such an impairment.
3. The individual is regarded as having an impairment.

SOCIAL SECURITY DISABILITY INSURANCE

SSDI is the primary federal insurance program that protects workers from loss of income as a result of disability. SSDI provides monthly cash benefits to disabled workers younger than age 65 and to certain of their dependents. SSDI is intended for workers who retire before age 65 because of a disability.

History of the Social Security Disability Insurance Program

The 1935 Social Security Act established the federal Social Security system to provide old-age benefits for retired workers. The SSDI program was enacted in 1956 to provide benefits to workers age 50 through 64 years who retired early because of a disability. Subsequent amendments broadened SSDI coverage to include certain dependents and workers younger than age 50.

Administration and Funding

SSDI is federally administered by the Social Security Administration. Funding is provided through the disability insurance (SSDI) portion of the Social Security payroll tax on wages. As of 2006 the payroll tax was 7.65% of earnings, of which 5.6% was for the Old-Age and Survivors Insurance portion of Social Security, 0.62% for the SSDI portion, and 1.45% for the hospital insurance portion of Medicare. A matching 7.65% tax is contributed by employers. Self-employed individuals must contribute the entire 15.3% because they pay the employer and employee shares. As of 2006, the wage base limits for Social Security (Old-Age and Survivors Insurance and disability insurance parts) was $94,200. There is no wage base limit for the Medicare (hospital insurance) payroll tax.

Eligibility

To become eligible for SSDI, individuals must meet two criteria:

1. They must have worked enough Social Security–covered work quarters.
2. They must have a severe impairment that makes them unable to do their previous work or any other kind of substantial financially gainful activity.

Social Security–covered work quarters are credited annually for the years during which an individual works, is covered by Social Security, and earns a specified amount, which is adjusted upward each year. No more than four quarters can be credited per year. Workers must be fully insured (based on Social Security contributions) and (except for individuals who are blind or who are more than 31 years old) must have at least 20 quarters of coverage during the 40-quarter period up to the time of disability to receive SSDI. Individuals who are fully insured under Social Security have at least one quarter of coverage for every four quarters up to the time of disability. Individuals who have 40 quarters are fully insured for life. Workers younger than age 31 and individuals who are blind need fewer quarters, but a minimum of six quarters is required. Disability for SSDI is defined as the inability to do any substantial gainful activity by reason of any medically determinable physical or mental impairment that can be expected to result in death or that has lasted or can be expected to last for a continuous period of not less than 12 months.

After it has been established that the applicant has enough quarters and is not earning more than the "substantial gainful activity amount," a State Disability Determination unit examines medical evidence to determine if the applicant's mental or physical impairment is severe enough to have more than a minimal effect on the applicant's ability to work. If so, the applicant's medical condition is compared with a Social Security Administration listing of more than 100 impairments (e.g., loss of two limbs; fracture of vertebra with spinal cord involvement, substantiated by appropriate sensory and motor loss; vision of 20/200 or less after correction).

Applicants whose medical conditions are at least as severe as those in the Social Security Administration listing are considered disabled. Applicants who are not found disabled at this point are evaluated two additional steps. First, a determination is made as to whether or not the applicant can do his or her past work. This decision is based on assessments of factors such as physical abilities (e.g., strength, walking, standing) or mental abilities (e.g., the ability to carry out and remember instructions or to respond appropriately in work settings).

For applicants who cannot perform past work, an assessment is done to determine their ability to perform other jobs that exist in the national economy. This assessment is based on the individual's functional capacity, age, education, and work experience. In general, individuals younger than age 50 are considered to be able to adapt to new work situations.

Imagine This!

After teacher Louise Carson had her workers' compensation claim denied, she quit her job and filed for SSDI. SSDI found Louise to be disabled at her teaching position; however, they determined that she could perform at a "new work" situation that was less stressful and suggested that Louise use her education and training to work in a library or become a private tutor.

Dependent coverage and survivor benefits are offered through SSDI to certain qualifying individuals. Disabled individuals can receive SSDI in three ways:

1. On their own as disabled workers (described previously)
2. As widows or widowers (who are age 50 to 59) of insured individuals
3. As adults age 18 through 64 who became disabled in childhood whose parents receive SSDI, are Social Security retirees, or who are deceased (but had been insured under Social Security)

SUPPLEMENTAL SECURITY INCOME

The **SSI** program provides monthly cash payments to low-income aged, blind, and disabled individuals. The SSI program was established by the 1972 amendments to the Social Security Act, which replaced earlier federal grants to the states for old-age assistance, aid to the blind, and aid to the permanently disabled.

Administration and Funding

The SSI program is administered by the Social Security Administration. Funding comes from general federal revenues. Many states have chosen the option to supplement federal SSI payments with their own funds.

Eligibility

In contrast to SSDI, individuals receiving SSI because of blindness or disability have no work requirements, but must meet a **financial means test**, a detailed and comprehensive questionnaire that establishes financial need. The SSI means test depends on income and resources. Individuals younger than age 65 must meet disability and financial criteria, whereas individuals age 65 or older need to meet only the financial means test. Individuals may receive SSI payments either as individuals or as couples. Both members of a couple must be aged, blind, or disabled and must meet the financial means test to collect payments. Aside of these provisions for couples, there are no dependent or survivor benefits in SSI.

The determination of disability under SSI for adults is identical to the one used in the SSDI program. For children younger than age 18, the determination of disability is based on a standard of comparable severity. Their methods of counting various types of income and resources are complex, but, in general, the maximum monthly income in 2006 for individuals applying for SSI was $603 and $904 for couples if they received only Social Security and $1291 for individuals and $1893 for couples if their income was only from wages. Countable resources are limited to $2000 for individuals and $3000 for couples (Table 11-3).

TABLE 11-3 SSI and SSDI Similarities and Differences

	SSI	SSDI
Also Known As	Supplemental security income	Social Security Disability Insurance
Eligibility Criteria	Needs based—must have little or no income and resources	Insured status as a worker, or a child, widow, or widower of an insured worker No resource limits, no limits on unearned income
Monthly Benefit Amounts	Designed to bring income up to federal benefit rate of $603 (2006) Check amount depends on (1) living situation, (2) earnings, and (3) unearned income Some states supplement the federal amount for some or all living situations	Either eligible for full benefit checks or ineligible and receive no benefits Amount based on: (1) earnings history of wage earner, (2) age when benefits begin, and (3) number of people in addition to the wage earner who are receiving benefits If benefit amount is less than SSI federal benefit rate ($603 in 2006), may also be eligible for SSI
When Checks Arrive	1st of the month; if the 1st is a holiday or weekend, the check arrives on the business day before the 1st	People who qualified for SSDI before May 1997, arrives 3rd of the month Qualified after May 1997 and birthday between (1) 1st-10th, arrives 2nd Wednesday; (2) 11th-20th, arrives 3rd Wednesday; (3) 21st-31st, arrives 4th Wednesday
Funding Source	Annual congressional appropriation from the "General Fund"	Social Security Trust Fund, FICA taxes
Laws and Regulations	Title XVI (16) of the Social Security Act (Title 42 US Code, the Public Health and Welfare, Chapter 7, Subchapter XVI) Regulations in 20 CFR; Part 416	Title II (2) of the Social Security Act (Title 42 US Code, the Public Health and Welfare, Chapter 7, Subchapter II) Regulations in 20 CFR, Parts 400-499
Medical Benefits	Medicaid eligible in 32 states In other states, must apply separately for Medicaid Eligible the month of SSI application and possibly 3 months retroactively	Medicare eligible (Parts A and B), 24 months after person qualifies for SSDI
Monthly Cost (Premium)	None	SSDI recipients have $88.50 (2006) deducted from their check each month. If SSDI recipient also has SSI, Medicaid pays the monthly Medicare premium
Deductible	None, but there may be cost sharing instituted by states for various services	Yes—in 2006, the Part B deductible is $124/year. If person also receives SSI, Medicaid pays the deductible
Copay	Possibly none; however, states may elect to have small copays for medications, services, hospitalization	20% of costs deemed allowable by Medicare; 100% of costs not deemed allowable by Medicare. If person also receives SSI, Medicaid pays all copays

TABLE 11-3	SSI and SSDI Similarities and Differences—cont'd	
	SSI	SSDI
Range of Coverage	Comprehensive. Generally covers physician visits, prescriptions, dentures, glasses, hospital and hospice care, home help services/personal care, and other costs. Pays Medicare premium for concurrent recipients. Pays premiums for private insurance when cost-effective. Coverage may vary from state to state	Hospital costs primarily. Some home health care and durable medical equipment. Usually does not cover prescriptions, glasses, dentures, day-to-day medical costs, and physician visits. Recent changes in Medicare coverage pay for comprehensive care at select clinics
Proof of Coverage	Card comes monthly. Lists person(s) covered, their recipient ID number for billing, managed care provider, and contract number of other insurance (e.g., Medicare) that should be billed first	Permanent wallet-sized card—white with red and blue stripe. Names person covered, coverage, and date coverage began

Available at: http://ruralinstitute.umt.edu/training/publications/fact_sheets/ssi_ssdi.asp.

 HIPAA Tip

As a "covered entity" under HIPAA, the Social Security Administration, which oversees the federal disability programs such as SSDI and SDI, must comply with HIPAA's medical information standards.

STATE DISABILITY PROGRAMS

A few states (California, Hawaii, New Jersey, New York, and Rhode Island) and Puerto Rico currently have disability programs that provide short-term benefits for employees. These state programs are set up to supplement Social Security disability benefits. Because Social Security disability benefits do not cover the first 6 months of the disability, these state plans provide benefits to qualifying disabled individuals until Social Security payments begin. The funds are financed by a combination of the employees' payroll deductions and employer contributions. An employee's contributions are based on his or her earnings and are withheld from wages by the employer and transferred to the state fund. There are severe penalties for failing to withhold the contributions. With the exception of Rhode Island, an employer can opt out of the state plan and put the employee's contributions into a private plan. Private plans must meet state requirements regarding coverage, eligibility, contribution amounts, and employee approval.

CENTERS FOR DISEASE CONTROL AND PREVENTION DISABILITY AND HEALTH TEAM

The **Disability and Health Team** is part of the new National Center on Birth Defects and Developmental Disabilities at the Centers for Disease Control and Prevention (CDC) located in Atlanta, Georgia. The team's focus is promoting the health of individuals who are living with disabilities. The CDC Disability and Health Team activities include the following:

- Assessing and monitoring disability prevalence
- Assessing the health status and quality of life for individuals with disabilities
- Describing risk factors and costs associated with secondary conditions and poor health
- Developing health promotion interventions to reduce secondary conditions and evaluate intervention effectiveness and costs
- Offering training to healthcare professionals interested in the field of disability and public health
- Supporting conferences to facilitate and encourage discussion, circulate and exchange information, establish research and policy priorities, and outline and undertake further action

In spring 2002, the Disability and Health Team gave out 16 competitive awards to individual states to implement effective state-level health promotion and wellness programs for individuals with disabilities. The program period began in 2002 and will continue for 3 to 5 years. The anticipated outcome of this program is improved health of state residents with disabilities.

TICKET TO WORK PROGRAM

The **Ticket to Work program** was created with passage of the federal Ticket to Work and Work Incentives Improvement Act of 1999. Ticket to Work is a *voluntary* program that gives certain individuals with disabilities greater choice in selecting the service providers and rehabilitation services they need to help them keep working or get back to work.

Purpose

Ticket to Work was created to help individuals who receive SSDI or SSI benefits find and keep employment by offering them more options for services and supports. Many individuals receiving SSDI or SSI choose not to work because they are concerned about losing their benefits. Ticket to Work gives these individuals an opportunity to choose services to meet their unique needs and obtain benefits-planning assistance so they can make informed choices about employment. Individuals receiving SSDI or SSI disability benefits may participate in Ticket to Work.

How the Program Works

Ticket to Work participants receive a paper document or "ticket" that explains the program and includes some personal information about them. They can take their ticket to an approved **employment network** to receive the services they want. An employment network can be a public agency or private organization that has agreed to provide services under the Ticket to Work program guidelines.

FILING SUPPLEMENTAL SECURITY INCOME AND SOCIAL SECURITY DISABILITY INSURANCE DISABILITY CLAIMS

Patient's Role

The patient initiates the SSI or SSDI claim. The best way to begin the process is to file a Social Security disability claim at the nearest Social Security office in person. An alternative method is to contact Social Security by telephone and arrange for a telephone interview to file the claim.

A claim for Social Security disability benefits may be filed on the same day that an individual becomes disabled. There is no reason to file a Social Security disability claim for a minor illness or one that is unlikely to last 1 year or more. An individual who has a serious illness or injury and expects to be out of work for 1 year or more should not delay in filing a claim for Social Security disability benefits.

Unless the disability is catastrophic (e.g., terminal cancer, a serious heart condition requiring transplant, total paralysis of both legs), there is no easy way to tell whether an individual would be found disabled by Social Security. Individuals should make the decision about whether or not to file for Social Security disability based on their own belief regarding their condition. If the individual believes that he or she is truly disabled and is not going to be able to return to work in the near future, that individual should file for Social Security disability benefits.

After a Social Security disability claim is filed, the case is sent to a disability examiner at the Disability Determination Agency in that state, who works with a physician to make the initial decision on the claim based on a thorough clinical examination and interviews. If the claim is denied and the individual requests reconsideration, the case is sent to a second disability examiner at the Disability Determination Agency, where it goes through much the same process. If a claim is denied at reconsideration, the individual may request a hearing. At this point, the case is sent to an administrative law judge who works for Social Security. The administrative law judge makes an independent decision on the claim, which is usually final.

An individual can hire an attorney to represent him or her on Social Security disability claim denials. The National Organization of Social Security Claimants' Representatives offers a referral service at 1-800-431-2804 during regular Eastern Standard Time business hours.

Applicants for SSI or SSDI benefits should get the free booklet *Social Security Disability Benefits* (Social Security Administration Publication No. 05-10029). This booklet suggests ways to help shorten the process by knowing what documents to include when applying for benefits.

Role of the Healthcare Provider

The disability determination process relies on the participation of the medical community in many ways. One of the most important ways is as a **treating source** that provides the long-term medical information (called medical evidence of record that is normally required in every claim for disability benefits. In addition to providing treating source evidence, the medical community can assist the disability programs in the following ways:

- As a member of the state Disability Determination Services disability evaluation team that makes the initial or continuing disability determination
- As a reviewer of the state decision
- As a consultative examiner for the Disability Determination Services
- As a medical expert for an administrative law judge

Healthcare providers who serve as medical experts may be asked to give verbal testimony or provide answers to questions on claim reviews. Frequently, the final decision to allow or deny a Social Security disability claim rests on the advice and medical opinions provided by these medical experts.

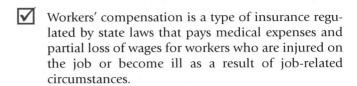

HIPAA Tip

HIPAA protects against gaps in insurance coverage, allowing the freedom to move from one job to another or the freedom to move from SSI or SSDI status to the ranks of the employed.

Role of the Health Insurance Professional

The health insurance professional needs to know the Social Security regulations so that he or she is able to provide the exact information needed for evaluation of an individual's disability. There are many steps in the application process, which can be time-consuming and confusing, and a knowledgeable healthcare team should do all they can to facilitate this process.

Similar to workers' compensation claims, there is no standard form for billing disability claims. When a patient comes to the medical facility for the purpose of getting the physician's medical opinion regarding disability, the health insurance professional should advise the patient to bring the necessary forms provided by the Social Security office. Additional responsibilities of the health insurance professional include

- procuring the patient's authorization to release information,
- acquiring the necessary information for claims processing,
- ensuring that the attending physician forms are complete and signed,
- photocopying all forms for the patient's health record,
- maintaining a well-documented health record, and
- answering the patient's questions.

● Stop and Think

Amy Turner, a health insurance professional for Dr. Laura Nelson, wants to be able to help patients through the often complicated process of filing for SSI/SSDI benefits. What would you suggest Amy do to become knowledgeable in this area?

What Did You Learn?

1. List six federal disability programs.
2. How do federal programs define disability?
3. ADA considers disability present if an individual meets what three criteria?
4. What is the difference between SSI and SSDI?
5. List the five states that provide short-term disability benefits

SUMMARY CHECK POINTS

- ☑ Workers' compensation is a type of insurance regulated by state laws that pays medical expenses and partial loss of wages for workers who are injured on the job or become ill as a result of job-related circumstances.

- ☑ Any employee who injures himself or herself on the job or develops an employment-related illness that prevents the individual from working is usually eligible to receive workers' compensation benefits. A spouse and dependents of an employee who dies or gets killed because of a job-related accident or illness also are eligible for benefits.

- ☑ Most employers must purchase workers' compensation insurance coverage for their workers; however, there are certain classifications of exemptions, depending on state statutes. Common types of exemptions include the following:
  - Employers with a *minimum* number of full-time employees (individual states determine this number)
  - Executive officers
  - Individuals who are business partners
  - Sole proprietors
  - Casual employees

- ☑ The four major benefit components to workers' compensation are as follows:
  - *Medical expense*—pays expenses involved for hospitalization, physicians' visits, and any necessary medical treatment
  - *Disability pay*—can be temporary or permanent if it is determined that the worker will never fully recover
  - *Vocational rehabilitation*—if the injury/illness results in the worker being unable to perform the usual duties of his or her occupation, retraining may be necessary for the worker to enter into a new trade or business; also, physical therapy may be needed
  - *Death benefits*—paid to surviving dependents

- ☑ The reporting requirements for filing a workers' compensation claim include the following steps:
  - Employee notifies a supervisor of the incident immediately and provides the names of any witnesses.
  - Employee completes a detailed accident report on a form furnished by the employer.
  - Employer reports the incident to the company's workers' compensation carrier.

- Employee is sent to a medical facility for treatment or diagnosis. (In emergencies, this should be the first step.)
- Attending physician completes statement and distributes copies.
- Follow-up progress reports are submitted until the employee returns to work, after which a final report is filed.

☑ When the injured or ill worker visits the healthcare facility for treatment, the attending physician takes a history, performs an examination, makes a diagnosis, and completes a statement indicating any physical or mental impairments resulting from the incident. Disability is determined based on these reports.

☑ The purpose of disability income insurance is to replace a portion of salary or wages earned income when an individual is unable to perform the requirements of his or her job because of injury or illness that is not work related.

☑ SSDI is a federal insurance program that pays monthly cash benefits to disabled workers younger than age 65 and to certain dependents who have lost their income because of disability. Individuals applying for SSDI must meet two criteria:
- They must have worked a specific number of Social Security–covered work quarters.
- They must have a severe impairment that makes them unable to perform their previous work or any other kind of financially gainful activity.

☑ SSI provides monthly cash payments to low-income aged, blind, and disabled individuals. There are no work requirements for SSI, but individuals must answer a detailed and comprehensive questionnaire that establishes financial need, called a financial means test. Disability determination for adults is the same under SSDI and SSI.

☑ The CDC Disability and Health Team activities include the following:
- Assessing and monitoring the occurrence of disabilities
- Assessing the health status and quality of life for individuals with disabilities
- Describing risk factors and costs associated with secondary conditions and poor health
- Developing and evaluating effectiveness of health promotion interventions
- Offering training to interested health professionals
- Supporting conferences to facilitate and encourage team activities

☑ Ticket to Work was created to help SSDI/SSI recipients find and keep employment by offering them more options. The program gives individuals an opportunity to choose services to meet their unique needs and obtain benefits-planning assistance so that they can make informed choices about employment. Participants receive a paper document (ticket) that explains the program and includes some personal information about them. They can take their ticket to an approved employment network to receive the desired services.

☑ The patient initiates an SSI/SSDI claim by going to the nearest Social Security office in person or by telephoning and arranging for a telephone interview to file the claim. After the claim is filed, the case is sent to a disability examiner who works with a physician to make the initial decision on the claim based on a thorough clinical examination and interviews.

☑ The health insurance professional's responsibilities for facilitating disability claims processing include the following:
- Obtaining the patient's authorization to release information
- Acquiring the necessary information and forms for claims processing
- Ensuring that the attending physician reports are complete and signed
- Photocopying all forms and correspondence for the patient's health record
- Maintaining a well-documented health record
- Answering the patient's questions

CLOSING SCENARIO

Jim and Tammy had discussed their individual areas of interest before beginning the chapter. Tammy visited with her Uncle Niles on several occasions to learn all she could about disability income insurance, and she shared what she learned with Jim. Meanwhile, Jim researched the workers' compensation websites available on the Internet. By the end of the chapter, the two students thought that they had acquired a good knowledge base for workers' compensation and private and federal disability income insurance. Jim now has a better understanding of the payment system that kept his family going after his father's death.

Jim and Tammy realize that acquiring a solid foundation in all areas of insurance is a benefit, not only to health insurance professionals, but also to the entire healthcare team. By becoming well informed, health insurance professionals can help educate patients to alleviate the cumbersome task of filing and maintaining all of the documents necessary for workers' compensation and disability insurance.

WEBSITES TO EXPLORE

For live links to the following websites, please visit the Evolve® site at http://evolve.elsevier.com/Beik/today/

- To find out about the workers' compensations laws in your state, log on to
http://www.workerscompensation.com/

- For an overview of *State Workers' Compensation Laws*, the U.S. Department of Labor provides one in PDF (Portable Document Format) at
http://www.dol.gov/ (*Note:* You must download and install a *free Adobe Acrobat Reader* to view and print PDF files)

- To keep up-to-date changes in both the SSDI and SSI programs, log on to http://www.ssa.gov/

- For more information on the CDC Disability and Health Team Program, log on to the CDC website at
http://www.cdc.gov

UNIT III

Cracking the Codes

Diagnostic Coding

Chapter Outline

CHAPTER OBJECTIVES

After completion of this chapter, the student should be able to

- Discuss the history and development of diagnostic coding.
- Outline the format of the ICD-9-CM manual.
- Describe the organization and use of Volume 2, the Alphabetic Index.

CHAPTER TERMS

- adjectives
- category
- code set
- coding
- combination code
- conditions
- diagnosis
- diseases
- E codes
- eponyms
- essential modifiers
- etiology
- hypertension
- in situ

CHAPTER OBJECTIVES

- Explain what "main terms" are and how to locate them.
- Differentiate between an "essential" and "nonessential" modifier.
- Discuss the importance of understanding coding conventions.
- Explain the organization of codes in Volume 1, the Tabular List.
- List the essential steps to diagnostic coding.
- Give an overview of the ICD-10.

CHAPTER TERMS

International Classification of Diseases, 9th Revision, Clinical Modification (ICD-9-CM)
International Classification of Diseases, 10th Revision (ICD-10)
main term

manifestation
morbidity
mortality
neoplasm
nonessential modifiers
notes
noun
subcategory
subclassification
V codes

OPENING SCENARIO

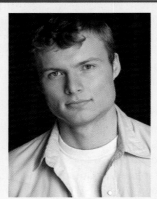

Since Park Chalmers was a little boy, he had wanted to be a doctor; however, when he fainted after witnessing a bicycle accident that severely injured his best friend's arm, Park realized that the clinical side of medicine was not for him. Still, the field of medicine intrigued him. After high school, Park moved from one dead-end job to another. He soon faced the fact that without specialized career training, the prospect of living comfortably in an apartment of his own appeared grim.

In his search for more meaningful employment, Park noticed an advertisement in the classified section of the newspaper for a coder at a local medical clinic. The position required coursework or on-the-job experience in ICD-9-CM and CPT coding. The pay range noted in the ad was enticing to Park; however, he had no idea what ICD-9-CM or CPT coding was. The terms themselves were "codes" to Park.

Curious about the meaning of ICD-9-CM and CPT coding, Park made inquiries when he attended a job fair at the community college. He was directed to the health careers booth where current health insurance students, along with the aid of an instructor, answered all his questions and gave a brief demonstration on diagnostic coding.

"I think I can learn this coding stuff," Park decided, and headed for the Student Services Department to enroll in the upcoming health insurance program.

HISTORY AND DEVELOPMENT OF DIAGNOSTIC CODING

Dorland's Illustrated Medical Dictionary defines **diagnosis** as "the determination of the nature of a cause of disease," or "the art of distinguishing one disease from another." **Coding**, as it applies to this topic, is the process of assigning a series of numbers or alphanumeric characters to a diagnosis for the purpose of identification or classification or both.

Diagnostic coding dates back to 17th century England, where statistical data were collected through a system called the *London Bills of Mortality*. By 1937, this method of tracking information had evolved into the International List of Causes of Death. The World Health Organization (WHO) published a statistical listing in 1948 that tracked **morbidity** (the presence of illness or disease) and **mortality** (the deaths that occur from a disease). This statistical WHO listing was called the International Classification

of Diseases (ICD) and ultimately became the book used worldwide today for coding diagnoses—the *International Classification of Diseases, 9th Revision* (ICD-9).

Use of ICD-9 began in the United States when the U.S. National Center for Health Statistics modified the system in 1977 with clinical information. This modification provided a way to classify morbidity data for the indexing of medical records, medical case reviews, ambulatory and other medical care programs, and basic health statistics. The result was the ***International Classification of Diseases, 9th Revision, Clinical Modification*** (**ICD-9-CM**). This modified version precisely describes the clinical picture of each patient and provides exact information above and beyond that needed for statistics and analysis of healthcare trends.

In 1988, Congress passed the Medicare Catastrophic Coverage Act. This act mandated the use of ICD-9 coding for all Part B Medicare Claims. A portion of this act was later revoked, but the part requiring use of ICD-9 codes for Medicare claims was upheld and became effective in April 1989. Basic guidelines regarding the use of ICD-9 codes were published by the Centers for Medicare and Medicaid Services (CMS), previously known as the Health Care Financing Administration (HCFA). Soon after Medicare began using ICD-9 codes, other insurance companies followed. Today, most third-party payers require the use of these diagnosis codes on all claims.

The ICD-9-CM currently comprises three volumes:
• Volume 1, Tabular List
• Volume 2, Alphabetical List
• Volume 3, Used for Hospital Inpatient Procedure Coding

In general, most publishers combine Volumes 1 and 2 in the same manual. Although most insurance companies do not require the use of Volume 3 for physician billing, Volume 3 is still used for hospital inpatient coding. (Medicare Part B does not accept codes from Volume 3; if they are used, the claim is denied.) It is important that the health insurance professional obtain and use the most recent version of the ICD-9 for effective and accurate coding. Any questions regarding which volume to use should be addressed to the appropriate carrier, fiscal intermediary, or billing consultant.

What Did You Learn?

1. When did diagnostic coding get its start in the United States?
2. How did the Medicare Catastrophic Coverage Act affect diagnostic coding?
3. Name the three volumes that make up the ICD-9-CM.
4. What ICD-9-CM volumes are generally used for physician billing?

ICD-9-CM MANUAL

Before any attempt is made to code a diagnosis, the health insurance professional must become familiar with the contents and structure of the ICD-9 manual. The format of the ICD-9 differs from one publisher to the next as far as how the material is arranged; however, the basic information is the same. The prefacing instructions given here are somewhat generic, as the ICD-9-CM manual is available from several different publishers in a variety of formats. The information, coding instructions, and codes were current at the time of this writing. For up-to-date information, the health insurance professional should consult the most recent ICD-9-CM coding manual.

The first several pages of the ICD-9 manual constitute an introduction and guide to using the ICD-9. Informational items typically include (but are not limited to) the following:

• Introduction
A discussion of the history and future of the ICD-9-CM system
The background of the ICD-9-CM
Characteristics of ICD-9-CM
The disease classification
• Instructional steps for using Physicians Volumes 1 and 2 correctly
Ten steps to correct coding
Organization
• A listing of ICD-9-CM Official Conventions, footnotes, symbols, and instructional notes
• A summary of code changes
• Valid 3-digit ICD-9 codes
• General coding guidelines

No matter which ICD-9-CM manual is used, it is important that the health insurance professional thoroughly study the prefacing information contained in the introductory pages because it serves as a basic foundation for diagnostic coding and aids in assigning diagnosis codes correctly. The following sections complete a typical format of ICD-9-CM manual:

• Volume 2, Index to Diseases
• Volume 1, Tabular List
• Appendix A, Morphology of Neoplasms
• Appendix B, Glossary of Mental Disorders
• Appendix C, Classification of Drugs by American Hospital Formulary Service List
• Appendix D, Industrial Accidents According to Agency
• Appendix E, Three-Digit Categories (Infectious and Parasitic Diseases)

VOLUME 2, THE ALPHABETIC LIST (INDEX)

Volume 2, the Alphabetical List, typically is located in the front half of the ICD-9-CM and is presented before Volume 1, the Tabular List. Volume 2 contains an alphabetical listing that provides detailed instructions that can help the coder determine if a diagnosis requires the use of additional or alternate codes. A diagnosis should *never* be coded strictly from the Alphabetical List.

A diagnosis code consists of at least three and up to five characters, depending on whether a 3-, 4-, or 5-digit code best represents the patient's diagnosis. ICD-9-CM codes range from 001 to V85.4 (2006) and identify symptoms, conditions, problems, complaints, or other reasons for the procedure, service, or supply provided. It is crucial that a diagnosis is coded to the "highest level of specificity." By consulting the Alphabetic List first, the health insurance professional can determine more accurately whether a 3-digit code sufficiently describes the diagnosis or whether additional numbers are required to attain the needed specificity. Diagnoses that are coded inadequately or inappropriately can result in a claim being underpaid, overpaid, delayed, or denied.

THREE SECTIONS OF VOLUME 2

Section 1, the Index to Diseases

Volume 2 contains three separate sections or indexes. The largest one, the Index to Diseases, is organized by **main terms**, which are always printed in boldface type for ease of reference. Main terms include the following:

- **Diseases**, such as influenza or bronchitis
- **Conditions**, such as fatigue, fracture, or injury
- **Nouns**, such as disease, disturbance, syndrome, or eponyms
- **Adjectives**, such as double, large, or kinked

Anatomic sites are not listed as main terms. If a patient has a diagnosis of deviated nasal septum, it would be found in Volume 2 under the main term "deviation," rather than "nasal." Ankle sprain would be located under "sprain," rather than "ankle." Figure 12-1 shows a sample page from Volume 2.

● Stop and Think

Marlee Davis is employed as a health insurance professional for cardiologist Ferris Barnes. Marlee is in charge of all the billing, coding, and insurance. While preparing to submit an insurance claim for patient Eloise Hardy, Marlee notes that the patient's healthcare record documents a diagnosis of "congestive heart failure." Identify the "main term" in this diagnosis.

Many conditions can be found in more than one place in the Alphabetic Index, which can be confusing sometimes. Obstetric conditions can be found under the name of the condition and under the entries for "delivery," "pregnancy," and "puerperal" (after delivery). Figure 12-2 provides examples of how each of these three terms are shown in Volume 2. Complications of medical and surgical care are indexed under the *name of condition* and under *complications*.

Eponyms. **Eponyms** are diseases, procedures, or syndromes named for individuals who discovered or first used them. They typically are located alphabetically by the individual's name and by the common name. Vincent's disease (trench mouth) can be found under "Vincent's," "disease," and "trench" (Fig. 12-3).

Essential Modifiers. **Essential modifiers** are indented under the main term as shown in the example in Figure 12-4. They modify the main term describing different sites, **etiology** (the cause or origin of a disease or condition), and clinical types. Essential modifiers must be a part of the documented diagnosis.

Nonessential Modifiers. **Nonessential modifiers** are terms in parentheses following the main terms. They typically give alternate terminology for the main term and are provided to assist the coder in locating the applicable main term. Figure 12-5 shows an example of how nonessential modifiers are depicted in Volume 2. Nonessential modifiers are usually not a part of the diagnostic statement.

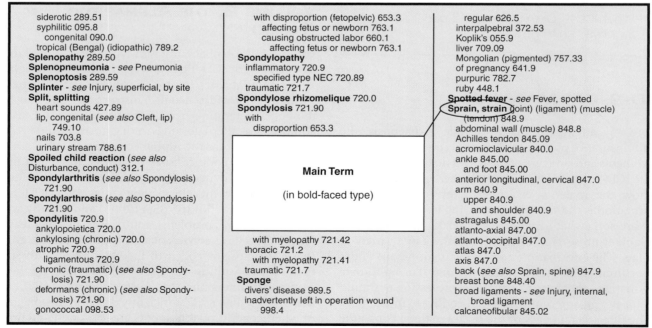

Fig. 12-1 Section of the ICD-9 Volume 2 showing sample page. (Data from International Classification of Diseases, 9th Revision. U.S. Department of Health and Human Services, Public Health Service, Centers for Medicare and Medicaid Services.)

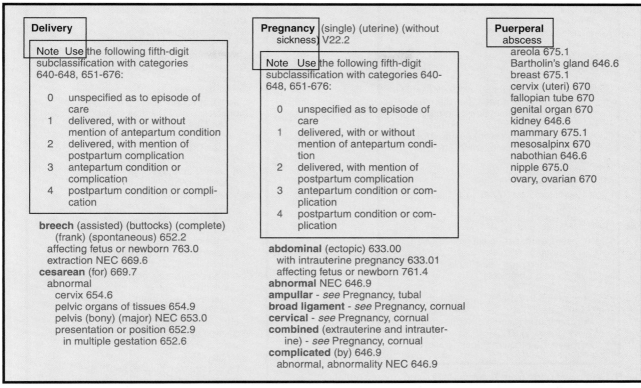

Delivery

Note Use the following fifth-digit subclassification with categories 640-648, 651-676:

0   unspecified as to episode of care
1   delivered, with or without mention of antepartum condition
2   delivered, with mention of postpartum complication
3   antepartum condition or complication
4   postpartum condition or complication

breech (assisted) (buttocks) (complete) (frank) (spontaneous) 652.2
affecting fetus or newborn 763.0
extraction NEC 669.6
cesarean (for) 669.7
abnormal
    cervix 654.6
    pelvic organs of tissues 654.9
    pelvis (bony) (major) NEC 653.0
    presentation or position 652.9
        in multiple gestation 652.6

Pregnancy (single) (uterine) (without sickness) V22.2

Note Use the following fifth-digit subclassification with categories 640-648, 651-676:

0   unspecified as to episode of care
1   delivered, with or without mention of antepartum condition
2   delivered, with mention of postpartum complication
3   antepartum condition or complication
4   postpartum condition or complication

abdominal (ectopic) 633.00
with intrauterine pregnancy 633.01
affecting fetus or newborn 761.4
abnormal NEC 646.9
ampullar - *see* Pregnancy, tubal
broad ligament - *see* Pregnancy, cornual
cervical - *see* Pregnancy, cornual
combined (extrauterine and intrauterine) - *see* Pregnancy, cornual
complicated (by) 646.9
abnormal, abnormality NEC 646.9

Puerperal
abscess
areola 675.1
Bartholin's gland 646.6
breast 675.1
cervix (uteri) 670
fallopian tube 670
genital organ 670
kidney 646.6
mammary 675.1
mesosalpinx 670
nabothian 646.6
nipple 675.0
ovary, ovarian 670

Fig. 12-2 Example showing how each of the above 3 terms is shown in Volume 2. (Data from International Classification of Diseases, 9th Revision. U.S. Department of Health and Human Services, Public Health Service, Centers for Medicare and Medicaid Services.)

VIN II (vulvar intraepithelial neoplasia I) 624.8
VIN III (vulvar intraepithelial neoplasia I) 233.3
Vincent's
angina 101
bronchitis 101
disease 101
gingivitis 101
infection (any site) 101
laryngitis 101
stomatitis 101
tonsillitis 101
Vinson-Plummer syndrome (sideropenic dysphagia) 280.8
Viosterol deficiency (*see also* Deficiency, calciferol) 268.9
Virchow's disease 733.99
Viremia 790.8

Fig. 12-3 Example of an eponym listing. (Data from International Classification of Diseases, 9th Revision. U.S. Department of Health and Human Services, Public Health Service, Centers for Medicare and Medicaid Services.)

traumatic - *see* Injury, nerve, spinal
nontraumatic - *see* Myelitis
stomach 536.9
psychogenic 306.4
sympathetic nerve NEC (*see also* Neuropathy, peripheral, autonomic) 337.9
ulnar nerve 354.2
vagina 623.9
Isambert's disease 012.3
Ischemia, ischemic 459.9
→ basilar artery (with transient neurologic deficit) 435.0
bone NEC 733.40
bowel (transient) 557.9
    acute 557.0
    chronic 557.1
    due to mesenteric artery insufficiency 557.1
brain - *see also* Ischemia, cerebral
    recurrent focal 435.9
cardiac (*see also* Ischemia, heart) 414.9

Fig. 12-4 Example of an essential modifier. (Data from International Classification of Diseases, 9th Revision. U.S. Department of Health and Human Services, Public Health Service, Centers for Medicare and Medicaid Services.)

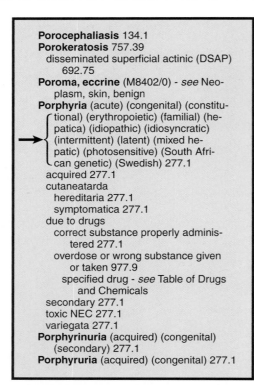

Porocephaliasis 134.1
Porokeratosis 757.39
   disseminated superficial actinic (DSAP)
   692.75
Poroma, eccrine (M8402/0) - see Neoplasm, skin, benign
Porphyria (acute) (congenital) (constitutional) (erythropoietic) (familial) (he-
   patica) (idiopathic) (idiosyncratic)
   (intermittent) (latent) (mixed hepatic) (photosensitive) (South Afri-
   can genetic) (Swedish) 277.1
   acquired 277.1
   cutaneatarda
      hereditaria 277.1
      symptomatica 277.1
   due to drugs
      correct substance properly adminis-
         tered 277.1
      overdose or wrong substance given
         or taken 977.9
      specified drug - see Table of Drugs
         and Chemicals
   secondary 277.1
   toxic NEC 277.1
   variegata 277.1
Porphyrinuria (acquired) (congenital)
   (secondary) 277.1
Porphyruria (acquired) (congenital) 277.1

Fig. 12-5 Section of page from Volume 2 showing nonessential modifiers using porphyria. (Data from International Classification of Diseases, 9th Revision. U.S. Department of Health and Human Services, Public Health Service, Centers for Medicare and Medicaid Services.)

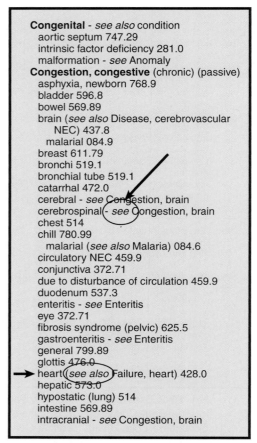

Congenital - see also condition
   aortic septum 747.29
   intrinsic factor deficiency 281.0
   malformation - see Anomaly
Congestion, congestive (chronic) (passive)
   asphyxia, newborn 768.9
   bladder 596.8
   bowel 569.89
   brain (see also Disease, cerebrovascular
      NEC) 437.8
      malarial 084.9
   breast 611.79
   bronchi 519.1
   bronchial tube 519.1
   catarrhal 472.0
   cerebral - see Congestion, brain
   cerebrospinal - see Congestion, brain
   chest 514
   chill 780.99
      malarial (see also Malaria) 084.6
   circulatory NEC 459.9
   conjunctiva 372.71
   due to disturbance of circulation 459.9
   duodenum 537.3
   enteritis - see Enteritis
   eye 372.71
   fibrosis syndrome (pelvic) 625.5
   gastroenteritis - see Enteritis
   general 799.89
   glottis 476.0
   heart (see also Failure, heart) 428.0
   hepatic 573.0
   hypostatic (lung) 514
   intestine 569.89
   intracranial - see Congestion, brain

Fig. 12-6 Section from Volume 2 using congestive heart failure. (Data from International Classification of Diseases, 9th Revision. U.S. Department of Health and Human Services, Public Health Service, Centers for Medicare and Medicaid Services.)

Notes. **Notes** such as *see* or *see also* typically refer the coder to continue the search under another main term. Referring back to the patient with a diagnosis of *congestive heart failure,* the main term "congestive" and the essential modifier "heart" are located in the Alphabetic Index, and there is a parenthetical notation (*see also* Failure, heart 428.0). This notation guides the coder to an alternate page in the Index, where the main term "failure, failed" is located. After the essential modifiers (heart and congestive) code 428.0 is located, the coder must cross-reference this code to the Tabular List to determine if 428.0 describes this diagnosis to its "greatest specificity" or if a 5th digit is needed. Figure 12-6 shows an example of how *see also* is used in Volume 2.

Imagine This!

Tricia Lorber, a health insurance professional, was preparing a claim for patient Arthur Renteria, whose health record documented "hemorrhoids, internal and external." Tricia used a diagnosis code of 455.3, but if she had coded to the "greatest specificity," two codes should have been reported: 455.0 and 455.3. This error cost the practice $100.

Hypertension and Neoplasm Tables. Also listed within the Alphabetic Index to Diseases are two tables: (1) Hypertension Table and (2) Neoplasm Table. If a patient is diagnosed with a type of **hypertension** (high blood pressure), the health insurance professional must locate the specific type in the hypertension table and make the determination if it is "malignant," "benign," or "unspecified" as indicated in the columnar codes (Fig. 12-7). If the patient's diagnosis is essential benign hypertension, the ICD-9 code would be 401.1. As with other code searches, hypertension and **neoplasm** (new growth) coding does not stop with the indexed tables in Volume 2.

Section 2, Table of Drugs and Chemicals

Section 2 of Volume 2 consists of the Table of Drugs and Chemicals, which contains the Alphabetic Index to Poisoning and External Causes of Adverse Effects of Drugs and Other Chemical Substances. Codes in this table are used when documentation in the health record indicates a poisoning, overdose, wrong substance given or taken, or

	Malignant	Benign	Unspecified
Hypertension, hypertensive (arterial) (arteriolar) (crisis) (degeneration) (disease) (essential) (fluctuating) (idiopathic) (intermittent) (labile) (low renin) (orthostatic) (paroxysmal) (primary) (systemic) (uncontrolled) (vascular)	401.0	401.1	401.9
with			
chronic kidney disease	403.01	403.11	403.91 ◄
heart involvement (conditions classifiable to 429.0-429.3, 429.8, 429.9 due to hypertension) (*see also* Hypertension, heart)	402.00	402.10	402.90
with kidney involvement-see Hypertension, cardiorenal			
renal involvement (only conditions classifiable to 585, 586, 587) (excludes conditions classifiable to 584) (*see also* Hypertension, kidney)	403.00	403.10	403.90
with heart involvement-see Hypertension, cardiorenal			
failure (and sclerosis) (*see also* Hypertension, kidney)	403.01	403.11	403.91
sclerosis without failure (*see also* Hypertension, kidney)	403.00	403.10	403.90
accelerated (*see also* Hypertension, by type, malignant)	401.0	-	-
antepartum-see Hypertension, complicating pregnancy, childbirth, or the puerperium			
cardiorenal (disease)	404.00	404.10	404.90
with			
chronic kidney disease	403.01	403.11	403.91 ◄
and heart failure	404.03	404.13	404.93 ◄
heart failure	404.01	404.11	404.91
and chronic kidney disease	404.03	404.13	404.93 ◄
and renal failure	404.03	404.13	404.93
renal failure	404.02	404.12	404.92
and heart failure	404.03	404.13	404.93
cardiovascular disease (arteriosclerotic) (sclerotic)	402.00	402.10	402.90
with			
heart failure	402.01	402.11	402.91
renal involvement (conditions classifiable to 403) (*see also* Hypertension, cardiorenal)	404.00	404.10	404.90
cardiovascular renal (disease) (sclerosis) (*see also* Hypertension, cardiorenal)	404.00	404.10	404.90
cerebrovascular disease NEC	437.2	437.2	437.2
complicating pregnancy, childbirth, or the puerperium	642.2	642.0	642.9
with			
albuminuria (and edema) (mild)	-	-	642.4
severe	-	-	642.5
edema (mild)	-	-	642.4
severe	-	-	642.5
heart disease	642.2	642.2	642.2
and renal disease	642.2	642.2	642.2
renal disease	642.2	642.2	642.2
and heart disease	642.2	642.2	642.2
chronic	642.2	642.0	642.0
with pre-eclampsia or eclampsia	642.7	642.7	642.7
fetus or newborn	760.0	760.0	760.0
essential	-	642.0	642.0
with pre-eclampsia or eclampsia	-	642.7	642.7
fetus or newborn	760.0	760.0	760.0
fetus or newborn	760.0	760.0	760.0
gestational	-	-	642.3
pre-existing	642.2	642.0	642.0

Fig. 12-7 Section from hypertension table. (Data from International Classification of Diseases, 9th Revision. U.S. Department of Health and Human Services, Public Health Service, Centers for Medicare and Medicaid Services.)

intoxication. The table also lists external causes of adverse effects resulting from ingestion or exposure to drugs or other chemical substances. A section of a page from the Table of Drugs and Chemicals is shown in Figure 12-8.

Section 3, Index to External Causes of Injury and Poisoning (E Codes)

Section 3 is the Alphabetic Index to External Causes of Injury and Poisoning, which contains **E codes** (Fig. 12-9). Codes in this section are used to classify environmental events, circumstances, and other conditions that are the cause of injury and other adverse effects. E codes are organized by main terms that describe the accident, circumstance, event, or specific agent causing the injury or adverse effect.

● Stop and Think

Twenty-year-old Bob Timmerman was driving his 1978 Trans-Am on a two-lane country road at dusk when he accidentally struck a slow-moving Amish carriage, injuring a 4-year-old child. The child sustained a fractured ulna and multiple lacerations and contusions. In what section of ICD-9 would the health insurance professional look to begin the search for the appropriate diagnostic code?

TABLE OF DRUGS AND CHEMICALS / Antibiotics

Substance	Poisoning	External Cause (E-Code) Accident	Therapeutic Use	Suicide Attempt	Assault	Undetermined
Antibiotics *(Continued)*						
specified NEC	960.8	E856	E930.8	E950.4	E962.0	E980.4
tetracycline (group)	960.4	E856	E930.4	E950.4	E962.0	E980.4
Anticancer agents NEC	963.1	E858.1	E933.1	E950.4	E962.0	E980.4
antibiotics	960.7	E856	E930.7	E950.4	E962.0	E980.4
Anticholinergics	971.1	E855.4	E941.1	E950.4	E962.0	E980.4
Anticholinesterase (organophosphorus) (reversible)	971.0	E855.3	E941.0	E950.4	E962.0	E980.4
Anticoagulants	964.2	E858.2	E934.2	E950.4	E962.0	E980.4
antagonists	964.5	E858.2	E934.5	E950.4	E962.0	E980.4
Anti-common cold agents NEC	975.6	E858.6	E945.6	E950.4	E962.0	E980.4
Anticonvulsants NEC	966.3	E855.0	E936.3	E950.4	E962.0	E980.4
Antidepressants	969.0	E854.0	E939.0	E950.3	E962.0	E980.3
Antidiabetic agents	962.3	E858.0	E932.3	E950.4	E962.0	E980.4
Antidiarrheal agents	973.5	E858.4	E943.5	E950.4	E962.0	E980.4
Antidiuretic hormone	962.5	E858.0	E932.5	E950.4	E962.0	E980.4
Antidotes NEC	977.2	E858.8	E947.2	E950.4	E962.0	E980.4
Antiemetic agents	963.0	E858.1	E933.0	E950.4	E962.0	E980.4
Antiepilepsy agent NEC	966.3	E855.0	E936.3	E950.4	E962.0	E980.4
Antifertility pills	962.2	E858.0	E932.2	E950.4	E962.0	E980.4
Antiflatulents	973.8	E858.4	E943.8	E950.4	E962.0	E980.4
Antifreeze	989.89	E866.8	-	E950.9	E962.1	E980.9
alcohol	980.1	E860.2	-	E950.9	E962.1	E980.9
ethylene glycol	982.8	E862.4	-	E950.9	E962.1	E980.9
Antifungals (nonmedicinal) (sprays)	989.4	E863.6	-	E950.6	E962.1	E980.7
medicinal NEC	961.9	E857	E931.9	E950.4	E962.0	E980.4
antibiotic	960.1	E856	E930.1	E950.4	E962.0	E980.4
topical	976.0	E858.7	E946.0	E950.4	E962.0	E980.4

Fig. 12-8 Section from Table of Drugs and Chemicals. (Data from International Classification of Diseases, 9th Revision. U.S. Department of Health and Human Services, Public Health Service, Centers for Medicare and Medicaid Services.)

What Did You Learn?

1. Name four items that are typically found in the ICD-9-CM introductory pages.
2. List the five appendices of Volume 1, and tell what each contains.
3. How is the Index to Diseases organized?
4. Define an "eponym," and give an example.
5. Name the two tables contained within the Alphabetic Index to Diseases.

PROCESS OF CLASSIFYING DISEASES

Coding involves transforming verbal descriptions of a diagnosis into numbers or a combination of alphanumeric characters. In the insurance and billing department of a medical facility, coding might be done by a professional certified coder; however, in smaller offices, this task may fall under the responsibilities of the health insurance professional. In assuming the latter, the first thing that the health insurance professional must do in the coding process is to locate the diagnosis in the health record. This can be relatively straightforward sometimes because many encounter forms list the more frequently used diagnoses within a certain medical specialty along with their corresponding ICD-9 codes (Fig. 12-10). Other times, the health insurance professional may have to refer back to the clinical notes to locate the diagnosis. If the notes are written, deciphering the healthcare professional's handwriting can sometimes be challenging (Fig. 12-11). With practice and experience, locating the diagnosis within the clinical notes and translating a physician's handwriting become easier.

After the diagnosis has been determined, the health insurance professional should identify the main term within the diagnosis. If the diagnosis is "breast mass," the main term would be "mass." (The anatomic site "breast" is not used in the Alphabetical Index to Diseases.) Figure 12-12 illustrates how the main term "mass" appears in Volume 2.

RAILWAY ACCIDENTS (E800-E807)

Note: For definitions of railway accident and related terms see definitions (a) to (d).

Excludes *accidents involving railway train and:*
aircraft (E840.0-E845.9)
motor vehicle (E810.0-E825.9)
watercraft (E830.0-E838.9)

The following fourth-digit subdivisions are for use with categories E800-E807 to identify the injured person:

.0 Railway employee
Any person who by virtue of his employment in connection with a railway, whether by the railway company or not, is at increased risk of involvement in a railway accident, such as:
catering staff of train
driver
guard
porter
postal staff on train
railway fireman
shunter
sleeping car attendant

.1 Passenger on railway
Any authorized person traveling on a train, except a railway employee.

Excludes *intending passenger waiting at station (8)*
unauthorized rider on railway vehicle (8)

●**E803 Railway accident involving explosion, fire, or burning**
Requires fourth digit. See beginning of section E800-E845 for codes and definitions.

Excludes *explosion or fire, with antecedent derailment (E802.0-E802.9)*
explosion or fire, with mention of antecedent collision (E800.0-E801.9)

●**E804 Fall in, on, or from railway train**
Requires fourth digit. See beginning of section E800-E845 for codes and definitions.

Includes: fall while alighting from or boarding railway train

Excludes *fall related to collision, derailment, or explosion of railway train (E800.0-E803.9)*

●**E805 Hit by rolling stock**
Requires fourth digit. See beginning of section E800-E845 for codes and definitions.

Includes: crushed by railway train or part
injured by railway train or part
killed by railway train or part
knocked down by railway train or part
run over by railway train or part

Excludes *pedestrian hit by object set in motion by railway train (E806.0-E806.9)*

ICD-9-CM E800-E899 Vol. 1

Fig. 12-9 Section from Index to External Causes. (Data from International Classification of Diseases, 9th Revision. U.S. Department of Health and Human Services, Public Health Service, Centers for Medicare and Medicaid Services.)

					Chlamydia / GC Screen	86631	
					Digoxin	80162	
					Dilantin	80185	
DIAGNOSIS: Chk or 1 = Primary		**2 = Secondary**			MSAFP	82105	
Abdominal Pain	789.00	COPD	496	Hypothyroidism	244.9	Pap Smear	88150
Allergies	995.3	CVA, Old	438.9	Long term med use	V58.69	RA	86430
Anemia	285.9	Depression	311	Nasopharyngitis	460	T-4, Free-RIA	84439
Anticoagulation Therapy	V58.61	Dermatitis	692.9	Otitis Media	382.00	Sensitivity	87186
Anxiety	300.00	Diabetes (Non-Insulin)	250.00	Pharyngitis	462	Theophylline	80198
Arthritis	716.90	Diabetes (Insulin-Depend.)	250.01	Physical Exam	V70.0	Urine Culture	87086
Arthritis, degen.	715.90	Dizziness	780.4	Physical, Athletic	V70.3	Cash ☐ Credit Card	INITIALS
Arthritis, Rheumatoid	714.0	Elevated BP	796.2	Physical, Preemployment	V70.5		GSM
Asthma	493.90	Fatigue	780.79	Pneumonia	486	Check # 3204	
Atrial Fibrillation	427.31	Gastroenteritis, viral	008.8	Pregnancy	V22.2		
Backache, unspec.	724.5	Gastroesophageal Reflux	530.81	Routine Child Exam	V20.0	PREVIOUS BALANCE	.00
Bronchitis	490	GYN Exam w/Pap	V72.3	Sinusitis, Acute	461.9		.00
CAD	414.00	Headaches	784.0	Sinusitis, Chronic	473.9	CREDIT BALANCE	
Chest Pain	786.50	Hypercholesterolemia	272.0	Tonsillitis	463	TODAY'S	
CHF	428.0	Hyperlipidemia	272.4	URI	465.9	CHARGES	47.00
Conjunctivitis	372.30	✓ Hypertension, Benign	401.1	UTI	599.0		

OTHER DIAGNOSIS (NOT LISTED)   CODE

PAYMENT ON TODAY'S CHARGES   47.00

PAYMENT ON PREVIOUS BALANCE

OFFICE RETURN
10   15   20   30   40   OTH_____
_____ _____ _____ FU_____
DAYS   WEEKS   MONTHS
WITH: PE

LAB RETURN
DAYS   WEEKS   MONTHS
TESTS:

NEW BALANCE

Fig. 12-10 Portion of an encounter form showing list of diagnoses.

Imagine This!

Marlee Davis, the health insurance professional in Dr. Barnes' office, deciphered one of the physician's handwritten diagnoses as "atrophic arthritis," rather than "aortic arteritis." The error was not caught before the submission of the claim, and the insurance company rejected the claim because the procedures listed on the claim form did not coincide with the diagnosis. When the patient received an explanation of benefits from his insurance carrier that the claim was denied, he phoned the office with a complaint. Marlee had to apologize to the patient and resubmit the CMS-1500 claim form.

Masochism 302.83
Masons' lung 502
Mass
  abdominal 789.3
  anus 787.99
  bone 733.90
  breast 611.72
  cheek 784.2
  chest 786.6
  cystic - *see* Cyst
  ear 388.8
  epigastric 789.3
  eye 379.92
  female genital organ 625.8
  gum 784.2
  head 784.2
  intracranial 784.2
  joint 719.60
    ankle 719.67
    elbow 719.62
    foot 719.67
    hand 719.64
    hip 719.65
    knee 719.66

Fig. 12-12 Section of Volume 2 showing Mass, breast. (Data from International Classification of Diseases, 9th Revision. U.S. Department of Health and Human Services, Public Health Service, Centers for Medicare and Medicaid Services.)

Note the numbers 611.72 following "breast" shown in the portion of Volume 2 in Figure 12-13. This is the 5-digit diagnosis code for breast mass. The number one cardinal rule in coding is *never* to code from the Alphabetic Index (Volume 2) alone. Before assigning this code, it is important to read any special notes or instructions, after which we turn to Volume 1, the Tabular Index, and locate the code 611.72.

● 611.7 Signs and symptoms in breast

611.71 Mastodynia
  Pain in breast

611.72 Lump or mass in breast

❑ 611.79 Other
  Induration of breast
  Inversion of nipple
  Nipple discharge
  Retraction of nipple

❑ 611.8 Other specified disorders of breast
  Hematoma (nontraumatic) of breast
  Infarction of breast
  Occlusion of breast duct
  Subinvolution of breast (postlactational) (postpartum)

❑ 611.9 Unspecified breast disorder

Fig. 12-13 Portion of Volume 2 showing the above code. (Data from International Classification of Diseases, 9th Revision. U.S. Department of Health and Human Services, Public Health Service, Centers for Medicare and Medicaid Services.)

HIPAA Tip

HIPAA requires that ICD-9-CM diagnosis codes be included on all Medicare claims billed to Part B carriers, with the exception of ambulance claims. Providers and suppliers rely on physicians to provide a diagnosis code or narrative diagnostic statement on orders/referrals.

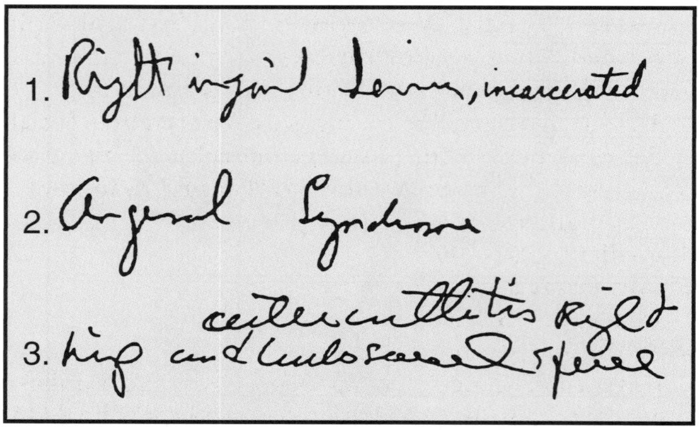

Fig. 12-11 Examples of handwritten diagnoses.

VOLUME 1, THE TABULAR LIST

Volume 1, the Tabular List, comprises 17 sections (Fig. 12-14). These 17 sections represent anatomic systems or types of conditions. The titles describe the content of the section followed by the range of codes in a specific category.

1. Infectious and Parasitic Diseases (001-139)
2. Neoplasms (140-239)
3. Endocrine, Nutritional & Metabolic Diseases & Immunity Disorders (240-279)
4. Diseases of the Blood & Blood-Forming Organs (280-289)
5. Mental Disorders (290-319)
6. Nervous System and Sense Organs (320-389)
7. Diseases of the Circulatory System (390-459)
8. Diseases of the Respiratory System (460-519)
9. Diseases of the Digestive System (520-579)
10. Diseases of the Genitourinary System (580-629)
11. Complications of Pregnancy, Childbirth, and the Puerperium (630-677)
12. Diseases of the Skin & Subcutaneous Tissue (680-709)
13. Diseases of the Musculoskeletal System & Connective Tissue (710-739)
14. Congenital Anomalies (740-759)
15. Certain Conditions Originating in the Perinatal Period (760-779)
16. Symptoms, Signs, and Ill-Defined Conditions (780-799)
17. Injury and Poisoning (800-999)

Fig. 12-14 List of 17 sections in Volume 1.

Organization of Volume 1 Codes

There are three types of codes in Volume 1:

- 3-digit **category** codes (e.g., 220, "benign neoplasm of ovary")
- 4-digit **subcategory** codes (e.g., 370.0, "corneal ulcer")
- 5-digit **subclassification** codes (e.g., 370.00, "corneal ulcer, unspecified")

Study the section of a page from Volume 1 that illustrates these three types of codes (Fig. 12-15).

To clarify further the 4- and 5-digit necessity, let's say that a patient's diagnosis in the health record is *coronary atherosclerosis*. Note in the example shown in Figure 12-16 that the color coding (bullet) of category 414 (other forms of chronic ischemic heart disease) indicates a 4th digit is needed, and the subcategory 414.0 (coronary atherosclerosis) needs a 5th digit to describe the patient's diagnosis

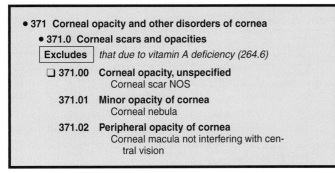

Fig. 12-15 Section of a page from Volume 1 showing 1-, 2-, and 3-digit codes. (Data from International Classification of Diseases, 9th Revision. U.S. Department of Health and Human Services, Public Health Service, Centers for Medicare and Medicaid Services.)

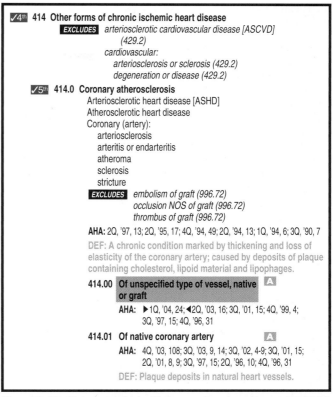

Fig. 12-16 Category 414. (Color codes from Ingenix: 2006 Expert ICD-9-CM, 2006, Ingenix, Eden Prairie.)

to the greatest specificity. It must be determined which of the subclassifications (414.00 through 414.06) best describes the patient's heart condition. If the 4-digit code (414.0) is indicated in Block 21 of the CMS-1500 form, it no doubt would be rejected and returned unpaid because a 5th digit is needed.

Color Coding

Most ICD-9 manuals use color coding in Volume 1 to alert the coder to special edits and other important issues. In the AMA publication, a 4th color-coded notation preceding a 3-digit code category indicates that a 4th digit is required. Other publications use a circle with either a 4 or a 5 inside to indicate additional digits are needed.

Another type of color coding is the age symbols (used in the AMA publication). Age-related color-coded alpha characters are white on a yellow background as follows:

N—newborn age, 0
P—pediatric age, 0-17
M—maternity age, 12-55
A—adult age, 15-124
MSP—Medicare secondary payer

Unspecified Code, Other Specified Code, and Manifestation Code also have special color coding in the AMA ICD-9 manual. Figure 12-17 illustrates how the AMA ICD-

Bottom right
Bottom left

N Newborn Age: 0	P Pediatric Age: 0-17	M Maternity Age: 12-55	A Adult Age: 15-124	MSP Medicare Secondary Payer

16 – Volume 1 *2005 ICD•9•CM*

✓4ᵗʰ ✓5ᵗʰ Additional Digit Required	Unspecified Code	Other Specified Code	Manifestation Code	▶◀ Revised Text	● New Code	▲ Revised Code Title

2005 ICD•9•CM **Volume 1 – 17**

Fig. 12-17 Section at bottom of Volume 1 pages showing color coding notes. (Color codes from Ingenix: 2006 Expert ICD-9-CM, 2006, Ingenix, Eden Prairie.)

9-CM manual uses color coding in Volume 1 to help guide the individual in selecting the right code and coding to the greatest specificity.

Remember: The health insurance professional must *not* use a 3-digit code if a 4-digit code is available and must *not* use a 4-digit code if a 5-digit code is available.

SUPPLEMENTARY SECTIONS OF VOLUME 1
V Codes

The **V Codes**, Supplementary Classification of Factors Influencing Health Status and Contact with Health Services (V01-V83), follow the aforementioned 17 sections. Codes in this section are used when circumstances other than a disease or injury are recorded as a diagnosis or problem. This can appear in the health record as one of three ways:

1. When an individual who is not sick visits the medical facility for a specific purpose, such as donating a tissue sample or to receive a vaccination.
2. When an individual with a known disease or injury comes in for specific treatment for that problem, such as dialysis for kidney disease, chemotherapy for cancer, or a cast change.
3. When a problem is present that influences the individual's health status, but is not, in itself, a current illness or injury. An example is an individual history of a certain disease or an individual who has an artificial heart valve, which may affect his or her present condition.

When the following terms are seen as the diagnosis in a health record, it is usually a clue that a V code is needed:
• Aftercare
• Examination
• Problem with
• Attention to

• Observation
• Screening for
• Admission
• Test(s)
• Vaccination(s)

Some V codes can be used alone, and some require a medical diagnosis from the main ICD-9 sections. Examples of common V code diagnoses include the following:
• Family history of malignant neoplasm
• Health supervision of infant or child
• Normal pregnancy
• Supervision of high-risk pregnancy

E Codes

The Supplementary Classification of External Causes of Injury and Poisoning, referred to as E Codes (codes E800 through E999), follows the section on V Codes. Codes in this section classify external causes of environmental events, circumstances, or conditions that caused the injury, condition, poisoning, or adverse effect being described, such as how an accident occurred or whether a drug overdose was accidental or intentional. Figure 12-18 shows a section from a page in this section to illustrate how codes in this portion of the ICD-9-CM manual are structured.

E codes are never used alone or as the primary diagnosis on a claim. They typically are combined with a code from one of the main chapters of the ICD-9 that indicates the nature of the condition. Healthcare providers usually are not required to assign E codes, unless there is an adverse reaction to a medication that has been taken according to directions. A typical example of this might be as follows:
    780.4 Dizziness due to
    E939.4 Valium, correct dose
Also, some third-party payers prefer that E codes not be used at all on claims. The health insurance professional should contact the carrier or fiscal intermediary to determine if E codes are allowed.

TABLE OF DRUGS AND CHEMICALS / Antibiotics

Substance	Poisoning	External Cause (E-Code)				
		Accident	Therapeutic Use	Suicide Attempt	Assault	Undetermined
Unna's boot	976.3	E858.7	E946.3	E950.4	E962.0	E980.4
Uracil mustard	963.1	E858.1	E933.1	E950.4	E962.0	E980.4
Uramustine	963.1	E858.1	E933.1	E950.4	E962.0	E980.4
Urari	975.2	E858.6	E945.2	E950.4	E962.0	E980.4
Urea	974.4	E858.5	E944.4	E950.4	E962.0	E980.4
topical	976.8	E858.7	E946.8	E950.4	E962.0	E980.4
Urethan(e) (antineoplastic)	963.1	E858.1	E933.1	E950.4	E962.0	E980.4
Urginea (maritima) (scilla) - *see* Squill	—	—	—	—	—	—
pertussis component	978.6	E858.8	E948.6	E950.4	E962.0	E980.4
rickettsial component	979.7	E858.8	E949.7	E950.4	E962.0	E980.4
yellow fever	979.3	E858.8	E949.3	E950.4	E962.0	E980.4
Vaccinia immune globulin (human)	964.6	E858.2	E934.6	E950.4	E962.0	E980.4
Vaginal contraceptives	976.8	E858.7	E946.8	E950.4	E962.0	E980.4
Valethamate	971.1	E855.4	E941.1	E950.4	E962.0	E980.4
Valisone	976.0	E858.7	E946.0	E950.4	E962.0	E980.4
Valium	969.4	E853.2	E939.4	E950.3	E962.0	E980.3
Valmid	967.8	E852.8	E937.8	E950.2	E962.0	E980.2
Vanadium	985.8	E866.4	—	E950.9	E962.1	E980.9
Vancomycin	960.8	E856	E930.8	E950.4	E962.0	E980.4

Fig. 12-18 Section from E code pages. (Data from International Classification of Diseases, 9th Revision. U.S. Department of Health and Human Services, Public Health Service, Centers for Medicare and Medicaid Services.)

The steps for selecting the correct E Code for adverse effects are as follows:

1. Locate the drug in the index on the table of Drugs and Chemicals.
2. Search for the code in the column entitled "Therapeutic Use"
3. Verify the code.
4. Do not use an E Code as the first diagnosis.
5. Note the corresponding code under "Poisoning," and use this as the primary code.

 HIPAA Tip

Always protect the confidentiality of all ICD-9 codes because these codes are part of the patient's record. HIPAA addresses coding issues and sets standards for their use, along with other issues regarding confidentiality in dealing with patient health records.

LOCATING A CODE IN THE TABULAR LIST (VOLUME 1)

Codes in Volume 1 are arranged numerically, so they are relatively easy to find. Use the numerical range descriptors at the top corners of each page to narrow down your search (Fig. 12-19). First, locate the 3-digit code that defines the category. Using the breast mass example, this would be 611, "other disorders of breast." The color coding indicates that a 4th digit is required for each subcategory. Read down through the subcategory entries until 611.7 is found, "signs and symptoms in breast." Note that a 5th digit is required. Locate the subclassification entry 611.72, "lump or mass in breast." If no other notes, symbols, or special editing codes are shown, it can be reasonable to assume that this diagnosis has been coded to its greatest specificity (Fig. 12-20).

What Did You Learn?

1. Briefly explain what coding involves.
2. List and identify the 17 main sections in Volume 1.
3. List and give an example of the three types of codes in the 17 sections of Volume 1.
4. What is the purpose of color coding?
5. Give four examples of common V Code diagnoses.
6. When are E codes used?

CONVENTIONS USED IN ICD-9-CM

The conventions used in Volumes 1 and 2 of the ICD-9 manual include abbreviations, punctuation, symbols,

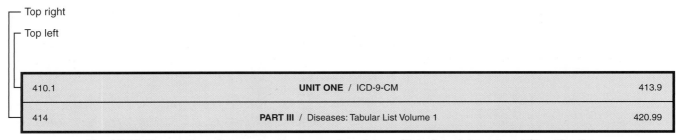

Top right

Top left

410.1	UNIT ONE / ICD-9-CM	413.9
414	PART III / Diseases: Tabular List Volume 1	420.99

Fig. 12-19 Top portion of page showing range descriptors. (Data from International Classification of Diseases, 9th Revision. U.S. Department of Health and Human Services, Public Health Service, Centers for Medicare and Medicaid Services.)

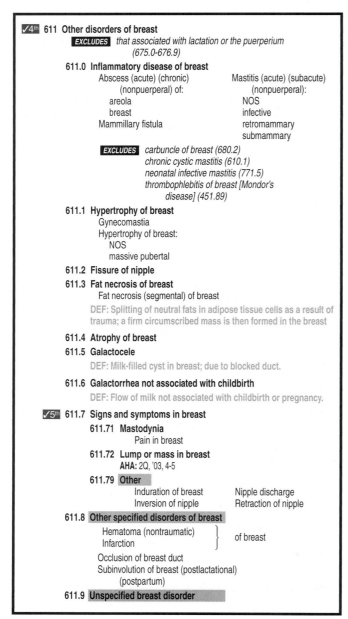

Fig. 12-20 Section of ICD-9 showing the above. (Color codes from Ingenix: 2006 Expert ICD-9-CM, 2006, Ingenix, Eden Prairie.)

footnotes, and other instructional notes. Many of these conventions are used in all three volumes; however, some are used only in Volumes 1 and 2. Although each publication typically has its own special list of conventions, the ones discussed subsequently are the ones used in the AMA publication and are basically the same as those used in the government's official version. Codes on health insurance forms must conform to the standards that are published in the *Federal Register*. The *Federal Register* is a daily publication that provides a uniform system for publishing federal regulations, legal notices, presidential proclamations, and executive orders. See Websites to Explore at the end of this chapter for the *Federal Register* website. To code accurately, the health insurance professional must understand what each of these elements means (Fig. 12-21).

● Stop and Think

Marlee, the health insurance professional in Dr. Ferris Barnes' office, was searching for a particular code in the ICD-9, when she noticed a blackened triangle (▲) in front of the diagnosis code that she sought. What does this symbol indicate to Marlee?

TYPEFACES

The AMA (and other publications) ICD-9-CM manual varies the format of the type to indicate other conventions, as follows:
- *Boldface:* Boldface type is used for main terms in the Alphabetic Index (Volume 2) and all codes and titles in the tabular list.
- *Italics:* Italicized type is used for all exclusion notes and to identify codes that should not be used for describing the primary diagnosis.

Examples of these two typeface formats are shown in Figure 12-22.

INSTRUCTIONAL NOTES

In addition to abbreviations, punctuation, and symbols, the ICD-9 uses instructional notes to help the health insurance professional further choose the correct code (Fig. 12-23).

What Did You Learn?

1. What is the function and purpose of boldface type?
2. What does NOS mean?
3. What does it mean when a colon (:) is used?
4. What does the bullet symbol (●) preceding a code indicate?
5. What does italicized type indicate?

ESSENTIAL STEPS TO DIAGNOSTIC CODING

Now that the basic background for ICD-9 coding has been presented, let's look at the essential steps of diagnostic coding.

1. Locate the diagnosis in the patient's health record (or on the encounter form).
2. Determine the "main term" of the stated diagnosis.
3. Find the main term in the Alphabetic Index (Volume 2) of the most recent version of the ICD-9-CM manual.
4. Read and apply any notes or instructions contained in the Alphabetic Index. *Reminder: Never code directly from the Alphabetic Index.*
5. Cross-reference the code found in the Alphabetic Index (Volume 2) to the Tabular List (Volume 1).
6. Read and be guided by the conventions and symbols, paying close attention to any footnotes or cross-references.
7. Read through the entire category, and code to the *highest level of specificity,* taking special care to assign a 4th or 5th digit to the code if the color coding indicates it is necessary.

Refer to Box 12-1 for a list of ICD-9 coding compliance tips. In addition, the AMA has published "The Ten Commandments of Diagnosis Coding," which are shown in Box 12-2.

NEC	**Not elsewhere classifiable.** NEC tells the coder that a specified form of the listed condition is classified differently. The category number for the term including NEC is to be used only when the coder lacks the information necessary to code to a more specific category. 244.8 **Other specified acquired hypothyroidism** Secondary hypothyroidism NEC

NOS	**Not otherwise specified.** This abbreviation is the equivalent of "unspecified" and is used only when there is not enough information available to code to a more specific, 4-digit subcategory.
	
	✔4th **410 Acute myocardial infarction**
	
	✔5th **410.1 Of other anterior wall**
	                Infarction (wall) ⎫ NOS with contiguous portion
	                anterior ⎭ of intraventricular septum

[ ]	**Square brackets are used to enclose synonyms, alternative terminology, or explanatory phrases.** They may appear within code descriptions or within instructional notes.
	
	✔4th **483 Pneumonia due to other specified organism**
	
	        483.0 Mycoplasma pneumoniae
	                Eaton's agent
	                Pleuropneumonia-like organism [PPLO]

( )	**Parentheses enclose supplementary words, called *nonessential modifiers*** that serve as guides in finding the correct code. These words may or may not be present in the narrative description of a disease and do not affect the code assignment.
	
	✔4th **626 Disorders of menstruation and other abnormal bleeding from female genital tract**
	
	        626.0 Absence of menstruation
	                Amenorrhea (primary) (secondary)

Fig. 12-21 List of conventions and symbols.

:	A colon is used in the tabular list after an incomplete term that needs one or more modifiers to make it a complete statement. (An exception to this rule pertains to the abbreviated NOS.)
	
	✔4th **415 Acute Pulmonary Heart Disease**
	
	    ✔5th **415.1 Pulmonary embolism and infarction**
	        Pulmonary (artery) (vein):
	          apoplexy
	          embolism
	          infarction (hemorrhagic)
	          thrombosis

{ }	Braces are used to connect a series of terms to a common step. Each term to the left of the brace is incomplete and must be completed by a term to the right of the brace.
	
	✔4th **Arthropathy associated with infections**
	
	  Includes arthritis associated with
	              arthropathy conditions
	              polyarthritis classifiable
	              polyarthropathy below

§	When the section mark (§) precedes a code, it indicates there is a footnote on the page. The section mark is only used in the Tabular List (Volume 1). § ✔4th **E812 Other motor vehicle traffic accident involving collision with motor vehicle** The footnote indicates that this code requires a fourth-digit. See beginning of section E810-E819 for codes and definitions.
•	This symbol is referred to as a "bullet." The bullet indicates that the code is new to this revision of the ICD-9. The 2003 ICD-9 added several new E-codes associated with terrorism.
▲	A triangle in the Tabular List (Vol. 1) indicates that the code title is revised. In the Alphabetic Index (Vol. 2), the triangle indicates that a code has been changed.
► ◄	These "sideways triangles" appear at the beginning and end of a section of new or revised text. The right-facing triangle appears at the beginning of the text; the left-facing one at the end.

Fig. 12-21—cont'd

What Did You Learn?

1. List the seven essential steps of diagnostic coding.
2. What should the health insurance professional do if he or she thinks a diagnosis documented in a health record can be worded better?

SPECIAL CODING SITUATIONS

CODING SIGNS AND SYMPTOMS

If a patient's condition has not been specifically diagnosed, the health insurance professional must code the signs or symptoms. Section 16 of the ICD-9 (codes 780 through 799) contains a list of codes classifying symptoms, signs, abnormal results of laboratory tests or other investigative procedures, and ill-defined conditions for which no diagnosis classifiable elsewhere is recorded. Some common examples of signs and symptoms include

• dizziness,
• fever,
• insomnia,
• nausea,
• shortness of breath, and
• headache

If a patient visits the medical facility with the chief complaint of nausea, but the healthcare provider has not yet determined what is causing the nausea, the code for nausea must be used. Looking in the Alphabetic Index (Volume 1) under "nausea," we find 787.02 for nausea

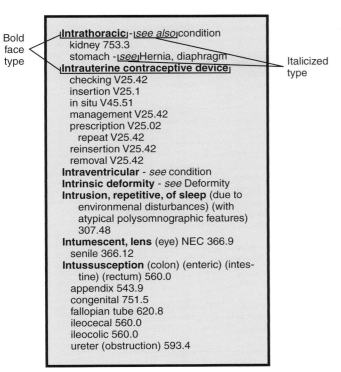

Bold face type

Italicized type

Intrathoracic - *see also* condition
   kidney 753.3
   stomach - *see* Hernia, diaphragm
Intrauterine contraceptive device
   checking V25.42
   insertion V25.1
   in situ V45.51
   management V25.42
   prescription V25.02
     repeat V25.42
   reinsertion V25.42
   removal V25.42
Intraventricular - *see* condition
Intrinsic deformity - *see* Deformity
Intrusion, repetitive, of sleep (due to
   environmenal disturbances) (with
   atypical polysomnographic features)
   307.48
Intumescent, lens (eye) NEC 366.9
   senile 366.12
Intussusception (colon) (enteric) (intestine) (rectum) 560.0
   appendix 543.9
   congenital 751.5
   fallopian tube 620.8
   ileocecal 560.0
   ileocolic 560.0
   ureter (obstruction) 593.4

Fig. 12-22 Example of boldface and italicized type. (Data from International Classification of Diseases, 9th Revision. U.S. Department of Health and Human Services, Public Health Service, Centers for Medicare and Medicaid Services.)

without vomiting and 787.01 for nausea with vomiting. Cross-referencing to the Tabular Index, we first locate the 3-digit category: "787, symptoms involving digestive system." Reading down through the subcategory and subclassification sections, note that 5 digits are needed. For accurate coding, it must be determined if the patient has nausea with vomiting, nausea alone, or vomiting alone. This should be documented in the clinical notes. If the clinical notes are nonspecific as to whether or not there is vomiting, it should be assumed there is not vomiting unless it is documented.

ETIOLOGY AND MANIFESTATION CODING

When the notation "code first underlying disease" is seen, this indicates that the etiology (cause or origin of the disease) is coded before the **manifestation** (sign or symptom of the disease). If the patient's diagnosis is diabetic ulcer of the heel, the disease process (diabetes) is coded first before the heel ulcer.

PROBABLE, QUESTIONABLE, RULE OUT, OR SUSPECTED CONDITIONS

Choosing the most specific code means coding only what is *known to be a fact and documented* in the health record.

Patients often have ill-defined complaints, such as back pain. Although the healthcare provider may suspect a specific condition—perhaps a herniated disk or a urinary tract infection—and order laboratory tests to confirm the diagnosis, the health insurance professional should code *only the sign or symptom* that brought the patient to the office until test results or other diagnostic procedures lead to a definitive diagnosis. If the suspected condition is diagnosed as such, it may inadvertently label the patient with an incorrect diagnosis, and as a result the patient may have difficulty obtaining health and disability insurance or may end up paying higher insurance premiums in the future. Use ICD-9 codes 780 to 789 to describe symptoms, signs, and ill-defined conditions that are not linked to a specific disease.

● Stop and Think

Lonny Chadwick noticed a suspicious-looking mole on his lower right leg and went to his dermatologist. Lonny's father died of malignant melanoma, and Lonny was concerned that his mole also was malignant. The dermatologist examined the mole and removed a section of tissue for a biopsy. When the biopsy results were returned, the laboratory report stated that the tissue sample was "abnormal, but inconclusive." Documentation in Mr. Chadwick's health record noted the fact that his father had died of malignant melanoma. The diagnosis stated "suspicious lesion, lower right leg, rule out melanoma." Subsequently, the health insurance professional submitted the claim with the diagnosis of "melanoma." What problems might arise from this incorrect coding process?

Imagine This!

Referring back to Lonny Chadwick (the patient with the suspicious lesion on his lower leg), when the health insurance professional resubmitted the claim, she used the V code V10.82. Mr. Chadwick's insurance carrier returned it stating they do not pay based on V codes. Subsequently, the claim had to be corrected and resubmitted a second time with the appropriate ICD-9 code. As a result of the two incorrectly coded claims, reimbursement for Mr. Chadwick's procedure took nearly 3 months.

INCLUDES	The instructional note INCLUDES further defines or clarifies the content of the category, subcategory, or subclassification.
EXCLUDES	Terms following the instructional note **EXCLUDES** are not classified to the category, subcategory, or specific subclassification code under which it is found. The note may also provide the location of the excluded diagnosis.
Use additional code	When this note appears, an additional code(s) must be used to provide a more complete description of the diagnosis.
Code first underlying disease	This italicized note indicates that the description given should not be used for coding the primary diagnosis. The italicized notation is followed by the code(s) for the most common underlying disease. These codes, referred to as manifestation codes, should not be used alone or indicated as the primary diagnosis (i.e., sequenced first). They must always be preceded by another code. Record the code for the primary disease first, and then record the italicized manifestation code
Unspecified Code	In the AMA ICD-9, these codes are highlighted yellow: Unspecified Code Use these codes only when neither the diagnostic statement nor the documentation provides enough information to assign a more specific code. (Note: Check with the carrier or FI to see if unspecified codes are acceptable on the claim form.)
Code, if applicable, any causal condition first	A code with this notation may be principal if no causal condition is applicable or known.
"And" and "with"	"and" means and/or; "with" indicates another condition is included in the code.

Fig. 12-23 Example of boldface and italicized type. (Color codes from Ingenix: 2006 Expert ICD-9-CM, 2006, Ingenix, Eden Prairie.)

Box 12-1

ICD-9 Coding Compliance Tips

1. Maintain access to and be versed in federal, state, and private payer requirements.
2. Review medical documentation to ensure the health record supports the codes selected to avoid claim denials.
3. Use only the most recent ICD-9 coding manual.
4. Conduct self-audits of coded claims.
5. When updates occur, perform audits to identify invalid or old codes, avoiding potential claim rejection problems.
6. Avoid abbreviated coding "cheat sheets," which can cause improper coding.
7. Do not code based on assumptions. Never assume that because a patient is receiving a specific treatment or is on a certain medication that the diagnosis must always be the same.
8. Never alter documentation. Making changes because something sounds "better" could lead to serious problems in the future. Always check with the healthcare professional when questions arise regarding documentation, and always document the discussion for any changes made to the claim.
9. Know all qualified and licensed personnel. Establish procedures to ensure that everyone has the qualifications they should have and renew their licenses on time.
10. Review all claims rejected because of improper coding. This step should be done by an experienced coder and should be part of a medical facility's internal coding practices.
11. Recognize and use the official HIPAA Guidelines in coding.

Imagine This!

Jane Thiele went to an ophthalmologist for a routine eye examination. After the examination, she went to the reception area to pay the $150 charge. "I know my insurance won't pay for routine exams, so I'll just write you a check today," Jane told the medical receptionist. "Oh, don't worry," the receptionist replied, "Dr. Packston often finds a way to help people out, so why don't you just wait to pay." Jane was surprised and pleased when a few weeks later she received a check from her insurance company for 80% of the charge. A few years later, Jane took early retirement from her job. Because of the high cost of converting her group insurance to a COBRA policy, she applied for less costly private insurance coverage. While Jane was in the process of applying for a private policy, she was told that any problems with her eyes would not be covered. When she asked why, she was told that her medical records from Dr. Packston had indicated a diagnosis of "early cataract," which was not the case at all. Because the new insurance policy excludes all procedures involving eyes, owing to Dr. Packston's diagnosis, Jane either will have to pay for any medical services involving her eyes if problems develop or will have to pay a much higher premium for total coverage.

COMBINATION CODES

A **combination code** is used when more than one otherwise individually classified disease is combined with another disease and one code is assigned for both, or when a single code is used to describe conditions that frequently occur together. An example of this is the code 034.0, "streptococcal sore throat," because a sore throat is often caused by the streptococci bacteria. If a patient has hypertensive heart and renal disease, these conditions are combined under one code (category 404), rather than assigning codes from the 402 and 403 categories.

CODING NEOPLASMS

A neoplasm results when abnormal cells grow uncontrollably, usually resulting in a tumor. Neoplasms may be classified as
• benign,
• malignant,
• **in situ** (confined to the site of origin without invasion),
• uncertain behavior, or
• unspecified behavior.
The anatomic site of the neoplasm may be the organ or area of the body where the tumor originated (primary) or the organ or area of the body where the tumor has spread (secondary).

To code neoplasms, first find the main term in the Alphabetic Index (Neoplasm Table). Using "fibroadenoma of the breast" as an example, assign the correct code using the following steps:

1. Locate the main term ("fibroadenoma") in the Alphabetic Index (Volume 2, Neoplasm Table, "by site, benign").
2. We know the site, so we cross-reference to the Neoplasm Table.
3. Locate the anatomic site (listed alphabetically).
4. If there is no additional information available, the code is 217.

If a detailed diagnosis is given, such as "malignant adenoma of the colon, primary," the resulting code is more specific:

1. Locate the main term ("adenoma") in the Alphabetic Index. (See also "neoplasm, by site, benign.")
2. Cross-reference to the Neoplasm Table.
3. Cross-reference "colon" to "intestine, intestinal, large, colon."
4. Assign the correct code under the "malignant, primary" column heading (153.9).

V codes are sometimes used if there is a family or personal history of malignant neoplasms.

CODING HYPERTENSION

One of the most common conditions coded is that of hypertension (high blood pressure). If a patient has a documented diagnosis of "hypertension, essential, benign," the steps to follow for coding this condition are as follows:

1. Locate the main term "hypertension" in the Alphabetic Index.
2. Note the three column headings in the Table: "malignant," "benign," and "unspecified."
3. The various terms in parentheses (nonessential modifiers) listed behind the main terms in boldface type (hypertension, hypertensive) include the word "essential."
4. Because "essential" is a nonessential modifier included under main term category, cross-reference it to the "benign" column.
5. Assign the code 401.1.

What Did You Learn?

1. List four common examples of signs and symptoms.
2. Which should be coded first, the etiology or the manifestation?
3. What is a combination code?
4. Compare a "primary" neoplasm site with a "secondary" site.

Box 12-2

AMA's "The Ten Commandments of Diagnosis Coding": An Irreverent Summary of Rules with Practical Coding Hints

I. The largest number of digits wins.
    Do not report three if there are four; do not report four if there are five.
II. Numeric codes win over alphanumeric.
    If the code is listed twice, once with a letter and once with all numbers, use the one with all numbers, if possible.
III. Watch out for punctuation.
    Do not even think it. Do not think "427 point 0" or 250 point 00." These codes are 4270 and 25000. Many claim form scanners and electronic claim programs cannot process the punctuation mark.
IV. Use only the codes related to the services performed.
    A patient with acute bronchitis and heart disease is seen for the bronchitis. The chart indicates it is time for an electrocardiogram. If you code the electrocardiogram for bronchitis, it may not pay. With Medicare, it could result in a "not medically necessary" rejection.
V. Diagnosis coding does not increase the payment; it only allows it.
VI. Do not code in greater specificity than the information provided.
    Do not code "rule out" and "suspected" as if the condition existed. The patient is seen because she thinks she broke her hand. Code "pain" or "contusion" if the x-ray does not confirm the fracture.
VII. Neoplasms are always benign, unless stated to be malignant. If malignant, they are always primary, unless stated to be secondary or in situ.
    Some lesion codes are general; others are found in the neoplasm table. When using the table, be certain to select the correct column and verify that code with the Tabular List. Do not give the patient something he or she does not have.
VIII. Always verify codes selected from the Alphabetic Index with the Tabular List.
IX. Diagnosis codes in the Tabular List, in italics, cannot be used as the primary diagnosis.
    These codes are listed as "excludes" or "code also the underlying disease." Be certain the correct code is selected and verified.
X. Sometimes the best diagnosis code is going to be the one that is least incorrect.

HIPAA AND CODING

Code sets for medical data are required for data elements in the administrative and financial healthcare transaction standards adopted under Health Insurance Portability and Accountability Act (HIPAA) for diagnoses, procedures, and drugs. Under HIPAA, a **code set** is any set of codes used for encoding data elements, such as tables of terms, medical concepts, medical diagnosis codes, or medical procedure codes. Medical data code sets used in the healthcare industry include coding systems for

- diseases, impairments, other health-related problems, and their manifestations;
- causes of injury, disease, impairment, or other health-related problems;
- actions taken to prevent, diagnose, treat, or manage diseases, injuries, and impairments; and
- any substances, equipment, supplies, or other items used to perform these actions.

 HIPAA Tip

Although the HIPAA requirements apply only to electronic claims, to maintain consistency in claims processing, CMS has mandated that ICD-9-CM requirements be applied to paper claims and electronic claims.

CODE SETS ADOPTED AS HIPAA STANDARDS

The following code sets have been adopted as the standard medical data code sets:

- ICD-9-CM, Volumes 1 and 2 (including *The Official ICD-9-CM Guidelines for Coding and Reporting*), as updated and distributed by the Department of Health and Human Services (HHS), for the following conditions:

Diseases

Injuries

Impairments

Other health-related problems and their manifestations

Causes of injury, disease, impairment, or other health-related problems

- ICD-9-CM, Volume 3 Procedures (including *The Official ICD-9-CM Guidelines for Coding and Reporting*), as updated and distributed by HHS, for the following procedures or other actions taken for diseases, injuries, and impairments in hospital inpatients reported by hospitals:

Prevention

Diagnosis

Treatment

Management.

- National Drug Codes, as updated and distributed by HHS, in collaboration with drug manufacturers, for certain drugs and biologics.
- Codes on Dental Procedures and Nomenclature, as updated and distributed by the American Dental Association, for dental services.
- The combination of CMS (formerly known as Health Care Financing Administration) *Common Procedure Coding System* (HCPCS), as updated and distributed by HHS, and *Current Procedural Terminology, 4rth Edition* (CPT-4), as updated and distributed by the AMA, for physician services and other health-related services. These services include, but are not limited to, the following:

Physician services

Physical and occupational therapy services

Radiologic procedures

Clinical laboratory tests

Other medical diagnostic procedures

Hearing and vision services

Transportation services including ambulance

- The HCPCS, as updated and distributed by CMS and HHS, for all other substances, equipment, supplies, or other items used in healthcare services. These items include, but are not limited to, the following:

Medical supplies

Orthotic and prosthetic devices

Durable medical equipment

HCPCS LEVEL 3 CODES

HCPCS Level 3 codes are known as local codes. Under the intent of HIPAA, the Level 3 codes were to be eliminated; however, some payers still require Level 3 codes for payment and reimbursement. As always, if questions arise, contact your local carrier or fiscal intermediary for guidelines for using Level 3 codes.

☑ HIPAA Tip

HIPAA compliant claims cannot contain ICD-9 Volume 3 procedure codes on claims submitted by physicians' offices.

What Did You Learn?

1. Explain what a "code set" is under HIPAA.
2. List the standard code sets adopted by HIPAA.

ICD-10

WHO typically releases an updated version of the ICD manual approximately every 10 years. The *International Classification of Diseases, 10th Revision* (ICD-10) was issued in three volumes from 1992 to 1994 and is now being used in some parts of the world. The intent of this revision was to address some of the problems that had been identified in the current ICD-9 and to improve classification of mortality and morbidity data.

ICD-10 provides increased clinical detail and addresses information regarding previously classified diseases and new diseases discovered since the ninth revision. Conditions are grouped according to those most appropriate for general epidemiologic purposes and the evaluation of healthcare. Although the format and conventions of the classification remain, for the most part, unchanged, ICD-10 differs from ICD-9-CM in the following ways:

- ICD-10 is printed in a three-volume set compared with the physician's ICD-9 two-volume set.
- ICD-10 has alphanumeric categories rather than numeric categories.
- Some chapters have been rearranged, some titles have changed, and conditions have been regrouped.
- ICD-10 has almost twice as many categories as ICD-9.
- Some fairly minor changes have been made in the coding rules for mortality.

THREE VOLUMES OF ICD-10

Volume 1, the Tabular List

The first volume (which is more than 1000 pages) contains the classification at the three-character and four-character levels, the classification of the morphology of neoplasms, special tabulation lists for mortality and morbidity, definitions, and the nomenclature regulations. The volume also reproduces the report of the International Conference for the Tenth Revision, which indicates the many complex considerations behind the revisions.

Volume 2, Instruction Manual

The second volume consolidates notes on certification and classification formerly included in Volume 1, supplemented by a great deal of new background information, instructions, and guidelines for users of the tabular list. Historical information about the development of the classification, which dates back to 1893, also is included.

Volume 3, Alphabetical Index

The final volume presents the detailed alphabetical index. Expanded introductory material is complemented by practical advice on how to make the best use of the index. To facilitate efficient coding, the index includes numerous diagnostic terms commonly used as synonyms for the terms officially accepted for use in the classification.

Hard copy and electronic versions of the three-volume set of ICD-10 are available through the WHO Publications Center USA. There is also an ICD-10 homepage at the WHO website.

ICD-10-PCS

The International Classification of Diseases 10th Revision Procedure Classification System (ICD-10-PCS) has been developed as a replacement for Volume 3 of the ICD-9. The CMS has developed a training manual that can be downloaded and reviewed using the Adobe Acrobat System. (See Websites to Explore at the end of this chapter for the URL.)

IMPLEMENTATION OF ICD-10

Revisions have been made to the initial version of ICD-10-CM based on the comments received from reviewers. An updated edition of ICD-10-CM was made available in late 2003 for public viewing. As of this writing, however, the codes in ICD-10-CM are not currently valid for any purpose or uses. Testing of ICD-10-CM will occur using this pre-release version. It is anticipated that updates to this draft will occur before implementation of ICD-10-CM.

No deadline has been established as yet for the mandatory use of the ICD-10 in the United States. Implementation will be based on the process for adoption of standards under HIPAA. There will be a 2-year implementation window when the final notice to implement has been published in the *Federal Register*. In the meantime, it might be prudent to download and view a version of this manual for the purpose of keeping up with coming changes in diagnostic coding.

What Did You Learn?

1. What is the intent of the ICD-10 revision?
2. List three ways ICD-10 differs from ICD-9.
3. Name the three volumes of ICD-10.
4. What does the ICD-10-PCS replace?
5. What date has been established for the mandatory use of ICD-10 codes in the United States?

SUMMARY CHECK POINTS

☑ Diagnostic coding got its start in 17th century England. In 1948, WHO developed and published a listing of morbidity and mortality statistics that eventually evolved into what is now known as the ICD. This publication is now in its ninth revision (ICD-9). The U.S. National Center for Health Statistics modified the ICD further, providing a way to use these data for indexing medical information, which precisely describes every patient's clinical picture (diagnosis). This revised version, by adding these *clinical modifications*, resulted in the ICD-9-CM. The CMS adopted the ICD-9-CM in 1988 and mandated that this coding system be used on all Medicare Part B claims. Today, most third-party payers also require ICD-9-CM diagnostic codes on health insurance claims.

☑ The ICD-9-CM manual comprises three volumes: Volume 1, the Tabular List; Volume 2, the Alphabetic List; and Volume 3, Inpatient Procedural Coding. (Typically, Volumes 1 and 2 are combined into one book.) Although there are various publications available, most follow a similar format. The first several pages of the manual consist of an introduction, providing a guide for using the ICD-9. The following sections complete the format:
   • Volume 2, the Index to Diseases
   • Volume 1, the Tabular List
   • Appendix A, Morphology of Neoplasms
   • Appendix B, Glossary of Mental Disorders
   • Appendix C, Classification of Drugs by American Hospital Formulary Service List
   • Appendix D, Industrial Accidents According to Agency
   • Appendix E, Three-Digit Categories (Infectious and Parasitic Diseases)

☑ Volume 2, the Alphabetic Index (typically presented before Volume 1, the Tabular List) contains three separate sections (indexes). The first section, the Index to Diseases, contains diagnostic terms for illnesses, injuries, and reasons for encounters with healthcare professionals. Within this section are two tables—the Hypertension Table and the Neoplasm Table. Section 2 contains the Table of Drugs and Chemicals, and Section 3 is the Alphabetic Index to External Causes of Injury and Poisoning.

☑ Main terms consist of diseases, conditions, nouns, adjectives, and eponyms. (Anatomic sites are not considered main terms in diagnostic coding.) Main terms are printed alphabetically in boldface type in Volume 2. The health insurance professional first must determine the main term within a clinical diagnosis and locate that term in the Index to Diseases. Some conditions can be found in more than one place. Obstetric main terms can be found under the name of the condition and under individual entries, such as delivery, pregnancy, and puerperal.

☑ Modifiers are words added to main terms that supply more specific information about the patient's clinical picture. *Essential* modifiers are the indented terms listed under a main term. They describe different anatomic sites, etiology, and clinical types. To be considered essential, a modifier must be a part of the documented diagnosis. *Nonessential* modifiers are terms in parentheses immediately following a main term. They give alternate terminology and are provided simply to assist the health insurance professional in locating the correct main term. Nonessential modifiers usually are not part of the documented diagnostic statement.

☑ ICD-9-CM uses a variety of coding conventions, which include abbreviations, punctuation, symbols, typefaces, footnotes, and other instructional notes. It is important that the health insurance professional understand what each one means because each has a significant impact on the process of accurate coding. The ultimate goal of coding is to "code to the greatest level of specificity." Coding conventions provide a means for accomplishing this goal by guiding the coder through this intricate process.

☑ Volume 1, the Tabular List, comprises 17 sections plus a section listing V Codes (Supplementary Classification of Factors Influencing Health Status and Contact with Health Services) followed by the section containing E codes (Supplementary Classification of External Causes of Injury and Poisoning). Five appendices, A through E, complete Volume 1. There are three types of codes used in the main part of Volume 1: 3-digit codes, 4-digit codes, and 5-digit codes. Codes are organized first by category (3-digit codes), then by subcategory (4-digit codes), and finally by subclassification (5-digit codes). The health insurance professional must follow all notes and conventions and code to the greatest level of specificity to ensure accurate coding. A 3-digit code must not be used if a 4-digit or 5-digit code more precisely describes the patient's diagnosis.

☑ The essential steps in accurate diagnostic coding are as follows:
- Step 1—Locate the diagnosis in the patient's health record (or on the encounter form).
- Step 2—Determine the "main term" of the stated diagnosis.
- Step 3—Find the main term in the Alphabetic Index (Volume 2) of the most recent version of ICD-9-CM.
- Step 4—Read and apply any notes or instructions contained in the Alphabetic Index. *Remember: Never code directly from the Alphabetic Index.*
- Step 5—Cross-reference the code found in the Alphabetic Index (Volume 2) to the Tabular List (Volume 1).
- Step 6—Read and be guided by the conventions and symbols, paying close attention to any footnotes or cross-references.
- Step 7—Read through the entire category and code to the *highest level of specificity*, taking special care to assign a fourth or fifth digit to the code if the color coding indicates it is needed.

☑ ICD-10 was issued in three volumes from 1992 to 1994 and is now being used in some parts of the world. The intent of this revision was to correct some of the problems contained in the ICD-9 and to improve classification of mortality and morbidity data. It is published in three volumes: Volume 1, the Tabular List; Volume 2, the Instruction Manual; and Volume 3, the Alphabetic Index. Although the format and conventions remain basically the same, the major differences (in addition to those already mentioned) include the following:
- ICD-10 has alphanumeric categories rather than numeric categories.
- Some chapters have been rearranged, some titles have changed, and conditions have been regrouped.
- ICD-10 has almost twice as many categories as ICD-9.

CLOSING SCENARIO

Park Chalmers found this introductory chapter on ICD-9-CM coding extremely interesting; he was convinced coding would meet his need for a challenging and meaningful career. Park thought he needed a "structured" approach to learning, and the clear-cut steps to coding enhanced his ability to comprehend the process. After completing the chapter on ICD-9-CM coding, Park decided that his search for a meaningful career might be over. With a career in coding, he could realize both of his goals—a challenging career and an opportunity to work in the field of medicine. Although becoming a health insurance professional was not the same as becoming a doctor, the anticipation of becoming an expert in insurance and coding spurred Park on, and he already was looking forward to the next chapter.

WEBSITES TO EXPLORE

For live links to the following websites, please visit the Evolve® site at http://evolve.elsevier.com/Beik/today/

- Central Office for ICD-9-CM website:
  http://www.icd-9-cm.org/

- Information abut the *Federal Register* and how the documentation found in the *Federal Register* affects the coding process can be found on their website at http://www.archives.gov/federal-register/

- For more information on ICD-10, log on to http://www.who.int/en/ and use "ICD-10" as your search word

- For more information about the HIPAA standardized code sets, search the following websites:
  http://cms.hhs.gov
  http://www.fda.gov/cder/ndc/index.htm

- The American Association of Medical Assistants (AAMA) website provides information about coding in the medical office and details about various educational workshops pertaining to this subject:
  http://www.aama-natl.org/

- For information on becoming a certified professional coder, log on to the American Academy of Professional Coders website:
  http://www.aapc.com/

Chapter 13

Procedural, Evaluation and Management and HCPCS Coding

Chapter Outline

CHAPTER OBJECTIVES

After completion of this chapter, the student should be able to

- Discuss the purpose and development of the CPT-4 Manual.
- Explain the format of CPT.
- Interpret the symbols used in CPT.
- Explain the significance of the semicolon in CPT.
- List the basic steps in CPT coding.
- Differentiate between a "new" and "established" patient in E & M coding.
- List and explain the three key components that establish the level in E & M coding.
- Name the four contributing factors that can affect the level of E & M coding.
- Explain how time can be measured in E & M coding.
- Compare and contrast the main differences in the 1995 versus 1997 E & M documentation guidelines.
- Explain the HCPCS coding system.
- Discuss HIPAA's requirements in relation to standardizing procedural coding.

CHAPTER TERMS

category
Category III codes
Centers for Medicare and Medicaid Services (CMS)
chief complaint (CC)
concurrent care
consultation
counseling
critical care
crosswalk
emergency care
established patient
Evaluation and Management (E & M) codes
face-to-face time
HCFA's Common Procedure Coding System (HCPCS)
HCPCS codes
Health Care Financing Administration (HCFA)
history of present illness (HPI)
indented code
inpatient
key components

Level I (codes)
Level II (codes)
Level III (codes)
modifier
modifying term
neonates
new patient
observation
outpatient
past, family, and social history (PFSH)
Physicians' Current Procedural Terminology, 4th Edition (CPT-4)
Physicians' Current Procedural Terminology, 5th Edition (CPT-5)
review of systems (ROS)
section
see
special report
stand-alone code
subheading
subjective information
subsection
unit/floor time

OPENING SCENARIO

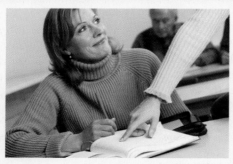

Park Chalmers found that ICD-9 coding met his needs for a chance at a challenging career and his desire to work in the medical field. He hoped that he also would find CPT coding to his liking. Melanie Sanders, another student in Park's medical insurance class, had struggled with diagnostic coding, and she confessed to Park that the chapter on CPT intimidated her. "If I don't get this coding stuff," Melanie confided to Park, "I'm going to have to drop the course." Melanie is not interested in becoming a professional coder—her career goal is to work in the clinical side of medical assisting. "I don't know why I have to know this stuff anyway," she tells Park, "I won't have to deal with coding once I've finished the program."

"Being familiar with all facets of administrative work in the medical office, including billing, insurance, and coding, makes you more employable," Park reminded her. "For instance, if you and one other applicant are competing for a job, and you know how to code, but the other individual doesn't, you'd have the edge. If you stick with it, I'll help you," Park promised.

Park gave Melanie an important tip: "The secret to coding is in its structure. There is a very systematic method for finding the appropriate code," he explained. "The most important thing is to follow the steps outlined in the chapter, and *never* code from the Alphabetic Index alone." Melanie, encouraged by Park's positive outlook toward coding and his pledge to help her, decides to give coding a second chance. With Park's help, she determined that perhaps she could understand CPT coding well enough to pass the course.

OVERVIEW OF CURRENT PROCEDURAL TERMINOLOGY (CPT) CODING

The *Physicians' Current Procedural Terminology, 4th Edition* (CPT-4), is a manual containing a list of descriptive terms and identifying codes used in reporting medical services and procedures performed and supplies used by physicians and other professional healthcare providers in the care and treatment of patients. The codes were developed by the **Health Care Financing Administration (HCFA)**, now called the **Centers for Medicare and Medicaid Services (CMS)**, and published by the American Medical Association (AMA) to help establish a more uniform payment schedule for Medicare carriers to use when reimbursing providers.

Since the early 1970s, HCFA has asked the AMA to work with physicians of every specialty to determine appropriate definitions for CPT codes and to try to determine accurate reimbursement amounts for each code. Two committees within AMA act on these issues: the CPT Committee, which updates the definitions of the codes, and the Relative Value Update Committee, which recommends reimbursement values to the CMS based on data collected by medical societies on the current rate of services described in the codes.

Because the world of medicine is constantly changing, the AMA publishes an updated version of the CPT manual every year. The health insurance professional must use the most recent edition of CPT when coding professional procedures and services for claims submissions.

Today, not just Medicare and Medicaid, but most managed care and other insurance companies base their reimbursements on the values established by CMS. As with ICD-9-CM diagnostic coding, it is important that the health insurance professional have a thorough understanding of CPT coding to facilitate accurate claims completion for maximum reimbursement. The main reason for this is because CPT codes are used instead of a narrative description in Block 24d of the CMS-1500 form to describe what services or procedures were rendered or what supplies were used during the patient encounter.

HIPAA Tip

Providers submitting claims for professional services on the CMS-1500 form should use the current ICD-9-CM diagnosis codes, current CPT procedural codes, and current Point-of-Service codes.

Purpose of CPT

The purpose of CPT coding is to provide a uniform language that accurately describes medical, surgical, and diagnostic services, serving as an effective means for reliable nationwide communication among physicians, insurance carriers, and patients. CPT codes also are used by most third-party payers and government agencies as a record of an individual healthcare provider's activities.

Development of CPT

As mentioned previously, the AMA developed and published the first CPT in 1966. This first edition

- helped encourage the use of standard terms and descriptors to document procedures in the health record,
- helped communicate accurate information on procedures and services to agencies concerned with insurance claims,
- provided the basis for a computer-oriented system to evaluate operative procedures, and
- contributed basic information for actuarial and statistical purposes.

The first edition of CPT contained primarily surgical procedures, with limited sections on medicine, radiology, and laboratory procedures. The second edition was published in 1970 and presented an expanded system of terms and codes to designate diagnostic and therapeutic procedures in surgery, medicine, and other specialties. At that time, the 5-digit coding system was introduced, replacing the former 4-digit classification. Another significant change was a listing of procedures relating to internal medicine. The third and fourth editions of CPT were introduced in the mid to late 1970s. The fourth edition, published in 1977, presented significant updates in medical technology, and a system of periodic updating was introduced to keep pace with the rapidly changing medical environment.

In 1983, CPT was adopted as part of **HCFA's Common Procedure Coding System (HCPCS**, pronounced "hick-picks"). With this adoption, HCFA mandated the use of HCPCS to report services for Part B of the Medicare Program. In October 1986, HCFA also required state Medicaid agencies to use HCPCS in the Medicaid Management Information System. In July 1987, as part of the Omnibus Budget Reconciliation Act, HCFA mandated the use of CPT for reporting outpatient hospital surgical procedures. Today, in addition to use in federal programs (Medicare and Medicaid), CPT is used extensively throughout the United States as the preferred system of coding and describing healthcare services.

What Did You Learn?

1. What is CPT?
2. What is the purpose of CPT?
3. Why were CPT codes developed?
4. Who publishes CPT-4?
5. How often is CPT updated?

THREE LEVELS OF PROCEDURAL CODING

HCPCS codes are descriptive terms with letters or numbers or both used to report medical services and procedures for reimbursement. As discussed earlier, they provide a uniform language to describe medical, surgical, and diagnostic services. HCPCS codes are used to report procedures and services to government and private health insurance programs, and reimbursement is based on the codes reported. A code, rather than a narrative description, can summarize the services or supplies provided when billing a third-party payer. HCPCS codes are grouped into three levels, as follows:

Level I. Level I contains the AMA Physicians' CPT codes. These are 5-digit codes, accompanied by descriptive terms, used for reporting services performed by healthcare professionals. Level I codes are developed and updated annually by the AMA.

Level II. Level II consists of the HCPCS National Codes used to report medical services, supplies, drugs, and durable medical equipment not contained in the Level I codes. These codes begin with a single letter, followed by 4 digits. Level II codes supersede Level I codes for similar encounters, evaluation and management (E&M) services, or other procedures and represent the portion of procedures involving supplies and materials. National Level II Medicare Codes are not restricted to Medicare as their title may suggest. An increasing number of private insurance carriers are encouraging, and some are even requiring, the use of HCPCS National Codes. HCPCS Level II codes are in a separate manual from Level I codes (CPT). Level II codes are developed and updated annually by the CMS and their contractors.

Level III. In preparation of standardization for the full implementation of Health Insurance Portability and Accountability Act (HIPAA), CMS has instructed carriers to eliminate local procedures and modifier codes from their claim processing systems. Official HCPCS Level III procedure and modifier codes are defined as codes and descriptors developed by local Medicare contractors for use by physicians, practitioners, providers, and suppliers in completion of claims for payment.

 HIPAA Tip

The combination of HCPCS and CPT-4 (including codes and modifiers) is the HIPAA adopted standard for reporting physician services and other healthcare services on standard transactions.

CPT MANUAL FORMAT

INTRODUCTION AND MAIN SECTIONS

Similar to the ICD-9-CM manual, CPT-4 is composed of several sections beginning with an introduction, identified by lower case Roman numerals. The main body of the manual follows the introduction and is organized in six sections. Within each section are subsections with anatomic, procedural, condition, or descriptor subheadings. Table 13-1 provides a list of the CPT sections and their number range sequence. The listed procedures and services, along with their identifying 5-digit codes, are presented in numeric order except for the Evaluation and Management (E & M) section. Because E & M codes are used by most physicians for reporting key categories of their services, this section is presented first.

Five-digit CPT codes may be defined further by modifiers to help explain an unusual circumstance associated with a service or procedure. As mentioned previously, the right coding modifiers are crucial to getting claims paid promptly and for the correct amount. Conversely, missing or incorrect modifiers are one of the most common reasons that claims are denied by payers. It is easy to get confused on how to use modifiers correctly, especially because, similar to CPT codes, they are constantly changing. The most important thing to remember when using modifiers is that the health record must contain adequate documentation to support the modifier (Fig. 13-1).

When coding procedures, it is important always to have the most recent edition of the CPT book available to look up current modifier codes. (Modifiers are listed in Appendix A at the back of the CPT manual.) Also, it is advisable for healthcare providers and their billing staff to read Medicare (and other) coding newsletters and periodically attend coding workshops.

Each main section of the CPT is preceded by guidelines specific to that section. These guidelines define terms that are necessary to interpret correctly and report the procedures and services contained in that section. The health insurance professional should read and study these guidelines before attempting to assign a code.

CATEGORY III CODES

Following the six sections listed in the main body of the CPT manual are the **Category III codes** (Fig. 13-2). Category III codes were established by the AMA as a set of temporary CPT codes for emerging technologies, services,

TABLE 13-1	**CPT Section Numbers and Their Sequence**
SECTION TITLE	**NUMBERING SEQUENCE**
Evaluation and Management	99201 to 99499
Anesthesiology	00100 to 01999, 99100 to 99140
Surgery	10021 to 69990
Radiology (Including Nuclear Medicine and Diagnostic Ultrasound)	70010 to 79999
Pathology and Laboratory	80048 to 89356
Medicine (except Anesthesiology)	90281 to 99199, 99500 to 99602

Modifier - 22 is used to indicate that there was "something unusual about the procedure, it took longer than usual or was harder than usual. The only way you'll get consideration for additional payment is if you use the modifier and have good documentation."

Modifier - 59 is used to indicate that a procedure or service was distinct or independent from other services performed on the same day (e.g., not normally reported together), but are appropriate under the circumstances, as documented.

Fig. 13-1 Examples of correct modifier use

and procedures for which data collection is needed to substantiate widespread use or for the Food and Drug Administration's approval process. If a Category III code has not been proposed and accepted into the main body of CPT (referred to as Category I codes) within 5 years, it is archived, unless a demonstrated need for it develops.

In the introduction of the CPT book, users are instructed not to select a code that merely approximates the service provided. The code should identify the service performed accurately. If a Category III code is available and accurately describes the service provided, it should be used instead of a Category I code. Category III codes are updated semiannually in January and July, and new codes are posted on the AMA website.

APPENDICES A THROUGH L

As with ICD-9-CM, CPT-4 contains several appendices, which follow the Category III codes. These appendices and their contents are as follows:

Appendix A—Modifiers
Appendix B—Summary of Additions, Deletions, and Revisions
Appendix C—Clinical Examples
Appendix D—Summary of CPT Add-On Codes
Appendix E—Summary of CPT Codes Exempt from Modifier -51
Appendix F—Summary of CPT Codes Exempt from Modifier -63
Appendix G—Summary of CPS Codes that Include Moderate (Conscious) Sedation

Appendix H—Alphabetic Index of Performance Measure by Clinical Condition by Topic
Appendix I—Genetic Testing Code Modifiers
Appendix J—Electrodiagnostic Medicine Listing of Sensory, Motor, and Mixed Nerves

Category III codes	0052T—0071T
0062T	Percutaneous intradiscal annuloplasty, any method, unilateral or bilateral including fluoroscopic guidance; single level
	🔵 *CPT Assistant* Mar 05:2-3, Apr 05:14, 16; *CPT Changes: An Insider's View* 2005
+ 0063T	one or more additional levels (List separately in addition to 0062T for primary procedure)
	🔵 *CPT Assistant* Mar 05:2; *CPT Changes: An Insider's View* 2005
	(For CT or MRI guidance and localization for needle placement and annuloplasty in conjunction with 0062T, 0063T, see 76360, 76393)
0064T	Spectroscopy, expired gas analysis (eg, nitric oxide/carbon dioxide test)
	🔵 *CPT Assistant* Mar 05:3; *CPT Changes: An Insider's View* 2005
0065T	Ocular photoscreening, with interpretation and report, bilateral
	🔵 *CPT Assistant* Mar 05:3-4; *CPT Changes: An Insider's View* 2005
	(Do not report 0065T in conjunction with 99172 or 99173)
0066T	Computed tomographic (CT) colonography (ie, virtual colonoscopy); screening
	🔵 *CPT Assistant* Mar 05:4; *CPT Changes: An Insider's View* 2005
	🔵 *Clinical Examples in Radiology* Winter 05:8, 12
0067T	diagnostic
	🔵 *CPT Assistant* Mar 05:4; *CPT Changes: An Insider's View* 2005
	🔵 *Clinical Examples in Radiology* Winter 05:8

Fig. 13-2 Example of Category III codes. (From American Medical Association: CPT 2006 Current Procedural Terminology, 2006, Professional Edition. Chicago, 2006, American Medical Association.)

Appendix K—Products Pending FDA Approval
Appendix L—Vascular Families

CPT INDEX
Main Terms

In the CPT manual, the index is presented last. As with the ICD-9-CM, the CPT index is organized by main terms (Fig. 13-3). Each main term can stand alone, or it can be followed by up to three modifying terms. There are four primary classes of main term entries:

1. Procedure or service (e.g., colonoscopy, anastomosis, debridement)
2. Organ or other anatomic site (e.g., fibula, kidney, nails)
3. Condition (e.g., infection, pregnancy, tetralogy of Fallot)
4. Synonyms, eponyms, and abbreviations (e.g., ECS, Pean's operation, Clagett procedure)

● Stop and Think

Surgeon Milford Tramen saw Patrick Lovell, a 34-year-old Illinois farmer, in his office on February 19 for the repair of an injury to the patient's mouth. The chief complaint in the medical record documents that the patient was "kicked in the mouth while vaccinating hogs." The surgeon stitched up the 3.4-cm cut, and the nurse administered a tetanus shot. What would be the main term for the procedure performed by the surgeon?

```
      Endoscopy.............. 45337
Ultrasound
      Endoscopy......... 45341-45342
Colonna Procedure
See Acetabulum, Reconstruction
Colonography
CT Scan............ 0066T, 0067T
Colonoscopy
Biopsy ............. 45380, 45392
Collection Specimen ........ 45380
   via Colotomy ............. 45355
Destruction
   Lesion .................. 45383
   Tumor .................. 45383
Dilation.................. 45386
Hemorrhage Control ........ 45382
```

Fig. 13-3 Example of main terms. (From American Medical Association: CPT 2006 Current Procedural Terminology, 2006, Professional Edition. Chicago, 2006, American Medical Association.)

Modifying Terms

As mentioned previously, each main term can stand alone, or it can be followed up by up to three **modifying terms** (Fig. 13-4). Modifying terms are indented under the main term. All modifying terms should be examined closely because these subterms often have an effect on the selection of the appropriate procedural code.

Code Layout

A CPT code can be displayed one of three ways:

1. A single code (Proetz therapy, nose 30210)
2. Multiple codes (prolactin 80418, 80440, 84146)
3. A range of codes (prostatotomy 55720-55725)

SYMBOLS USED IN CPT

The CPT manual uses several symbols that help guide the health insurance professional in locating the correct code.

```
Delay of Flap
Skin Graft........... 15600-15630
Deligation
Ureter.................... 50940
Deliveries, Abdominal
See Cesarean Delivery
Delivery
See Cesarean Delivery, Vaginal Delivery
Delorme Operation
See Pericardiectomy
Denervation
Hip
   Femoral................. 27035
   Obturator ............... 27035
   Sciatic .................. 27035
Denervation, Sympathetic
See Excision, Nerve, Sympathetic
Denis-Browne Splint ....... 29590
Dens Axis
See Odontoid process
Denver Developmental
Screening Test ...... 96101-96103
Denver Krupic Procedure
See Aqueous Shunt, to Extraocular Reservoir
Denver Shunt
Patency Test .............. 78291
Denver-Krupin Procedure .. 66180
```

Fig. 13-4 Example of main term with modifying terms. (From American Medical Association: CPT 2006 Current Procedural Terminology, 2006, Professional Edition. Chicago, 2006, American Medical Association.)

Accurate procedural coding cannot be accomplished without understanding the meaning of each of these symbols (Table 13-2).

MODIFIERS

Modifiers are important to ensuring appropriate and timely payment. A health insurance professional who understands when and how to use them reduces the problems caused by denials and expedites processing of claims.

A modifier provides the means by which the reporting healthcare provider can indicate that a service or procedure performed has been altered by some specific circumstance, but has not changed its definition or code. The judicious application of modifiers tells the third-party payer that this case is unique. By using appropriate modifiers, the office may be paid for services that are ordinarily denied. In addition, modifiers can describe a situation that, without the modifier, could be considered inappropriate coding.

Modifiers are not universal; they cannot be used with all CPT codes. Some modifiers may be used only with E & M codes (e.g., modifier -24 or modifier -25), and others are used only with procedure codes (e.g., modifier -58 or modifier -79). Check the guidelines at the beginning of each section for a listing or description of the modifiers that may be used with the codes in that section. Appendix A of the CPT manual contains a comprehensive list of modifiers.

UNLISTED PROCEDURE OR SERVICE

A healthcare provider may perform a service or procedure for which a code is unavailable in the CPT manual. When this happens, specific codes have been designated for reporting these unlisted procedures. At the end of each subsection or subheading in question, a code is provided under the heading "other procedures," which typically ends in "-99." In the surgery section, note the "other procedures" code 39499 at the end of the "mediastinum" subsection. This would be the code of choice for any unlisted procedures of the mediastinum.

SPECIAL REPORTS

When a rarely used, unusual, variable, or new service or procedure is performed, many third-party payers require a **special report** to accompany the claim to help determine the appropriateness and medical necessity of the service or procedure. Items that should be addressed in the report, if applicable, include
- a definition or description of the service or procedure;
- the time, effort, and equipment needed;
- symptoms and final diagnosis;
- pertinent physical findings and size;
- diagnostic and therapeutic services;
- concurrent problems; and
- follow-up care.

☑ **HIPAA Tip**

HIPAA does not mandate the use of modifiers. According to the adopted HIPAA implementation guide, use of modifiers is not required. Their usage is "situational," meaning that the use of a modifier is required only when a modifier clarifies or improves the reporting accuracy of the associated procedure code.

What Did You Learn?

1. List the six main sections of CPT.
2. What is the purpose of the guidelines that appear at the beginning of each main section of CPT?
3. What are Category III codes?
4. Name the five appendices contained in CPT.
5. What are the four primary classes of main term entries?
6. What is the function of a "modifier"?

TABLE 13-2	Symbols Used in the CPT Manual
SYMBOL	**EXPLANATION**
Bullet (●)	A bullet (●) before a code means the code is **new** to the CPT book for that particular edition
Triangle (▲)	A triangle (▲) means the description for the code has been **changed** or **modified** since the previous revision of the CPT book
Horizontal triangles (►◄)	Horizontal triangles ►◄ placed at the beginning and end of a descriptive entry indicates that it contains **new or revised wording**
Plus Sign (+)	Add-on codes are annotated by a + symbol
Ø	This symbol is used to identify codes that are exempt form the use of modifier -51
➔	Reference to *CPT Assistant, Clinical Examples in Radiology* and *CPT Changes* book
⚡	The lightening bolt indicates codes for vaccines that are pending Food and Drug Administration approval
⊙	This symbol is used to identify codes that include conscious sedation

FORMAT OF CPT

There are two types of CPT codes: stand-alone and indented. The terminology of a **stand-alone code** is complete in and of itself. It contains the full description of the procedure without additional explanation. Some procedures do not contain the entire written description, however. These are known as **indented codes**. Indented codes refer back to the common portion of the procedure listed in the preceding entry, and correct code selection requires careful attention to the punctuation in the description.

IMPORTANCE OF THE SEMICOLON

In the CPT, the semicolon is used to separate main and subordinate clauses in the code descriptions. This symbol was adopted to save space in the manual where a series of related codes are found. CPT code "38100 splenectomy; total (separate procedure)" is a stand-alone code. The code immediately following it, 38101, is indented and reads "partial (separate procedure)." The semicolon after splenectomy in code 38100 becomes part of the indented code 38101. The full description of code 38101 in effect would read "splenectomy; partial (separate procedure)." See Figure 13-5 for an example of a stand-alone code followed by an indented code used in the above-mentioned example.

SECTION, SUBSECTION, SUBHEADING, AND CATEGORY

Codes in the tabular section of CPT are formatted using four classifications: **section, subsection, subheading,** and **category**. To illustrate this, locate the code "51000 aspiration of bladder by needle" in the Tabular List. At the top left, note the code range on that particular page (50970 through 51610), followed by the words "surgery/urinary system." "Surgery" is the *section,* and "urinary system" is the *subsection.* Moving down the page, note the word "bladder" in large font bold. Bladder is the *subheading.* Immediately under bladder, note the word "incision," which indicates the *category* (Fig. 13-6).

CROSS-REFERENCING WITH SEE

When searching for the correct main term, the word "*see*" is frequently seen. "*See*" is used as a cross-reference term in the CPT alphabetic index and directs the coder to an alternate main term (Fig. 13-7).

What Did You Learn?

1. Explain the significance of the semicolon in CPT coding.
2. How is a "stand-alone" code different from an "indented code"?
3. What does the cross-referencing term *see* indicate?

| 37799 | Unlisted procedure, vascular surgery |
| | ◗ *CPT Assistant* Spring 93:12, Fall 93:3, Feb 97:10, Sep 97:10, May 01:11, Oct 04:16 |

Hemic and Lymphatic Systems

Spleen

Excision

38100	Splenectomy; total (separate procedure)
	➲ *CPT Assistant* Jul 93:9, Summer 93:10
38101	partial (separate procedure)
	➲ *CPT Assistant* Summer 93:10
+ 38102	total, en bloc for extensive disease, in conjunction with other procedure (List in addition to code for primary procedure)
	➲ *CPT Assistant* Summer 93:10

Repair

| 38115 | Repair of ruptured spleen (splenorrhaphy) with or without partial splenectomy |
| | ◗ *CPT Assistant* Summer 93:10 |

Laparoscopy

Surgical laparoscopy always includes diagnostic laparoscopy. To report a diagnostic laparoscopy (peritoneoscopy) (separate procedure), use 49320.

Fig. 13-5 Example of a stand-alone code followed by an indented code used in the example of Figure 13-4. (From American Medical Association: CPT 2006 Current Procedural Terminology, 2006, Professional Edition. Chicago, 2006, American Medical Association.)

BASIC STEPS OF CPT CODING

CPT coding is a structured process, and it is important for the health insurance professional to follow a few basic steps so that the correct code is identified and assigned.

1. *Identify the procedure, service, or supply to be coded.* These are typically found on the ledger card, on the encounter form, or in the patient data in the computerized accounting software.
2. *Determine the main term.* The index is located at the back of the CPT manual. Main terms are in boldface type and are listed alphabetically with headings located in the top right and left corners, similar to a dictionary (Fig. 13-8). For the purpose of review, main terms are organized by four primary classes of main entries: a procedure or service; an organ or other anatomic site;

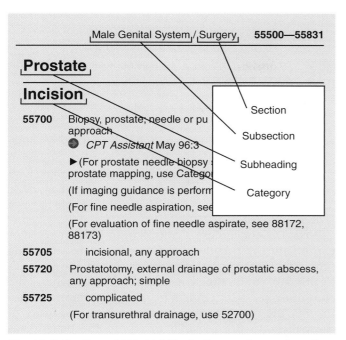

Male Genital System / Surgery   55500—55831

Prostate

Incision

55700   Biopsy, prostate; needle or pu
        approach
        ● *CPT Assistant* May 96:3
        ▶ (For prostate needle biopsy
        prostate mapping, use Catego
        (If imaging guidance is perform
        (For fine needle aspiration, se
        (For evaluation of fine needle aspirate, see 88172, 88173)

55705   incisional, any approach

55720   Prostatotomy, external drainage of prostatic abscess, any approach; simple

55725   complicated

        (For transurethral drainage, use 52700)

Section
Subsection
Subheading
Category

Fig. 13-6 Section of Tab List illustrating section, subsection, subheading, and category. (From American Medical Association: CPT 2006 Current Procedural Terminology, 2006, Professional Edition. Chicago, 2006, American Medical Association.)

a condition; or a synonym, eponym, or abbreviation.) Subterms (if applicable) are indented under main terms.

Reminder! Do not select the final code from the alphabetic index alone.

3. Locate the main term in the alphabetic index and note the code or codes.
4. Cross-reference the single code, multiple codes, or the code range numerically in the tabular section of the manual.
5. Read and follow any notes, special instructions, or conventions associated with the code.
6. Determine and assign the appropriate code.

Before assigning an indented code, refer to the stand-alone code above it. Read the words that *precede* the semicolon, ensuring that the combined description (the portion of the stand-alone code *up to* the semicolon *plus* the wording included in the indented description) corresponds to the documented procedure or service.

What Did You Learn?

1. What is the first step in CPT coding?
2. What factors should be considered before assigning an "indented code"?

Dermatology
Actinotherapy 96900
Examination of Hair
   Microscopic 96902
Ultraviolet A Treatment 96912
Ultraviolet B Treatment
   96910-96913
Ultraviolet Light Treatment
   96900-96913
Unlisted Services and
   Procedures 96999
Dermatoplasty
Septal 30620

Dermoid
See Cyst, Dermoid
Derrick-Burnet Disease
See Q Fever
Descending Abdominal Aorta
See Aorta, Abdominal
Desipramine
Assay 80160
Desmotomy
See Ligament, Release
Desoxycorticosterone 82633
Desoxycortone
See Desoxycorticosterone
Desoxyephedrine
See Methamphetamine
Desoxynorephedrin
See Amphetamine

Fig. 13-7 Example of *see* used as a cross-reference. (From American Medical Association: CPT 2006 Current Procedural Terminology, 2006, Professional Edition. Chicago, 2006, American Medical Association.)

EVALUATION AND MANAGEMENT (E & M) CODING

The E & M codes (99201 and 99499) are found at the beginning of the CPT manual. The E & M section of the CPT is divided into broad categories, including office visits, hospital visits, and consultations. Most of the categories are divided further. There are two subcategories of office visits (new versus established patients), and two categories of hospital visits (initial versus subsequent visits).

The subcategories list codes that describe differing levels of service provided, ranging from low levels of service to higher and more intense levels of service. Initially, these codes were based on highly subjective factors that were applied inconsistently among carriers. In 1992, new uniform, national criteria were established to determine the appropriate level code to be used. Under these criteria, every visit regardless of location must include at least two of

Fig. 13-8 Example of header words at top of page in CPT manual. (From American Medical Association: CPT 2006 Current Procedural Terminology, 2006, Professional Edition. Chicago, 2006, American Medical Association.)

the following three components—history, examination, and medical decision making.

E & M codes represent the services provided directly to the patient during an encounter that do not involve an actual procedure. If a patient has an appointment in the office, only the office visit receives an E & M code. If any procedures take place (e.g., a urinalysis or an electrocardiogram), those procedures receive a CPT code. E & M codes are designed to classify services provided by a healthcare provider and are used primarily in outpatient settings. E & M codes are technically CPT codes (Level I HCPCS); however, they are referred to as E & M instead of CPT to distinguish the difference between evaluation and management services and procedural coding (Fig. 13-9). The level of service code selected for an office visit is given a numerical level (1 to 5). The code level assigned depends on the complexity of the history, examination, and medical decision making and usually is not affected by the time the provider spends with the patient. The range of codes for office or other outpatient services are 99201 to 99205 for new patients and 99211 to 99215 for established patients. There is a specific distinction between new and established patients associated with E & M coding. The exact definitions are discussed in the next section.

VOCABULARY USED IN E & M CODING

To understand E & M coding more fully, the coder must become acquainted with several terms, as follows:
- **New patient**—an individual who is new to the practice, regardless of location of service, or one who has not received any medical treatment by the healthcare provider or any other provider in that same office *within the past 3 years.*
- **Established patient**—an individual who has been treated previously by the healthcare provider, regardless of location of service, within the past 3 years. If the provider saw the patient for the first time in a hospital, and that individual comes to the office for a follow-up visit after discharge, the patient is considered an established patient to the practice because health record documentation was generated from the hospital visit.
- **Outpatient**—a patient who *has not* been officially admitted to a hospital, but receives diagnostic tests or treatment in that facility or a clinic connected with it.
- **Inpatient**—a patient who *has* been formally admitted to a hospital for diagnostic tests, medical care and treatment, or a surgical procedure, typically staying overnight.

- **Consultation**—when the attending healthcare provider recommends that the patient see another physician (often a specialist) for a problem usually associated with one major body system. A family practitioner may advise a patient who presents with a suspicious mole to see a dermatologist.

Note: Do not confuse a consultation with a referral. A consultation is usually a one-time visit; the attending physician (or provider) retains control of the patient's healthcare, and the consultation ends when the consulting provider renders his or her opinion. With a referral, the original provider relinquishes total care of the patient to the provider to whom the patient has been referred.
- **Counseling**—a discussion with the patient or the patient's family or both. Counseling typically includes one or more of the following:
  - Discussing diagnostic test results, impressions, or recommended studies
  - prognosis
  - explaining the risks or benefits of recommended treatment or instruction for management of care
  - patient or family education
- **Concurrent care**—when a patient receives similar services (e.g., hospital visits) by more than one healthcare provider on the same day.
- **Critical care**—the constant attention (either at bedside or immediately available) by a physician in a medical crisis.
- **Emergency care**—care given in a hospital emergency department.

● Stop and Think

Tom Galliger was in the Air Force for 4 years. During that time, he did not see Dr. Boker, his physician in his hometown of Gaithersville. Dr. Boker's office policy is to place any inactive files on microfilm after 2 years of inactivity. After Tom finished his tour of duty, he returned home to Gaithersville. Soon after returning home, he sprained his ankle hiking in the mountains and subsequently scheduled an appointment with Dr. Boker. Would Tom be considered a new or established patient?

Evaluation and Management

Office or Other Outpatient Services

The following codes are used to report evaluation and management services provided in the physician's office or in an outpatient or other ambulatory facility. A patient is considered an outpatient until inpatient admission to a health care facility occurs.

►To report services provided to a patient who is admitted to a hospital or nursing facility in the course of an encounter in the office or other ambulatory facility, see the notes for initial hospital inpatient care (page 12) or initial nursing facility care (page 22).◄

For services provided by physicians in the emergency department, see 99281-99285.

For observation care, see 99217-99220.

For observation or inpatient care services (including admission and discharge services), see 99234-99236.

New Patient

99201   **Office or other outpatient visit** for the evaluation and management of a new patient, which requires these three key components:

■ **a problem focused history;**

■ **a problem focused examination;**

■ **straightforward medical decision making.**

Counseling and/or coordination of care with other providers or agencies are provided consistent with the nature of the problem(s) and the patient's and/or family's needs.

Usually, the presenting problem(s) are self limited or minor. Physicians typically spend 10 minutes face-to-face with the patient and/or family.

➲ *CPT Assistant* Winter 91:11, Spring 92:13, 24, Summer 92:1, 24, Spring 93:34, Summer 93:2, Fall 93:9, Spring 95:1, Summer 95:4, Fall 95:9, Jul 98:9, Sep 98:5, Jun 99:8, Feb 00:3, 9, 11, Aug 01:2, Oct 04:11, Apr 05:3

99202   **Office or other outpatient visit** for the evaluation and management of a new patient, which requires these three key components:

■ **an expanded problem focused history;**

■ **an expanded problem focused examination;**

■ **straightforward medical decision making.**

Counseling and/or coordination of care with other providers or agencies are provided consistent with the nature of the problem(s) and the patient's and/or family's needs.

Fig. 13-9 Portion from E & M coding section. (From American Medical Association: CPT 2006 Current Procedural Terminology, 2006, Professional Edition. Chicago, 2006, American Medical Association.)

DOCUMENTATION REQUIREMENTS

Because the level of the E & M codes is based on the complexity of the history, examination, or medical decision making performed during the visit, the key to

---

Imagine This!

Vancil Allen, a 73-year-old white man, was admitted to the hospital with chest pain and shortness of breath after a minor automobile accident. His cardiologist, Marcus Walters, was the admitting physician. While hospitalized, Vancil complained of severe pain in his right lower back. Further examination revealed a kidney stone. Subsequently, Dr. Marta Tomi, a urologist, was called in to take over the care of Vancil's kidney problems.

---

reimbursement is being able to prove the level of complexity of the performed services. The only valid source of proof is the documentation in the patient's medical record.

Coding E & M services should be based on the extent of documentation in the patient's medical record (Fig. 13-10). The criteria for E & M services must be well understood by the treating provider and documented in the record. Each record needs to show elements of the history, such as the history of present illness (HPI) (e.g., location, severity, frequency, duration); the review of systems (ROS); and past, family, and social history (PFSH). The physical examination should list all systems or organs examined. Medical decision making should discuss the number of options or diagnoses considered in the decision, the amount of data or complexity of data reviewed, and the risk to the patient of the decision made.

THREE FACTORS TO CONSIDER

The health insurance professional must determine three factors that will direct him or her to the proper category in the E & M coding section:

1. *Place of service* (where the service was provided)
   - Physician's office
   - Hospital
   - Emergency department
   - Nursing home
   - Other

2. *Type of service* (the reason the service was rendered)
   - Office visit
   - Consultation
   - Admission
   - Newborn care

3. *Patient status* (type of patient)
   - New patient
   - Established patient
   - Outpatient
   - Inpatient

6/10/2004

HX: This 27-year-old white male presents to the clinic today for chief complaint of an abrasion on the right knee following a fall yesterday. According to the patient, he had this soft tissue lesion prior to the fall; and when he fell, he basically abraded the lower half of the lesion. He is here for reevaluation and possible excision of the lesion.

PAIN ASSESSMENT: Scale 0-10, one.
ALLERGIES: DEMEROL
CURRENT MEDS: None

PE: NAD. Ambulatory. Appears well.
VS: BP: 120/74   WT: 150#
RIGHT KNEE EXAMINATION: The patient has a tibial prominence and just above that, there is what appears to be a 1.5 cm epidermal inclusion cyst with an abraded area inferiorly. There is mild erythema and serous drainage but no purulence. There is no appreciable edema. Just lateral to that lesion is a small superficial abrasion. The knee examination was totally within normal limits.

IMP: Epidermal inclusion cyst measuring 1.5 to 2 cm of the right knee, traumatized with abrasion

PLAN: The patient was empirically started on Keflex 500 mg 1 p.o. b.i.d. He was given instructions on home care and is to follow up this week for excision of the lesion. Routine follow up as noted. RTN PRN.

Frederick Mahoney, MD

Fig. 13-10 Sample documentation.

When these three factors are determined, the health insurance professional can move on to determining the key components, the next step in E & M coding.

For example, Cindy Carlson recently moved to Jackson City because of a job transfer. Shortly after arriving in Jackson City, Cindy sprained her ankle while jogging in the park. She scheduled an appointment with Dr. Allen Schubert, a family practitioner, for medical treatment. In this scenario
• the place of service would be the physician's office,
• the type of service would be an office visit, and
• the patient status would be "new" because Cindy has never been seen in Dr. Schubert's office before.

Now that the first three factors have been established, the next step is to determine the three key components of the encounter.

KEY COMPONENTS

The health insurance professional must establish what level of service the patient received. Levels of service are based on three **key components**:
• History
• Examination
• Complexity of medical decision making
In addition to these three key components, there may be contributing factors that affect the E & M coding level reported, including
• counseling,
• coordination of care,
• nature of presenting problem, and
• time.

History

A patient history is **subjective information**. The essentials of the history are based on what the patient tells the healthcare provider in his or her own words. An experienced health insurance professional should be able to identify the various elements and levels of a history by reading the clinical notes entered into the health record.

Elements of a Patient History. A patient history is based on four elements:

1. **Chief complaint (CC)**—the reason the patient is seeing the physician, usually in the patient's own words; the CC might be "I feel awful, and I can't keep anything down."

2. **HPI**—details of the severity and duration of signs and symptoms regarding the CC (e.g., fever for 2 days, severe cough, chest pains on and off since breakfast). The HPI typically consists of eight qualifiers:
   • *Location* (describes where the symptom is occurring, such as neck, stomach, or ankle)
   • *Quality* (burning, stabbing, throbbing)
   • *Severity* (8 on a scale of 1 to 10)
   • *Duration* (how long symptom has been present or how long it lasts when it occurs)
   • *Timing* (constant, after meals, during exercise)
   • *Context* (the situation associated with symptom, such as began after altercation at work, after a big meal, while exercising)

- *Modifying factors* (cold rag to back of neck helps)
- *Associated signs and symptoms* (nausea, vomiting, jagged lights in field of vision)

Using the Cindy Carlson scenario described earlier, the HPI might be: "Patient describes pain and swelling in the right ankle area. Applying weight on the ankle increases the pain. Ibuprofen and ice packs relieve the pain and swelling temporarily."

Note: The HPI is typically written in present tense.

3. **ROS**—involves a series of questions the provider asks the patient to identify what body parts or body systems are involved, for example:
   - Constitution: denies recent weight gain/loss
   - Eyes: jagged lights in peripheral vision
   - Ear, nose, throat: denies sore throat or ear pain
   - Cardiovascular: denies chest pain, orthopnea
   - Respiratory: denies hemoptysis
   - Gastrointestinal: negative
   - Genitourinary: denies nocturia or frequent urinary tract infections
   - Musculoskeletal: denies joint pain
   - Skin: denies rashes, skin lesions
   - Neurologic: denies seizures or tremors
   - Psychological: denies suicidal ideation
   - Endocrine: denies polydipsia, polyphagia
   - Hematologic/lymph: denies easy bruising
   - Allergy/immunologic: allergic to citrus fruit/strawberries

Typical documented ROS notation would be as follows:
Pulmonary: cough × 4 weeks; otherwise negative
Cardiac: negative except for complaints of fatigue
All other systems negative

The ROS for Cindy Carlson's condition would be limited to one body part (right ankle) or one organ system (musculoskeletal).

4. **PFSH**—includes the patient's past illnesses, operations, injuries, and treatments and any diseases or conditions other members of the patient's family have, which could be hereditary. A social history includes a review of the patient's past and current activities, such as marital status, employment, drug and alcohol use, and any other pertinent social factors that might affect the current problem.

These history-taking elements, with the exception of PFSH, are involved to some degree in all patient encounters. The extent or level of history is determined by these elements.

History Levels. The first element to consider is the level of patient history:

- *Problem-focused history*—provider concentrates on the CC and takes a *brief* history (HPI) centering around the severity, duration, or symptoms with regard to the CC. Typically, there would be no PFSH or ROS conducted.
  - *Example:* A 6-month old infant presents with diaper rash.
- *Expanded problem focused history*—provider considers the CC, obtains a brief history of the problem, and performs a problem-pertinent ROS centered around the organ system involved.
  - *Example:* A 13-year-old girl presents with chronic otitis media and a draining ear.
- *Detailed history*—provider concentrates on the CC and obtains an extended HPI, but this time an extended ROS is conducted, and a relevant PFSH is taken. With a detailed history, the ROS might involve multiple organ systems.
  - *Example:* A 56-year-old man presents with a stasis ulcer of 3 months' duration.
- *Comprehensive history*—this is the most complex of the four levels of history taking. Besides the CC, the provider obtains an extended HPI, does a complete ROS, and takes a detailed PFSH.
  - *Example:* A 73-year-old man presents with chest pain and shortness of breath on exertion.

Cindy Carlson's examination would fall into the problem-focused history level.

Examination

The second component in determining the correct E & M level is the patient examination. As with history taking, there are four degrees, or detailed intensities, involved in a patient examination:

- *Problem focused*—limited to the affected body part or organ system identified in the CC. Considering the previous example of the infant with diaper rash, the examination would typically involve only the diaper area.
- *Expanded problem focused*—examination would involve the affected body area or organ system and any other related areas or organ systems. Considering the patient with otitis media (from the aforementioned example), the body areas and organ systems involved would be the ear, nose, and throat system and possibly the eyes.
- *Detailed*—extended examination is performed, which would include the affected body area and all related organ systems. Considering the previous example of the patient with a stasis ulcer, the examination typically would involve the lower extremities and possible various body systems.
- *Comprehensive*—a comprehensive examination—the most extensive type—is required for this level, encompassing all affected body areas and organ systems. For the 73-year-old man with chest pain and shortness of breath (see earlier example), the examination would need to be extensive because the physician must consider an impending cardiac episode.

Cindy Carlson's examination would be limited to the affected body part, resulting in the problem-focused category.

Medical Decision Making

The last of the three key components is medical decision making. The level of medical decision making is determined by weighing the complexity involved in the healthcare provider's assessment of and professional judgment regarding the patient's diagnosis and care. In determining the complexity of decision making, the health insurance professional must consider three elements:

1. How many diagnostic and treatment options were considered
2. The amount and complexity of data reviewed
3. The amount of risk for complications, morbidity, or mortality.

The degree to which each of these three elements is considered determines the level of complexity in medical decision making. There are four medical decision making levels:

- *Straightforward*
  - Minimal number of (typically only one) diagnoses and management options to consider
  - Minimal or no data to be reviewed
  - Minimal risk of complications or death if the condition remains untreated
- *Low complexity*
  - Limited number of diagnoses or management options
  - Limited amount of data to be reviewed
  - Low risk of complications or death if the condition is left untreated
- *Moderate complexity*
  - Multiple diagnoses and management options to consider
  - Moderate amount or complex data to be reviewed
  - Moderate risk of complications or death if problem is left untreated
- *High complexity*
  - Extensive diagnoses and management options
  - Extensive amount and complex data to be reviewed
  - High risk for complications or death if the condition remains untreated

Dr. Schubert's extent of medical decision making for his patient Cindy Carlson would be straightforward. There is a minimal number of (only one) diagnoses and management options to consider, minimal or no data to be reviewed, and minimal risk of complications or death if the condition remains untreated. For a new patient, three of the three criteria must be met or exceeded for that level code to be reported.

HPI, ROS, PFSH—Level 2
Examination—Level 2
Medical decision making—Level 2
The E & M code would be 99202.

Imagine This!

Sarah Perez, a 55-year-old restaurant manager, was diagnosed with benign essential hypertension in June 2001. On doctor's orders, Sarah comes to Heartland Medical Clinic every week to have her blood pressure checked. Elizabeth Allen, a medical assistant at Heartland, takes and records Sarah's blood pressure reading in her health record. Sarah does not see a physician for these encounters. Francis Bentley, Heartland's health insurance professional, reports this encounter as 99211, or Level 1, in E & M coding. The visit is documented in the progress notes with the medical assistant's signature or initials, but no further documentation is needed.

Stop and Think

New patient Erin Kole, a 15-year-old lifeguard, comes to Mountain View Family Practice with a severely sunburned nose. Considering history, examination, and medical decision making, what E & M level would this encounter fall under?

CONTRIBUTING FACTORS

In addition to the three key components in assigning an E & M code, contributing factors sometimes enter into the picture. Contributing factors help the healthcare provider determine the extent of the three key components (history, examination, and medical decision making) necessary to treat the patient effectively. These contributing factors are as follows:

1. *Counseling*—A service provided to the patient or his or her family that involves the following:
   - Impressions and recommended diagnostic studies
   - Discussion of diagnostic results
   - Prognosis
   - Risks and benefits of treatment
   - Instructions

2. *Coordination of care*—A healthcare provider often must arrange for other services to be provided to a patient, such as being admitted to a long-term care facility or home healthcare.

3. *Nature of presenting problem*—The presenting problem (CC) is what guides the healthcare provider in determining the level of care necessary to diagnose the problem accurately and treat the patient effectively. There are five types of presenting problems:

Minimal—Services typically are provided by a member of the medical staff other than the physician, but a physician must be on the premises at the time the service is rendered. This type may be used only if the patient does not see the physician.

Example: A 10-year-old girl comes in for an injection based on charted orders by the physician. A medical assistant gives the injection.

Self-limiting—Problem runs a definite or prescribed course, is transient in nature, and is not likely to affect the health status of the patient permanently.

Example: A patient with a sore throat is examined.

Low severity—Risk of morbidity is low, and there is little to no risk of mortality without treatment. Patient is expected to recover fully without functional impairment.

Example: A 16-year-old boy comes in with a case of severe acne.

Moderate severity—There is moderate risk of morbidity or mortality without treatment and an increased probability of prolonged functional impairment without treatment.

Example: A 40-year-old woman with a 3-month history of severe, recurrent headaches undergoes an initial evaluation.

High severity—Patient has a high to extreme risk of morbidity or mortality without treatment and a high probability of severe, prolonged functional impairment without treatment.

Example: A 10-year-old girl presents with severe coughing fits with wheezing that affect her sleep and other activities.

The healthcare provider should document the complexity of the patient's presenting problem in the health record. The health insurance professional must identify the words that correctly indicate the type of presenting problem.

4. *Time*—There are two ways time is measured in E & M coding:

   - **Face-to-face time**—This is the time the healthcare provider spends in direct contact with a patient during an office visit, which includes taking a history, performing an examination, and discussing results.
   - **Unit/floor time**—This includes time the physician spends on bedside care of the patient and reviewing the health record and writing orders.

Note: Time is not considered a factor unless 50% of the encounter is spent in counseling. Time is *never* a factor for emergency department visits.

Time typically is noted in the E & M section in statements such as the one located under code 99203 shown in Figure 13-11.

| **Imagine This!** |

Dr. Markov is asked to see a 56-year-old factory worker for dyspnea related to cirrhosis of the liver and ascites. Dr. Markov spends 60 minutes on the unit reviewing the chart and interviewing and examining the patient and an additional 20 minutes writing notes and conferring with the attending physician. Most (more than 50%) of Dr. Markov's interaction with the patient was related to eliciting his values and goals of care, clarifying his understanding of his diagnosis and prognosis, giving information, and counseling. There were some specific suggestions about the use of morphine to relieve the patient's dyspnea. For this initial consultation in the hospital that lasted 80 minutes, you would choose E & M code 99254.

99203	**Office or other outpatient visit** for the evaluation and management of a new patient, which requires these three key components:

- a detailed history;
- a detailed examination;
- medical decision making of low complexity.

Counseling and/or coordination of care with other providers or agencies are provided consistent with the nature of the problem(s) and the patient's and/or family's needs.

> Usually, the presenting problem(s) are of moderate severity. Physicians typically spend 30 minutes face-to-face with the patient and/or family.

Fig. 13-11 Example from E & M Section showing how time is noted. (From American Medical Association: CPT 2006 Current Procedural Terminology, 2006, Professional Edition. Chicago, 2006, American Medical Association.)

PROLONGED SERVICES

When considering the applicable E & M coding level for a patient encounter, the health insurance professional looks at the history, examination, and medical decision making. Occasionally, the amount of time the healthcare provider spends face-to-face with the patient exceeds the usual length of service associated with the corresponding level in the inpatient or outpatient setting (Fig. 13-12). When this happens, this extra time is reported in addition to other physician services. The reason for the extra time spent must be documented.

Total Duration of Prolonged Services	Code(s)
less than 30 minutes (less than 1/2 hour)	Not reported separately
30-74 minutes (1/2 hr. - 1 hr. 14 min.)	99354 × 1
75-104 minutes (1 hr. 15 min. - 1 hr. 44 min.)	99354 × 1 AND 99355 × 1
105-134 minutes (1 hr. 45 min. - 2 hr. 14 min.)	99354 × 1 AND 99355 × 2
135-164 minutes (2 hr. 15 min. - 2 hr. 44 min.)	99354 × 1 AND 99355 × 3
165-194 minutes (2 hr. 45 min. - 3 hr. 14 min.)	99354 × 1 AND 99355 × 4

Fig. 13-12 Example of extra time scenario. (From American Medical Association: CPT 2006 Current Procedural Terminology, 2006, Professional Edition. Chicago, 2006, American Medical Association.)

What Did You Learn?

1. Explain the difference between a "new" and "established" patient.
2. How does an "outpatient" differ from an "inpatient"?
3. What are the three factors to consider before assigning an E & M code level?
4. Name the three key components in E & M coding.
5. What is "subjective" information?
6. Name the four "contributing factors" that assist the coder in assigning an E & M code.

SUBHEADINGS OF THE MAIN E & M SECTION

Following the Office or Other Outpatient Services codes of the main E & M section are additional subheadings. The codes in these various subheadings are used to report services provided to patients who are admitted to a hospital or nursing facility resulting from an encounter in the physician's office or other ambulatory facility.

OUTPATIENT OR OTHER OUTPATIENT SERVICES

The first subheading under the main E & M section deals with reporting professional services provided in the physician's office or in an outpatient or other ambulatory facility. (An individual is considered an outpatient unless he or she has been admitted to a hospital.) In this section, codes are differentiated between "new" and "established" patients. Codes for new patient services range from 99201 through 99205, and codes for established patients begin with 99211 through 99215. As the codes increase numerically, the patient's problem becomes more complex or life-threatening or both. Also, for new patients, all three key components (history, examination, and medical decision making) must be met or exceeded; however, only two must be met for established patients (Table 13-3).

HOSPITAL OBSERVATION STATUS

Observation is a classification for a patient who is not sick enough to qualify for the acute inpatient status, but requires hospitalization for a brief time. Patients typically are admitted for observation to determine what and how severe their problem or condition is. Codes in this category are used to report services provided to a patient designated as under "observation status" in a hospital.

TABLE 13-3   Elements Needed to Substantiate Code Choice

LEVELS OF E & M SERVICE	PROBLEM FOCUSED	EXPANDED PROBLEM FOCUSED	DETAILED	COMPREHENSIVE
History	CC	CC	CC	CC
	Brief HPI	Brief HPI	Extended HPI	Extended HPI
		Problem-focused ROS	Extended ROS	Complete ROS
			Pertinent PFSH	Complete PFSH
Examination	Limited to affected body area or organ system	Limited to affected body area or organ system and related organ systems	Extended to all affected body areas and any related organ systems	Multisystem examination or examination of complete single organ system
Medical decision making	Straightforward	Low	Moderate	High
Diagnosis/management	0-1 element	2 elements	3 elements	>3 elements
Data	0-1 element	2 elements	3 elements	>3 elements
Risk	Minimal	Low	Moderate	High

1. *Initial Observation Care* (codes 99218 through 99220)—Use the codes from this category to report services for the first (or additional) day of a multiple-day observation stay. The two higher level codes require a comprehensive history and physical examination. The lowest level code requires a detailed or comprehensive history and physical examination.
2. *Observation Discharge Care* (code 99217)—Report this service only for the final day of a multiple-day stay.
3. *Observation or Inpatient Care Services* (codes 99234 through 99236)—Use codes to report observation or inpatient services where the patient is admitted and discharged on the same date of service. The two higher level codes require a comprehensive history and physical examination. The lowest level code requires a detailed or comprehensive history and physical examination.

When observation status services are initiated at another site, such as the emergency department, physician's office, or nursing facility, all E & M services provided by the supervising physician in conjunction with initiating the "observation status" are considered part of the initial observation care, if performed on the same day.

Imagine This!

Billy Marshall, a 6-year-old boy, was brought to the emergency department after a fall from a jungle gym at the school playground. Billy did not lose consciousness; however, he complained of headache, and his teacher reported an episode of vomiting. Billy was admitted for 24-hour observation to rule out head injury.

HOSPITAL INPATIENT SERVICES

- *Initial hospital care:* The codes in this category are for reporting services provided only by the admitting physician. Other physicians providing initial inpatient E & M services should use consultation or subsequent hospital care codes, as appropriate.
- *Subsequent hospital care:* The codes in this category are for reporting inpatient E & M services provided after the first inpatient encounter (for the admitting physician) or for services (other than consultative) provided by a physician other than the admitting physician.

A hospitalized patient may require more than one visit per day by the same physician. Group the visits together and report the level of service based on the total encounters for the day. Third-party payers vary in their requirements for reporting this service.

- *Hospital discharge services:* Use these codes for reporting services provided on the final day of a multiple-day stay.

Time is the controlling factor for assigning the appropriate hospital discharge services code. Total duration of time spent by the physician (even if the time spent is not continuous) should be documented and reported. These codes include final examination, discussion of hospital stay, instructions to caregivers, preparation of discharge records, prescriptions, and referral forms, if applicable.

CONSULTATIONS

By definition, a physician may not bill for a consultation unless another physician formally requests his or her opinion about the patient's present or future course of treatment. In addition, the consulting physician must communicate that opinion in either a letter or a dictated report. The patient's medical record should include the request by the physician who initiated the consultation and any information (letter, report, or dictation) that was communicated back to this physician.

If a specialist has a patient transferred to his or her care and is going to assume ongoing responsibility for that portion of the patient's care, this is a referral and office visit or hospital visit codes should be used, not consultation codes. An example would be a referral from another oncologist for ongoing treatment because of patient choice or geographic transfer.

There are two consultation subheadings in E & M coding:
- Office or other outpatient
- Initial inpatient

These two subheadings define the location where the consultation was rendered—physician's office; outpatient (or other ambulatory facility), codes 99241 through 99245; or inpatient hospital, codes 99251 through 99255. Only one initial consultation is reported by a consultant for the patient on each separate admission. Any subsequent service is reported with applicable codes from Subsequent Hospital Care codes 99231 to 99233 or Subsequent Nursing Facility Care 99307 to 99310. A follow-up consultation includes monitoring the patient's progress, recommending management modifications, or advising on a new plan of care in response to the patient's status.

● Stop and Think

Dr. Toledo, a family practitioner, has been treating patient Alma Cahill for a rash on her face; however, the medication she has prescribed is not helping the problem, and the rash is spreading to the neck. Dr. Toledo, with Alma's approval, makes an appointment with Dr. Farmer, a dermatologist, for continued treatment of the rash. Is this a consultation or a referral?

EMERGENCY DEPARTMENT SERVICES

E & M codes 99281 through 99288 are used for new and established patients who have been treated in an emergency department that is part of a hospital. To qualify, the facility must be available for immediate emergency care 24 hours a day for patients not on "observation status."

The "Other Emergency Services" subheading's single code, 99288, is used in physician-directed emergency care, advanced life support, when the physician is located in a hospital emergency or critical care department and is in two-way voice communication with ambulance or rescue personnel outside the hospital. The physician directs the performance of necessary medical procedures.

Pediatric critical care patient transport codes (99289 and 99290) are "time-based" codes used when a physician, located in a hospital or other facility, directs emergency treatment of a pediatric patient (24 months old or younger) to the transporting staff via two-way communication. Code 99289 is used for the first 30 to 74 minutes of hands-on care during transport. Code 99290 is used in addition to 99289 to report each additional 30 minutes of care.

CRITICAL CARE SERVICES

- Critical care services can be provided in any setting.
- The physician must provide constant attendance or constant attention to a critically ill or injured patient. The physician need not be constantly at bedside per se, but is engaged in physician work directly related to the individual patient's care.
- Time is the controlling factor for assigning the appropriate critical care code. Total duration of time spent by the physician (even if the time spent is not continuous) should be documented and reported.
- Critical care codes should not be used for less than 30 minutes' duration.
- Services in critical care units must meet CPT guidelines to be billed as critical care.

NEONATAL INTENSIVE CARE SERVICES

Services are provided to **neonates** (newborns 28 days old or younger) admitted to the intensive care unit. Infants older than 28 days who are admitted to an intensive care unit should be assigned the appropriate critical care or E & M codes. Neonatal codes are global 24-hour codes and not reported as hourly services. When the neonate is not critically ill and attains a body weight exceeding 1500 g, the initial hospital care codes (99221-99223) should be used. The same definitions for critical care services apply for adults, children, and neonates. Subsequent intensive care codes (99299 and 99300) were new codes added in 2003. These per-day codes are used for the evaluation and management of recovering low-birth-weight infants with a present body weight of 1500 to 2500 g and 2501-5000 g, respectively.

ADDITIONAL CATEGORIES OF THE E & M SECTION

The categories that follow Neonatal and Pediatric Critical Care Services are as follows:
- Nursing Facility Services (99304 through 99318)
- Domiciliary, Rest Home (e.g., Boarding Home), or Custodial Care Services (99324 through 99337)
- Domiciliary, Rest Home (e.g., Assisted Living Facility), or Home Care Plan Overnight Services (99339 andd 99340)
- Home Services (99341 through 99350)
- Prolonged Services (99354 through 99360)
- Case Management Services (99361 through 99373)
- Care Plan Oversight Services (99374 through 99380)
- Preventive Medicine Services (99381 through 99429)
- Newborn Care (99431 through 99440)
- Special Evaluation and Management Services (99450 through 99456)
- Other Evaluation and Management Services (99499)

What Did You Learn?

1. What does "observation status" mean in E & M coding?
2. What is a "confirmatory consultation?"
3. Which of the four contributing factors has the most impact on critical care?
4. What is the term given to a newborn less than 30 days old?

Note: These categories and code ranges are based on the 2006 CPT-4 Manual.

E & M MODIFIERS

Before assigning a final E & M code, it is important to check for potential modifiers that should be assigned to report an altered service or procedure (e.g., an unusual or special circumstance that affects the service or procedure). Attaching modifiers to codes provides additional information regarding the services performed. Leaving off a needed modifier can result in denial of payment. The following is a list of the modifiers used most often with the codes in the E & M section. (Appendix A in the CPT manual contains a complete list of modifiers.)
- Prolonged Evaluation and Management Services: Modifier -21 or 09921.
  - This modifier is used only with the highest level of each E & M category when the service provided is greater than that usually designated for that code.

- Documentation should be provided to describe the circumstances.
  - This modifier does not affect reimbursement under Medicare's physician fee schedule.
- Unrelated Evaluation and Management Service by the Same Physician During a Postoperative Period: Modifier -24 or 09924
  - This modifier is used to differentiate between a related and unrelated service during the postoperative period. (Documentation must be submitted to the carrier when this modifier is assigned.) The ICD-9-CM code must substantiate that the care was provided for a condition unrelated to the condition that required surgery.
- Significant, Separately Identifiable Evaluation and Management Service by the Same Physician on the Same Day of a Procedure or Other Service: Modifier -25 or 09925
  - This modifier is used to differentiate services associated with global payment from services to be considered separately for payment. (Sending supporting documentation with the claim is not required when this modifier is applied.) This modifier should not be used to indicate that the visit or consultation resulted in the decision to perform major surgery.
- Mandated Services: Modifier -32 or 09932
  - This modifier is used to inform the third-party payer that the service is required or mandated (e.g., PRO, governmental, legislative, or regulatory requirement, or third-party payer).
- Reduced Services: Modifier -52 or 09952
  - In some instances, a service or procedure may be partially reduced or eliminated at the physician's discretion.
- Decision for Surgery: Modifier -57 or 09957
  - This modifier identifies an E & M service provided by the physician on the day before or the day of a surgery during which the initial decision to perform surgery was made.

nations, tests, treatments, and outcomes. The health record chronologically documents the care of the patient and is an important element contributing to high-quality care. The appropriately documented health record facilitates

- the ability of the physician and other healthcare professionals to evaluate and plan the patient's immediate treatment and to monitor his or her healthcare over time,
- communication and continuity of care among physicians and other healthcare professionals involved in the patient's care,
- accurate and timely claims review and payment,
- appropriate utilization review and quality of care evaluations, and
- collection of data that may be useful for research and education.

An appropriately documented health record can reduce many of the challenges associated with claims processing and may serve as a legal document to verify the care provided, if necessary. Figure 13-13 is a list of the top 10 coding errors.

E & M DOCUMENTATION GUIDELINES: 1995 VERSUS 1997

In addition to the guidelines found in the CPT manual, HCFA (now CMS) published two sets of documentation guidelines. The first set of guidelines became effective in 1995, and the second set became effective in 1997. The goal was to develop and refine a way to assign a "score" accurately for each level of medical services in the E & M categories. The guidelines specifically identify the elements that must be documented in the medical record to support a particular level or service and a workable method to determine the level of medical decision making.

1995 Guidelines

The history and medical decision-making criteria outlined in the 1997 guidelines are basically the same as the 1995 guidelines. The main difference in the two sets of guidelines is in the criteria needed for the examination compo-

---

What Did You Learn?

1. What is the function of a modifier?
2. Why is it important to attach a needed modifier to a code?
3. Where are modifiers found in the CPT manual?

IMPORTANCE OF DOCUMENTATION

Health record documentation is required to record pertinent facts, findings, and observations about a patient's health history including past and present illnesses, exami-

---

1. No documentation for services billed.
2. No signature or authentication of documentation.
3. Always assigning the same level of service.
4. Billing of consult vs. outpatient office visit.
5. Invalid codes billed due to old resources.
6. Unbundling of procedure codes.
7. Misinterpreted abbreviations.
8. No chief complaint listed for each visit.
9. Billing of service(s) included in global fee as a separate professional fee.
10. Inappropriate or no modifier used for accurate payment of claim.

Fig. 13-13 Top 10 coding and billing errors.

nent. The 1995 guidelines criteria required less information to be documented for the examination than the 1997 guidelines, but the examination criteria are vague and generally leave much to the opinion of an auditor, easily opening the door for differing opinions between auditor and physician.

1997 Guidelines

In the 1997 guidelines, the examination criteria are detailed and require more documentation. The advantage with this approach is that the 1997 guidelines criteria leave little room for an auditor to form an opinion different from that of the physician, and it becomes easier for auditors to verify that a higher level of service reported was correctly coded. Although the 1997 guidelines criteria may require a little more time to learn for some health insurance professionals, templates are available to make this task easier. Because of various problems encountered with the 1997 guidelines, mandatory implementation of this newer set of rules was postponed, and CMS currently allows either set of rules (1995 or 1997) to be used.

As mentioned previously, the principal difference between these two sets of rules is the examination portion. The 1997 guidelines has a series of detailed examinations with required items indicated by shaded areas or bullets, whereas the 1995 guidelines have a more general counting of body areas and systems. The health insurance profes-

sional may choose either the 1995 or 1997 rules. Table 13-4 compares the 1995 versus 1997 guidelines.

DECIDING WHICH GUIDELINES TO USE

Although it is acceptable to use either the 1995 or the 1997 E & M documentation guidelines, it is unacceptable to use them interchangeably on the same document. An extended history may be documented under the 1997 guidelines by identifying three chronic or inactive conditions and the current status of those conditions. The 1995 guidelines *do not* permit this documentation practice. Under the 1995 guidelines, an extended history requires documentation of at least four HPI elements. The HPI elements include *location, quality, severity, duration, timing, context, modifying factors, and associated signs/symptoms.*

What Did You Learn?

1. Name three ways a well-documented health record contributes to high-quality healthcare.
2. What is the principal difference between the 1995 E & M documentation guidelines compared with the guidelines published in 1997?
3. Which set of guidelines does CMS prefer a medical office use?

TABLE 13-4 Comparison Physical Examination

1995 REQUIREMENTS	1997 REQUIREMENTS
Problem-Focused Examination	**Problem-Focused Examination**
Limited to affected body area or organ system	1-5 element(s) in one or more organ system(s) or body area(s)
Expanded Problem-Focused Examination	**Expanded Problem-Focused Examination**
Limited examination of the affected body area or organ system and other symptomatic or related organ system(s) Two to seven body areas or organ systems	6 elements in one or more organ system(s) or body area(s)
Detailed Examination	**Detailed Examination**
Extended examination of the affected body area(s) and other symptomatic or related organ system(s) Two to seven body areas or organ systems	At least six organ systems or body area(s) For each of the six organ systems or body areas, at least 2 elements identified by a bullet is expected; *or* At least 12 elements identified by a bullet in two or more organ systems or body areas
Comprehensive Examination	**Comprehensive Examination**
A general multisystem examination or a complete examination of a single organ system* Eight or more organ systems	At least nine organ systems or body areas For each organ system/body area, *all* elements identified by a bullet should be performed For each organ system/body area, documentation of at least 2 elements identified by a bullet is expected

*1995 criteria do not define documentation elements for a single organ system examination.

OVERVIEW OF THE HCPCS CODING SYSTEM

HCPCS is a coding system that is composed of Level I (CPT) codes, Level II (National) codes, and formerly Level III (local) codes. CPT codes are composed of 5 digits that describe procedures and tests. CPT codes are developed and maintained by the AMA with annual updates. Level II (National) codes are 5-digit alphanumeric codes consisting of one alphabetic character (a letter between A and V) followed by 4 digits. HCFA created Level II codes to supplement CPT, which does not include codes for nonphysician procedures, such as ambulance services, durable medial equipment, specific supplies, and administration of injectable drugs. Level II codes are developed and maintained by CMS with quarterly updates. The following are examples of Level II codes:

A4646—Supply of low osmolar contrast material (300 to 399 mg of iodine)

J0150—Injection, adenosine (Adenocard), 6 mg

J2250—Injection, midazolam hydrochloride (Versed), 1 mg

If a CPT code and HCPCS Level II code are available for the service provided, CMS requires that the HCPCS Level II code be used.

HCPCS Level II Format

HCPCS Level II codes are organized into 17 sections (Fig. 13-14). The D codes, which include dental procedure codes D0000 through D9999, represent a separate category of codes from the Current Dental Terminology (CDT-4) code set, which is copyrighted and updated by the American Dental Association.

Index of Main Terms

An index of main terms, arranged in alphabetical order similar to the Level I CPT-4 codes, follows the 17 alphabetized sections. Codes are located in the index using similar guidelines as CPT-4 codes: locate the main term, turn to the alphanumeric listing, and find the applicable code (Fig. 13-15).

Table of Drugs

The Level II (National) code manual also contains a table of drugs, which the health insurance professional should use to locate appropriate drug names that correspond with the generic names listed in the J code subsection.

MODIFIERS

As with CPT-4, HCPCS Level II code sets contain modifiers. Modifiers in HCPCS Level II are alphabetic or alphanumeric. They are used to indicate that a service or procedure that has been performed has been altered by some

- **A Codes:** Transportation Services Including
  - Ambulance
  - Medical and Surgical Supplies
  - Respiratory Durable Medical Equipment, Inexpensive and Routinely Purchased
  - Administrative, Miscellaneous and Investigational
- **B Codes:** Enteral and Parenteral Therapy
- **C Codes:** Hospital Outpatient Prospective Payment System (OPPS)
- **E Codes:** Durable Medical Equipment
- **G Codes:** Temporary Codes for Professional Services Procedures
- **H Codes:** Alcohol and/or Drug Services
- **J Codes:** Drugs Administered Other Than Oral Method
- **K Codes:** Temporary Codes for Durable Medical Equipment
- **L Codes:** Orthotic Procedures
- **M Codes:** Medical Services
- **P Codes:** Pathology and Laboratory Tests
- **Q Codes:** Temporary Codes
- **R Codes:** Domestic Radiology Services
- **S Codes:** Temporary National Codes
- **T Codes:** National Codes for State Medicaid Agencies
- **V Codes:** Vision/Hearing/Speech-Language Pathology Services

Fig. 13-14 17 Sections of HCPCS Level II (National) codes.

specific circumstances, but not changed in its definition or code. The HCPCS manual contains a complete listing of modifiers and their meaning.

What Did You Learn?

1. How are HCPCS Level II codes structured?
2. What do "J" codes represent in HCPCS coding?
3. What is the function of a HCPCS Level II code modifier?

HIPAA AND HCPCS CODING

CMS has taken steps to prepare for the full implementation of HIPAA. HIPAA requires that there be standardized procedure coding. For CMS to meet this requirement, they have produced an instructional guide to assist the health insurance professional in eliminating local procedure and modifier codes from their system. Official HCPCS Level III procedure and modifier codes are defined as codes and descriptors developed by Medicare contractors for use by physicians, practitioners, providers, and suppliers on a local level for the completion of insurance claims. Level

HCPCS 2004 INDEX / Hair analysis

H

Hair analysis (excluding arsenic), P2031
Hallus-Valgus dynamic splint, L3100
Hallux prosthetic implant, L8642
Haloperidol, J1630
    decanoate, J1631
Halo procedures, L0810–L0860
Halter, cervical head, E0942
Hand finger orthosis, prefabricated,
    L3923
Hand restoration, L6900–L6915
    partial prosthesis, L6000–L6020
    orthosis (WHFO), E1805, E1825,
        L3800–L3805, L3900–L3954
    rims, wheelchair, E0967
Handgrip (cane, crutch, walker), A4636

Hydrocollator, E0225, E0239
Hydrocolloid dressing, A6234–A6241
Hydrocortisone
    acetate, J1700
    sodium phosphate, J1710
    sodium succinate, J1720
Hydrogel dressing, A6242–A6248,
    A6231–A6233
Hydromorphone, J1170
Hydroxyzine HCl, J3410
Hyland G-F 20, J7320
Hyoscyamine Sulfate, J1980
Hyperbaric oxygen chamber, topical, A4575
Hypertonic saline solution, J7130

I

pump, heparin, dialysis, E1520
pump, implantable, E0782, E0783
pump, implantable, refill kit, A4220
pump, insulin, E0784
pump, mechanical, reusable, E0779, E0780
pump, uninterrupted infusion of Epi-
    prostenol, K0455
supplies, A4221, A4222, A4230–A4232
therapy, other than chemotherapeutic
    drugs, Q0081
Inhalation solution (*see also* drug name),
    J7608–J7699
Injections (*see also* drug name), J0120–J7320
    contrast material, during MRI, A4643
    supplies for self-administered, A4211
Insertion, indwelling catheter, G0002
Insertion tray, A4310–A4316

Fig. 13-15 Example page from HCPCS Index. (Data from U.S. Department of Health and Human Services, Centers for Medicare and Medicaid Services.)

III codes that were approved by CMS through the official process were incorporated into the HCPCS manual. Unapproved local procedure and modifier codes that were not approved by CMS were dropped.

ELIMINATION OF UNAPPROVED LOCAL CODES AND MODIFIERS

In anticipation of implementation of HIPAA, CMS has required medical offices to eliminate any unapproved local procedure or modifier codes that they are currently using. To accomplish this, medical offices must do the following:

- Identify all unapproved local procedure and modifier codes that were established or that are being used
- "Crosswalk" any unapproved local procedure and modifier codes to a temporary or permanent national code
- Submit any unapproved local procedure or modifier codes that the medical facility believes should be retained, along with a request for a temporary national code with a justification, to the regional office representative by April 1, 2002
- Delete all other unapproved local procedure and modifier codes by October 16, 2002

✓ HIPAA Tip

Payers and providers alike must go over the HCPCS codes they use and determine how to best replace their "local" HCPCS codes with the new national codes.

WHAT IS A CROSSWALK?

A **crosswalk** is a procedure by which codes used for data in one database are translated into the codes of another

database, making it possible to relate information between or among databases. In coding, a crosswalk is a "link" that refers to a relationship between a medical procedure (CPT code) and a diagnosis (ICD code). Medicare uses CPT/ICD crosswalks to validate or substantiate medical necessity under LCD/LMRP (Local Medicare Review Policy). Third-party payers also establish crosswalk tables for validating and auditing medical claims. In brief, physicians dealing in Medicare Part B claims are paid by CPT procedure code, not diagnosis. To validate proper coding (e.g., the reason for the procedure), providers must specify a diagnosis. If the diagnosis does not support the procedure, the claim may not get paid.

What Did You Learn?

1. What does HIPAA require of HCPCS coding?
2. Which level of HCPCS codes did HIPAA eliminate?
3. What is a "crosswalk?

CURRENT PROCEDURAL TERMINOLOGY, 5TH EDITION (CPT-5)

The AMA is in the process of developing the next generation of *Physicians Current Procedure Terminology, Fifth Edition* (**CPT-5**). Ideally, this updated version will improve existing CPT features and correct deficiencies. CPT-5 is structured to respond to challenges presented by emerging user needs and HIPAA. Changes to CPT have been oriented toward the need to preserve the core of CPT, while encouraging progress. Transition into the changes proposed for CPT-5 will be gradual, and all enhancements and modifications will occur through the traditional CPT Editorial process. To avoid disruption in medical offices, it is planned that changes will be phased-in over several years.

The AMA states that CPT-5 "is intended to preserve the core elements that define CPT as the *language to communicate clinical information for administrative and financial purposes.*" CPT-5 will continue to include
- descriptions of clinically recognized and generally accepted healthcare services,
- five-character core codes (5 digits for regular CPT codes for the foreseeable future) with concept extenders (modifiers), and
- professional responsibility for a mechanism for periodic review and updating.

The AMA further states that "CPT-5 encourages progress so that CPT *evolves with changes in healthcare delivery and services to accommodate the needs of users.*" To stimulate change, CPT will continue to
- maximize user input while continuing to maintain an editorially rigorous update process;
- provide accurate and up-to-date communication of clinical services; and
- respond to the requirements of healthcare professionals, payers, and researchers for tools to support evidence-based clinical practice.

What Did You Learn?

1. What well-known organization is developing CPT-5?
2. Name two things CPT-5 is predicted to accomplish.

SUMMARY CHECK POINTS

☑ The *purpose* of CPT is to provide a uniform language accurately describing medical, surgical, and diagnostic services, serving as an effective means for reliable communication among physicians, third-party payers, and patients nationwide.

☑ CPT was developed and published by the AMA in 1966. Originally, it contained mainly surgical procedures, with limited sections on medicine, radiology, and laboratory procedures. The second edition, published in 1970, expanded codes to designate diagnostic and therapeutic procedures in surgery, medicine, and other specialties. In 1970, the 5-digit system was introduced, replacing the former 4-digit codes, and internal medicine procedures were added.

☑ In 1983, CPT was adopted as part of HCPCS. HCFA (now CMS) mandated the use of HCPCS to report

services for the Medicare Part B Program. In 1986, HCFA required state Medicaid agencies to use HCPCS. In 1987, as part of the Omnibus Budget Reconciliation Act, HCFA mandated the use of CPT for reporting outpatient hospital surgical procedures.

☑ Today, CPT is the preferred system of coding and describing healthcare services.

☑ The CPT manual begins with an introduction, followed by six sections in the main body of the manual. Category III Codes follow the main section, after which there are 12 appendices—A through L. The CPT Index of main terms appears at the back of the manual.

☑ A bullet (●) before a code means the code is "new" to the CPT book for that particular edition.

☑ A triangle (▲) means the description for the code has been "changed or modified" since the previous edition of the CPT book.

☑ Horizontal triangles (▶◀) placed at the beginning and end of new or revised guidelines indicates changes in wording.

☑ Add-on codes are annotated by a + symbol.

☑ The Ø symbol is used to identify codes that are exempt form the use of modifier -51.

☑ The semicolon is used to separate main and subordinate clauses in the CPT code descriptions. The complete description listed *before* the semicolon applies to that code plus any additional succeeding, indented codes. The complete description *after* the semicolon applies only to that code.

☑ The basic steps for CPT coding are
- Step 1—identify the procedure, service, or supply to be coded.
- Step 2—determine the main term.
- Step 3—locate the main term in the alphabetic index and note the code.
- Step 4—cross-reference the single code, multiple codes, or the code range numerically in the tabular section of the manual.
- Step 5—read and follow any notes, special instructions, or conventions associated with the code.
- Step 6—determine and assign the appropriate code.

☑ A new patient is someone who is new to the practice, regardless of location of service, or one who has not received any medical treatment by the healthcare provider or any other provider in that same office *within the past 3 years.*

☑ An established patient is an individual who has been treated previously by the healthcare provider, regardless of location of service, within the past 3 years. If the provider saw the patient for the first time in a hospital, and that individual comes to the office for a follow-up visit after discharge, the patient is considered an established patient to the practice because health record documentation was generated from the hospital visit.

☑ The three key components that establish the level in E & M coding are as follows:
  • *History*—subjective information based on four elements: CC (in the patient's own words), HPI, ROS, and PFSH. There are four levels of history: (1) problem focused, (2) expanded problem focused, (3) detailed, and (4) comprehensive.
  • *Examination*—deals with the degree to which the healthcare provider examines various body areas and organ systems that are affected by the CC. There are four levels of examination: (1) problem focused, (2) expanded problem focused, (3) detailed, and (4) comprehensive.
  • *Medical decision making*—this component is determined by weighing the complexity involved in the healthcare provider's assessment of and the professional judgment made regarding the patient's diagnosis and care. The three elements considered are how many diagnostic and treatment options are considered; the amount and complexity of data reviewed; and the amount of risk for complications, morbidity, or mortality. There are four levels in medical decision making: (1) straightforward, (2) low complexity, (3) moderate complexity, and (4) high complexity.

☑ Besides the above-mentioned three key components, the four contributing factors that may affect the level of E & M Coding are as follows:
  • Counseling
  • Coordination of care
  • Nature of presenting problem—minimal, self-limiting, low severity, high severity
  • Time

☑ Time can be measured two ways in E & M coding:
  • *Face-to-face time*—time the physician spends in direct contact with the patient during an office visit, which includes taking a history, performing an examination, and discussing results.
  • *Unit floor time*—time the physician spends on patient bedside care and reviewing the health record and writing orders.

☑ The history and medical decision-making criteria outlined in the 1995 guidelines are the same as the 1997 guidelines. The main difference in the two sets of guidelines is the criteria for the examination. The 1995 guidelines criteria require less information to be documented for the examination than does the 1997 guidelines. The 1997 guidelines have a series of detailed examinations with required items indicated by shaded areas or bullets, whereas the 1995 rules have a more general counting of body areas and systems.

☑ The HCPCS is a coding system that is composed of Level I (CPT) codes, Level II (national) codes, and formerly Level III (local) codes. CPT codes are composed of 5 digits that describe procedures and tests. Level II (national) codes are 5-digit alphanumeric codes that describe pharmaceuticals, supplies, procedures, tests, and services. HCFA created Level II codes to supplement CPT, which does not include codes for nonphysician procedures, such as ambulance services, durable medical equipment, specific supplies, and administration of injectable drugs. If there are a CPT code and HCPCS Level II code for the service provided, CMS requires that the HCPCS Level II code be used.

☑ HIPAA requires that there be standardized procedure coding. In anticipation of implementation of HIPAA, CMS has required medical offices to eliminate any unapproved local procedure or modifier codes that they are currently using. To accomplish this, medical offices must:
  • Identify all unapproved local procedure and modifier codes that were established or that are being used.
  • "Crosswalk" any unapproved local procedure and modifier codes to a temporary or permanent national code.
  • Submit any unapproved local procedure or modifier codes that the medical facility believe should be retained, along with a request for a temporary national code with a justification, to the regional office representative by April 1, 2002.
  • Delete all other unapproved local procedure and modifier codes by October 16, 2002.

CLOSING SCENARIO

Park and Melanie have finished the chapter on CPT coding. Although they agree it was more challenging than the chapter on ICD-9 coding (particularly the E & M coding), Melanie believes that Park's help was extremely beneficial. She is now convinced that she will finish the course on time and with an acceptable grade. Meanwhile, Park still believes that coding is the right career move for him. He has researched the websites at the end of the chapter to learn all he can about coding. He has even located a website bulletin board where practicing coders write in questions and answers on coding issues. After he finishes the medical insurance course, Park plans to take a coding course over the Internet. He is looking forward to continuing his pursuit of a career in coding.

WEBSITES TO EXPLORE

For live links to the following websites, please visit the Evolve® site at http://evolve.elsevier.com/Beik/today/

- AMA at http://www.ama-assn.org/

- Medicare Learning Network (Medlearn) at http://www.cms.hhs.gov/medlearn/

- CMS at http://www.cms.hhs.gov/

- US Department of Health & Human Services at http://www.hhs.gov/

REFERENCES AND RESOURCES

American Medical Association. Current Procedural Terminology, CPT (2004) Standard Edition. Chicago, 2006, AMA Press.

American Medical Association. HCPCS, 2005. Chicago, 2005, AMA Press.

Buck CJ: Step-by-Step Medical Coding, 5th ed. Philadelphia, 2004, Saunders.

Covell A: Coding Workbook for the Physician's Office. 2003, Delmar/Thomson Learning, Clifton Park, NY.

Davis JB: CPT and HCPCS Coding Made Easy! A Comprehensive Guide to CPT and HCPCS Coding for Health Care Professionals. 2000, PMIC, Downer's Grove, IL.

Fordney MT: Insurance Handbook for the Medical Office, 7th ed. Philadelphia, 2002, Saunders.

Rowell JC, Green MA: Understanding Health Insurance, A Guide to Professional Billing, 7th ed. 2004, Delmar/Thomson Learning.

UNIT IV

The Claims Process

Chapter 14

The Patient

Chapter Outline

I. Patient Expectations
   - A. Professional Office Setting
   - B. Relevant Paperwork and Questions
   - C. Honoring Appointment Times
   - D. Patient Load
   - E. Getting Comfortable with the Healthcare Provider
   - F. Privacy and Confidentiality
   - G. Financial Issues

II. Future Trends
   - A. Aging Population
   - B. The Internet as a Healthcare Tool
   - C. Patients as Consumers

III. HIPAA Requirements
   - A. Authorization to Release Information
   - B. HIPAA and Covered Entities
   - C. HIPAA Requirements for Covered Entities
   - D. Patient's Right of Access and Correction
   - E. Accessing Information Through Patient Authorization
   - F. Accessing Information Through De-identification

IV. Billing Policies and Practices
   - A. Assignment of Benefits
   - B. Keeping Patients Informed
   - C. Accounting Methods
     - 1. "One-Write" or Pegboard Accounting System
     - 2. Electronic Patient Accounting Software

V. Billing and Collection
   - A. Billing Cycle
   - B. Arranging Credit or Payment Plans
     - 1. Self-Pay Patients
     - 2. Establishing Credit
   - C. Problem Patients
     - 1. Five Categories of Problem Debtors
     - 2. Collecting from Problem Debtors

VI. Laws Affecting Credit and Collection
   - A. Truth in Lending Act
   - B. Fair Credit Billing Act
   - C. Equal Credit Opportunity Act
   - D. Fair Credit Reporting Act
   - E. Fair Debt Collection Practices Act

VII. Collection Methods
   - A. Collection by Telephone
     - 1. Timetable for Calling
     - 2. Selecting Which Patients to Call
   - B. Collection by Letter

VIII. Billing Services

IX. Collection Agencies

X. Small Claims Litigation
   - A. Who Can Use Small Claims
   - B. How the Small Claims Process Works

CHAPTER OBJECTIVES

After completion of this chapter, the student should be able to

- List and discuss various patient expectations.
- Name two future trends in the patient-practice relationship.
- Explain what a "HIPAA covered entity" is.
- Define "identifiable information," and list the various elements that make it so.
- Explain how personal health information can be "de-identified."
- List the elements that a HIPAA-approved release of information must contain.
- Discuss two methods of accounting used in today's healthcare facilities.
- Describe how a healthcare practice can increase its financial success.
- List the five federal laws that affect collections.
- Outline the steps involved in the small claims litigation process.

CHAPTER TERMS

accounts receivable
alternate billing cycle
assignment of benefits
billing cycle
collection agency
collection ratio
daily journal
defendant
de-identified
disbursements journal
Equal Credit
    Opportunity Act
Fair Credit Billing Act
Fair Credit Reporting
    Act
Fair Debt Collection
    Practices Act

general journal
general ledger
HIPAA-covered entities
identifiable health
    information
"one-write" systems
patient information
    form
patient ledger
payroll journal
plaintiff
self-pay patient
small claims litigation
surrogates
Truth in Lending Act

OPENING SCENARIO

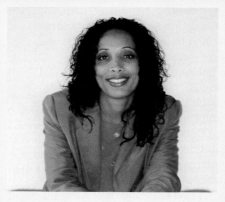

Callie Foster enrolled in the health insurance program not only because it offered interesting and challenging career opportunities, but also because of an incident she had recently experienced. Callie had had ear pain for several days, so she called for an appointment at ENT Dr. Susan Dayton's office. Callie took time off work to drive the 30 miles to the ENT clinic. When she arrived and signed in at the front desk, the medical receptionist asked for her insurance card; however, after searching in vain through her pockets and purse, Callie said she must have left it at home. "Then," said the receptionist brusquely, "you will have to reschedule. Dr. Dayton does not see patients who do not have insurance." Before Callie could confirm the fact that she had coverage through her employer, the receptionist turned away, ignoring her protests. Callie ended up in the emergency department later that day with a ruptured eardrum.

This experience was very upsetting, and Callie wants to find out what patients typically expect when they visit a healthcare office. She firmly believes that all members of the healthcare team should learn how to empathize and listen to what patients have to say. Callie was convinced that there is no excuse for impolite behavior and harsh treatment in a healthcare office.

Scott Tanner is a classmate of Callie Foster. Scott's interests lay not only in the patient side of medical insurance, but also in credit law and collections. Scott wants to learn about the small claims process; his parents own rental units and occasionally experience problems collecting rents. Scott and Callie look forward to having their questions answered in Chapter 14.

PATIENT EXPECTATIONS

When patients visit a healthcare practice they bring something with them that may not be obvious to the healthcare team. Besides their sore throats, broken legs, or heart palpitations, they bring with them a set of expectations.

These expectations were created by previous experiences with other healthcare providers, the media, and the opinions of their friends and family. If the healthcare provider and healthcare office staff are oblivious to those expectations, the entire practice risks being perceived as cold and unfeeling. If the healthcare office staff is successful in meeting or exceeding these expectations, the patient likely will be pleased with the care he or she receives.

The first step in creating a good patient-staff relationship begins when the individual telephones for an appointment. How this encounter is handled can have a lasting impression of how the patient perceives the entire practice—including the healthcare providers. If the rapport between the physicians and the medical team is strained and uneasy, patients pick up on this, and they are likely to feel tension also. The bottom line—overlooking patients' needs and expectations can be costly to the practice. Keep in mind that without patients, there is no practice.

It is also important to be up-front with office policies and procedures. When patients are sick or hurting, they usually do not feel up to questioning the medical staff about their policies or procedures. They usually are reacting from their physical symptoms, and their lack of questions or interest is caused by the fear of the unknown. Some conditions can be very frightening, such as a burning chest pain or a breast lump. It is the responsibility of the medical staff to find out what their patients' expectations are by asking questions. Being open with patients, anticipating their concerns, and helping create an atmosphere where patients feel they can discuss their needs safely are comforting and affirming.

Patient expectations vary from office to office. The following are some issues to consider when evaluating new patient protocol.

PROFESSIONAL OFFICE SETTING

When individuals walk into a hardware or clothing store, they are looking for physical items—tangible things they can pick up, examine, and put into their shopping cart. If they are unhappy with the hammer or sweater purchased, they can voice a complaint or return the item for a refund. The services offered by a healthcare facility are intangible—individuals cannot see or feel them. When individuals buy intangible services, they compensate by looking for **surrogates**—or substitutes to put their mind at ease. Surrogates that patients look for in a healthcare office may be the office location, size and layout, and staff enthusiasm; even the color of the walls can affect a new patient's initial judgment as to the quality of care that particular office provides. A shabby reception room suggests shabby care.

RELEVANT PAPERWORK AND QUESTIONS

A good deal of paperwork must be completed and many questions need to be answered when seeing a healthcare provider for the first time. Besides being brief and of high quality, paperwork should seem relevant to the reason the patient is there. Personal questions, such as whether a patient smokes or drinks, how many pregnancies a (female) patient has had, whether a patient is divorced or widowed, and whether a patient has some form of sexual dysfunction, should be asked privately out of hearing from office staff and other patients. It also might be necessary to explain how these forms and questions relate to the individual's care and treatment.

HONORING APPOINTMENT TIMES

Time is a valuable commodity in today's fast-paced lifestyle in the United States, and staying on schedule communicates respect for the patient's time. Because the encounter may be a new experience for some patients, when he or she phones for an appointment, time-management experts recommend that the medical receptionist explain approximately how long an initial visit will take and what to expect. If the healthcare provider gets behind schedule, as is often the case, patients can become annoyed, glancing at their watches, shifting in their seats, and looking at the receptionist expectedly for explanations. The reception staff should keep the patient advised as to the length of delay and the reason for the delay. The patient might be told, "Dr. Miller has been delayed because of an emergency, so you may have to wait another 10 or 15 minutes." The patient should be kept apprised of the anticipated time he or she will be seen: "Dr. Miller has just left the hospital and will be here in approximately 10 minutes." If it looks

Imagine This!

Jennifer Cooper had a 2 p.m. appointment with Dr. Shirley Bennet, a gynecologist. She arrived about 10 minutes early, as the receptionist recommended when she made the appointment. After completing all the necessary new patient forms, the reception staff advised Jennifer that Dr. Bennet had been called out on an emergency cesarean section, and that she would be about a half hour late. The staff gave Jennifer the options of waiting or rescheduling. Jennifer, already having waited nearly 2 weeks for an opening in Dr. Bennet's schedule, chose to stay. Dr. Bennet kept the reception staff informed periodically as to how things were progressing, and this information was quickly and quietly passed on to Jennifer. Additionally, she was offered a choice of coffee or a cold soda. The reception room atmosphere was comfortable with pleasant background music and had an assortment of recent issues of magazines to browse through. Although Jennifer ended up waiting nearly 45 minutes for her appointment with Dr. Bennet, she did not become irritated or impatient because she was kept apprised of Dr. Bennet's schedule and was treated courteously by the staff.

like the wait is going to be lengthy, the receptionist should offer to reschedule the patient's appointment or ask if the patient has a brief errand to run. Many individuals today believe that their time is equally as valuable as the physician's, especially if they have taken time off work for their appointment.

Imagine This!

Lurvis Burke, a civil engineer with a consulting engineering firm, took time out of his busy schedule to visit a cardiologist for a routine stress test, recommended by his family physician. Lurvis had a 9 A.M. appointment with Dr. Harlan Solomon and arrived shortly before his appointment time, filled out the new patient paperwork, and sat down to wait. Two hours later, his name was called and a member of the medical staff ushered him to an examination room without a word. When Dr. Solomon entered the examination room where Lurvis was waiting, he found an angry patient who informed him that he did not appreciate the long wait, and that he considered his time just as important as the physician's. Lurvis vowed not to return to Dr. Solomon's office in the future. Compare this patient's experience with that of Jennifer Cooper.

● Stop and Think

Reread the "Imagine This!" scenario featuring Lurvis Burke. Do you think Mr. Burke is justified in his decision to not return to this office? How would you have handled this situation if you were the front desk receptionist?

PATIENT LOAD

A new patient often draws conclusions as to the competency of the healthcare provider and the entire healthcare team by observing how many others are waiting in the reception area. If the reception area is empty when the patient enters, he or she may think, "Why aren't there more people here? Maybe this doctor isn't very good." To avoid this negative reaction, some practices schedule new patients during their busiest times. This can be a workable solution as long as it does not result in a longer wait for established patients.

Imagine This!

Juanita Lindo, the medical receptionist for Anthony Park, a neurosurgeon, informed new patients when scheduling appointments that Dr. Park preferred reserving an ample amount of time for the encounter. The physician allowed a half hour before the examination, an hour for the examination, and a half hour after to answer all questions and ensure the patient and family members were comfortable and well informed as to their options before leaving his office. When a patient arrived for an appointment, he or she was already aware of how long the encounter would take, explaining the absence of a reception room full of waiting patients.

GETTING COMFORTABLE WITH THE HEALTHCARE PROVIDER

It is human nature for patients to want to like their physicians as much as respect them. Perceptive patients expect their physicians to reveal enough information about themselves so that they can "identify" with them. That does not mean the physician and staff members need to discuss their personal lives with patients, but sharing of personal information does promote a good provider-patient relationship and often tends to relieve anxiety if the physician and staff members compare a personal experience that is relevant to what the patient is experiencing.

Imagine This!

Dottie Shrike visited Dr. Forrest Carpenter, her family practitioner, for treatment of an episode of anxiety and mild depression after being fired from her job as a teacher's aide. Dr. Carpenter, attempting to alleviate some of Dottie's angst, related a story about an experience he had had before becoming a physician. He was working for a trucking firm and had lost his job because of noncompliance with company policy. He was young then, like Dottie, and the experience left him feeling humiliated and vulnerable. Relating this story to Dottie allowed her to feel as if he really understood her problem, reinforcing the provider-patient relationship.

PRIVACY AND CONFIDENTIALITY

If the medical professional wants patients to reveal their most personal health-related secrets, patients must feel confident that this information will be kept private and confidential. If patients who are waiting in the reception room hear the front desk staff talking about other patients, it can lead them to believe that their own information will be treated casually, too. The office staff must make every effort possible to assure patients that any personal information they divulge will be held in the strictest confidence. When making and receiving telephone calls, speak quietly or close the glass partition (which is recommended by Health Insurance Portability and Accountability Act [HIPAA] regulations) so that conversations do not carry out into the reception area. Also, the entire medical staff should be cautioned when talking among themselves or to patients in examining rooms. Walls are often thin, allowing voices to carry into adjacent rooms.

FINANCIAL ISSUES

Most patients have an idea of what their medical care and treatment should cost before they make an appointment. Some even do some "comparison shopping." Although many patients may be embarrassed or uneasy discussing fees, especially ahead of time, it is good business practice to discuss the financial ramifications of the healthcare encounter. Most physicians prefer to leave the subject of fees to their reception staff. When a new patient telephones for an appointment and explains his or her condition or symptoms that prompted the call, giving the individual a range of what the initial fee will be is considered appropriate. Today's healthcare consumers expect the cost of their healthcare to be addressed up-front.

● Stop and Think

Mary Ellen Brown calls Dr. Bennet's office for an appointment. She explains that she is new in the area and is looking for a "good" OB-GYN because she thinks she may be pregnant. What kind of information might the medical receptionist give Mrs. Brown?

What Did You Learn?

1. Besides their health problems, what do patients bring with them to the healthcare office?
2. List four "issues" that affect patient expectations.
3. Why is a clean, well-kept reception room important?
4. What is the rationale of explaining policies and fees up-front to patients?

FUTURE TRENDS

Most healthcare experts agree that today's healthcare bears little resemblance to that of a decade ago. The United States is faced with a rapidly changing healthcare environment, and individuals who are involved in the healthcare field must identify and anticipate future trends—from new technology to changing directions and demographics.

AGING POPULATION

Over the next 30 years, as the baby boomer generation ages, the number of Americans older than age 65 will double. Healthcare facilities will need to be prepared to handle an increasing volume of elderly patients. Dealing with the geriatric population can be quite different from dealing with younger groups. The healthcare staff should be aware of, or even specially trained in, the particular skills for interacting with this demographic faction. Many local medical organizations or community colleges offer continuing education courses in the care and treatment of elderly patients.

THE INTERNET AS A HEALTHCARE TOOL

Individuals have found that the Internet offers access to a lot of relevant, quality healthcare information. Websites are delivering large amounts of healthcare knowledge to consumers, allowing them to form their own opinions and expectations. Individuals are involved in the relatively new process of self-education not possible before the advent of the Internet. Websites help individuals find physicians and hospitals that offer certain procedures, and other websites offer lifestyle advice plus educational details and references for a multitude of health conditions.

Imagine This!

Greg Manning was diagnosed with prostate cancer, and the options his physician gave him held a high probability of impotence, which was unacceptable to Greg. He logged onto the Internet and began an extensive search for possible alternatives. He found a clinic in another state where the medical staff offered a relatively new, noninvasive procedure that was highly successful in patients with similar malignancies. Greg traveled to the clinic and met with the staff physicians to discuss the procedure. Greg was very happy with the alternative they presented and subsequently underwent the new procedure successfully.

Internet tools that can be used to reach today's computer-oriented consumer can help healthcare facilities serve patients better. Some successful online patient-centered topics include

- physician-patient communication,
- online scheduling (e.g., examinations, procedures),
- online billing services,
- physician biographies, and
- procedural information.

It is predicted that future patients will rely more and more on the Internet, and healthcare providers will have to adapt their practices to meet these state-of-the-art electronic requirements.

PATIENTS AS CONSUMERS

As evidenced by the increase in medical news on television and in advertising, radio broadcasts, periodicals, and Internet sites, the healthcare industry must acknowledge a new type of patient—one who is more educated, more aware of choices, and more likely to take an active part in his or her own healthcare decisions. Experts say that today's patients should be considered "consumers," rather than "patients." Today, Americans are exposed to an enormous amount of medical information on a daily basis. Some of this information can be misleading and confusing. Whether or not patients are correctly informed, however, healthcare providers will be expected to take the time to satisfy their questions about diagnosis, treatment, and therapy options.

A new set of healthcare consumer essentials has been developed that experts believe should become mandatory for any healthcare facility that endeavors to provide patient-centered service. These essentials include

- choice,
- control (self-care, self-management),
- shared medical decision making,
- customer service, and
- information.

Today's patients, similar to other types of consumers, are likely to switch healthcare plans or healthcare providers if they believe they are not getting the quality service they desire.

What Did You Learn?

1. List three things that affect future trends in the healthcare office.
2. How might the Internet change the future of healthcare?
3. Name three medical services that currently are being offered over the Internet.
4. List four healthcare consumer "imperatives" that experts claim should be mandatory for "patient-centered" services.

HIPAA REQUIREMENTS

HIPAA has had a big impact on healthcare, particularly where confidentiality is concerned. What is contained in a patient's health record has always been confidential—dating back to the wording of the Hippocratic oath. HIPAA has refined the rules of confidentiality, however, for covered entities in a much more comprehensive way.

AUTHORIZATION TO RELEASE INFORMATION

The release of any information contained in a patient's health record to a third party, with certain exceptions, is prohibited by law. Civil and criminal penalties exist for the unauthorized release of such information. A healthcare provider can be allowed to release confidential information from an individual's health records only with the consent of the individual or the person authorized to give consent for that individual.

HIPAA AND COVERED ENTITIES

HIPAA is a federal law designed to protect the privacy of individuals' health information. A major component of HIPAA addresses this privacy by establishing a nationwide federal standard concerning the privacy of health information and how health information can be used and disclosed. This federal standard generally preempts all state privacy laws except for those that establish stronger protections. HIPAA privacy laws became effective April 14, 2003.

 HIPAA Tip

Covered entities, such as health plans, healthcare providers, and claims clearinghouses, must comply with HIPAA rules. Other businesses may comply voluntarily with the standards, but the law does not require them to do so.

HIPAA-covered entities consist of healthcare providers, health plans (including employer-sponsored plans), and healthcare clearing houses (including billing agents). These covered entities must comply with HIPAA rules for any health information of identifiable individuals. Protected health information under HIPAA is referred to as individually identifiable health information. **Identifiable health information** refers not only to data that are explicitly linked to a particular individual, but also includes health information with data items that reasonably could be expected to allow individual identification. Identifiable medical information includes medical records, medical billing records, any clinical or research databases, and tissue bank samples. Covered entities generally are unable to communicate or transfer protected health information to noncovered entities (who do not come under HIPPA rules) without violating HIPAA.

Potential identifiers that can link information to a particular individual include obvious ones, such as name and Social Security number, and the following:

- All geographic subdivisions smaller than a state, including street address, city, county, precinct, Zip Code (under certain circumstances, the initial 3 digits of a Zip Code can be used)
- All elements of dates (except year) directly related to an individual, including birth date, admission date, discharge date, and date of death
- Voice and fax telephone numbers
- E-mail addresses
- Medical record numbers, health plan beneficiary numbers, or other health plan account numbers
- Certificate/license numbers
- Vehicle identifiers and serial numbers, including license plate numbers
- Device identifiers and serial numbers
- Internet Protocol (IP) address numbers and Universal Resource Locators (URLs)
- Biometric identifiers, including finger and voice prints
- Full-face photographic images and any comparable images
- Any other unique identifying number, characteristic, or code

Note: The *covered entity* may assign a code or other means of identification to allow de-identified information, if it later may become necessary to re-identify the information. When the above-listed identifiable elements are removed, the information is, under most circumstances, considered **de-identified**.

HIPAA REQUIREMENTS FOR COVERED ENTITIES

Essentially, a HIPAA-covered entity cannot use or disclose protected health information for any purpose other than treatment, payment, or healthcare operations without either the authorization of the individual or an exception in the HIPAA regulations. In addition to limiting the use and disclosure of protected health information, HIPAA also gives patients the right to access their medical information and to know who the covered entity has disclosed this information to (including investigative research files). It also restricts most disclosures to the minimum amount possible to accomplish the intended purpose and establishes criminal and civil penalties and fines for improper use and disclosure by HIPAA-covered entities.

HIPAA requires covered entities to do the following:

- Institute a required level of security for health information, including limiting disclosures of information to the minimum required for the activity
- Designate a privacy officer and contact person

- Establish privacy and disclosure policies to comply with HIPAA
- Train all staff members on privacy policies
- Establish sanctions for staff members who violate privacy policies
- Establish administrative systems in relation to the health information that can respond to complaints, respond to requests for corrections of health information by a patient, accept requests not to disclose for certain purposes, and track disclosures of health information
- Issue a privacy notice to patients concerning the use and disclosure of their protected health information
- Establish a process through an international review or privacy board for a HIPAA review of research protocols
- Include consent for disclosures for treatment, payment, and healthcare operations in treatment consent form (optional)

HIPAA provides a limited public policy exception for protected health information disclosure involving public health issues, judicial and administrative proceedings, law enforcement purposes, and others as required by law.

PATIENT'S RIGHT OF ACCESS AND CORRECTION

A patient has the right to inspect or obtain copies of his or her protected health information from a healthcare provider or health plan, but not from clearinghouses. In contrast to other rules, exceptions to the right of access are limited. The primary exceptions are for circumstances considered reasonably likely to endanger the life or physical safety of that individual or another person (emotional health is excluded) and for clinical research.

The privacy rules introduce a new concept—the patient's right to correct or amend his or her medical record. This reflects an idea that has long been controversial: patient ownership of the medical record. Although under the new HIPAA rules, this right is limited by reasonable protections for the covered entity who controls the protected information, for the first time a patient has a right to ask for corrections or amendments to his or her medical record and to place an explanation into the record if that request is denied. The rules do not include, however, a requirement that incorrect information be removed from the record; rather it should be labeled as corrected, and the correction should be appended.

> ☑ **HIPAA Tip**
>
> Basic patient rights under HIPAA include the following:
> - Right to notice of information practices
> - Right to access to personal health information (PHI)
> - Right to an accounting of how PHI has been disclosed outside normal patient care channels
> - Right to request a amendment/correction to PHI

ACCESSING INFORMATION THROUGH PATIENT AUTHORIZATION

HIPAA states that when an authorization to release information (Fig. 14-1) is required from a patient, it must include the following elements:

- A description that identifies the information in a specific and meaningful fashion
- The name of the person authorized to make the requested use or disclosure
- The name of the person to whom the covered entity may make the requested use or disclosure
- A description of each purpose of the requested use or disclosure
- An expiration date or event that relates to the purpose of the use or disclosure
- A statement of the individual's right to revoke the authorization in writing and the exceptions to the right to revoke, together with a description of how the individual may revoke the authorization
- A statement that information used may be subject to re-disclosure by the recipient and no longer be protected by this rule
- Signature of the individual and date signed
- A description of a representative's authority to act for an individual if the authorization is signed by a personal representative of the individual.

 HIPAA Tip

Uses and disclosures *not* requiring patient consent:

- To carry out treatment, payment, or healthcare operations
- For public health, health oversight, judicial/administrative proceedings, coroners/medical examiners, and law enforcement

---

ACCESSING INFORMATION THROUGH DE-IDENTIFICATION

Covered entities can release de-identified health information without patient authorization. Protected health information can be de-identified through a general deletion of the identifiers listed in the section entitled HIPAA and Covered Entities. To release the information without patient authorization, the covered entity cannot have actual information that could be used alone or in combination with other information to identify an individual.

● Stop and Think

What information in the following documentation should be removed to "de-identify" this patient?
Frasier, Eric
DOB 1/13/1977
Patient #12112
6/10/2004

History: Eric presents to the clinic today for chief complaint of an abrasion on the right knee following a fall yesterday. According to the patient, he has had this soft tissue lesion for some time, and when he fell, he basically abraded the lower half of the lesion. He is here for re-evaluation and possible excision of the lesion.

   Pain assessment: Scale 0 to 10, 1
   Allergies: Meperidine (Demerol)
   Current medications: None
   Physical examination: NAD; ambulatory; appears well
   Vital signs: Blood pressure, 120/74 mm Hg; weight 150 lb
   Right knee examination: The patient has a tibial prominence, and just above that, there is what appears to be a 1.5-cm epidermal inclusion cyst with an abraded area inferiorly. There is mild erythema and serous drainage, but no purulence. There is no appreciable edema. Just lateral to the lesion is a small superficial abrasion. The knee examination was normal.
   IMP: Epidermal inclusion cyst measuring 1.5 to 2 cm of the right knee, traumatized with abrasion
   Plan: The patient was empirically started on cephalexin (Keflex) 500 mg 1 p.o. b.i.d. He was given instructions on home care and is to follow-up this week for excision of the lesion. Routine follow-up as noted. Return as needed.
   Frederick Mahoney, MD
   Friendly Family Clinic

What Did You Learn?

1. What are the three "entities" that are covered under HIPAA?
2. List at least six elements that make a patient health record "identifiable."
3. How does a patient health record become "de-identifiable?"
4. Name three exceptions to the confidentiality rule.

BILLING POLICIES AND PRACTICES

Billing policies and practices differ from one healthcare practice to another; however, they are basically the same.

Standard Authorization to Use or Disclose Protected Health Information (PHI)

Section A: The individual for whom this authorization is being requested. Please complete the following:

Name: First ___ M ___ Last ___ Group # ___ Identification # ___

Social Security Number ___ Date of Birth ___

Address ___ City ___ State ___ ZIP ___

Area Code & Telephone Number ___ E-mail Address (if available) ___

Section B: Please place an "X" in the box next to each category of specific Protected Health Information to disclose. (You may mark as many boxes as appropriate.)

☐ Any and All Information about my CHIP Coverage ☐ Claims ☐ Premium Payment/Billing History
☐ Eligibility and Enrollment ☐ Other (describe): ___

Section C: Describe the reason for the release or request of information.

☐ At my request ☐ Other (describe): ___

Section D: Who will provide this information?

Name: CHIP and its Plan Administrator
Address: 400 W. Monroe, Suite 202
Anytown, IL 08095
Relationship: Health Plan

Section E: Who will receive this information?

Name ___
Address ___
Relationship ___

Section F: Please place an "X" in the box next to the date or event that describes when your authorization will expire. (Please mark only one box.)

☐ Upon Revocation ☐ 1 year after my death ☐ 1 year after my CHIP coverage ends
☐ A specific date: ___ Month Day Year ☐ Other (describe): ___

Section G: I understand that:
- This authorization will expire on the date or event listed in Section F above.
- This authorization is voluntary.
- Payment, enrollment or eligibility for benefits for my health care will not be affected if I do not sign this form.
- I may revoke this authorization at any time by notifying in writing the company/individual listed in Section D from providing the PHI identified in this authorization, but if I do revoke this authorization, it won't have any affect on any actions the Comprehensive Health Insurance Plan took before they received the revocation.
- Information disclosed as a result of this authorization may no longer be protected by federal privacy laws and may be disclosed by the company or individual receiving the information.
- I should retain as my copy one of the duplicate authorization forms I received.

Section H: Signature.

I hereby authorize the use or disclosure of the Protected Health Information as described in Section B pertaining to the Individual listed in Section A.

Signature of Individual or Individual's Personal Representative ___ Date: month/day/year ___

Section I: If Section H is signed by a Personal Representative, please complete the information below:

Personal Representative's Name ___ Relationship to Individual ___

Personal Representative's Address ___ City ___ State ___ ZIP ___

Personal Representative's Area Code & Telephone Number ___ Personal Representative's E-mail Address (if available) ___

TPAuth Rev 6.03 — Page 1 of 1 (See Instructions on Next Page) — Standard Authorization–CHIP

Fig. 14-1 HIPAA-approved release of information form.

Most healthcare facilities anticipate that procedures and services provided to their patients will be paid for at the time of their occurrence. If the patient has insurance, most offices accept a partial payment or copay—typically 10% to 25% of the fee. Medical facilities are in business to make a profit; procedures and policies should be in place to protect the financial success of the practice.

ASSIGNMENT OF BENEFITS

An **assignment of benefits** is an arrangement by which a patient requests that his or her health insurance benefit payments be made directly to a designated person or facility, such as a physician or hospital. When new patients come to the healthcare office, they are typically requested to fill out a form providing name, address, employer, and health insurance information. Usually at the bottom of the page is a place for the patient's signature or, in the case of a minor or mentally handicapped individual, the signature of a parent or legal guardian. This form is commonly referred to as the **patient information form**.

On many patient information forms, in addition to the authorization to release information, there is nomenclature above the patient's signature that provides for the assignment of benefits, authorizing this transfer of payment from the insured to the healthcare provider. Some healthcare providers do not see a patient unless this assignment of benefits is signed.

Many healthcare providers today participate in a health maintenance organization, a preferred provider organization, or some similar organization. These practitioners are referred to as participating providers. When a provider is a participating provider, assigning benefits on the CMS-1500 or on the patient information form is unnecessary because there is a contractual agreement between the provider and the third-party carrier that payment automatically is sent directly to the provider. That is one of the benefits to becoming a participating provider.

KEEPING PATIENTS INFORMED

It is important that patients understand the healthcare practice's patient accounting policies and procedures, such as

- approximately how much the medical service or procedure will cost,
- when they are expected to pay for it, and
- what the practice is willing to do as far as claims submission to their insurance carrier.

Discussing professional fees with patients can be a delicate situation. The health insurance professional should not intimidate or offend patients when discussing fees and payment policies; however, he or she should ensure that patients are clear about their responsibilities. Most patients appreciate having billing information presented clearly and matter-of-factly, yet always in a pleasant and courteous manner. The healthcare office staff should encourage patients to ask questions about their bills or the payment/insurance process. Many offices have printed materials available, such as an informational brochure, for stating or reinforcing the practice's financial policies and procedures. This written information can be helpful in collecting fees.

Establishing sound billing practices is important in a healthcare office. Although healthcare practitioners are dedicated to the health and well-being of their patients, they are ultimately running a business for the purpose of making a profit. Keeping accurate financial records is equally as important as keeping accurate patient health records.

The ultimate goal in healthcare office billing is reimbursement or payment for the medical services provided to patients. A satisfactory **collection ratio** (the total amount collected divided by the total amount charged) can be challenging at times. Some healthcare offices display a sign that payment for services rendered is expected on the day services are provided. In other words, patients are expected to pay as they go, just as retail stores expect customers to pay for a tube of toothpaste or a can of soup at the time of purchase.

The front desk staff should request payment when the patient-provider encounter is concluded. Experts consider this the most effective payment policy. Patients who put off paying for their services are historically more difficult to collect from. It is common practice for the reception staff to ask for a particular percentage—often 20%—of the current charge; 20% is a common coinsurance amount.

● **Stop and Think**

The accounts receivable total of Dr. David Barclay's office was $231,500 for the first quarter of 2004. If $173,625 of this amount was successfully collected, what would be Dr. Barclay's collection ratio for this quarter?

ACCOUNTING METHODS

There is a good chance that the office where the health insurance professional finds employment uses a computerized medical accounting system for financial records. This is not always the case, however, and the health insurance professional should be aware of how paper accounting records are generated and maintained. A typical paper method of accounting includes a series of journals and ledgers, such as the following:

A **daily journal** (or day sheet) (Fig. 14-2) is a chronologic record of all patient transactions, including previous balances, charges, payments, and current balances for that day.

A **disbursements journal** (Fig. 14-3) is a listing of all expenses paid out to vendors, such as building rent, office supplies, and salaries. Some offices maintain a separate **payroll journal** (Fig. 14-4) for wages and salaries.

A **general journal**, the most basic of journals, is a chronologic listing of transactions. It has a specific

		DATE	PROFESSIONAL SERVICE	FEE	PAYMENT	ADJUST-MENT	NEW BALANCE	OLD BALANCE	PATIENT'S NAME
1									
2									
3									
4									
5									
6									
7									
8									
9									
10									
11									
12									
13									
14									
15									
16									Totals this page
17									Totals previous page
18									Totals to date

JOURNAL OF DAILY CHARGES, PAYMENTS & DEPOSITS

PLACE FIRST PEG HERE

COLUMN A   COLUMN B   COLUMN C   COLUMN D   COLUMN E

MEMO _____

DAILY - FROM LINE 31
ARITHMETIC POSTING PROOF
Column E	$
Plus Column A	
Sub-Total	
Minus Column B	
Sub-Total	
Minus Column C	
Equals Column D	

MONTH - FROM LINE 31
ACCOUNTS RECEIVABLE PROOF
Accts. Receivable Previous Day	$
Plus Column A	
Sub-Total	
Minus Column B	
Sub-Total	
Minus Column C	
Accts. Receivable End of Day	

Fig. 14-2 Example of a day sheet.

format for recording each transaction. Each transaction is recorded separately and consists of
- a date,
- all accounts that receive a debit entry (these are typically listed first with an amount in the appropriate column),
- all accounts that receive a credit entry (these are indented and listed next with an amount in the appropriate column), and
- a clear description of each transaction.

A **general ledger** is the core of the practice's financial records. The general ledger constitutes the central "books" of an accounting system, and every transaction flows through the general ledger. These records remain as a permanent track of the history of all financial transactions from day 1 of the life of a practice. The general ledger can be used to prepare a range of periodic financial statements, such as income statements and balance sheets.

A **patient ledger** (Fig. 14-5) is a chronologic accounting of a particular patient's (or family's) activities, including

FEBRUARY 2006

DATE	DESCRIPTION	CHECK NUMBER	AMOUNT	PER CAPITA	RENT	PHONE	OFFICE SUPPLIES	POSTAGE	OFFICERS' EXPENSE	NEWS LETTER
1-FEB	ABC Realty	291	475.00		475.00					
1-FEB	AFT	292	2,301.60	2,301.60						
1-FEB	State Fed	293	1,288.60	1,288.60						
1-FEB	Central Labor Council	294	75.60	75.60						
1-FEB	Bell Telephone	295	131.00			131.00				
7-FEB	State Fed	296	1,828.60	1,828.60						
21-FEB	Sue Smith, Sec'y	297	50.00						50.00	
28-FEB	Mary Jones, Petty Cash	298	18.50				16.00	2.50		
			6,168.90	5,494.40	475.00	131.00	16.00	2.50	50.00	0.00

Fig. 14-3 Sample cash disbursements journal.

Date	Employee	Hourly Rate	Regular Hours	Overtime Hours	Net Pay	Check Number	Federal Withholding	OASI	Insurance	Retirement	Other	Gross Pay	Fund	Account

Fig. 14-4 Payroll journal.

all charges and payments. The entire group of patient ledgers is referred to as the **accounts receivable**.

"One-Write" or Pegboard Accounting System

Paper accounting systems, such as "one-write" or "write-it-once" systems, have been widely used in physicians' offices over the years. **One-write systems** (Fig. 14-6) (also known as the pegboard system) are a useful method of accounting for small practices. A one-write system captures information at the time the transaction takes place. These systems are efficient because they eliminate the need for recopying the data, and many are compatible with electronic data processing if the office decides to computerize. Many small businesses rely totally on the one-write system for simplicity and versatility. One-write systems are popular for several reasons; they are

• accurate,
• relatively inexpensive,
• easy to learn, and

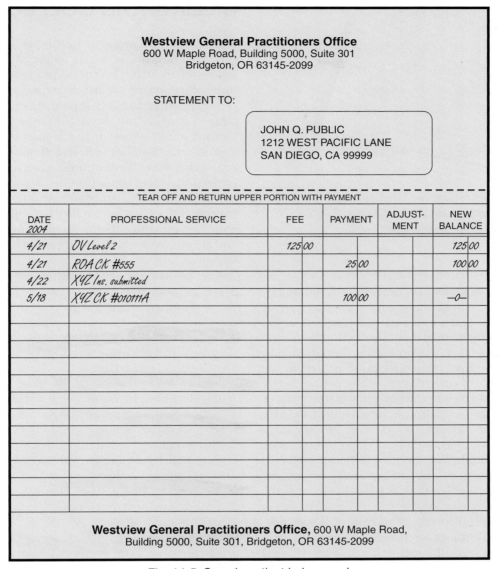

Fig. 14-5 Sample patient ledger card.

- use a write-it-once process for recording daily office transactions.

Electronic Patient Accounting Software

Increasingly, healthcare offices are using electronic patient accounting software programs, and most healthcare practices are computerized to some extent. Previous barriers to computerization have been largely overcome by the introduction of effective and user-friendly systems for the management of clinical records and appointments. Computerized patient billing software typically includes accounts receivable, appointment scheduling, insurance billing, and practice management modules.

Computerized patient accounting typically begins with inputting the demographic patient data and creating a patient "account" within the software program. When all patient data have been entered into the system, patient lists and many other documents can be generated in

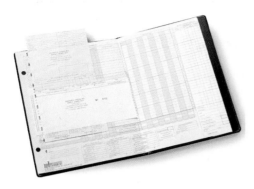

Fig. 14-6 Front office "one-write" (pegboard) billing example. (Courtesy Bibbero Systems, Inc., Petaluma Calif., (800) 242-2376; Fax (800) 242-9330; www.bibbero.com)

several ways. A list of patient appointments by day and by provider and an encounter form for each one can be printed. When the patient encounter is concluded, the health insurance professional inputs the information from the encounter form—date, diagnosis code, procedure code, and charges. Also, any payments can be posted to the computer program. A current copy of the patient ledger can be printed and given to the patient as a statement or as a receipt. Appointments also can be scheduled, deleted, and adjusted within the accounting system. Periodic statements, aging reports, and CMS-1500 claim forms can be generated. The computer program performs all phases of the accounting process quickly and accurately. Any system, computerized or manual, is only as good, however, as the individual who inputs the information. Accuracy is crucial. A back-up system is also crucial in case of power fluctuations or failure. Without a dependable back-up system, all electronic data could be lost as a result of electrical problems or human error. Daily back-ups should be made and stored in a fireproof vault to prevent loss of patient records.

What Did You Learn?

1. What is an "assignment of benefits"?
2. Name three things that are important for patients to know about a healthcare practice.
3. What are the four elements that must be included in each transaction in a general journal?
4. Name three advantages to the "one-write" pegboard accounting system.
5. A computerized patient accounting system can generate many kinds of documents. Name four.

BILLING AND COLLECTION

Individuals who work in healthcare offices claim that collecting past due accounts is one of the least pleasant aspects of the job. Healthcare practices that maintain a high collection ratio say that the most effective way to collect money is to establish a formal financial policy that is clear to patients and the healthcare staff and enforce it. Patients need to know that it is important to pay in full and on time, and the medical staff needs to know what is expected of them. There are times when the health insurance professional must take a firm stand, and the situation can get uncomfortable. An aggressive approach to account collection does not have a negative effect on developing good rapport with patients. A collection policy that is fair and clear to patients and staff results in fewer misunderstandings (Fig. 14-7).

The following is a list of suggestions some healthcare practices use that aid in their financial success. These items are often included in the practice's policy manual.

- *Have a written payment/credit policy.* Give a copy to each patient, and discuss it with him or her and ensure that each point is understood.
- *Do not ignore overdue bills.* The older the bill, the more uncollectible it becomes. Begin a plan of action as soon as the account becomes 30 days old.
- *Rebill promptly.* Some experts suggest rebilling every 15 days, rather than the traditional 30 days. Stamp or place a sticker on the second statement with the words *Second Notice.*
- *Telephone or write a letter.* This can be effective if the second statement does not get a response from the patient.
- *Do not apologize when telephoning or writing about delinquent bills.* Simply ask the customer to write a check today for the full amount owed.
- *Be pleasant and courteous.* There is never a reason to get into an argument, even if the patient becomes hostile. Listen patiently to what the patient has to say without interrupting; try to be understanding.
- *Ask for the full amount, not just a partial payment.* If a patient owes $500, ask for the full $500. If the patient says he or she will send a partial payment, ask what the exact amount will be and exactly what date the payment will be sent. Avoid vagueness, such as, "I'll send you something in a couple of days."
- *Negotiate the terms, but not the amount.* If you believe the patient truly has a problem paying, offer to work out a payment plan, but do not make this offer right away, only as a last resort. Also, always adhere to the office policy when negotiating terms.
- *Use the services of a small claims court.* If patient promises are not kept or if the account ages past a certain time period (e.g., 60 days, depending on office policy), small claims litigation is an alternative.

Payment Policy

Thank you for choosing our practice! We are committed to the success of your medical treatment and care. Please understand that payment of your bill is part of this treatment and care.

For your convenience, we have answered a variety of commonly-asked financial policy questions below. If you need further information about any of these policies, please ask to speak with a Billing Specialist or the Practice Manager.

How May I Pay?
We accept payment by cash, check, VISA, Mastercard, American Express and Discover.

Do I Need A Referral?
If you have an HMO plan with which we are contracted, you need a referral authorization from your primary care physician. If we have not received an authorization prior to your arrival at the office, we have a telephone available for you to call your primary care physician to obtain it. If you are unable to obtain the referral at that time, you will be rescheduled.

Which Plans Do You Contract With?
Please see attached list.

What Is My Financial Responsibility for Services?
Your financial responsibility depends on a variety of factors, explained below.

Office Visits and Office Services

If you have:	You are Responsible for:	Our staff will:
Commercial Insurance Also known as indemnity, "regular" insurance, or "80%/20% coverage."	Payment of the patient responsibility for all office visit, x-ray, injection, and other charges at the time of office visit.	Call your insurance company ahead of time to determine deductibles and coinsurance. File an insurance claim as a courtesy to you.
Medicare HMO	All applicable copays and deductibles at the time of the office visit.	File the claim on your behalf, as well as any claims to your secondary insurance.
Workers' Compensation	If we have verified the claim with your carrier No payment is necessary at the time of the visit. If we are not able to verify your claim Payment in full is requested at the time of the visit.	Call your carrier ahead of time to verify the accident date, claim number, primary care physician, employer information, and referral procedures.
Workers' Compensation (Out of State)	Payment in full is requested at the time of the visit.	Provide you a receipt so you can file the claim with your carrier.
Occupational Injury	Payment in full is requested at the time of the visit.	Provide you a receipt so you can file the claim with your carrier.
No Insurance	Payment in full at the time of the visit.	Work with you to settle your account. Please ask to speak with our staff if you need assistance.

Fig. 14-7 Payment policy. (Courtesy Karen Zupko & Associates.)

● Stop and Think

You notice that Theodore Simpson's account balance is $365, and he has not made a payment for 45 days. Office policy is to telephone patients 15 days after the last statement has been sent. How will you handle this? Create a telephone "scenario" of your conversation with Mr. Simpson.

BILLING CYCLE

Sending statements to patients on a regular basis is necessary to maintain cash flow for the practice and an acceptable collection ratio. Every healthcare office has its own routine for sending statements. Typically, statements are mailed periodically—usually every 30 days. This process is called a **billing cycle**. In large practices, one 30-day mass billing for all patients is a cumbersome task. Large healthcare offices often use an **alternate billing cycle**—a billing system that incorporates the mailing of a partial group of statements at spaced intervals during the month. With an alternate billing cycle, the breakdown of accounts frequently is determined by an alphabetical list of last names or by account numbers. Patients with last names ending in A through F would be sent statements on the first of the month; patients with last names ending with G through L would receive statements on the 10th day of the month. One advantage to an alternate billing cycle is that cash flow is distributed throughout the entire month, whereas billing only once a month generates a large amount of receipts at one time during the month. No one specific method is considered best for all healthcare practices. Each practice must establish its own system that works well.

ARRANGING CREDIT OR PAYMENT PLANS

The cost of some medical treatments or procedures can be thousands of dollars, and the patient might not have adequate insurance coverage (or may have no insurance at all) to pay the medical fees. Many healthcare facilities offer patient/client financing plans, which allow patients to get the treatment or procedures they need and want and pay for it in periodic installments—much the same as purchasing a car. A comprehensive range of plan options is available in healthcare facilities across the United States that offer a low, or at least a manageable, monthly payment to fit almost every budget.

Self-Pay Patients

Some patients may have inadequate health insurance coverage or no insurance at all. These are referred to as **self-pay patients**. Just because patients are self-pay does not mean they are "deadbeats." Some individuals who do not carry health insurance still are able to pay their medical bills in a timely manner.

As mentioned previously, the patient should be provided with the policies and expectations of the healthcare practice early on in the encounter. Under most state laws, full payment for medical services is due and payable at the time the service is provided. Healthcare providers often take the initiative, however, to temper this mandate as they see fit.

When a patient completes the patient information form, and there is no insurance listed, the health insurance professional should inquire as to the reason. It is possible that the insurance section was overlooked. If the patient has no insurance, it is prudent to inquire tactfully as to how he or she intends to pay for the service. Some healthcare offices ask the patient whether or not he or she has insurance when the appointment is made, and if not, the patient must make at least a partial payment in advance.

Ideally, the practice should have an established credit plan for self-pays because it is mandatory that every patient be treated equally. Equally as important, the healthcare office cannot refuse to see an established patient because of an outstanding debt. There is a procedure, however, where (if carried out within the confines of the law) a healthcare provider can terminate the patient-provider relationship. This involves sending a certified letter to the patient, with a return receipt to confirm the patient received the letter, communicating the fact that the patient can no longer be treated (for whatever reason spelled out in the letter), and giving the patient a specified amount of time to find alternative care. Following this structured method of notifying the patient that the practice will no longer accept him or her as a patient and spelling out the reason why limit the practice's liability in the event of legal action brought by the patient accusing the practice of "abandonment."

Establishing Credit

When patients cannot make payment in full, credit is sometimes arranged, and a payment plan is established (Fig. 14-8). Some medical facilities offer a credit arrangement whereby the patient can pay the fee, interest-free, in several installments. Other medical facilities allow more flexibility for self-paying patients by offering an installment plan with interest rates lower than most major credit cards.

It is important to keep in mind, however, that an installment payment plan of more than four payments comes under the Federal Truth in Lending Act of 1968, Regulation Z. Regulation Z applies to each individual or business that offers or extends consumer credit if the following four conditions are met:

1. The credit is offered to consumers.
2. Credit is offered on a regular basis.
3. The credit is subject to a finance charge (i.e., interest) or must be paid in more than four installments according to a written agreement.
4. The credit is primarily for personal, family or household purposes.

The Truth in Lending Act of 1968 and Regulation Z are discussed in more detail later in this chapter.

PROBLEM PATIENTS

There are times, for whatever reason, that the health insurance professional knows or has reason to believe that it may be difficult to collect fees from a particular patient. A policy should be in place for "problem" patients such as these or for patients who, for whatever reason, "send up a red flag." The following are some suggestions to maximize collection success from problem or questionable patients:

5   Financial Arrangements

Payment is expected at time of service.

For your convenience, we offer the following methods of payment. Please check the option which you prefer.

_____ Cash

_____ Personal Check

_____ Credit Card   _____ Visa _____ Mastercard

_____ I wish to make arrangements with an office manager today.

Late Charges

I realize that failure to keep this account current may result in you being unable to provide additional services except for emergencies or where there is prepayment for additional services. In the case of default on payment of this account, I agree to pay collection costs and reasonable attorney fees incurred in attempting to collect on this amount or any future outstanding account balances.

Thank you for filling out this form completely.
The information you have provided will help us serve your healthcare needs more effectively and efficiently.
If you have any questions at any time, please ask – we are always happy to help.

Fig. 14-8 Sample of financial arrangement plan.

- Contact a local credit bureau to find out if the patient is creditworthy.
- Discuss the credit policy with the patient before the encounter, and establish a payment that is affordable for the patient.
- Have the patient sign a written agreement.
- Ask the patient make a down payment of at least 20%.
- Arrange with the patient and his or her bank for automatic withdrawals if the patient has an account where that is a viable option.
- Charge interest (if that is practice policy) or a "carrying fee" to give the patient added incentive to make regular payments and pay off the balance promptly.
  Note: Even if the practice does not charge interest, if it is mutually agreed that the account will be paid off in more than four payments, the practice by law must provide the patient with a copy of the Truth in Lending Law.
- Arrange to have payments automatically deducted each month on a presigned credit card form.
- Do not allow the payments to extend past the treatment program, or 12 months, whichever is the lesser.
- Provide the patient with a self-addressed, stamped, return envelope in each bill.

Keep a copy of the signed agreement on file, so the office staff can refer to the agreement for specific monthly payments or fees for missed payments. Most healthcare offices keep these agreements in a separate file rather than in the patient's health record.

When setting up payment arrangements, be considerate but firm. The health insurance professional should explain the payment plan clearly, emphasizing that payments must not be missed, and that the payment must be received on or before the due date.

Five Categories of Problem Debtors

It takes experience and intuition to know the difference between patients who will not or tell you they cannot pay but who have sufficient funds to do so and the patients who genuinely cannot pay. Problem debtors fall into five categories:

- The *something-else-came-up debtors*—Unforeseen events cause delay payments, a common occurrence in most healthcare practices. The patient has had an emergency, had intended to pay the bill, but now is in a financial situation that prevents him or her from paying the bill on time.
- The *chronically slow debtors*—These patients have funds, but simply do not pay their bills on time.
- The *can't pay debtors*—These patients are over-extended; they have too many expenses and not enough income to pay them.
- The *forgetful debtors*—This type simply needs reminding.
- The *fraudulent debtors*—These are patients who had no intention of paying. These are the "deadbeats." The good news is they compose only a small percentage of the population.

It may be a waste of time to call patients who fall into this last category. Efforts should be concentrated on recovering dollars from patients who can or want to pay—the something-else-came-up, the chronically slow, the can't-pay, and the forgetful debtors. These are the individuals who will pay, but they may need prodding to collect.

Collecting from Problem Debtors

A recommended procedure for collecting from problem debtors is as follows:

- Ask for full payment on the day services are rendered.
- If the patient cannot or will not pay in full, request at least 20% of the bill.

- Send the patient a statement after 30 days.
- Send a second statement 15 to 30 days later with a "second reminder" sticker or note.
- Telephone the patient 15 days after the second statement has gone out if a substantial payment has not been received.
- Turn the account for collection or take the patient to small claims court.

What Did You Learn?

1. List five things a healthcare practice can do to aid in their financial success.
2. Explain how an "alternate billing cycle" can be used.
3. What is meant by a "self-pay" patient?
4. Name the four conditions that must be met under Regulation Z when a business extends credit.

LAWS AFFECTING CREDIT AND COLLECTION

Because healthcare offices typically extend credit to their patients/customers, they need to comply with federal consumer credit laws. Before we get too far into the collection process, it is important that the health insurance professional become acquainted with collection laws. The following is an introduction to the relevant federal laws dealing with consumer credit.

TRUTH IN LENDING ACT

The **Truth in Lending Act** helps consumers of all kinds know what they are getting into. It requires the person or business entity to disclose the exact credit terms when extending credit to applicants and regulates how they advertise consumer credit. Among the items that must be disclosed to a consumer who buys on credit are the following:

- The monthly finance charge
- The annual interest rate
- When payments are due
- The total sale price (the cash price of the item or service, plus all other charges)
- The amount of any late payment charges and when they'll be imposed.

FAIR CREDIT BILLING ACT

The **Fair Credit Billing Act** tells the business entity, in this case, the healthcare practice, what to do if a customer claims you made a mistake in their billing. The customer must notify the practice within 60 days after the first statement containing the claimed error was mailed. The practice must respond within 30 days unless the dispute already has been resolved. The practice also must conduct a reasonable investigation and, within 90 days of getting the customer's letter, explain why the bill is correct or else correct the error. If this procedure is not followed, the practice must give the customer a $50 credit toward the disputed amount—even if the statement was correct. Until the dispute is resolved, the practice cannot report to a credit bureau that the customer is delinquent.

State laws also may deal with billing disputes. Generally, if a state law on this subject conflicts with the federal statute, the federal statute will control, but there is one exception: A state law will prevail if it gives a consumer more time to notify a creditor about a billing error. As explained earlier, the federal law gives a consumer 60 days after receiving a bill to notify you of a billing error. If a state law gives a consumer 90 days to notify you, the consumer will be entitled to the extra 30 days. In addition to advising how to handle billing disputes, the Fair Credit Billing Act requires that the entity granting credit, in periodic mailings, must tell consumers what their rights are.

EQUAL CREDIT OPPORTUNITY ACT

The **Equal Credit Opportunity Act** states that a business entity may not discriminate against a credit applicant on the basis of race, color, religion, national origin, age, sex, or marital status. The act does allow freedom to consider legitimate factors in granting credit, such as the applicant's financial status (earnings and savings) and credit record. Despite the prohibition on age discrimination, you can reject a consumer who has not reached the legal age for entering into contracts.

FAIR CREDIT REPORTING ACT

The **Fair Credit Reporting Act** deals primarily with credit reports issued by credit reporting agencies. It is intended to protect consumers from having their eligibility for credit damaged by incomplete or misleading credit report information. The law gives consumers the right to a copy of their credit reports. If they see an inaccurate item, they can ask that it be corrected or removed. If the business entity reporting the credit problem does not agree to a change or deletion, or if the credit bureau refuses to make it, the consumer can add a 100-word statement to the file explaining his or her side of the story. This statement becomes a part of any future credit report.

FAIR DEBT COLLECTION PRACTICES ACT

The **Fair Debt Collection Practices Act** addresses abusive methods used by third-party collectors—bill collectors hired to collect overdue bills. Small businesses are more directly affected by state laws that apply directly to collection methods used by a creditor. The Fair Debt Collection Practices Act states that unless a debtor consents or a court order permits, debt collectors may not call to collect a debt

- at any time or place that is unusual or known to be inconvenient to the consumer (8 A.M. to 9 P.M. is presumed to be convenient),
- when the medical staff is aware that the patient/debtor is represented by an attorney with respect to the debt, unless the attorney fails to respond to the communication in a reasonable time period, and
- at work if the creditor is aware of the fact that the patient's employer prohibits such contacts.

What Did You Learn?

1. List the five federal laws that affect credit and collection.
2. Generally, if a state law allows more time for the debtor to notify the creditor about a billing error than does the federal statue, which prevails?
3. What does the Equal Credit Opportunity Act address?
4. Name the three telephone limitations upheld by the Fair Debt Collection Practices Act.

COLLECTION METHODS

No matter how careful, how cautious, or how capable the health insurance professional or collection manager is; no matter how experienced, how resourceful, or how persuasive the health insurance professional or collection manager is—there always will be some bad debts in a healthcare practice. There are two common methods healthcare offices use for collecting bad debts: collection by telephone and collection by letter.

COLLECTION BY TELEPHONE

Collecting overdue accounts by phone is a job that many healthcare office employees would prefer not to do. It is so much easier to write a collection letter than to call a patient about a delinquent account, but the collection call is considered far more effective. Many offices have even found that the collection call, when done correctly, is an inexpensive and effective collection technique. It costs money to continue sending statements and letters.

Healthcare practices that have experienced success with telephone collections call patients approximately 15 days after a second statement has been mailed out. The practice identifies the remaining accounts to be called and priori-

tizes them according to amount owed with the largest amount to be handled first. An alternative method is to work the accounts in alphabetical order, but if time runs out, the last half of the alphabet may not get called, which may include individuals who owe large amounts. Ideally, call the most recent and largest accounts first.

Making collection calls throughout the day with special emphasis from 5 P.M. to 8 P.M. is recommended whenever possible. Most offices report that more patients can be reached between 5 P.M. and 7 P.M. than at any other time during the day. The health insurance professional should be aware of the legal limits of telephone collection calls as spelled out in the Fair Debt Collection Practices Act. For more information on this act, see the listing in Websites to Explore.

Timetable for Calling

A workable telephoning timetable needs to be specific and must be followed consistently to get results. This may be one half of the list per week or per month, depending on the size of the practice. Random calling tends not to work as well.

Do not wait too long to get aggressive with collections. Many offices wait 4, 5, or 6 months before making the first collection call—a policy that yields a very low return. Collection specialists claim that calling closer to the time of service results in greater payoffs. The longer an account is left without follow-up calls, the less chance there is of collecting the fees.

Selecting Which Patients to Call

The next step is to select which patients to call. Some offices believe that it is not cost-effective to call accounts that are less than a certain amount—$30 to $45. A large practice with thousands of patient visits per month may not find it cost-effective to call accounts less than $100. Fig. 14-9 shows examples of typical conversation scenarios and how the health insurance professional may handle the situation.

COLLECTION BY LETTER

Collecting delinquent accounts by letter has been fairly successful for some healthcare practices. The timing and wording of written communications with patients should be based on numerous factors, including the size of the balance owing, the payment history of the patient, and the philosophy and policy of the practice.

When composing collection letters, be careful with the verbiage used so as not to anger or upset the patient. Be matter-of-fact and nonthreatening. Adopt the attitude that the patient has simply overlooked the bill and will make a payment because of this reminder letter. Fig. 14-10 shows a series of example collection letters. These letters

Patient:	"The check is in the mail."
HIP:	"Thank you for mailing your check. What day did you mail it? What was the amount of the check and the check number?"
Patient:	"I don't pay the bills. Talk to my wife."
HIP:	"Mr. Hughes, you're our patient. That is why I'm calling you regarding the account."
Patient:	"I'll have to discuss it with my husband. He's at work right now."
HIP:	May I call your husband at work and straighten this out? What is the phone number?"
Patient:	"I'll have to think about it and see if I can raise the money."
HIP:	"Mr. Hughes, credit was extended to you in good faith when it was needed. I'm sure you are a responsible person and want to meet your obligations."
Patient:	"I'm laid off work and can't pay anything now."
HIP:	"Mrs. Hughes, I'm sorry that you've been laid off. How long have you been out of work? Are you receiving unemployment compensation? Is your spouse working?"
Patient:	"But I can't pay all of it now."
HIP:	"We have a payment plan available, Mr. Williams, that will bring your account up-to-date without too much difficulty."

Fig. 14-9 Sample phone conversations.

can be tailored to fit the particular needs of the practice and the patients. Additional letters or phone calls can be added to extend the time between communications. The key is to stay in constant communication with overdue accounts, rather than adopting a "wait until tomorrow" attitude or assuming that the account will have to be written off or turned over for collection.

What Did You Learn?

1. Why might a telephone call be more effective in collecting delinquent accounts than a letter?
2. When does the text suggest the healthcare practice make its first collection call?
3. What minimum amount does the text say warrants a telephone call?

BILLING SERVICES

Some healthcare practices "outsource" their medical billing by hiring a separate professional medical billing service. A reputable medical billing service can provide comprehensive, cost-effective, HIPAA-compliant medical billing solutions for healthcare professionals nationwide. Medical billing services typically are organized and run by medical billing professionals who design, implement, and manage the accounts receivable portion of the healthcare practice. A well-run medical billing service can help a healthcare practice run more efficiently by eliminating staffing issues, undisciplined medical billing and collection processes, outdated medical billing systems, and archaic reporting

tools that result in poor collection ratios. Billing services can perform multiple functions for the healthcare practice, such as

- preparing and submitting insurance claims;
- providing data entry of patient demographics, insurance information, charges, payments, and adjustments;
- tracking payments from patients and third-party payers;
- producing practice management reports; and
- collecting delinquent accounts.

Usually, a computer, modem, and Internet access are all that is needed to access a billing service's network, after which the medical facility can retrieve up-to-the-minute patient information and practice management reports at any time on a secure server. Many billing services are available locally and nationwide. With the advent of the Internet, a healthcare office can interact with a professional billing service anywhere in the United States. Care should be taken, however, when choosing a billing service. The service should be thoroughly researched and references checked out with several of their current customers.

What Did You Learn?

1. What is a billing service?
2. List five functions of a billing service.

COLLECTION AGENCIES

A **collection agency** is an organization that obtains or arranges for payment of money owed to a third party—in this case, a healthcare office. Many healthcare practices use

Example Letter 1: Send when the account is past 30 days	Example Letter 2: Send 15 days after letter #1 if no payment is made
Dear Mrs. Williams: Your account balance of $340.50 is now overdue. Please send your payment to the above address at your earliest convenience. If you have questions, you can reach our bookkeeper at xxx-xxxx between 8 a.m. and 5 p.m. weekdays. Sincerely, XYZ Family Clinic	Dear Mrs. Williams: Despite several communications, we have not received payment for your overdue balance in the amount of $340.50. Your account is now seriously past due. Please send your payment to the above address or contact our bookkeeper at xxx-xxxx if you have questions. We will contact you by telephone if we do not hear from you within 7 days. Sincerely, XYZ Family Practice
Example Letter 3: Send 15 days after letter #2 if no payment is made.	**Example Letter 4:** Send 15 days after letter #3 if no payment is made.
Dear Mrs. Williams: We have made all reasonable attempts to work with you to reduce your seriously overdue balance with our clinic. You have not met the terms of the payment plan that we agreed upon. Professional services have been provided to your family in good faith, and payment of your account will protect your status as a family in good standing. We must hear from you within 15 days of the date of this letter. Our bookkeeper is available on weekdays between the hours of 8 a.m. and 5 p.m. Sincerely, XYZ Family Clinic	CERTIFIED MAIL RETURN RECEIPT REQUESTED Dear Mrs. Williams: You have failed to pay or satisfactorily reduce your severely delinquent balance despite our many efforts to work with you. Therefore, XYZ Family Clinic will no longer be providing medical care for you and your children. You should place your family under the care of another physician as soon as possible. You may contact XYZ Family Clinic or the County Medical Society for a referral to a new physician. When you have selected another physician, please send us a signed authorization so that we can provide a copy of your children's medical charts or a summary of its contents to your new physician. XYZ Family Clinic will remain available to treat your children for a short time, which will be no more than 30 days from the date of this letter. Please make the transfer to a new physician as soon as possible within that period. Sincerely XYZ Family Clinic

Fig. 14-10 Sample letter series for delinquent accounts.

collection agencies to help collect delinquent accounts. Collection agencies provide a service to businesses that
- are too small to have a collection department of their own,
- lack the expertise to collect delinquent accounts themselves,
- think a collection agency would get faster results, or
- simply do not want to deal with the hassle of collections.

Most collection agencies request at least 50% of the money they collect. Experts suggest that delinquent bills should be turned over for collection only when it is obvious that payment by any other means is a dead issue. When to go to collection is a business decision made within each healthcare practice.

If the decision is made to turn delinquent accounts over to a collection agency, care should be taken when choosing the agency. Experts say that a credible collection agency should be a member of a national trade association, such as Consumer Data Industry Association, formerly Associated Credit Bureaus, and American Collectors Association. These organizations provide all-important standards and training. When choosing a collector, choose one that specializes in collecting medical accounts. Also, use standard business practices such as talking with associates; checking references, credentials, and local professional or trade memberships; and touching base with state or local licensing authorities and perhaps the Better Business Bureau. In addition to checking references and credentials, the healthcare practice should ensure that the agency chosen

- employs trained, certified collectors who understand and abide by the Fair Debt Collection Practices Act and follow the requirements of state laws;
- is insured, licensed, and bonded; and
- is able to collect in other states.

 HIPAA Tip

The HIPAA Privacy Rule does not require consent from a patient before turning in his or her account for collection. Covered providers still must be cautious when using personal health information for collection purposes in determining just how much personal health information is needed to accomplish the specific goal of satisfying their account receivables.

What Did You Learn?

1. What is a collection agency?
2. List four reasons a healthcare practice might hire a collection agency.
3. What two trade organizations do experts suggest contacting when choosing a collection agency?
4. Name three things to look for in a reputable collection agency.

SMALL CLAIMS LITIGATION

Small claims litigation is an alternative to turning accounts over for collection. Filing a small claims suit can be effective for a healthcare practice to collect delinquent accounts. Before making the decision to take a delinquent patient to small claims court, however, the cost should be weighed against the monetary gain. The cost of generating a small claims lawsuit is typically between $30 and $50, so the account ideally should total enough to offset this expense. The process is administrated by the services at local county or district courts, but the individual initiating the small claims lawsuit must prepare the paperwork.

The small claims process is set up to make it easy for individuals or businesses to recover legitimate debts without using expensive legal advisors. The claim usually is heard by a judge in chambers (or, in some case, an appointed arbitrator), with the parties presenting their sides in person. The individual or business entity that initiates the legal process must pay the initial costs, such as filing and serving fees, but these fees usually can be recovered from the debtor. Small claims suits can be for any amount of money up to a limiting threshold, which varies by state, usually anywhere from $3000 to $5000; however, there is ongoing legislation in many states to raise this limit to $10,000.

WHO CAN USE SMALL CLAIMS

As a general rule, any person of legal age or any business entity can file a small claims lawsuit if there is a legitimate claim against someone who owes money and is refusing to pay. All that is needed is proof that the debt exists. In the case of a healthcare office, this is usually some sort of written evidence, such as a patient ledger. The important thing is that there is full and proper documentation. The most prolonged and expensive disputes generally result from inadequate paperwork and a lack of attention to detail.

Before a claim can proceed, the court expects the **plaintiff** (the party bringing the lawsuit) to have explored all other avenues of settlement. This means that the plaintiff should allow the other side (in this case, the patient) a "reasonable period of time" to make a payment before resorting to legal action.

HOW THE SMALL CLAIMS PROCESS WORKS

The procedure starts with the plaintiff filling out a standard form, which outlines details about the claim and the various parties. The following information needs to appear on the form:

1. Name of the party being sued
2. Current address of that party
3. Amount of the plaintiff's claim
4. Basis, or proof, of the claim.

The completed form is returned to the court office with the appropriate filing and serving fees. A copy of the form is "served" to the **defendant** (the party being sued), who may choose to pay the debt in full plus all accrued fees before the process goes any further. He or she also may dispute the claim in its entirety.

If the claim, or any part of it, is disputed, the matter goes to a court hearing where the evidence is heard in informal surroundings, usually around the table in a judge's chambers. The plaintiff and defendant are given an opportunity to introduce evidence, ask questions, and explain to the judge (or arbitrator) why judgment should be entered in his or her favor. The judge usually makes an immediate decision, and the parties involved get a full and final result on the day of the hearing. The judgment of the court is an official statement in the court's records that the defendant owes the plaintiff a certain amount of money with interest. The judgment must be enforced out of the defendant's assets. More simply put, if the judgment is in favor of the plaintiff, the defendant must pay immediately. If the defendant does not pay after judgment, the plaintiff can "attach," or gain ownership of the defendant's assets, such as a paycheck, a bank account, or a car.

Small claims litigation can be successful, but it is time-consuming and can be costly if there are a lot of claims. If the practice has someone on staff who is able and willing to prepare all the proper documents and attend court hearings, this process can have positive results. Filing and serving fees can be far less than the typical 50% of the outstanding debt kept back by a collection agency.

What Did You Learn?

1. What was the initial intent of the small claims process?
2. What is a typical monetary threshold for a small claims suit?
3. What is the first step in initiating a small claims suit?
4. List the four elements of information that must appear on the small claims form.

SUMMARY CHECK POINTS

☑ Patients typically come to a healthcare office expecting certain things, such as the following:
- *A professional office setting*—Because patients cannot see and touch an intangible service, such as healthcare, they look for substitutes to put their mind at ease. Substitutes include esthetics, such the office location, size and layout, and carpet, and staff enthusiasm.
- *Relevant paperwork and questions*—Patients prefer paperwork to be brief, of high quality, and relevant to the encounter. Personal questions should be asked privately, and patients should be given reasons as to why these forms and questions are important to their care and treatment.
- *Honoring appointment times*—Time has become a valuable commodity in *everyone's* life; the medical receptionist should indicate approximately how long an initial visit will take and briefly explain what to expect when the patient phones for an appointment. If the schedule lags, the patient should be told the reason for the delay and offered alternatives to waiting.

- *Patient load*—Negative conclusions as to the competency of the entire healthcare team can be offset by explaining to the patient why the reception room has no or few patients waiting.
- *Getting comfortable with the healthcare provider*—Sharing a relevant personal experience or information promotes a good provider-patient relationship and often tends to relieve an anxious patient.
- *Privacy and confidentiality*—Patients must feel confident that any personal information they divulge would be kept private and confidential. The staff should be discrete when talking to patients or among themselves because voices tend to carry.
- *Financial issues*—Discuss financial issues and practice policies up-front with patients so they know what to expect.

☑ Future trends in the patient-practice relationship include the following:
- *An aging population*—Over the next 30 years, the number of Americans older than age 65 will double, and healthcare facilities will need to be prepared to handle an increasing volume of elderly patients.
- *Using the Internet as a healthcare tool*—Individuals are using websites to find physicians and hospitals that offer opportunities for certain procedures, lifestyle advice, and educational details and references for a multitude of health conditions. Future patients will rely more on the Internet, and healthcare providers will have to adapt their practices to meet these state-of-the-art electronic requirements.
- *Seeing patients as consumers*—Treating patients as "consumers," rather than "patients," is recommended. Today's patients, similar to other types of consumers, are likely to switch healthcare plans or healthcare providers or both if they think they are not getting quality service.

☑ Any individual or any business involved in transferring data or carrying out transactions related to patient protected health information is a HIPAA-covered entity. The law applies to three groups:
- *Healthcare providers*—Any provider of healthcare services or supplies who transmits any health information in electronic form in connection with a transaction for which standard requirements have been adopted
- *Health plans*—Any individual or group plan that provides or pays the cost of healthcare

- *Healthcare clearinghouses*—Any public or private entity that transforms healthcare transactions from one format to another.

☑ Personally identifiable information includes information about an individual collected by the covered entity that reasonably could be used to identify the individual, regardless of the source of such information or the medium in which it is recorded. Personally identifiable information includes, but is not limited to, first and last name, residence or other physical address, electronic mail address, telephone number, birth date, credit card information, and Social Security number.

☑ When all identifiable elements are removed, the information is, under most circumstances, considered de-identified.

☑ A HIPAA-approved release of information must contain the following elements:
  - A specific and meaningful description of the information sought
  - The name of the person or persons authorized to make the request
  - The name of the person or persons to whom the covered entity may make the request
  - A description of each purpose of the requested use or disclosure
  - An expiration date that relates to the purpose of the use or disclosure
  - A statement of the right (and exceptions to this right) to revoke the authorization in writing and saying how this may be accomplished
  - A statement that information used may be subject to re-disclosure by the recipient and no longer be protected by this rule
  - Signature of the individual and date signed
  - A description of the covered entity's authority to have a representative act for the individual (if applicable)

☑ Two common methods of accounting are used in today's healthcare facilities.
  - *"One-write" pegboard accounting system*—This system, made up of several accounting forms and carbonized shingled receipts, captures information at the time the transaction occurs with a single writing and eliminates the need for recopying the data. One-write systems are popular because they are accurate, are easy to learn, and use a write-it-once process for recording daily office transactions.
  - *Electronic patient accounting software*—A computer software program can perform all phases of the accounting process quickly and accurately. It allows the input of demographic data and creates a patient "account" from which many documents can be generated, such as a list of appointments by day and by provider and an encounter form for each one. A current copy of the patient ledger can be printed showing dates, diagnosis and procedure codes, charges, payments, and current balances. Appointments also can be scheduled, deleted, and adjusted within the accounting system. Periodic statements, aging reports, and CMS-1500 claim forms can be generated.

☑ Some things a healthcare practice might do to increase its financial success include, but are not limited to, the following:
  - Establish a written credit policy
  - Discuss payment and practice policies up-front with patients
  - Bill promptly
  - Plan an action for bills more than 30 days old
  - Telephone (or send a letter) after the second statement
  - Use the services of a small claims court

☑ Laws affecting credit and collection include
  - the Truth in Lending Act,
  - the Fair Credit Billing Act,
  - the Equal Credit Opportunity Act,
  - the Fair Credit Reporting Act, and
  - the Fair Debt Collection Practices Act

☑ The steps involved in small claims litigation are as follows:
  - Acquire the proper forms from the local county or district court, along with instructions on how to fill them out properly.
  - Include the following information on the original form: (1) the name of the defendant, (2) the current address of the defendant, (3) the amount of the plaintiff's claim, and (4) the basis of the claim.
  - Attach documentation that provides proof that the money is owed.
  - Return the completed form (and the required number of copies) to the court office with the appropriate filing and serving fees.
  - Appear in court on the date indicated to substantiate the case.

CLOSING SCENARIO

Before Callie Foster completed Chapter 14, her goal was to learn how to be considerate, patient, and empathetic to patients because of a recent negative incident she had experienced at a healthcare office. Her confrontation had been very upsetting, and she firmly believed that no one should be treated so rudely. Callie thought that what other patients expect when they come to a healthcare office is what she herself expected when she went to Dr. Dayton's office. It became obvious, however, as she progressed through the chapter, that although consideration, patience, and empathy are important during the actual patient-staff encounter; when it comes to collections, sometimes a fair but firm and pragmatic attitude is necessary.

Scott found the section on consumer credit laws especially interesting and informative. To him, the steps involved in the small claims litigation process were straightforward and manageable—a fair and economical way to collect outstanding accounts.

WEBSITES TO EXPLORE

For live links to the following websites, please visit the Evolve® site at http://evolve.elsevier.com/Beik/today/

- For information on HIPAA regulations, go to http://www.hipaadvisory.com/regs/

- For more information on financial policies for healthcare offices, go to http://www.pcc.com/pub/pm/finpol.html

- For more information on laws regarding credit and collection, log on to http://www.consumerlaw.com/debt.html http://www.fair-debt-collection.com/

- For more information on the Consumer Data Industry Association, log on to http://www.cdiaonline.org/index.cfm

- For more information on the American Collectors Association, log on to http://www.debtmarketplace.com/

- For more information on small claims procedures, log on to http://www.peopleslawyer.net/smallclaims/

REFERENCES AND RESOURCES

A HIPAA security overview: practice brief. Journal of AHIMA 75, 2004.
How to "HIPAA"—top 10 tips. AMA, 2003.
Burton B: Quick Guide to HIPAA for the Physician's Office. Philadelphia, 2004, Saunders.

The Claim

Chapter Outline

CHAPTER OBJECTIVES

After completion of this chapter, the student should be able to
- List and explain the six keys to successful claims.
- List and explain the six steps of the adjudication process.
- Discuss time limits for submitting insurance claims and appeals.
- Outline the process for submitting secondary claims.
- Discuss the process for appealing incorrect payments and denied claims.
- Explain the Medicare multilevel appeals process.

CHAPTER TERMS

adjudication
birthday rule
clean claim
coordination of benefits
correct code initiative
downcoding
employer identification number (EIN)

hearing on record
insurance claims register (log)
Medicare secondary payer claims
personal hearing
secondary claim
suspension file
telephone hearing

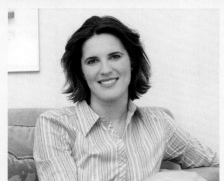

Zoey Edwards, confined to a wheelchair after an automobile accident at the age of 12, was looking for a career opportunity where she could work out of her home. She noticed an article in a flyer from a local community college about a healthcare billing and insurance program. The article listed the career possibilities for graduates of this program, along with testimonials from several former students who had established successful home-based businesses in healthcare billing and insurance. Zoey decided that a career in this field might meet her needs. Through a state-of-the-art communications network, and with the help of the student services staff at the college, Zoey was able to "attend class" in the comfort of her own home, traveling to campus only for major examinations.

Kristin Underwood also was looking for an opportunity to work at home and still care for her two preschool children. Kristin had a friend who worked as a health insurance professional in a local healthcare office, so she was aware of the challenges and rewards this career area offered. Kristin thought she had the personal traits and work ethic to make a home business successful, so she enrolled in a career school in her neighborhood and signed up for a healthcare insurance course.

GENERAL GUIDELINES FOR COMPLETING THE CMS-1500 FORM

In earlier chapters, we discussed the steps for completing the universal CMS-1500 claim form for generic commercial carriers and the major payers—Medicaid, Medicare, and TRICARE/CHAMPVA. For the purpose of review, Box 15-1 lists some general guidelines for preparing all paper claims. Earlier chapters also stressed the importance of strict adherence to payer-specific guidelines when preparing claims.

What Did You Learn?

List five important guidelines for submitting paper claims.

KEYS TO SUCCESSFUL CLAIMS

Claims processing involves many steps, and each step must be performed thoroughly and accurately to receive the maximum payment that the health record documentation substantiates. This process begins with the patient appointment and ends with the carrier's subsequent payment. Understanding how this process works allows the health insurance professional to file claims properly, resulting in full and timely reimbursement. Fig. 15-1 illustrates the six "keys" to successful claims processing.

FIRST KEY: COLLECT AND VERIFY PATIENT INFORMATION

Unless a patient visits the healthcare facility on a regular basis (e.g., weekly allergy shots or blood pressure checks), the health insurance professional should reverify the patient's information each time he or she visits the office. New patients must complete a patient information form on the first visit. Established patients should be required to update the form at least annually because within a year's time, the patient could have remarried, moved to a new address, changed jobs, or, most important, changed insurance companies. In addition to demographic data, the patient information form should include basic items such as the insurance carrier's name, policy and group numbers (if applicable), the insured's name (if different from the patient), effective date of coverage, and any secondary insurance information. It is not unusual for some practices with a high volume of Medicare patients to have a separate information form for those patients.

After the patient information form is completed, the health insurance professional should check it over to ensure that the correct information has been entered in the required blanks, and that all information is legible. One key to successful claims submission is to have the patient provide as much information as possible, and the health insurance professional should verify this information.

In some situations, more than one insurer is involved. Such cases might occur when the patient and his or her spouse are covered under separate employer group plans or when the parents of a minor patient are divorced, and each parent has his or her own insurance policy. In the case of the latter, if the primary carrier is not designated on the information form, the health insurance professional

Box 15-1

General Guidelines for Completing the CMS-1500 Form

- Use the preprinted red and white CMS-1500 claim form only.
- Follow OCR guidelines.
- Submit claims that are legible using computer-generated or typed entries.
- Submit only six line items per claim. Do not compress two lines of information on one line.
- Send paper claims unfolded in large envelopes.
- Use standard fonts (preferably Courier) in 10-point or 12-point size.
- Type within each block and not outside the block. Characters out of alignment would cause the claim to be returned as misaligned.
- Follow payer guidelines as to where to type the insurance carrier's name and address. Some carriers stipulate that the area to the right of the bar code be left blank.
- Do not submit a narrative description of the ICD-9 code in Item 21.
- Do not submit procedure codes with negative charges in Item 24d.
- Do not type a telephone number in the NPI(a) or NON-NPI(b) portion of the field in Item 33.
- Do not highlight information. Instead, underline information on attachments that you want to bring to the payer's attention.
- Remove pin-feed strips on pin-fed claims at the perforations only. Do not cut the strips because it may alter the document size.
- Do not tape, glue, or staple attachments to the CMS-1500 claim form. Do not tear, bend, or fold corners of the claim form with attachments.
- Attachments should be the same size as the paper claim form ($8\frac{1}{2} \times 11$ inches).

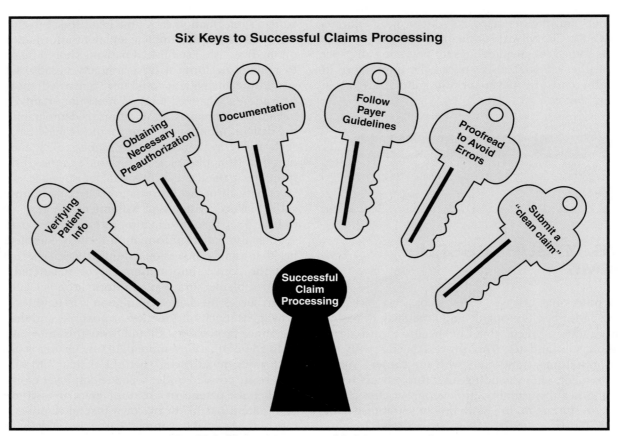

Fig. 15-1 Six keys to successful claims processing.

should obtain this information from the parent who accompanies the child to the office.

In addition to the standard demographic and insurance questions asked on the patient information form, many healthcare practices include a section (often positioned at the bottom of the form) for the patient to sign a release of information and an assignment of benefits. Other practices use separate forms for these functions. A signed and dated release of information is necessary before the health insurance professional can complete and submit an insurance claim. When a patient signs an assignment of benefits, he or she is authorizing the insurance carrier to send payment directly to the healthcare provider.

After obtaining a complete and accurate patient information form, the health insurance professional should make a photocopy of the patient's insurance card and place it in an easily accessible location in the patient's health record, such as inside the front cover. Some insurance identification (ID) cards also have information on the back. If this is the case, the health insurance professional should be sure to copy the back of the card also.

☑ HIPAA Tip

Patients have certain rights and protections against the misuse or disclosure of their health records. All patients should receive a Notice of Privacy Practices that informs individuals of their rights and of the healthcare practice's legal duties with respect to protected health information.

Imagine This!

Shirley Gibson, a health insurance professional for Westlawn Family Medical Center, updates all demographic and insurance information when patients come to the office for an appointment. Additionally, she checks to ensure that the release of information is signed, dated, and current, as is the assignment of benefits. After the patient completes the new information form, Shirley checks it for accuracy and legibility. If two insurance companies are listed, she asks the patient which is primary. In some cases, Shirley has to call either the employer or the insurance carrier to verify which is the primary carrier. "It is important for smooth, efficient, and timely claims processing," Shirley says, "to have all information current and accurate before the claim is prepared for submission. It is surprising," she continues, "how much people move around, change jobs, and change insurers these days."

SECOND KEY: OBTAIN THE NECESSARY PREAUTHORIZATION AND PRECERTIFICATION

The health insurance professional should be familiar with the rules regarding preauthorization and precertification. Some third-party payers reject certain types of claims if they do not know about and approve the services beforehand. Services that most often require preauthorization or precertification include inpatient hospitalizations, new or experimental procedures, and certain diagnostic studies. Emergency services typically do not need prior authorization, but they often require some type of follow-up with the insurance company—typically within 24 to 48 hours. Ultimately, it is the patient's responsibility to know when and how to notify the insurance company for preauthorization or precertification; however, the health insurance professional should advise the patient when this process is necessary to avoid denied claims. Also, if the patient is incapacitated in any way, the health insurance professional or a member of the healthcare staff should notify the patient's insurer to acquire the necessary preauthorization. Telephone numbers for contacting the carrier are usually on the back of the patient's ID card. Fig. 15-2 shows the back of an insurance ID card with a toll-free number to call when precertification is needed. Some carriers issue a "prior authorization" number, which should be placed in Block 23 of the CMS-1500 form.

● Stop and Think

Helen Rigdon was admitted as an inpatient to Memorial East Hospital after a visit to the emergency department for a bleeding ulcer. After Helen was discharged, she received an EOB from her insurance carrier stating that they were denying the claim because there had been no preauthorization for the hospital admission. In this case, whose responsibility was it to contact the insurance company to obtain the required preauthorization?

IMPORTANT PHONE NUMBER INFORMATION

For pre-admission certification, OB and emergency admissions call 1-800-558-xxxx.

To locate a participating provider call 1-800-810-xxxx or access BlueCard website @ www.bcbs.com.

Providers - Please submit all claims to your local Blue Cross and Blue Shield Plan.

Pharmacists - Pharmacy Benefits Manager (PBM) is AdvancePCS. For assistance call 1-800-600-xxxx.

Wellmark Blue Cross and Blue Shield of Iowa, an independent licensee of the Blue Cross and Blue Shield Association.

Fig. 15-2 Back of insurance ID card.

Reminder: Medicare (fee-for-service) does not need prior authorization to provide services.

THIRD KEY: DOCUMENTATION

It is the healthcare provider's responsibility to document the appropriate comments in the patient's health record. Each entry must indicate clearly the history, physical examination, and medical decision making for the patient. The provider also fills out an encounter form, indicating the proper procedure codes (CPT or HCPCS level II) and diagnosis codes (ICD-9-CM) to describe the patient's condition and the services that were rendered. These codes should be checked before transferring to the claim because some practitioners when in a hurry may indicate the wrong ones. The health insurance professional places the appropriate diagnosis codes, procedure codes, charges, and any other pertinent information in the proper boxes on the claim. Claims may be in paper or electronic format. Each required field on the claim helps to determine if that claim is clean. Claims that are not clean are returned for more information or are denied. It is important that the claim show the exact diagnosis that is documented in the health record.

FOURTH KEY: FOLLOW PAYER GUIDELINES

As pointed out in previous chapters, some major payers (Medicaid, Medicare, Blue Cross and Blue Shield, TRICARE/CHAMPVA) have slightly differing guidelines for completing the CMS-1500 claim form. The health insurance professional must obtain the most recent guidelines from each of these major payers to complete the claim exactly to their specifications.

FIFTH KEY: PROOFREAD CLAIM TO AVOID ERRORS

Claims are commonly denied. Being aware of some common mistakes can help the health insurance professional avoid delays, denials, or rejections. It is good practice to proofread the claim carefully when it is completed, paying particular attention to code entries and dollar amounts. Make sure the claim is dated, and the proper signature is affixed. When the claim is completed and signed, make a photocopy for the file. Box 15-2 lists some common errors that cause a claim to be denied.

SIXTH KEY: SUBMIT A CLEAN CLAIM

The most important document in the healthcare insurance process is the insurance claim form—the CMS-1500—and the most important thing about the CMS-1500 is that, when completed and submitted to the third-party insurer, it is a **clean claim**. A clean claim means that all of the information necessary for processing the claim has

---

Box 15-2
Common Errors Made on Claims

- Patient's insurance ID number is incorrect.
- Patient information is incomplete.
- Patient/insured name and address do not match the insurer carrier's records.
- Physician's EIN number, provider number, NPI, or Social Security number is incorrect or missing.
- There is little or no information regarding primary or secondary coverage.
- Physician's (or authorized person's) signature has been omitted.
- Dates of service are incorrect or do not correlate with information from other providers (e.g., hospital, nursing homes).
- The fee column is blank, not itemized, and not totaled.
- The CPT or ICD-9 codes are invalid, or the diagnostic codes are not linked to the correct services or procedures.
- The claim is illegible.
- Preauthorization/precertification was not obtained before services rendered.

● Stop and Think

Silver River Medical Center has a higher than average number of denied paper claims. The billing and insurance staff consists of four health insurance professionals, and each handles approximately 50 to 55 claims per day. Many of the claims are denied because of simple errors—transposed numbers, misspelled patient names, incorrect charges, or the provider signature has been omitted. What might the billing/insurance staff do to resolve this problem?

---

been entered on the claim form, and the information is correct. Clean claims are usually paid in a timely manner; paying careful attention to what should appear in each of the boxes helps produce clean claims.

What Did You Learn?

1. Why is it important to update the patient information form with each patient visit?
2. What is the result of failing to obtain preauthorization/precertification for certain procedures, such as inpatient hospitalization?
3. Whose responsibility is it to document appropriate comments in the health record?
4. What is a "clean claim"?

HIPAA AND THE NATIONAL STANDARD EMPLOYER IDENTIFIER NUMBER

The Secretary of the Department of Health and Human Services (HHS) proposed that the **employer identification number (EIN)** that is assigned by the Internal Revenue Service (IRS) be used as the employer identifier standard for all electronic healthcare transactions as required by HIPAA. The ruling requires the following:

- Health plans must accept the EIN on all electronic transactions that require an employer identifier.
- Healthcare clearinghouses must use the EIN on all electronic transactions that require an employer identifier.
- Healthcare providers must use the EIN on all transactions, wherever required, that are electronically transmitted.
- Employers must disclose their EIN when requested to do so by an entity that conducts standard electronic transactions requiring that employer's identifier.

An EIN consists of 9 digits with the first 2 digits separated by a hyphen (e.g., 00-1234567). The IRS assigns EINs to employers who can obtain an EIN by submitting IRS Form SS-4 (Application for Employer Identification Number). Business entities that pay wages to one or more employees are required to have an EIN as their taxpayer identifying number; most employers already have an EIN assigned to them.

In May 2002, HHS issued a final rule to standardize the identifying numbers assigned to employers in the health care industry by using the existing EIN (this EIN should appear in Block 25 of the CMS-1500 form with a space replacing the hyphen). Most covered entities were to have been in compliance with the EIN standard by July, 30, 2004; however, small health plans were allowed an additional year to comply.

What Did You Learn?

1. What is the format of an EIN?
2. How does a provider acquire an EIN?

CLAIM PROCESS

After a claim has been received by a third-party payer, it is reviewed, and the carrier makes payment decisions. This process is referred to as **adjudication**. If the claim is clean, it continues on through several more steps to the reimbursement process, and, ideally, the insurance carrier pays up to the allowed amount (according to the patient's policy) for the services that have been billed. The carrier can reduce payment, however, or deny the claim completely. If any information is missing, or if there are errors on the claim, the process is stopped, and the claim is returned to the healthcare office where it originated. Fig. 15-3 is a flow chart that illustrates how a paper claim progresses through the various steps after it is received at the payer's facility. The steps discussed in the following sections and listed in Fig. 15-4 are for a paper claim. (The steps for processing an electronic claim are discussed in Chapter 16.)

STEP ONE: CLAIM IS RECEIVED

When the insurance carrier receives the claim, it is dated, and the claim is processed through an optical recognition scanner (OCR). If any attachments accompanied the claim, the practice name, provider/group number, address, and telephone number should appear on each attached document. This helps prevent claim denial in case the attachments get separated from the claim during the adjudication process. Box 15-3 lists the general guidelines for OCR scanning.

STEP TWO: CLAIMS ADJUDICATION

After the data are entered into the payer's computer system, if the claim is clean, it is approved and proceeds on to be paid. It first must pass through a series of edits, however, to verify the patient's coverage and eligibility and check for medical necessity, exclusions, preexisting conditions, and noncovered services contained in the patient's policy. If the claim requires additional information, the insurer contacts the healthcare practice or the patient. In the case of a paper claim, this contact usually is accomplished by mail, but it also can be by telephone. If the claim is not clean, it is denied and returned to the provider.

When a claims error is discovered that could result, or already has resulted, in inaccurate reimbursement, a corrected claim should be prepared and submitted. The health insurance professional should mark the corrected claim as a *"corrected billing"* and *"not a duplicate claim."* It is also advisable to include a note describing the error, plus any additional documentation necessary to support the correction. Some practices use a claims correction form (Fig. 15-5) for submitting corrected claims. The form is filled out, attached to a corrected claim, and resubmitted to the payer.

☑ HIPAA Tip

A new transaction currently being developed by HIPAA will allow payers to request additional information to support claims. This transaction will use Logical Observation Identifiers Names and Codes (LOINC) to request the clinical information that is required to process healthcare claims.

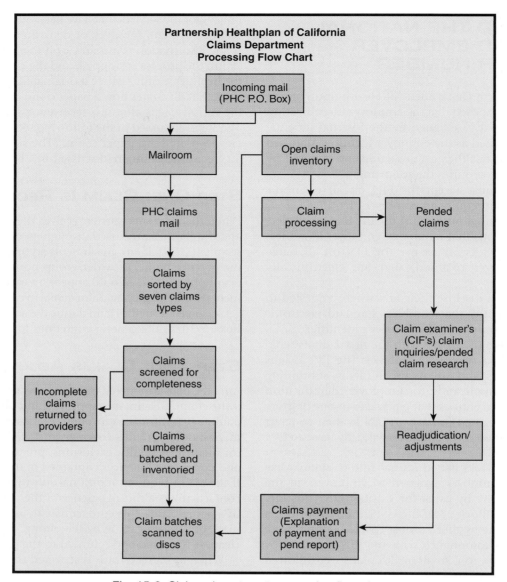

Fig. 15-3 Claims department processing flow chart.

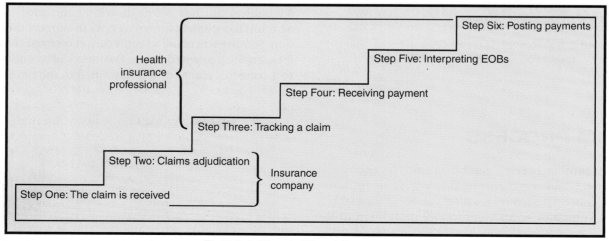

Fig. 15-4 Steps of the claim process.

Box 15-3

General Guidelines for Optical Character Recognition Scanning

- Use only the original preprinted red and white CMS-1500 claim form. This form is designed specifically for OCR systems. The scanner cannot read black and white (copied, carbon, faxed, or laser printer–generated) claim forms.
- Do not use red ink pens, highlighters, "post-it" notes, stickers, correction fluid, or tape anywhere on the claim form. The red ink or highlighter would not be picked up in the scanning process and would black out information.
- Do not write or use stamps or stickers that say "Rebill," "Tracer," or "Second Submission" on claim form.
- Use standard fonts that are 10 to 12 characters per inch. Do not mix character fonts on the same claim form. Do not use italics or script. Handwritten entries should be avoided.
- Use upper case (capital letters) for all alpha characters.
- Do not use punctuation marks, slashes, dashes, or any special characters anywhere on the claim form.
- Use black printer ribbon, ink-jet, or laser printer cartridges. Ensure ink is not too light or faded.
- Ensure all claim information is entirely contained within the proper field on the claim form and on the same horizontal plane. Misaligned data would delay processing and may even be missed.
- If corrections need to be made, reprinting the claim is preferred. Correction fluid should not be used.

STEP THREE: TRACKING CLAIMS

The healthcare practice should have a mechanism in place for tracking claims. Typically, it takes a paper claim 4 to 6 weeks to complete the entire claims process; however, this varies by carrier and geographic location. Sometimes a claim may be clean, but some question arises, which results in a delay. Carefully tracking the progress of claims alerts the health insurance professional to the claims that remain unpaid past the normal payment time.

Imagine This!

Laurence Benson visits his family physician, Myron Peters, yearly for annual wellness examinations. Every 3 years, Dr. Peters orders an electrocardiogram for Myron as part of his routine examination. Normally, Laurence's insurance carrier, XYZ Health Indemnity, pays within 2 to 3 weeks. It is Dr. Peters' office policy to send a statement to the patient if the insurance carrier does not pay within 60 days. When Laurence received an overdue statement, he called Dr. Peters' office and asked the health insurance professional to check into the matter. When she did, she was told that the claim was "pending" because the individual who reviewed it saw something on the attached electrocardiogram that required further assessment by the medical review committee, but the committee was "bogged down" with a backlog of claims to review.

If, at the end of a set time period, the claim is not paid, and no communication has been received explaining the delay, the health insurance professional should follow-up on the claim. Many offices use a form similar to the one in Fig. 15-6 for claims follow-up.

● Stop and Think

Re-read Imagine This! concerning Dr. Peters. How might Dr. Peters' health insurance professional modify her routine to avoid future problems similar to the one experienced by Mr. Benson?

Creating a Suspension File System

For offices filing paper claims, some sort of claims tracking system is recommended, such as a **suspension file**. A suspension file is a series of files set up chronologically and labeled according to the number of days since the claim was submitted. Claims in a file labeled "current" might be 30 days or less; a second series might be labeled "claims over 30 days," and so forth. Another type of follow-up system that works well is the one pictured in Fig. 15-7, in which claims are filed according to the date they are submitted.

Claim copies should be removed systematically. Paid claims can be filed in a permanent folder or binder, under each major payer. If payment has not been received, some sort of follow-up procedure can be initiated. Claims follow-up should be given a high priority and become a

Claim Correction Form

Physician offices are encouraged to submit claims electronically. This form should be used in situations where the provider cannot submit corrected claims electronically or where electronic submissions would not adequately address the issue.

Submitted To:

Plan/Payer Name: _____ Date Submitted: _____

Plan/Payer Address: _____

City _____ State: _____ Zip: _____

Telephone: (____) _____ Fax: (____) _____ E-mail: _____

Patient Name: _____ D.O.B.: _____

First   M.I.   Last

Subscriber Name: _____ Date of Service: _____

Policy #: _____ Group #: _____ Original Claim #: _____

Submitted From:

Provider Name: _____ TIN or ID #: _____

Contact: _____ Telephone: (____) _____ Ext. _____

Fax: (____) _____ E-mail: _____

THE FOLLOWING WAS CORRECTED ON THIS CLAIM:

❑ The patient's policy/group number was incorrect. The correct number(s) are shown above.

❑ The correct CPT code is _____ instead of _____

❑ Wrong date of service was filed. The correct date is _____

❑ Visits were denied based on the diagnosis given. Proper diagnosis code is _____ instead of _____

❑ Visit: ❑ Procedure: denied as over carrier's utilization limits. Please see attached letter to justify extensions of these limits.

❑ Carrier indicated that the patient is covered by another plan that is Primary. This is incorrect. Patient indicates you are Primary.

❑ The secondary carrier is: _____ ❑ There is no secondary carrier.

❑ The procedure was denied as medically not necessary. Documentation to support the medical necessity of this service is attached.

❑ Our clerk: ❑ Carrier's clerk: failed to enter correct number of times (units) procedure was performed. Correct units are as follows:

     D.O.S.: _____ Code: _____ Units: _____ Charge Total $: _____

❑ Multiple Surgical Procedures:

     ❑ Carrier failed to approve any procedure at 100%.   ❑ Carrier approved incorrect procedure at 100%.

     Carrier should have approved code _____ @ 100%/50% instead of _____

     Carrier should have approved code _____ @ 100%/50% instead of _____

     Carrier should have approved code _____ @ 100%/50% instead of _____

❑ Modifiers should be attached to code(s)

	Code	Code			Code	Code
❑ -50	_____	_____		❑ -51	_____	_____
❑ -58	_____	_____		❑ -59	_____	_____
❑ -79	_____	_____		❑ -GA	_____	_____
❑ __	_____	_____		❑ __	_____	_____

❑ The following E/M visit was denied as included in the global surgical fee. In fact, the service was a significant separately identifiable service provided above and beyond the procedure and submitted with appropriate E/M modifier. Please reconsider with attached documentation:

     Code: _____ with modifier(s): ❑ -24 ❑ -25 Charge $: _____

❑ UPIN information for code _____ was omitted. Physician name: _____ UPIN: _____

❑ Plan specific provider I.D. omitted. The I.D. # is _____

❑ CLIA number was omitted. The CLIA number is _____

❑ The place of service was incorrect. The place of service should be _____

❑ The service was rendered at the physician's physical location listed in Box 32 of the claim form.

❑ Failed to attach EOB from Primary carrier. The EOB is attached to this form.

❑ Failed to enter correct information on indicated line of claim form.

     Line #: _____ Correct Information: _____

❑ Other reason for claim correction: _____

❑ Comment: _____

June 2003

Fig. 15-5 Example of a claims correction form.

Prompt Payment Tracking Form

Information Checklist

Please provide copies of the following:

- ☐ The claim form submitted to insurance company
- ☐ Electronic claim receipt if applicable
- ☐ Correspondence from the insurance company (EOBs, requests for additional information, etc.)
- ☐ Details of written/oral contacts with insurance company regarding this claim
- ☐ Other pertinent information

Note: Mark out all confidential patient information, such as name, date of birth or social security number.

Practice/Physician Information (complaint by)

Name: _____

Address:_____

City, Zip_____

Phone: _____   Fax: _____

E-Mail: _____

Insurance Company and Claim Information

Original Submission Date:_____

Company:_____   Phone: _____

Date(s) of Services:_____   Claims Rep(if known): _____

Submitted via: ☐ Paper   ☐ Electronic

Action by Insurance Company

Date of Initial Response from Ins. Co.: _____

☐Denied   ☐Requested Additional Information   ☐Reduced Payment   ☐ Other (see attached)

Insurance Company Response: _____

_____

_____

Current Status of Claim: _____

_____

_____

Fig. 15-6 Example of a claims tracking form.

regularly scheduled part of the health insurance professional's work week.

Experienced health insurance professionals who deal with Medicare and Medicaid carriers recommend making inquiries in writing or using the forms specifically created for follow-up. Inquiries to commercial carriers often are handled more efficiently by a telephone call. If a claim has been denied for a simple reason, without notification, a quick phone call is time well spent. In the case of resubmission, always attach a note with the date, the contact person's name, and a description of the conversation. Keep a copy of all correspondence as documented proof of response.

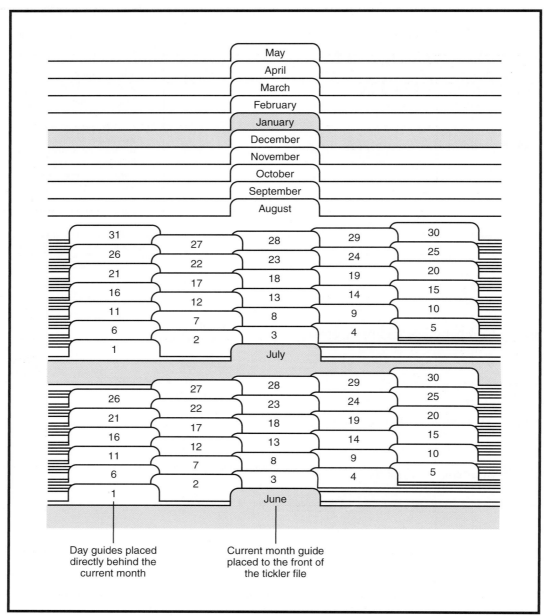

Fig. 15-7 Suspension file.

Creating an Insurance Claims Register System

An alternative to the suspension file is to record claims information on an **insurance claims register** or log (Fig. 15-8). When a claim is submitted, the health insurance professional records the filing date, the patient's name and chart number, name and address of the payer, and the amount billed. As payments are received, the original copy of the claim form is removed from the follow-up file and compared with the explanation of benefits (EOB). The amount paid is recorded in the applicable column

along with any difference from the amount billed as shown on the log sheet. Any notations, such as "claim sent to review" or "claim denied for additional information," should be recorded in the status column along with the date the notice was received. If a claim is resubmitted, that date also should be recorded on the log.

STEP FOUR: RECEIVING PAYMENT

The insurer sends the payment for services and the EOB—sometimes called a remittance advice (RA)—back

INSURANCE CLAIMS REGISTER

Filing Date	Chart Number	Patient's Name	Name & Address Where Claim Submitted	Amount Billed	Amount Paid	Difference	Status or Comment
10 /6	1221	Matthew Kramer	First Insurance 1st Avenue Newark, NJ 12345	$525			10/21 busy 10/30 busy 11/6 busy
10 /6	1350	Luke Myers	Better Insurance 3rd Avenue New York City, NY 0211	$1200	$700	$500	Requester Review 10/30
10 /6	1098	Christi Wilson	County Farm Ins 6th Avenue New Era, IA 45678	$125	$50	$75	$75 deductible. Bill Patient
10 /6	1352	Rose Larson	Last Insurance 7th Avenue New Hope, MS 56789	$1500	0		Sent to Medical Review 10/30

Fig. 15-8 Example of an insurance claim register.

to the provider's office. (Whether or not there is a payment, there is always an EOB or RA.) If the practice submits claims electronically, the EOB or RA may be in an electronic format as well. Each EOB should be checked thoroughly to ensure that the payment is consistent with the fee schedule or contracted amount from the insurance company (Table 15-1). Claims that have been denied or rejected for any reason or that have been reduced in payment should be reviewed to determine the source of the denial or payment reduction. It then must be decided whether to pursue the claim further.

STEP FIVE: INTERPRETING EXPLANATION OF BENEFITS

The EOB is the key to knowing how much of the claim was paid, how much was not, and why. Sometimes understanding what this document means can be challenging, however. To complicate this, every payer has a different EOB format. The EOB has a unique vocabulary, such as "applied to deductible," "above usual and customary," "patient copay," and "allowable." Often codes are used, and the health insurance professional must determine what each code means. Deciphering the EOB language and codes reveals the following:

TABLE 15-1	Common Payment Errors
RESULT	**REASON**
A service is reduced	The adjudicator may have downcoded the claim for lack of documentation
	The CPT code was converted to an RVS code that did not directly correlate with CPT
Reimbursement is made at a much reduced rate	Possibly a data entry error. Compare the CPT code submitted with the code paid
Low reimbursement	Precertification was not completed
	Insufficient documentation to establish medical necessity
Multiple units are paid as one unit	The insurer "missed" a number in the unit column
Reimbursement for a procedure or service suddenly drops	This could mean a recalculation of the allowable fee or an error. Phone the payer
Payment is not received	Claim is lost or "caught in the system." Begin your inquiry
Multiple procedures were not paid	The insurance company either ignored the additional procedures or lumped them in with the primary procedure

Available at: http://www.quadax.com/primer/Chap2.asp#CommonPaymentErrors.

- Date received
- Date processed
- Amount of billed charges
- Charges allowed by the carrier
- How much of the claim was applied to patient deductible
- How much of the patient's annual deductible has been met
- Why a service was reduced or denied

Knowing how to read the EOB is important because it aids in collecting full reimbursement, including any balance owed by the patient. Fig. 15-9 shows an EOB from a commercial insurance company and an explanation of what each code means.

Troubleshooting Explanation of Benefits

As discussed, an EOB explains the outcome of the claim that was submitted for payment processing. If the payment was reduced or rejected, the EOB itemizes the reason for doing so. By reading the EOB and following the instructions, the health insurance professional is able to analyze the situation. If an error has been made on the claim, and it is correctable, it should be done so in a timely manner. If it is believed that the insurance carrier made the error, it should be reported to them immediately.

Initially, there are several things to evaluate when looking over an EOB that indicates no payment or a reduced payment. The first thing is to compare the totals billed on the EOB and the CMS-1500 form. If they do not match, it is a good indication that the insurer missed a procedure. If the totals match, but the number of line items (actual procedure codes performed) do not, more than likely the insurer bundled one procedure into another, without listing them as "duplicate."

Imagine This!

Dr. Edwin Carter, a podiatrist, performed three arthroplasties on Priscilla Fortune's toes at $500 each procedure. When the EOB was received, the total charge was $1500, but there were only two codes of 28285 listed. This meant that Ms. Fortune's insurance carrier had bundled two of the procedures into one, but the fee schedule was considered for *only* one. To clear things up, Wayne Thomas, Dr. Carter's health insurance professional, had to contact the insurer and explain that there were three distinct procedures performed on three individual toes and not two, as the carrier had assumed.

The odds are that if a claim is reduced or rejected, the problem lies with the provider's office. This is not always the case, however, and the health insurance professional should be vigilant in analyzing the EOB. One billing professional suggests keeping copies of sample EOB for procedures the medical practice performs regularly for each payer. This way, a payment discrepancy stands out when compared with the file. This "example" file can be used for appealing claims, as long as all patient identification is deleted.

Downcoding

Downcoding by an insurance company occurs when claims are submitted with outdated, deleted, or nonexistent CPT codes. When this happens, the payer assigns a substitute code it thinks best fits the services performed. Often, the

EXPLANATION OF BENEFITS

EMPLOYEE BENEFIT PLAN ADMINISTRATION SERVICES

EMPLOYER/GROUP NAME	SOUTHEAST IOWA SCHOOLS	DATE PREPARED	08–06–06
PLAN/LOCATION NUMBER	10000000 14008020 02	SOCIAL SECURITY I.D. NUMBER	
EMPLOYEE/MEMBER NAME	BEIK JANET I	CONTROL #	8470.0
PATIENT NAME	BEIK JANET I	EOB #	9808060048

JANET I BEIK
545 IOWA CITY RD
SOMEWHERE IA 00506

SOUTHEAST IOWA SCHOOLS
SOMEWHERE IA 00506

PROVIDER NAME and TYPE OF SERVICE	DATES FROM/THRU	AMOUNT CHARGED	AMOUNT COVERED	EXPL. CODE	COVERED AT 100 %	COVERED AT %	COVERED AT %
HAYS, ANDERSON, DIAGNOSTIC LABORATORY	06–22–98	15.00	15.00	099 514	15.00		
ADJUSTMENTS TO BENEFITS TOTAL →		15.00	15.00		15.00		
			Less Deductible				
			Balance		15.00		
			Benefit %		AT 100%	AT %	AT %
			Plan Benefits		15.00		
			Total Benefit		15.00		

099   THIS PREFERRED PROVIDER ACCEPTS THE "AMOUNT COVERED" AND HAS AGREED NOT TO
099   BILL PATIENTS FOR MORE THAN DEDUCTIBLES, COPAYS & NONCOVERED CHARGES.
514   THIS WORKSHEET WAS PROCESSED BY JENNIFER

DEDUCTIBLE SATISFIED: 1000.00

PAYMENTS HAVE BEEN ISSUED TO THE FOLLOWING BASED ON ABOVE EXPENSES.

HAYS, ANDERSON,   15.00

Fig. 15-9 Example of EOB.

healthcare practice does not agree with the choice because the substituted code results in a lesser payment. Similar problems occur when an insurer's payment system is based on CPT codes, and an RVS (Relative Value System) code is submitted that does not directly translate to CPT. When these claims are reviewed by a claims adjuster, he or she assigns a valid CPT code. Coding accurately and knowing which coding systems payers use helps avoid these downcoding problems.

If the claims adjuster changes a valid procedure code that was submitted on the claim, the health insurance professional should contact them and ask for the reason. If the contact is by mail, documentation that supports the code submitted should be included. In some cases, a procedure is denied because the insurer states that it is considered "integral to the main procedure." In other cases, a modifier that was submitted on the claim was dropped, or the claim was subject to a **correct code initiative** edit.

Correct code initiative edits are the result of the National Correct Coding Initiative, which develops correct coding methods for CMS. The edits are intended to reduce overpayments that result from improper coding. If the denial was due to a correct code initiative edit, documentation supporting why the procedure was distinct and not related to another procedure must be submitted.

STEP SIX: POSTING PAYMENTS

After the EOB has been reconciled with the patient's account, the health insurance professional or other staff member posts the payment received from the insurance carrier to the patient ledger and bills the patient for any applicable outstanding copayments or deductible amounts. Participating providers cannot balance bill, but nonpartici-

pating providers for commercial claims are allowed to bill the patient for any balance the insurance carrier does not pay. It is against the law to waive Medicare copayments unless financial hardship has been established and documented. Fig. 15-10 illustrates a payment entry on a patient ledger. (*Note:* Contractual adjustments are discussed in Chapter 17.)

TIME LIMITS

As stated previously, claims should be submitted to the insurance carrier as soon as possible, ideally within 30 days or sooner of the conclusion of treatment. Claims for patients who receive ongoing treatment typically are submitted on a periodic basis—every 15 to 30 days, depending on the policy of the healthcare practice. Most

STATEMENT

Westlake Medical Clinic
2604 Spindle Center
Cherokee, XY 23133
231-555-1212

Stanley P. Grady
1234 Old Colony Road
Calamus City, XY 23232

DATE	REFERENCE	DESCRIPTION	CHARGES	CREDITS PYMNTS.	CREDITS ADJ.	BALANCE
2004		BALANCE FORWARD ⟶				26 00
1/10	Stanley	99214, ROA	135 00	8 00		153 00
3/21	Stanley	99214, ROA	135 00	8 00		280 00
5/18	Stanley	99214, ROA	135 00	8 00		407 00
5/20		XYZ Ins. Claim				
6/24		XYZ Ins. Ck 319116		324 00		83 00
6/24		Contr. Adj XYZ			50 00	33 00

B40BC-2   PLEASE PAY LAST AMOUNT IN BALANCE COLUMN ⟶

Fig. 15-10 Example of a patient ledger card with entries.

third-party payers have time limits for when claims can be submitted to be considered for payment. The time limit for each of the major carriers discussed in this book is addressed in the corresponding chapters.

When the time limit for claim submission has been exceeded, a claim cannot be paid. The time limit in which to file a claim varies from carrier to carrier and often depends on various circumstances, such as the following:

- Whether the provider of the services participates (or is contracted) with the insurer
- Whether the provider of services does not participate (or is not contracted) with the insurer
- The method in which the claim was submitted for payment (i.e., electronic or paper)
- The type of provider who is billing for services (e.g., physician, hospital)
- When coordination of benefits apply

Generally, an insurer allows a maximum of 1 year from the date of service for submitting a claim; however, this is not always the case because some commercial carriers allow 180 days. If there is any question as to time limits, the health insurance professional should contact the carrier. It is a good idea to include each major payer's time limits in the same file containing their claims submission guidelines.

Most insurance companies also have a time limit for filing appeals. The time limit varies from carrier to carrier, and it is important that the health insurance professional keep this information on file so that it is readily available when and if needed.

The health insurance professional should establish a routine for completing and submitting insurance claims, such as at the end of every week or on the 15th and 30th of each month. How often claims are submitted varies depending on

- the size of the practice,
- office staffing,
- the type of claim (e.g., workers' compensation, supplemental security income, Medicare),
- how the claims are submitted (electronically or paper),
- whether claims are sent directly or a clearinghouse is used, and
- the major carriers involved.

What Did You Learn?

1. What is typically the first thing that happens to a claim when it is received by the insurer?
2. If the insurer determines a claim is "unclean," what happens to it?
3. Name the two suggested methods for tracking claims.
4. List four common payment errors.
5. Why is it important for the health insurance professional to know how to interpret EOBs?

Imagine This!

Maise Smyth is employed as a billing and insurance clerk for family practice physician, Dr. Isaac Finnes, at the Gulf Coast Medical Clinic. Dr. Finnes sees approximately 25 patients a day. The clinic is not yet computerized, so all of the claims are submitted on paper. To accomplish this challenging workload, Maise has set up a routine for submitting preparation. At the end of each day, she sorts the health records by insurer name. The following is Maise's schedule for claims preparation:

Monday—Blue Cross and Blue Shield
Tuesday—Medicare and Medicaid
Wednesday—TRICARE/CHAMPVA
Thursday—Magna Insurance (a major carrier in the area)
Friday—all miscellaneous carriers/claims follow-up

By the end of the day on Friday, all claims for patients seen that week have been prepared and submitted. Because there are only a few miscellaneous carriers, Maise has time on Friday afternoon to do any necessary claims tracking.

PROCESSING SECONDARY CLAIMS

Occasionally, patients may be covered under two insurance plans. When this happens, the health insurance professional may have to prepare and submit a primary claim and a **secondary claim**. The insurer who pays first is the primary payer, and that payer receives the first claim. The insurance company who pays after the primary carrier is referred to as the secondary insurer. This second carrier receives a claim after the primary carrier pays its monetary obligations.

As mentioned previously, the health insurance professional must determine which coverage is primary and which is secondary. If it is not immediately obvious which payer is primary, the health insurance professional should ask. If the patient does not know, a telephone call to one of the insurance companies should answer the question quickly and easily. If there is a second insurance policy, it is important to check "yes" in Block 11d on the CMS-1500 form and complete Blocks 9a through 9d (Fig. 15-11).

Occasionally, a patient and spouse (or parent) are covered under two separate employer group policies, resulting in what is referred to as **coordination of benefits**. When a coordination of benefits situation exists, the health insurance professional should

- verify which payer is primary and which is secondary, and
- send a copy of the EOB from the primary payer along with the claim to the secondary carrier (if the EOB is

9. OTHER INSURED'S NAME (Last Name, First Name, Middle Initial)
XYZ INSURANCE COMPANY

a. OTHER INSURED'S POLICY OR GROUP NUMBER
123456

b. OTHER INSURED'S DATE OF BIRTH	SEX
MM DD YY	
11 03 1978	M [X] F [ ]

c. EMPLOYER'S NAME OR SCHOOL NAME
ACME DRYGOODS INC

d. INSURANCE PLAN NAME OR PROGRAM NAME
CERTIF EMPLOYEE BENEFITS

Fig. 15-11 Section of CMS-1500 form showing Blocks 9 through 9d.

not included, the claim is likely to be denied or delayed pending coordination of benefits determination).

The rule of thumb for dependent children covered under more than one policy is as follows: The payer whose subscriber has the earlier birthday in the calendar year generally is primary. This is referred to as the **birthday rule**.

● Stop and Think

Fran and Ted Washburn and their two children have been coming to Gulf Coast Clinic on a regular basis for nearly 2 years. Shortly before the last office visit, Fran and Ted divorced; Ted changed jobs and moved to a different address in a nearby town. Fran and Ted are both employed, and each is covered under a separate employer group policy. Ted's date of birth is 09/06/65 and Fran's is 08/16/66. Which parent's policy should be considered primary?

Medicare secondary payer claims are claims that are submitted to another insurance company *before* they are submitted to Medicare. When a Medicare beneficiary has other insurance coverage that is primary to Medicare, the other insurer's payment information must be included on the claim that is submitted to Medicare; otherwise, Medicare may deny payment for the services. In some instances, as with Medicare/Medicaid, there is an automatic crossover, and a second claim does not have to be submitted. The health insurance professional should check the current guidelines of the specific payer in questions when a secondary policy is involved.

What Did You Learn?

1. What is a secondary claim?
2. What document typically must accompany a secondary claim?
3. Explain what is meant by the "birthday rule."

APPEALS

An appeal, as defined in insurance language, is the process of calling for a review of a decision made by a third-party carrier. Providers of service and patients have the right to appeal a rejected insurance claim or a payment made that the provider or patient (or both) believes is incorrect.

INCORRECT PAYMENTS

Before appealing a payment or a claim, whether with Medicare or a private commercial insurer, the health insurance professional should notify the insurer in writing that there has been an error. Many payers have a set time limit for claim appeals and often print it on their EOB.

A basic rule for appealing a claim is always to include a copy of the original claim, EOB or RA, and any additional documentation necessary to provide evidence for the appeal. Cover letters also are effective for appeals and provide the claims reviewer all of the necessary information regarding the reason for the appeal. If the payer does not responded to an appeal, the health insurance professional can pursue other alternatives, such as contacting the state's insurance commissioner and sending a clear, well-documented account of the discrepancy. See the website at the end of this chapter for links to individual state insurance departments.

DENIED CLAIMS

If the health insurance professional believes a claim has been wrongly denied, an appeal can be filed. The appeal process differs from carrier to carrier; however, appeals generally must be in writing and initiated within a specified number of days—usually 30 to 60. The appeal letter should identify the claim and the reason the health insurance professional believes the claim should be approved. The appeal usually is sent directly to the carrier along with any written comments, documents, records, or other information relating to the claim, even if they were not submitted with the original claim. The carrier typically reviews the appeal within 30 calendar days. Sometimes the insurance carrier's review committee allows the provider (or their representative) to present the case in person or over the telephone, which allows the individual or committee members conducting the review to ask questions to clarify the reason why the provider (or the provider's representative) thinks the claim is valid. The outcome of the appeal is determined, and the provider is notified verbally or in writing of the decision. This decision is usually final; however, some carriers allow second-level or even third-level appeals. The health insurance professional should consult the individual carrier's guidelines regarding the steps to take when initiating an appeal.

If the claim remains unpaid after all levels of appeal are exhausted, there are still some options open. If there have been repeated problems with a particular carrier, the state insurance commission can be contacted and the problem case outlined in a letter. A second option is to file a complaint with HIPAA. Also, it may be important to get the patient involved because he or she often can make helpful contributions.

HIPAA Tip

HIPAA provides an online health plan complaint form so that healthcare providers and their staff members can report administrative and payment disputes with health insurers and third-party payers. The form is designed to collect information from physicians on health plan and third-party payer noncompliance with the provisions of the HIPAA Transaction and Code Set Standards.

APPEALING A MEDICARE CLAIM

The Medicare program has a multilevel appeal process in place to challenge denied or underpaid claims. There are five different levels of the Medicare appeals process:
- Level I—appeal request
- Level II—hearing
- Level III—administrative law judge (ALJ) hearing
- Level IV—appeals council hearing
- Level V—judicial review

Level I: Appeal Request

The Medicare appeal process begins when either the healthcare provider or the beneficiary disagrees with the carrier's determination as explained on the EOB or RA. If the claim was assigned, only the provider can initiate the review. If the claim was unassigned, the beneficiary usually initiates the review or can stipulate in writing that the physician is authorized to act on his or her behalf.

The review request must come within 20 days from the date of the original determination for Part A appeals and 120 days for Part B appeals. A Part B appeal can be submitted on the HCFA-1964 Request for Review Form (Fig. 15-12). If a fully completed HCFA-1964 Request for Review Form is not used to express disagreement with the initial determination, a written appeal request must contain the following information:
- Beneficiary name
- Medicare health insurance claim number
- Name and address of provider/supplier of item/service
- Date of initial determination

- Date of service for which the initial determination was issued
- Which item, if any, or service is at issue in the appeal

The health insurance professional should forward the request to the local fiscal intermediary or carrier and clearly mark it *"review"* to avoid denial as a duplicate claim. As with any review, always include a copy of the claim, the EOB or RA, and any information that would aid in the review determination (e.g., a statement that the payment error was due to a clerical mistake or any documentation to support payment at the appropriate level, such as chart notes, operative report, or hospital records).

HIPAA Tip

According to HIPAA's privacy regulations, documents relating to uses and disclosures, authorization forms, business partner contracts, notices of information practice, responses to a patient who wants to amend or correct their information, the patient's statement of disagreement, and a complaint record must be maintained for 6 years.

Level II: Fair Hearing

If the claim has gone through the basic review steps and the health insurance professional still disagrees with the payer's determination, a Request for Hearing—Part B Medicare Claim form may be filed. To qualify for a fair hearing, the amount in question must be at least $100. Medicare allows a practice to "batch" claims with the same problem and procedure to equal the required $100 base. The hearing must be requested within 6 months of the date the informal review decision was made. The request must be in writing and sent to the Medicare Hearing Officer or Coordinator. A request for a fair hearing is pursued in one of three ways:

1. **Hearing on record**—a hearing officer investigates all aspects of the claim, but the physician does not testify unless oral testimony is determined to be necessary. A hearing on record is often the most productive fair hearing procedure. The physician is advised of the officer's decision, and a copy of the decision is forwarded to the local Medicare carrier for appropriate action.
2. **Telephone hearing**—the provider (or his or her representative) presents the case to a hearing office. Before the scheduled hearing, the physician is provided with information in the hearing officer's file. The

DEPARTMENT OF HEALTH AND HUMAN SERVICES
HEALTH CARE FINANCING ADMINISTRATION

FORM APPROVED
OMB NO. 0938-0033

REQUEST FOR REVIEW OF PART B MEDICARE CLAIM
Medical Insurance Benefits – Social Security Act

NOTICE – Anyone who misrepresents or falsifies essential information requested by this form may upon conviction subject to fine and imprisonment under Federal Law.

1. Carrier's Name and Address

2. Name of Patient

3. Health Insurance Claim Number

4. I do not agree with the determination you made on my claim as described on my Explanation of Medicare Benefits dated:

5. MY REASONS ARE: (Attach a copy of the Explanation of Medicare Benefits, or describe the service, date of service, and physician's name–NOTE–If the date on the Explanation of Medicare Benefits mentioned in Item 4 is more than six months ago, include your reason for not making this request earlier.)

6. Describe illness or injury:

7. □ I have additional evidence to submit. (Attach such evidence to this form.)
   □ I do not have additional evidence.

COMPLETE ALL OF THE INFORMATION REQUESTED. SIGN AND RETURN THE FIRST COPY AND ANY ATTACHMENTS TO THE CARRIER NAMED ABOVE. IF YOU NEED HELP, TAKE THIS AND YOUR NOTICE FROM THE CARRIER TO A SOCIAL SECURITY OFFICE, OR TO THE CARRIER. KEEP THE DUPLICATE COPY OF THIS FORM FOR YOUR RECORDS.

8. SIGNATURE OF EITHER THE CLAIMANT OR HIS REPRESENTATIVE

Claimant | Representative

Address | Address

City, State and Zip Code | City, State and Zip Code

Telephone Number | Date | Telephone Number | Date

Form HCFA-1964 (9/91)

CARRIER COPY

Fig. 15-12 Request for Review of Part B Medicare Claim.

REQUEST FOR HEARING
PART B MEDICARE CLAIM
Medical Insurance Benefits - Social Security Act

NOTICE—Anyone who misrepresents or falsifies essential information requested by this form may upon conviction be subject to fine and imprisonment under Federal Law.

CARRIER'S NAME AND ADDRESS

1 NAME OF PATIENT

2 HEALTH INSURANCE CLAIM NUMBER

3 I disagree with the review determination on my claim, and request a hearing before a hearing officer of the insurance carrier named above.

MY REASONS ARE: (Attach a copy of the Review Notice. NOTE: If the review decision was made more than 6 months ago, include your reason for not making this request earlier.)

4 CHECK ONE OF THE FOLLOWING

☐ I have additional evidence to submit. (Attach such evidence to this form or forward it to the carrier within 10 days.)

☐ I do not have additional evidence.

CHECK **ONLY ONE** OF THE STATEMENTS BELOW:

☐ I wish to appear in person before the Hearing Officer.

☐ I do not wish to appear and hereby request a decision on the evidence before the Hearing Officer.

5 EITHER THE CLAIMANT OR REPRESENTATIVE SHOULD SIGN IN THE APPROPRIATE SPACE BELOW

SIGNATURE OR NAME OF CLAIMANT'S REPRESENTATIVE	CLAIMANT'S SIGNATURE
ADDRESS	ADDRESS
CITY, STATE, AND ZIP CODE	CITY, STATE, AND ZIP CODE
TELEPHONE NUMBER DATE	TELEPHONE NUMBER DATE

(Claimant should not write below this line)

ACKNOWLEDGMENT OF REQUEST FOR HEARING

Your request for a hearing was received on _____ . You will be notified of the time and place of the hearing at least 10 days before the date of the hearing.

SIGNED

DATE

Form CMS-1965 (05/03)

Fig. 15-13 Request for Hearing Part B Medicare Claim.

provider is advised of the decision, and a copy is forwarded to the Medicare carrier for action.

3. **Personal hearing**—when the provider believes a hearing is best done in person, the Medicare hearing officer may agree to schedule a face-to-face meeting to discuss the case. Complete and well-organized records help present the best case possible.

Fig. 15-13 shows the form used to request a hearing on Part B Medicare claims.

Level III: Administrative Law Judge Review

To pursue the third level of appeal, the claim must have completed the fair hearing process, the dollar amount in question must be at least $500, and the appeal must be requested within 60 days of the fair hearing judgment.

Level IV: Departmental Appeals Board Review

If the provider (or beneficiary) is dissatisfied with the ALJ's decision, he or she may request a review by the Departmental Appeals Board (DAB). There are no requirements at this level regarding the amount of money in controversy. The request for a DAB review must be submitted within 60 days of receipt of the ALJ's decision, and should specify the issues and findings by the ALJ being contested.

Level V: Judicial Review in United States District Court

After a decision by the DAB, if $1000 or more is still in controversy, a judicial review before a US District Court judge can be considered. The provider must request a US District Court hearing within 60 days of receipt of the DAB's decision. Medicare's appeals process was amended in 2002. Table 15-2 compares the former requirements with current ones.

What Did You Learn?

1. If a payer does not respond to an appeal, what alternative does the health insurance professional have?
2. Who initiates an appeal on unassigned Medicare claims?
3. What is the time limit for a Medicare review request?
4. Name the three ways a Fair Hearing request may be pursued.

SUMMARY CHECK POINTS

☑ The six keys to successful claims are as follows:

- *Verify patient information*—It is important to keep patient information and a signed release of information current to generate clean claims, process them expeditiously, and minimize claim delay or denial because of misinformation. Also, if there is a second insurance carrier, primary status must be determined.
- *Obtain necessary preauthorization and precertification*—Most insurance carriers have a rule that when a patient is to be hospitalized or undergo certain procedures or diagnostic studies, preauthorization or precertification must be acquired beforehand. If this is not done, the claim is likely to be denied. Medicare does not require preauthorization for medically necessary services.
- *Documentation*—The healthcare provider must document accurate and appropriate information in the patient's health record to substantiate the procedures and diagnoses listed on the claim form.
- *Follow payer guidelines*—Because every third-party payer has slightly different guidelines for completing and submitting claims, the

---

TABLE 15-2	Changes to Medicare's Appeals Process	
MEDICARE'S APPEAL PROCESS	**FORMER REQUIREMENTS**	**CURRENT REQUIREMENTS**
Filing time limit—part A appeals	60 days from initial determination	20 days from initial determination
Filing time limit—part B appeal	180 days from initial determination	120 days from initial determination
Monetary threshold for AJL hearing	$500 (remaining in controversy)	$100 (remaining in controversy)
Medicare summary notices sent to Medicare beneficiaries	No filing date specified	Specified a filing date

Adapted from Lash Group Healthcare Consultants, 2002.

health insurance professional should create and maintain a file for each payer's current guidelines and follow those guidelines to the letter when preparing claims.
- *Proofread the claim to avoid errors*—It is important to proofread paper claims carefully before submitting them. Most errors that result in denial are simple mistakes, such as typos, transpositions, or omissions, resulting from carelessness and failure to double check each entry on the claim form.
- *Submit a clean claim*—The ultimate goal in the healthcare insurance process is to submit a clean claim, meaning all of the necessary, correct information appears on the claim. Clean claims typically are processed quickly.

☑ The claim process includes several steps, as follows:
- When the claim is received by the third-party payer, the claim is dated, attachments (if any) are confirmed, and the claim is processed through an OCR scanner.
- The claim passes through a series of edits and is compared with the patient's policy to verify coverage, eligibility, medical necessity, exclusions, preexisting conditions, and noncovered services. If the claim is "clean," it is approved and proceeds on for payment, if payment is due. If there is a problem with the claim, the provider is notified by mail or by telephone.
- At the end of a set time period (4 to 6 weeks for paper claims), if a claim is not paid, and no communication has been received explaining the delay, the claim needs to be followed up. The healthcare facility should have a mechanism in place for "tracking" claims so that no claim "falls through the crack." This tracking mechanism could be a suspension filing system or an insurance claims log system.
- Whether or not a payment is made against a claim, there is *always* an EOB. Each EOB should be checked to ensure no error has been made by the insurance carrier. If the claim is denied, or there has been a payment reduction, a decision must be made whether or not to appeal.
- Interpreting the EOB is the "key" to understanding how the claim was adjudicated. Accurately deciphering an EOB aids in collecting full reimbursement, including any balance owed by the patient.
- After the EOB has been reconciled, the payment is posted to the patient's account ledger. Participating providers of commercial claims cannot balance bill beyond

deductibles and copayments; nonparticipating providers can. Medicare copayments cannot be waived, unless a financial hardship case has been established.

☑ The time limits for submitting claims vary with insurance carriers; however, most allow 1 year after the date of service. It is important to follow specific payer guidelines because some demand claims submission within 90 days. The health insurance professional should endeavor to file all claims in a timely manner for the benefit of the practice and the patient.

☑ The most important consideration with patients who are covered under more than one insurance policy is to establish which one is primary. After that, complete the claim for the primary carrier, checking "yes" in Block 11d on the CMS-1500 form and completing Blocks 9a through 9d. Usually, the process for sending a claim to the secondary carrier is to include the EOB from the primary carrier with the claim. It is important to check the guidelines of the secondary carrier for submission rules.

☑ The first step in appealing a denied claim (or a claim where the payment has been reduced) is to notify the insurance carrier. Most payers have time limits for appealing claims and for submitting claims—typically 30 to 60 days. The health insurance professional should check the payer-specific guidelines for appealing claims. If all efforts of appeal are exhausted without success, and the health insurance professional is certain the claim is valid, a remaining option is to contact the state insurance commissioner's office.

☑ The Medicare program has a multilevel appeals process in place to challenge the determination on a claim.
- *Level I: appeal request*—A party who is dissatisfied with an initial Medicare coverage determination may request that the carrier review such determination. The request for an appeal must be filed within the time limit allowed (see Table 15-2). The request also must meet the requirements for the contents of an appeal request.
- *Level II: hearing*—If the claim has gone through the basic review steps and the issue is still unresolved, a Fair Hearing request form (Request for Hearing—Part B Medicare Claim form) may be filed with the time limit specified in the Medicare guidelines. A Fair Hearing can be conducted one of three ways: (1) hearing on record, (2) telephone hearing, or (3) personal hearing.

- *Level III: ALJ hearing*—The following criteria must be met when requesting an ALJ hearing: (1) The ALJ hearing must be requested in writing, and (2) the amount in controversy must be $500 or more (appeals may be combined to meet the $500 limit).
- *Level IV: DAB review*—If the provider (or beneficiary) is dissatisfied with the ALJ's decision, he or she may request a review by the DAB. There are no requirements regarding the amount of money in controversy.

The request for a DAB review must be submitted within 60 days of receipt of the ALJ's decision and should specify the issues and findings by the ALJ being contested.
- *Level V: judicial review in U.S. District Court*— If $1000 or more is still in controversy after the decision by the DAB, a judicial review before a U.S. District Court judge is the last level. The provider/beneficiary must request a U.S. District Court hearing within 60 days of receipt of the DAB's decision.

CLOSING SCENARIO

Zoey and Kristin felt confident that what they had learned about healthcare billing and filing insurance claims would give them a solid foundation for an "at-home" career. Learning the keys to successful claims was an important concept in the overall health insurance process. If a claim was not clean, the bottom line was that submitting it was a waste of time, effort, and money for all parties involved. Understanding what happens to a claim after it reaches the payer's office also was interesting and enlightening for these two students. Until now, where the claim went after it left the healthcare office and what was done with it were basically mysteries to them, and the term "adjudication" was simply another perplexing word with ambiguous meaning. After completing Chapter 15, the entire claim process and meaning of adjudication became clear.

Appealing claims, especially Medicare claims, also was a learning experience. Zoey and Kristin already were aware that learning the intricacies associated with Medicare could be demanding, but becoming educated with the various levels of appeal and studying the forms lessened their apprehension. Overall, Zoey and Kristin knew they were on their way to an exciting and rewarding home career.

WEBSITES TO EXPLORE

For live links to the following websites, please visit the Evolve® site at http://evolve.elsevier.com/Beik/today/

- For more information on HIPAA, log on to http://www.cms.hhs.gov/hipaa/

- For general information on claims processing, log on to http://www.ama-assn.org/

- For links to individual state insurance offices, log on to http://www.naic.org/state_web_map.htm

- To learn more about the Medicare appeals process, check the following websites:
  http://www.cms.hhs.gov/
  http://www.gpoaccess.gov/fr/index.html
  http://www.cms.hhs.gov/medlearn/
  http://www.medicare.gov

UNIT V

Advanced Application

Chapter 16

The Role of Computers in Health Insurance

Chapter Outline

CHAPTER OBJECTIVES

After completion of this chapter, the student should be able to

- Explain how computers have affected health insurance.
- Define electronic data interchange.
- List the essential elements of electronic data interchange.
- Compare and contrast submitting claims through a clearinghouse versus direct data entry.
- Discuss the advantages of submitting claims electronically.
- Explain how the Department of Health and Human Services final "rule" affects Medicare.
- List and explain three additional electronic services available to the health insurance professional.

CHAPTER TERMS

Administrative Simplification and Compliance Act (ASCA)
billing services
code sets
direct data entry (DDE) claims
electronic claims clearinghouse
electronic data interchange (EDI)
electronic funds transfer (EFT)
electronic medical record (EMR)
electronic remittance advice (ERA)
enrollment process
identifiers
privacy standards
security standards
small provider of services
small supplier
telecommunication
unusual circumstances

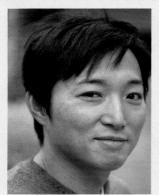

Student Ellie Farnsworth has an associate's degree in computer technology. She enrolls in the medical insurance course to be able to apply her computer skills to medical billing and health insurance claims. Ellie realizes that HIPAA has changed the face of not only electronic claims transmission, but also world healthcare in general. Ellie wonders why so much emphasis is being placed on HIPAA. "Every chapter talks about HIPAA," Ellie complains. "It's like we eat, sleep, and drink HIPAA."

Benji Yutsuki is also computer literate. He understands the vulnerability of electronic transmissions, but agrees with Ellie that there is a lot to understand with HIPAA. "My aunt works in a medical office, and she said they call it the 'HIPAA hippo,'" he says with a laugh. Benji tries to convince Ellie to be patient, however. "I believe HIPAA is more important than we might think," Benji adds, "especially as far as patients and the general public are concerned."

After the two students discuss HIPAA and how this act affects electronic healthcare transactions, they agree that it is in their best interest to attempt to understand why it was created and its importance to healthcare in general.

IMPACT OF COMPUTERS ON HEALTH INSURANCE

Just a few years ago, it was unusual to find a medical office where computers were used for patient accounting and insurance claims submission. As the age of technology advanced, however, the use of computers became more widespread. From a health insurance perspective, computers are now used for

- enrolling an individual in a health plan,
- paying health insurance premiums,
- checking eligibility,
- obtaining authorization to refer a patient to a specialist,
- processing claims, and
- notifying a provider about the payment of a claim.

As computer technology advanced, however, it became clear that the health information being transmitted through computers and the Internet had to be monitored and laws enacted to protect the security of health information and the privacy of individuals. The U.S. government, under Health Insurance Portability and Accountability Act (HIPAA) regulations, now mandates that all healthcare information that is electronically transmitted follow specific rules and guidelines to provide this needed security and protection.

HIPAA'S ROLE IN ELECTRONIC TRANSMISSIONS

HIPAA was intended to reform health insurance and simplify the healthcare administrative processes. Provisions of HIPAA's **Administrative Simplification and Compliance Act (ASCA)** require health plans and healthcare clearinghouses to use certain standard transaction formats and

code sets for the electronic transmission of health information. These requirements also apply to healthcare providers who transmit health information in electronic form in connection with the transactions covered in the rule. As usage of electronic transmissions of healthcare information increased, privacy and security regulations were adopted to enhance the privacy protections and security measures directed at health information.

One of the goals of ASCA was to reduce the number of forms and methods of completing claims and other payment-related documents and to use a universal identifier for providers of healthcare. Another goal was to increase the use and efficiency of computer-to-computer methods of exchanging standard healthcare information. The five specific areas of administrative simplification addressed by HIPAA are as follows:

- **Electronic data interchange (EDI)** is the electronic transfer of information in a standard format between two entities. EDI allows business entities to exchange information and transact business in a rapid and cost-effective way. The transactions that are included within HIPAA consist of standard electronic formats for enrollment, eligibility, payment and remittance advice, claims, health plan premium payments, health claim status, and referral certification and authorization.
- **Code sets** include data elements used to document uniformly the reasons why patients are seen and procedures or services are provided to them during their healthcare encounters.
- **Identifiers** are the numbers used in the administration of healthcare to distinguish individual healthcare providers, health plans, employers, and patients. Over time, identifiers are intended to simplify the administrative processes, such as referrals and billing; improve accuracy of data; and reduce costs.

- **Security standards** need to be developed and adopted for all health plans, clearinghouses, and providers to follow and to be required at all stages of transmission and storage of healthcare information to ensure integrity and confidentiality of the records at all phases of the process, before, during, and after electronic transmission.
- **Privacy standards** are intended to define what are appropriate and inappropriate disclosures of individually identifiable health information and how patient rights are to be protected.

ASCA made it compulsory for all Medicare claims to be submitted electronically effective October 16, 2003, with certain exceptions (see section on Medicare and Electronic Claims Submission). These electronic claims are to be in a format that complies with the appropriate standard adopted for national use. ASCA allowed extra time for medical facilities to implement and test HIPAA-compliant software.

What Did You Learn?

1. Name five things that computers are used for in relation to health insurance.
2. List the five specific areas of administrative simplification addressed by HIPAA.

ELECTRONIC DATA INTERCHANGE

EDI may be most easily defined as the replacement of paper-based documents with electronic equivalents. More specifically, EDI is the exchange of documents in standardized electronic form, between business entities, in an automated manner, directly from a computer application in one facility to an application in another. EDI offers the prospect of easy and inexpensive communication of information throughout the healthcare community.

HISTORY OF ELECTRONIC DATA INTERCHANGE

The early applications of what later became known as EDI can be traced back to the 1948 Berlin Airlift, where the task of coordinating air-freighted consignments of food and other consumables (which arrived with differing manifests and languages) was facilitated by creating a standard shipping manifest. Electronic transmission began during the 1960s, initially in the transportation industries, when standardization of documents became necessary, and the U.S. Transportation Data Coordinating Committee (TDCC) was

formed to coordinate the development of translation rules among four existing sets of industry-specific standards. A further step toward standardization came with the creation of standards for the American National Standards Institute (ANSI), which gradually extended and replaced those created by the Transportation Data Coordinating Committee.

EDI can be compared and contrasted with electronic mail (e-mail). E-mail enables free-format, textual messages to be electronically transmitted from one person to another. EDI supports structured business messages (expressed in hard-copy, preprinted forms or business documents) and transmits them electronically between computer applications, rather than between people. The essential elements of EDI are

- the use of an *electronic transmission medium*, rather than physical storage media, such as magnetic tapes and disks;
- the use of *structured, formatted messages based on agreed standards* (such that messages can be translated, interpreted, and checked for compliance with an explicit set of rules);
- *relatively fast delivery* of electronic documents from sender to receiver (generally meaning receipt within hours or even minutes); and
- *direct communication between applications* (rather than merely between computers).

EDI depends on a sophisticated information technology communications system. This system must include data processing, data management, and networking capabilities, to enable the efficient capture of data into electronic form, the processing and retention of data, controlled access to it, and efficient and reliable data transmission between remote sites.

A common connection point is needed for all participants, together with a set of electronic "mailboxes" (so that the organizations' computers are not interrupted by one another) and security and communications management features. It is feasible for organizations to implement EDI directly with one another, but it generally proves advantageous to use a third-party network services provider.

BENEFITS OF ELECTRONIC DATA INTERCHANGE

EDI leads to faster transfer of data, fewer errors, and less time wasted on exception handling, resulting in a more streamlined communication process. Benefits of EDI can be achieved in such areas as inventory management, transport, and distribution; administration and cash management; and, in this case, transmission of healthcare information data. EDI offers the prospect of simple and inexpensive communication of structured information throughout the healthcare community.

HIPAA Tip

HIPAA has set standards for the electronic transmission of healthcare data. As of October 16, 2003, any healthcare service provider has the option of sending client medical billing data electronically to a health plan (or payer), but if they do, the data must be in a HIPAA-compliant format. The health plan must be able to receive and process the data and respond electronically, likewise in a HIPAA-compliant format.

What Did You Learn?

1. What is EDI?
2. Name the four essential elements of EDI.
3. List three benefits of EDI.

ELECTRONIC CLAIMS PROCESS

The electronic claims process incorporates the use of EDI. In the case of electronic insurance claims, EDI is the exchange of information between the provider's office and a third party. There are essentially two ways to submit claims electronically: through an electronic claims clearinghouse or directly to an insurance carrier. To send claims electronically, the medical practice needs a computer, modem, and HIPAA-compliant software.

ENROLLMENT

Whether the medical practice chooses to use a clearinghouse or submit claims directly to the insurance carrier, it needs to go through an **enrollment process** before submitting claims. The enrollment process typically involves completing and returning EDI setup requirement forms. This process is necessary so that the business that receives the claims can create a compatible information file about the practice in their computer system so that claims can be processed. Most government and many commercial carriers require enrollment. Some also require that the practice sign a contract before sending any claims. The enrollment process typically takes several weeks to complete. The biggest obstacle to getting set up for electronic claims processing is the time that it takes for approval from state, federal, and in some cases commercial or health maintenance organization carriers.

ELECTRONIC CLAIMS CLEARINGHOUSE

An **electronic claims clearinghouse** is a business entity that receives claims from several medical facilities and consolidates these claims so that one transmission containing multiple claims can be sent to each insurance carrier. More specifically, a clearinghouse serves as an intermediary between medical practices and the insurance companies, facilitating the electronic exchange of information between the facilities.

A clearinghouse works as follows. When received, claims are edited and validated to ensure they are error-free and are checked for completeness. If an error is discovered or information is missing, the issuing facility is notified that there is a problem with a claim. Often, the claim can be repaired quickly and resubmitted to the clearinghouse, eliminating the costly delay associated with mailing back an incorrectly submitted paper claim. If the claim is "clean," the clearinghouse translates the data elements into a format that is compatible with the format required by the target insurance carrier. (The data are not changed, but the order in which they are presented may be changed to accommodate the sequence required by a particular insurance company's claims processing software system.) When reformatted, the data are sent electronically (usually overnight) to the target insurance company for processing. The insurance company prepares an explanation of benefits or a remittance advice, which is sent electronically to the clearinghouse. The data are reformatted (back into the original format) and transmitted back to the originating medical facility. Fig. 16-1 is a flow chart of electronic claims transmission through a clearinghouse.

Imagine This!

Clark Emmerson, a health insurance professional with Loveland Health Center, sends all of the center's insurance claims to RapidServ Clearinghouse. RapidServ performs an edit check on each claim and redistributes them in batches to the appropriate carrier. On one particular batch, a computer error resulted in the employer identification number being left off the claims. RapidServ caught the error, corrected it, and sent the claims on without having to return them to Clark for completion.

DIRECT DATA ENTRY CLAIMS

Submitting claims directly to an insurance carrier, referred to as **direct data entry (DDE) claims,** is a little more complex. As with a claims clearinghouse, most government carriers and many commercial carriers require enrollment before submitting DDE claims electronically. The

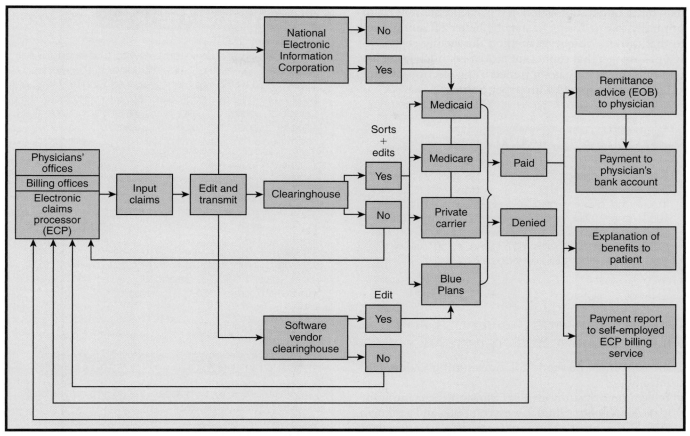

Fig. 16-1 Example of a flow chart of claim sent to clearinghouse.

medical facility also needs software from each insurance carrier to whom it will be submitting claims. Most carriers have their own software or can recommend someone who supports direct transmissions within range of the medical facility. The most common direct claims submission method is done by creating a "print image" file of the insurance claim and using the direct claims software to send the claims to the insurance carrier; however, the method used in DDE claims can vary from carrier to carrier.

CLEARINGHOUSE VERSUS DIRECT

When deciding which method is better for a medical facility to use—a clearinghouse or direct to the carrier—there are several things to consider:

- Submitting claims directly to the carrier is normally the less expensive method of the two if the practice submits claims primarily to one carrier. If the practice submits claims electronically to multiple carriers, however, it may be more expensive than using a clearinghouse. If the direct method is chosen, the practice will need to enroll and become compatible with each carrier's software to which claims are submitted.
- With a clearinghouse, the practice needs to deal with only one business entity, and claims for multiple carriers can

be submitted in one transmission. The simplicity of sending all claims to one location should not be underestimated when considering which method to use. Submitting claims to multiple carriers requires the health insurance professional to become expert in each of the claims submission modules that are used because each one is unique.

- Some carriers accept claims only at certain times, whereas a clearinghouse accepts claims any time.
- Telephone expense is often overlooked when comparing direct transmission with a clearinghouse. Many clearinghouses support toll-free lines for claims transmissions.
- Updates to an insurance carrier's transmission software are usually free when using the clearinghouse. When using a direct submission module, updates typically take place at the customer's site and often require a skilled programmer, which can be costly.
- With a clearinghouse, a single confirmation report is produced for all insurance carriers. Separate confirmation reports are produced for each carrier where claims are submitted directly.

The bottom line—unless the medical facility submits insurance claims to primarily one carrier and has well-trained staff members to handle multiple carrier software, an electronic claims clearinghouse might be a better choice than direct carrier submission. If the practice submits claims primarily to one carrier, it may be better off going direct to that carrier. Whichever method the facility chooses, it is a proven fact that claims are processed much faster and reimbursement time is shortened using electronic claims submission compared with paper claims.

> ● **Stop and Think**
>
> Fairview Geriatric Care Center sees only patients on Medicare. Hattie Carmichael, the health insurance professional at Fairview, must make a recommendation at the next staff meeting whether to submit claims through a clearinghouse or use DDE. Which methods of claims submission do you think Hattie should choose?

OTHER METHODS AVAILABLE FOR FILING CLAIMS ELECTRONICALLY

There are other methods for transmitting claims electronically:
- **Telecommunication** involves transmitting claim information over phone lines using a computer and a modem. This is the most common form of electronic claim transmission.
- **Billing services** are companies that file claims for a fee, usually a per-copy charge. In addition, billing services usually take on the responsibility of keeping up with rapidly changing Medicare laws.

ADVANTAGES OF FILING CLAIMS ELECTRONICALLY

There are numerous advantages to filing claims electronically. EDI transmissions typically
- result in faster, more efficient claim submissions, and with fewer errors;
- provide immediate notification if a claim has been accepted or rejected and why;
- allow faster processing (and ultimately payment) of claims;
- generate electronic remittance advices (ERAs) from health plans and quickly and accurately posts them to the practice's accounting system automatically;
- provide claims status information reports;
- use a universal set of codes with all health plans;
- obtain faster and more accurate eligibility information;
- reduce claim denials owing to eligibility;
- conduct prior authorization and referral requests electronically;
- acquire prior authorizations and referral requests; and
- reduce claim denials because of authorization or referral issues.

> ● **Stop and Think**
>
> After making the decision to switch from paper to electronic claims, the office manager at the Genesis Health and Wellness Center asked Garner Polk, a health insurance professional with Genesis, to conduct research and prepare a report for the next staff meeting recommending a list of equipment needed for the switchover. If you were Garner, what would you recommend?

> ☑ **HIPAA Tip**
>
> Under the new rules set forth in HIPAA, electronic claims may include only "standard medical code sets" (e.g., the ICD-9 diagnostic codes, CPT codes, and Medicare's HCPCS codes).

> **What Did You Learn?**
>
> 1. What are the two essential ways to submit claims electronically?
> 2. Name the process that needs to be completed before sending claims electronically.
> 3. How does the claims clearinghouse process work?
> 4. When might direct carrier submission be a better choice than a clearinghouse?
> 5. List five advantages of filing claims electronically.

GETTING STARTED

HIPAA encourages physicians, hospitals, and other healthcare professionals to submit claims electronically. Electronic submission increases the accuracy of claims payment. Electronic submission also offers advantages such as faster turnaround, lower administrative costs, and elimination of mail delays and postage.

OBTAINING ELECTRONIC CLAIM CAPABILITY

There are several ways to obtain electronic claims capability:
- *Install an office automation system.* Numerous software and hardware suppliers have computer systems available for filing claims electronically.
- *Hire a billing service or clearinghouse.* Either can assist the health insurance professional in getting started and do all testing necessary to ensure successful transmissions.

- *Have a system custom designed.* If the practice is unable to locate a system that meets its needs, it may want to hire a computer programmer to custom design a special system.
- *Obtain electronic billing software.*

When a medical practice makes the changeover from paper to electronic claims, specific steps must be taken. The staff needs to do the following:

- Determine the weekly claim volume and decide which transmission alternative adapts best to that particular facility. (It is important to consider the possible future expansion of the practice.)
- Research the products and services of software vendors, billing services, and clearinghouses. Request client lists from each vendor, and contact offices in the same specialty to compare and rate customer satisfaction.
- Contact the carriers to whom claims will be submitted. There is usually a testing and approval process when beginning EDI submission. Most carriers and clearinghouses monitor and troubleshoot the first few transmissions.

TYPICAL HARDWARE AND SOFTWARE REQUIREMENTS

Following is a list of equipment and software programs that are required for electronic claims transmission. This list is not absolute; it includes just typical examples.

- Pentium PC running the latest version of Windows or Macintosh
- Internet service provider
- Netscape Navigator or Internet Explorer
- Word processing software
- A 56K modem, a DSL line, or cable modem
- Adobe Acrobat or PDF Factory Software to convert documents to Portable Document Format (PDF)
- Adobe Acrobat Reader to view documents online
- Scanner for documents that are not in a word processing format (optional).

What Did You Learn?

1. Name two ways that a medical facility can obtain electronic claim capability.
2. What steps must be taken when switching from paper claims to electronic claims submission?
3. List the equipment typically needed for electronic claims transmission.

MEDICARE AND ELECTRONIC CLAIMS SUBMISSION

Congress enacted ASCA to improve the administration of the Medicare program by taking advantage of the effi-

ciencies to be gained through electronic claim submission. The Department of Health and Human Services (HHS) published the final "rule" for the electronic submission of Medicare claims mandated under ASCA. With certain exceptions, ASCA requires that all claims sent to the Medicare Program on or after October 16, 2003, be submitted electronically. This "rule" is applicable only to providers, practitioners, and suppliers who submit claims under Part A or Part B of Medicare. It does not apply to claims submitted by providers to Medicare Advantage (Medicare+ Choice) organizations.

The move from paper to electronic submissions is expected to result in significant savings for Medicare physicians, practitioners, suppliers, and other healthcare providers and for the Medicare program itself. (The Medicare program is considered a covered entity subject to HIPAA regulations because it falls within the definition of a "health plan.")

Electronic claims submission is required only for initial Medicare claims, including initial claims with paper attachments, submitted for processing by the medical fiscal intermediary or carrier that serves the physician, practitioner, facility, supplier, or other healthcare provider. The "rule" does not require any other transactions (e.g., changes, adjustments, or appeals to the initial claim) to be submitted electronically.

Claims submitted via DDE are considered to be electronic claims for purposes of the "rule." In addition, claims transmitted to a Medicare contractor using the free or low-cost claims software issued by Medicare fee-for-service plans are also electronic claims for purposes of the "rule." The only exceptions to the electronic claims submission requirement under the "rule" are as follows:

- The entity has no method available for submitting claims electronically. Three situations fall into this category:
  1. Roster billing of vaccinations covered by the Medicare program
  2. Claims for payment under Medicare demonstration projects
  3. Claims where more than one plan is responsible for payment before Medicare
- The entity submitting the claim is a small provider of services or small supplier. A **small provider of services** is a hospital, critical access hospital, skilled nursing facility, comprehensive outpatient rehabilitation facility, home health agency, or hospice program with fewer than 25 full-time equivalent employees. A **small supplier** is a physician, practitioner, facility, or supplier with fewer than 10 full-time equivalent employees.
- The Secretary of HHS finds that a waiver of the electronic submission requirement is appropriate because of **unusual circumstances**. Unusual circumstances exist in any one of the following situations:
  1. Submission of dental claims
  2. A service interruption in the mode of submitting the electronic claims that is outside of the control of the

submitting entity, but only for the period of the interruption and subject to the specific requirements set forth under the "rule"

3. On demonstration to the satisfaction of the Secretary of HHS that other extraordinary circumstances exist that preclude the submission of electronic claims

Other than the above-listed exceptions, ASCA states that no payment may be made under Parts A or B of the Medicare program for claims submitted in nonelectronic form. Entities that fail to comply with the "rule" may be subject to claim denial, overpayment recovery, and applicable interest on overpayments. HHS does not intend to broaden these limited exceptions.

● Stop and Think

Margaret Turner, a family practice physician, runs a health clinic in Flint County, which is located in a rural area of the Midwest. Besides herself, Dr. Turner employs a physician's assistant, a registered nurse, a laboratory technician, two full-time medical assistants, and a part-time bookkeeper. Dr. Turner hires a private billing service (which has 16 full-time employees) to handle all of the clinic's billing and insurance claims. Based on the HHS "rule," does Dr. Turner's facility qualify as an exempt entity?

Imagine This!

The computer system in the Fairview Geriatric Care Clinic was damaged during an electrical storm. Luckily, Hattie Carmichael, the health insurance professional, had made a tape backup, so no data were lost. The computer tech support staff informed her, however, that it would be a week or more before the system would be up and running again. This qualifying as an "unusual circumstance," Hattie informed InfoData, the local Medicare B carrier, that she would be submitting paper claims during the period of time the computer was not functional.

What Did You Learn?

1. To what entities is the HHS final "rule" applicable?
2. To what types of claims does the "rule" *not* apply?
3. Give an example of an "unusual circumstance" for which waiver of electronic submission might apply.

ADDITIONAL ELECTRONIC SERVICES AVAILABLE

In addition to submitting claims electronically, several other electronic services are available to the health insurance professional, which can streamline the insurance claims submission process.

ELECTRONIC FUNDS TRANSFER

Electronic funds transfer (EFT) is a system wherein data representing money are moved electronically between accounts or organizations. In the case of insurance claims, when claims are submitted electronically, many carriers transfer the payments directly into the provider's bank account rather than mailing a check, making the funds instantly usable. There are several advantages to receiving insurance payments via EFT rather than paper checks; EFT

- reduces the amount of paper;
- eliminates the risk of paper checks being lost or stolen in the mail;
- saves time and hassle of going to bank to deposit checks; and
- speeds funds to the provider's bank account, where they can be used or can start earning interest immediately, whereas paper checks can take 1 week to process.

To enroll in the Medicare direct deposit program or another carrier's direct deposit program, contact the specific payer and ask for an EFT enrollment form, fill it out, and mail it back. To help ensure the validity of deposit information, the form must have original signatures (no copies, facsimiles, or stamped signatures) and include a copy of a canceled or voided check for the bank and the account in which you want your monies to be deposited. Fig. 16-2 shows a typical form used to authorize EFT.

ELECTRONIC REMITTANCE ADVICE

In addition to EFT, Medicare and other carriers offer an **electronic remittance advice (ERA)**. An ERA allows the provider's office to receive explanation of benefits or remittance advices electronically. With ERA, payments can be posted automatically to patient accounts, allowing the health insurance professional to update accounts receivable much more quickly and accurately than if he or she had to post the payments manually. Fig. 16-3 is an example form authorizing the carrier to transmit a remittance advice electronically.

If a medical facility chooses to receive a Medicare ERA, it first needs to have its computer system programmed. A programmer needs the Health Care Financing Administration (HCFA) National Standard Format or ANSI 835 specifications (available on the HCFA website). When a practice begins receiving payment reports electronically, they may choose to discontinue receiving the paper copy.

Electronic Funds Transfer (EFT) Form

Please choose one of these options:

☐ Elect EFT payments   ☐ Change EFT information   ☐ Terminate EFT payments

Name of Brokerage Firm: _____

Name of Broker: _____

Business Address: _____

City: _____ State: _____ Zip Code: _____

Phone Number: _____

Please attach a voided check, if available. When providing the Account and Routing/Transit Numbers, please refer to the series of numbers located at the bottom of your check and insert those numbers located between the symbols shown. For your reference, please see the sample check on the reverse side of this form.

Type of Account: ☐ Business Account   or   ☐ Personal Account   *(check one)*
                   ☐ Checking   or   ☐ Savings   *(check one)*

Name(s) on Account: _____
Please list all names that appear on the account

Account Number: ⑆ _____ ⑈

Name of Financial Institution: _____

City: _____ State: _____

Routing/Transit Number: ⑆ ☐☐☐☐☐☐☐☐☐ ⑆

<u>IMPORTANT NOTE:</u> **It is the applicant's responsibility to ensure that the information provided on this form is complete and accurate.**   **will not be responsible and shall be held harmless for errors made in EFT payments that are a result of inaccurate or incomplete information provided on this form. In no event and under no circumstances will**   **liability exceed the amount of the EFT payments in question.**

_____   _____   _____   _____
Signature of Account Owner   Date   Signature of Brokerage Firm Authorized Representative   Date

_____   _____
Print Name   Print Name

_____   _____
Title   Title

To protect the privacy of your financial information, please do not fax or e-mail completed forms. Please mail your signed and completed forms to the following address: **Health Care, Inc., Treasury Department, 93 Fourth Street, Anytown, MA 09080**

For Internal Use Only:	Vendor ID #

Fig. 16-2 Example of an EFT form.

Authorization for Electronic Transmission
Of AHCCCS Fee-For-Service Remittance Advice

I Hereby request and authorize the AHCCCS Administration to transmit my Fee-For-Service Remittance Advice via the Internet to the electronic mail (email) address listed below. I understand that I will no longer receive a paper copy of my Remittance Advice once I begin receiving my Remittance Advice electronically.

I understand that although my Remittance Advice will be transmitted electronically, my reimbursement check(s) will continue to be delivered by the U.S. Postal Service to the pay-to address(es) on file with the AHCCCS Administration Provider Registration Unit.

I understand that it is my responsibility to notify the AHCCCS Administration Provider Registration Unit in writing of any change in my email address.

Provider/Group Name: _____

AHCCCS Provider Identification Number: _____

Street Address: _____

City: _____ State: _____ ZIP Code: _____

Telephone: ( ) _____ Fax: ( ) _____

Name of Contact Person: _____

Email address: _____

Signature of Provider
Or Authorized Representative: _____

Date: _____

Mail this form to: AHCCCS Provider Registration Unit
MD 8100
701 E. Jefferson St.
Anytown, XY 85034

or

Fax this form to: AHCCCS Provider Registration Unit
(602) 256-xxxx

Please allow 10 working days for implementation of this change.

Fig. 16-3 Example authorization for ERA.

The electronic capabilities of many third-party payers and clearinghouses include periodic claim status reports (Fig. 16-4), which give a detailed list of claims that have to be paid, are pending, or have been denied. These reports can be hard copies or electronic through the practice software.

What Did You Learn?

1. What occurs when funds are transmitted electronically?
2. List two advantages of ETF.
3. What is one advantage of receiving a remittance advice electronically over a paper remittance advice?

ELECTRONIC MEDICAL RECORD

An **electronic medical record (EMR)** is an electronic file wherein patients' health information is stored in a computer system. Synonymous terms for an EMR include EPR (electronic patient record), EHR (electronic health record), and CPR (computerized patient record).

The use of EMRs to store patient health information is becoming increasingly prevalent in today's healthcare environment. The information contained in EMRs varies greatly in type—ranging from simple and routine clinical data to sophisticated medical images. An EMR typically includes the following components:

- *Patient's history*—including past encounters, medications, procedures, referrals, and vital statistics
- *Transaction capability*—such as ordering of laboratory tests, medical procedures, and prescriptions
- *Administrative functionality*—including invoice generation, payment requests, payer documentation compliance, and clinical research data compilation

Fig. 16-4 Example of an electronic claims status information advice.

Imagine This!

Anthony Skovoski, a radiologist with Mt. Clair Hospital, has an in-house computer set up so that the hospital can transmit x-ray images electronically to him at home. On days that Dr. Skovoski is not at work, the hospital can transmit images directly to his house and he can read them and generate a written report within minutes, avoiding a 40-minute commute to the hospital. If Dr. Skovoski needs information from the patient's health record, he also can access that from his home computer.

There are obvious benefits to be gained from being able to store, ask questions of, and exchange medical information electronically among various healthcare sites.

Because EMRs contain clinical information about patients, they form a crucial part of a healthcare system. Currently, many physicians keep paper records about their patients. When clinical patient information is exchanged (e.g., between a hospital and a family practitioner), it is usually done manually through the mail, by some sort of delivery service, or by fax or phone. This practice makes it difficult to obtain accurate information in a timely fashion.

One of the most significant activities of the healthcare industry is information management. Because of the enormous amount of patient data in existence, computer technology can be an extremely useful tool for the healthcare industry. There are many obstacles that must be overcome, however, before computerized patient medical records are used universally in the healthcare environment, such as the issue of privacy, medicolegal requirements, and the effect of EMRs on existing medical practices.

FUTURE OF ELECTRONIC MEDICAL RECORDS

An intercommunicative EMR system, in which an emergency department physician in Florida can treat a vacationing heart patient from the Midwest effectively by "pulling up" his EMR on a computer, has the potential to improve the provision of heath care. In the "best-case scenario," it would allow clinicians to be able to access a more timely and complete picture of a patient's clinical history, allowing physicians to make better informed healthcare decisions for their patients. To be effective, however, the EMR system would have to integrate data from several sources through a linked collection of records and message capabilities. The system also would have to provide decision support, such as reminders, alerts, and clinical pathway information. The EMR must serve as the provider's primary source of information, including orders and test results.

With this approach, all the user would require to be fully operational are a browser, an Internet service provider, and a personal computer.

If an EMR system is to provide a comprehensive solution for today's practice environment, it should streamline workflow efficiency, improve adherence to treatment standards, provide detailed financial practice analysis, enhance patient education and interaction, and optimize compliance with regulatory and managed care guidelines.

Claims submission, physician referrals, patient records, and scheduling information are among the pieces of administrative data that providers could send through a secure central processing hub. This technology would guarantee that data transactions comply with all regulations mandating the privacy of medical data transfer and would allow a non–World Wide Web–enabled application to run centrally over an Internet connection. The software could be operated as though it were local on the remote user's computer.

The advantages of this process would be considerable. Users could employ a handheld device, PC, or laptop to input medical record information into a file held on a proprietary server. Some large medical centers already offer such services to their physician groups. This allows patients in an emergency to inform the emergency department physician where to find their chart or laboratory reports on the World Wide Web.

PRIVACY CONCERNS OF ELECTRONIC MEDICAL RECORDS

Providers and patients want assurances that transferred data would not become vulnerable and would not fall into the wrong hands. To address this, the American Medical Association together with microchip maker Intel have introduced an encrypted identification code that can keep Internet transactions private and patients' rights protected. As consumers explore online EMR possibilities and begin to trust that online healthcare can be kept as confidential as their banking accounts, the market can explore its full potential, and providers can realize its benefits.

Despite a strong inclination toward the adoption of Internet-based EMRs, significant obstacles remain. Software packages have been developed without the thorough knowledge of what is going on in the provider's office. One challenge for software engineers is to find ways to make it easier for providers to acquire information during the patient's visit, rather than making information gathering another step in the process. Software designers need to figure out how providers can feed data (e.g., temperature or blood pressure readings) into the medical record without the need to type in the data separately.

Another concern is the cost. Providers frequently purchase expensive state-of-the-art software only to realize additional expenses are incurred through training, installation, and upgrades. The EMR of the future will reside on the Internet server, however, whose cost of creating and maintaining can be reasonably priced (e.g., through an annual licensing fee and a nominal charge per transaction), and whose security is assured.

☑ HIPAA Tip

The HIPAA compliance security standards mandate safeguards for physical storage and maintenance, transmission, and access to individual health information. The standards apply not only to the transactions adopted under HIPAA, but also to all individual health information that is maintained or transmitted. HIPAA gives organizations the flexibility to choose the best security solutions to meet the security and privacy mandates.

What Did You Learn?

1. What are EMRs?
2. What are two important concerns regarding EMRs?

SUMMARY CHECK POINTS

☑ The age of technology has had a great impact on health insurance. Many functions that previously were performed manually now are done faster and with fewer errors using a computer. Processing claims electronically is one of the biggest changes the computer has brought to claims processing. Advanced technology also has created a concern for the security of privacy of health information, however.

☑ EDI is the exchange of documents in standardized electronic form, between business entities, in an automated manner, directly from a computer application in one facility to an application in another.

☑ The essential elements of EDI include the following:
  - *An electronic transmission medium*, such as magnetic tapes and disks
  - *Structured, formatted messages based on agreed standards* or set of rules
  - *Relatively fast delivery* of electronic documents from sender to receiver
  - *Direct communication between applications*

☑ A clearinghouse acts as an intermediary between the medical facility and the insurance carrier. A clearinghouse receives claims from several medical facilities, checks the claims for errors or omissions, consolidates the claims, and transmits them (usually in batches) to individual insurance carriers. With DDE, the medical facility typically installs software from each insurance carrier to whom it will be submitting claims and transmits the claim directly to the carrier without going through an intermediary. DDE often is accomplished by creating a "print image" file of the claim and using the direct claims software to send the claims to the insurance carrier; however, the method used in DDE claims varies from carrier to carrier.

☑ Some advantages of submitting claims electronically include, but are not limited to, the following:
- Faster, more efficient claim submissions, with fewer errors
- Immediate claim status notification
- Quicker processing (and ultimately faster payment) of claims
- Fast and accurate posting of ERAs automatically to the practice's accounting system
- Use of universal code sets with all health plans
- Reduction of claim denials because of eligibility, authorization, or referral issues

☑ The HHS published the final "rule" for electronic submission of Medicare claims mandated under ASCA. With certain exceptions, ASCA requires that all claims sent to the Medicare Program on or after October 16, 2003, be submitted electronically. This "rule" is applicable only to providers, practitioners, and suppliers who submit claims under Part A or Part B of Medicare. It does not apply to claims submitted by providers to Medicare+Choice organizations.

☑ Other electronic services available to the health insurance professional include the following:
- *EFT* allows data representing money to be moved electronically from one bank account to another. In the case of insurance, reimbursements to providers in the form of EFTs is instantaneous, allowing funds to be immediately available to the medical practice.
- *ERA* allows Medicare and other carriers to transmit the explanation of benefits or remittance advice to the provider electronically, and payments can be posted directly into patient accounts automatically.
- *EMR* is an electronic file stored in a computer or other electronic medium containing a patient's health information.

CLOSING SCENARIO

Now that they are finished with the chapter, Ellie and Benji realize that as health insurance professionals, they will no doubt receive and transmit protected health information on a daily basis. With the advent of HIPAA, patients will depend on people like them more than ever to ensure that their health information remains confidential and secure. By understanding and implementing the HIPAA administrative and technical requirements, health insurance professionals can assure patients that their electronic claims will be processed in a timely manner, and that their private health information will be safeguarded. Ellie and Benji realize that one of the important reasons HIPAA was created was to protect the privacy and security of healthcare information that is electronically transmitted; they also realize the importance of HIPAA to healthcare in general.

WEBSITES TO EXPLORE

For live links to the following websites, please visit the Evolve® site at http://evolve.elsevier.com/Beik/today/

- Guides providing formats for data exchanged by healthcare entities (HCFA-1500, UB92, ADA-94, and proprietary forms) may be obtained at http://www.wpc-edi.com/hipaa/

- For more information on individual code sets, browse the following websites:
http://cms.hhs.gov
http://www.cms.hhs.gov/providers/edi/

- Official versions of National Data Communications files are available on the Internet at http://www.fda.gov/cder/ndc/index.htm

REFERENCES AND RESOURCES

AHIMA e-HIM Work Group on Health Information in a Hybrid Environment: The complete medical record in a hybrid electronic health record environment. http://www.ahima.org, 2003.

Amatayakul M: Make your telecommuting program HIPAA compliant. J AHIMA 73:16A-C, 2002.

Bonewit-West K: Computer Concepts and Applications for the Medical Office. Philadelphia, 1993, Saunders.

Davis N. LaCour M: Introduction to Health Information Technology. Philadelphia, 2002, Saunders.

Fordney MT: Insurance Handbook for the Medical Office. Philadelphia, 2002, Saunders.

Gylya BA: Computer Applications for the Medical Office. Philadelphia, 1997, FA Davis.

Hagland M: Electronic record, electronic security. J AHIMA 75:18-22, 2004.

Keller C, Valerius J: Medical Insurance. 2002, Glencoe/McGraw-Hill, Columbus, OH.

Moisio M: Guide to Health Insurance Billing. 2001, Delmar.

Quinsey CA, Brandt MD: AHIMA practice brief: information security—an overview. 2003.

Rowell J, Green M: Understanding Health Insurance. 2004, Delmar.

Sanderson SM: Computers in the Medical Office. 1998, Glencoe/McGraw-Hill.

Sanderson SM: Patient Billing, Using MediSoft Advanced. 2002, Glencoe/McGraw-Hill.

Chapter 17

Reimbursement Procedures: Getting Paid

CHAPTER OBJECTIVES

After completion of this chapter, the student should be able to

- List and explain the various types of reimbursement.
- Discuss the prospective payment system.
- Explain the federal government's role in the prospective payment system.
- Describe diagnosis-related groups (DRGs), ambulatory payment classifications (APCs), and resource utilization groups (RUGs).
- Discuss peer review organizations' responsibilities as they relate to the prospective payment system.
- Identify the various functions most patient accounting software is capable of performing.
- Explain a "contractual write-off."
- List the advantages of HIPAA-compliant practice management software.

CHAPTER TERMS

accounts receivable aging report
activities of daily living
ambulatory payment classifications (APCs)
average length of stay (ALOS)
balance billing
business associate
capitation
comorbidity
contract write-off
cost outliers
covered entity
diagnosis-related groups (DRGs)
discounted fee-for-service
disproportionate share
DRG grouper
fee-for-service
geographic practice cost index (GPCI)
home health prospective payment system (HH PPS)

inpatient rehabilitation facility prospective payment system (IRF PPS)
labor component
long-term care hospital prospective payment system (LTCH PPS)
nonlabor component
peer review organization (PRO)
principal diagnosis
prospective payment system (PPS)
reimbursement
relative value scale (RVS)
residential healthcare facility
resource-based relative value scale (RBRVS)
resource utilization groups (RUGs)
short-stay outlier
skilled nursing facility
standardized amount
Tax Equity and Fiscal Responsibility Act (TEFRA)

OPENING SCENARIO

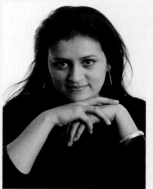

Dave Brown does not understand why it is important for a health insurance professional to learn about reimbursement systems and patient accounting systems. In his opinion, the important content in this course is the information regarding completing and submitting insurance claims forms. When that is mastered, he is prepared to start a successful medical billing career—or is he?

Janetta Karlowski has a different opinion. She had been working as a billing and insurance clerk in a medical office for the past 4 years and enrolled in the course because she did not know enough about these systems, and this lack of information was holding her back. "Reimbursement systems are constantly changing, and new ones are being added," she told Dave. "Granted, they may be complicated and confusing, but you have to stay on top of things to really do the job right, or you'll find yourself being replaced by someone who is better educated."

Dave is still skeptical as he looks over the objectives. PPS, APCs, RUGs, DRGs—it's like alphabet soup. How can anyone make sense of all these acronyms? "We'll work together," Janetta convinces him, "and we'll get through this chapter together. We've come this far; we can't quit now." She realized this information was more advanced than the previous chapters, and perhaps she should not have criticized Dave for being skeptical of its relevance to the average medical billing and insurance clerk. After 4 years of experience, however, Janetta is convinced that knowledge is power, and the more you know about your specialty, the better your chances are for advancement and higher pay.

UNDERSTANDING REIMBURSEMENT SYSTEMS

To understand fully the entire health insurance picture and how fees are established, the health insurance professional should be aware of the various reimbursement systems, their structure, and how they impact health insurance in general. Understanding reimbursement systems is important in making the most of payment opportunities. Every healthcare facility should assign someone the responsibility of being the "reimbursement expert." The health insurance professional might fit this role best, and he or she should be prepared to take on this responsibility. The rules are constantly changing with the frequent introduction of new payment formulas, and it takes diligence and dedication to keep up with these changes. Small adjustments in the payment rates can make a big difference in practice income. The following sections describe the various types of reimbursement and their fee structures.

TYPES OF REIMBURSEMENT

From an insurance standpoint, the term **reimbursement** means payment to the insured for a covered expense or loss experienced by or on behalf of the insured. More specifically in health insurance, reimbursement is a payment made to a provider or to a patient in exchange for the performance of healthcare services. In the healthcare office, there are several different types of reimbursement (Table 17-1).

Fee-for-Service

As we learned in Chapter 4, **fee-for-service** is a system of payment for healthcare services whereby the provider charges a specific fee (typically the usual, customary, and reasonable [UCR] fee) for each service rendered and is paid that fee by the patient or by the patient's insurance carrier.

Discounted Fee-for-Service

When a healthcare provider offers services at rates that are lower than UCR fees, that arrangement is called discounted fee-for-service. A typical example of discounted fee-for-service is when a provider is a participating provider with a preferred provider organization (PPO) and charges patients enrolled in that PPO lower rates in return for certain amenities from the PPO. (See Chapter 7 for details on a PPO.)

Prospective Payment System

A third type of reimbursement is the **prospective payment system (PPS)**. With PPS, reimbursement is made to the healthcare provider based on predetermined factors and not on individual services. PPS is Medicare's system for reimbursing Part A inpatient hospital costs. The amount of payment is determined by the assigned diagnosis-related group (DRG). PPS rates are set at a level intended to cover operating costs for treating a typical inpatient in a given DRG. Payments for each hospital are adjusted for differences in area wages, teaching activity, care to the poor, and other factors. PPS and DRGs are discussed in more detail later.

Capitation

Capitation is a method of payment for healthcare services in which a provider or healthcare facility is paid a fixed, per capita amount for each individual to whom services are provided without regard to the actual number or nature of the services provided to each individual patient. Capitation is a common method of paying physicians in health maintenance organizations.

MEDICARE AND REIMBURSEMENT

The **Tax Equity and Fiscal Responsibility Act (TEFRA)** was enacted by Congress in 1982. This legislation provided for, among other things, limits on Medicare reimbursement that applied to stays in long-term acute care hospitals. After TEFRA was passed, the fee-for-service–based payment system was replaced with a PPS.

Initially, only Medicare patients were included in the PPS system. Later, Medicaid patients were added on a state-to-state basis. In the PPS, a predetermined payment level is established based primarily on the patient's diagnoses

TABLE 17-1	Comparison of Reimbursement Methods
REIMBURSEMENT TYPE	**EXPLANATION**
Fee-for-service	Services/procedures are paid as charged from physician's fee schedule (typically UCR fees)
Discounted fee-for-service	Services/procedures are paid at contracted rates lower than UCR fees
PPS	Flat-rate reimbursement based on predetermined factors, such as diagnoses, procedures, or a combination of both
Capitation	Payment is based on a fixed, per capita amount for each person served without regard to the actual number or nature of services provided

and services performed. The hospital receives a set payment. If dollars spent to care for a patient are less than the PPS payment, the healthcare facility is allowed to keep the extra money and makes a profit on the care provided. If the dollars spent to care for a patient are more than the PPS payment, however, the healthcare organization loses money in caring for the patient.

Medicare presently has three primary reimbursement systems:

- *Prospective payment*—a system of predetermined prices that Medicare uses to reimburse hospitals for inpatient and outpatient services and skilled nursing facilities, rehabilitation hospitals, and home health services.
- *Fee schedules*—consisting of price lists that Medicare uses to reimburse healthcare providers for the services they provide and other healthcare providers for items and services that are not "bundled" into PPS; such as clinical laboratory tests, durable medical equipment, and some prosthetic devices.
- *Medicare+Choice* (now called Medicare Advantage)—Medicare's managed care program in which Medicare pays a set fee to managed care plans to provide care for Medicare beneficiaries.

Medicare's Prospective Payment System

Congress adopted the PPS to regulate the amount of resources the federal government spends on medical care for the elderly and disabled. The Social Security Amendments of 1983 mandated the PPS for acute hospital care for Medicare patients. The system was intended to encourage hospitals to modify the way they deliver services. Congress had four chief objectives in creating the PPS:

1. To ensure fair compensation for services rendered and not compromise access to hospital services, particularly for the seriously ill
2. To ensure that the process for updating payment rates would account for new medical technology, inflation, and other factors that affect the cost of providing care
3. To monitor the quality of hospital services for Medicare beneficiaries
4. To provide a mechanism through which beneficiaries and hospitals could resolve problems with their treatment

Congress gave primary authority for implementing the PPS to the Centers for Medicare and Medicaid Services (CMS). It also assigned responsibilities to outside, independent organizations to ensure that the medical profession, hospital industry, and Medicare beneficiaries had the opportunity to provide input on the creation and implementation of the system.

Prospective payment rates are set at a level intended to cover operating costs for treating a typical inpatient in a given **DRG**. The DRG system is an inpatient classification system based on several factors, including principal diagnosis, secondary diagnosis, surgical factors, age, sex, and discharge status. Under Medicare's PPS, hospitals are paid a set fee for treating patients in a single DRG category, regardless of the actual cost of care for the individual. DRGs are discussed in more detail later.

In addition to payment adjustments for differences in area wages, teaching activity, care to the poor, and other factors, hospitals also may receive additional payments to cover extra costs associated with atypical patients—those whose stays are either considerably shorter or considerably longer than average (referred to as **cost outliers**) in each DRG.

How Medicare's Prospective Payment System Works

Payment levels are set ahead of time, or prospectively, and are intended to pay the healthcare provider for a particular group of services. The established payment rate for all services that a patient in an acute care hospital receives during an entire stay is based on a predetermined payment level that is selected on the basis of averages. This means that some providers' actual costs will be above the average payment, and some will be below. Whatever the case, the provider receives only the preset amount, regardless of whether actual costs are more or less.

Several variations of payment systems have developed from the initial PPS currently being used by Medicare and other third-party payers in the United States. Understanding the differences between the various PPS can be challenging and confusing. These various PPS are known by their acronyms—DRGs, APCs, RUGs, LTC-DRGs, HH-PPS, and IRF-PPS. The following sections focus on these systems, their affected healthcare settings, and the methods employed in determining reimbursement.

 HIPAA Tip

HIPAA regulations *do not* mandate that all healthcare facilities become computerized.

SYSTEMS FOR DETERMINING REIMBURSEMENT

Until the latter part of the 20th century, fee-for-service was the usual method of determining reimbursement in the United States. As the nation faced a growth in the elderly population, and access to healthcare improved, the government stepped in with legislation enacted to control the increasing cost of healthcare associated with these factors. Out of these federal laws, several new systems of reimbursement appeared (Table 17-2).

Relative Value Scale

The **relative value scale (RVS)**, first developed by the California Medical Association in the 1950s, is a method of determining reimbursement for healthcare services based on establishing a standard unit value for medical and surgical procedures. RVS compares and rates each individual service according to the relative value of each unit and converting this unit value to a dollar value. RVS units are based on median (or average) charges for a same or similar procedure of all healthcare providers during the time period in which the RVS was established and published. The total relative value unit (RVU) consists of three components:

1. A relative value for *physician work*
2. A relative value for *practice expense*
3. A relative value for *malpractice risk*

Example: For CPT code 29530 (strapping, knee), the physician work RVU is .57, the practice expense RVU is .41, and malpractice risk .05.

According to the American Medical Association, the biggest challenge in developing an RVS-based payment schedule was overcoming the lack of any available method or data for assigning specific values to physicians' work. The Harvard University School of Public Health, in cooperation with the CMS, conducted a study that led to the initial relative work values. The central part of the study was a nationwide survey of physicians to determine the work involved in each of approximately 800 different medical services. More than half of the relative value estimates of almost 6000 services included in the 1992 Medicare RVS were based directly on findings from the Harvard RBRVS study.

Values for new and revised procedures that appear in the CPT manual are included in the updated RVS each year. The American Medical Association works in conjunction with national medical specialty societies to develop recommendations for CMS regarding values to be assigned to these new and revised codes.

Resource-Based Relative Value Scale

The Omnibus Budget Reconciliation Act of 1989 legislated a system to replace the UCR structure, which at that time was being used for the Medicare fee system. This new system, called the **resource-based relative value scale (RBRVS)**, was designed not only to address the increasing

TABLE 17-2	Prospective Payment Systems Comparison	
TYPE OF SYSTEM	APPLICABLE SETTING	REIMBURSEMENT BASED ON
DRG	Acute care	Diagnosis and procedures
APC	Ambulatory care	Procedures, using diagnoses to verify medical necessity
RUG	Skilled nursing facilities	Minimum data set, including activities of daily living index
HH PPS	Home health care	Outcome and assessment information set
IRF PPS	Inpatient rehabilitation facilities	Length of hospital stay and function-related group classification

cost of healthcare in the United States, but also to try to resolve the inequities between geographic areas, time in practice, and the current payment schedule. Also included in this new reimbursement system was the elimination of **balance billing**—the practice of billing patients for any balance left after deductibles, coinsurance, and insurance payments have been made.

At the base of this new system was the RVS discussed in the previous section. Similar to the RVS, there are three components of the RBRVS:

1. Total work
2. Practice costs
3. Malpractice costs

Total work is defined by six factors:

1. Time
2. Technical skill
3. Mental effort
4. Physical effort
5. Judgment
6. Stress

These six factors are measured before, during, and after the specific service or procedure. Practice costs are defined as overhead costs, including office rent, nonphysician salaries, equipment, and supplies. Malpractice costs are based on the average professional liability premiums healthcare providers have to pay each year.

Diagnosis-Related Groups

The DRG system classifies hospital inpatient cases into categories with similar use of the facility's resources. The DRG system is used as the basis to reimburse hospitals for inpatient services and was established to create an incentive for hospitals to operate more efficiently and more profitably. Under DRGs, a hospital is paid a predetermined, lump sum amount, regardless of the costs involved, for each Medicare patient treated and discharged. DRGs are organized into 25 major diagnostic categories, which are based on a particular organ system of the body (i.e., musculoskeletal system, nervous system). Only one DRG is assigned to a patient for a particular hospital admission. One payment is made per patient, and that payment is based on the DRG assignment.

The DRG grouping is based on diagnoses, procedures performed, age, sex, and status at discharge. DRGs are used for reimbursement in the PPS of the Medicare and Medicaid healthcare insurance systems. DRGs adopted by CMS are defined by diagnosis and procedure codes used in the ICD-9 manual.

The history, design, and classification rules of the DRG system and its application in patient discharge data and updating procedures are published in the *DRG Definitions Manual* (CMS, US Department of Health and Human Services [HHS]). Several refinements of DRGs and different national versions have been published. More detailed information about these different systems is available on the Internet using "HCFA DRG Definitions Manual" as search words.

How Diagnosis-Related Groups Work. A patient's DRG categorization depends on the coding and classification of the patient's healthcare information using the ICD-9-CM coding system. The key piece of information is the patient's **principal diagnosis**—the reason for admission to the acute care facility. The primary procedure to be performed also plays an important part in assigning DRGs. In addition to the coding of the patient's principal diagnosis, the healthcare organization codes and submits information about comorbidities and complications. (A **comorbidity** is the presence of more than one disease or disorder that occurs in an individual at the same time.) Also taken into consideration is the patient's principal procedure and any additional operations or procedures performed during the time spent in the hospital. The **DRG grouper** (a computer software program that takes the coded information and identifies the patient's DRG category) also considers the patient's age, gender, and discharge status. All this information together determines the DRG category, which sets the payment dollar amount for the acute inpatient hospital visit.

Imagine This!

Alvin Rictor, a 66-year-old construction worker, underwent a procedure at Mid-Prairie Acute Care Facility to reattach his severed left leg. The hospital's total incurred expense was $12,000 (e.g., staff time, operating room expenses, supplies, anesthesia); however, DRG 209 (major joint and limb reattachment procedures of lower extremity) was assigned, which reimbursed the hospital $9600. As a result, Mid-Prairie Acute Care Facility suffered a $2400 loss on Alvin Rictor's hospital stay.

Assigning a Diagnosis-Related Group to a Patient. As discussed in the previous section, the principal diagnosis and principal procedure determine the DRG assignment. Other factors that may play a role in DRG assignment are secondary diagnoses, patient age, the presence or absence of complications or comorbidities, patient sex, and discharge status. Each DRG is assigned a relative weight and an **average length of stay (ALOS)**. The relative weights indicate the relative resource consumption for the DRG. ALOS is the predetermined number of days of approved hospital stay assigned to an individual DRG. Referring back to the example in Imagine This!, DRG 209 at Mid-Prairie Acute Care Facility has a relative weight of 2.0782 and an ALOS of 5 days.

Calculating Diagnosis-Related Group Payments.

Calculating DRG payments involves a formula that accounts for the adjustments discussed in the previous section. The DRG weight is multiplied by a **standardized amount**, which is a figure representing the average cost per case for all Medicare cases during the year. The standardized amount is the sum of

- a **labor component**, which represents labor cost variations among different areas of the United States, and
- a **nonlabor component**, which represents a geographic calculation based on whether the hospital is located in a large urban or other area. The labor component is adjusted by a wage index.

If applicable, cost outliers, **disproportionate share** (payment adjustment to compensate hospitals for the higher operating costs they incur in treating a large share of low-income patients), and indirect medical education payments are added to the formula.

Imagine This!

Sara Mason, a 72-year-old widow, fell off her front porch. An ambulance transported her to Bay General Hospital, a Medicare-certified hospital in San Francisco. She was diagnosed with an open fracture of the left femur, requiring surgical intervention. In addition, the attending physician determined from her medical history that Sara has non–insulin-dependent diabetes with associated peripheral vascular disorder.

Step 1: Calculating the Standard Rate
The PPS rate calculation begins with the "standardized amounts." The standardized amounts are composed of a labor and a nonlabor component. The rates for large urban areas are used because San Francisco is in this category. Bay General Hospital's Standard Federal Rate at the time of Sara's hospitalization consists of the two categories of base operating costs, adjusted for large urban areas:
Labor related—$2809.18
Non–labor related—$1141.85

Step 2: Adjusting for the Wage Index Factor
The labor-related portion of the standardized amount is adjusted for area differences in wage levels by using the wage index factor. The wage index is calculated from a cost-of-living adjustment and earnings by occupational category. At the time of Sara's accident, the wage index for San Francisco was 1.4193.

Note: To locate the wage index factor for a particular area in the United States, log onto the CMS website, and key "Table 4a" in the advanced search box. This table provides the wage index for urban areas; Table 4b contains the wage index for rural areas.

The labor portion of the standardized federal rate is multiplied by the wage index factor to adjust Bay General Hospital's DRG base rate.

$$\$2809.18 \times 1.4193 = \$3987.07$$
(adjusted labor rate for San Francisco)
$$\$3987.07 + \$1141.85 = \$5128.92$$
(generic hospital's adjusted base rate)

Step 3: Adjusting for the DRG Weight
The DRG weight reflects the level of treatment expected for an average patient in this DRG. The relative weight for the hip and femur procedure is 1.8128. This weight is multiplied by the labor and nonlabor components calculated in Step 1. Based on the ICD-9 codes, this case was classified as surgical major diagnostic category 8, hip and femur procedure, except that the femur is not a major joint, Sara is older than age 17, and she has comorbidities or complications (diabetes).

$$(\$3987.07 + \$1141.85) \times (1.8128) = \$9297.71$$

Step 4: Disproportionate Share Payment
Medicare-contracted hospitals that provide a disproportionate percentage of care to Medicaid or Medicaid-eligible patients who are not eligible for Medicare Part A may qualify for PPS adjustments. The CMS applies this payment adjustment to the Bay General Hospital's DRG revenue for inpatient operating costs.

Step 5: Indirect Medical Education Payment
Teaching hospitals that have medical residents may receive an added payment. This payment is based on the number of full-time equivalent residents, number of hospital beds, and number of discharges. The base payment rate is multiplied by the adjustment factor for indirect medical education plus the disproportionate share hospital. Bay General qualifies as a disproportionate share hospital and receives additional funds. This rate is 0.1413. Their base payment rate is multiplied by this rate.

$$(\$9297.71) \times (1 + 0.1413) = \$10{,}611.47$$

The adjustment factor for indirect medical education is 0.0744. This rate is added to the disproportionate share hospital factor plus 1 to give the hospital an adjustment rate of

$$1 + 0.1413 + 0.0744 = 1.2157.$$

The payment the hospital can expect to receive for this case is

$$\$9297.71 \times 1.2157 = \$11{,}303.23$$

Step 6: Outlier Payments
The CMS provides an additional payment for beneficiaries whose lengths of stay or costs exceed the threshold rate. The hospital cost for Sara's care was $9983.64. She stayed in the hospital for 5 days. The hospital was paid $11,303.23 by Medicare. If the cost of her care had exceeded the payment rate by $14,050, Bay General could request an outlier payment.

http://oig.hhs.gov/oei/reports/oei-09-00-00200.pdf

Ambulatory Payment Classifications

In 2001, CMS was mandated through the Omnibus Budget Reconciliation Act of 1986 to develop a PPS for outpatient services. All services paid under this new PPS are classified into groups called **ambulatory payment classifications (APCs)**. APCs are a service classification system designed to explain the amount and type of resources used in an outpatient encounter. Under the APC system, Medicare pays hospitals for treating patients in outpatient clinics and pays physicians for treating patients in their offices.

Each procedure or treatment has an APC code. The APC codes 116, 117, and 118 are for chemotherapy, and APC 109 is for bone marrow transplantation. Services in each APC are similar clinically in terms of the resources they require. A fixed payment rate is established for each APC. Depending on the services provided, hospitals may be paid for more than one APC in a single encounter.

There are close to 500 APCs recognizing significant outpatient surgical procedures, radiology and other diagnostic services, medical visits, and partial hospitalizations. The key data in determining this fixed payment rate are the coding and classification of services provided to the patient based on the CPT coding system.

In July 2000, APCs replaced Medicare's cost-based reimbursement with a fixed payment for most hospital outpatient services. This changeover is similar to the one that occurred when the DRG system was implemented on the inpatient side of hospital care.

Resource Utilization Groups

The basic idea of **resource utilization groups (RUGs)** is to calculate payments to a **skilled nursing facility** according to severity and level of care. Under Medicare's PPS, patients are classified into 1 of 44 RUGs determining the per diem payment to a skilled nursing facility. A skilled nursing facility is a nursing home that provides skilled nursing or skilled rehabilitation services or both to patients who need skilled medical care that cannot be provided in a custodial level nursing home or in the patient's home.

When a patient is admitted to a **residential healthcare facility** or nursing home, his or her physician is required to prepare a written plan of care for treatment, including rehabilitative therapy. A physical therapist determines what specific type of rehabilitative therapy needs to be provided. Under the Medicaid reimbursement system, residential healthcare facilities are entitled to different rates of reimbursement depending in part on the type of care their patients require and receive. To determine the appropriate reimbursement rate, each patient is placed into an RUG category.

RUG categories are divided further into hierarchical groups based on the patient's ability to perform **activities of daily living**. Activities of daily living are behaviors related to personal care, including bathing or showering, dressing, getting in or out of bed or a chair, using the toilet, and eating. A qualified registered nurse assessor places each patient into an RUG category by completing a patient review instrument. Each RUG category is assigned a numerical value based on the resources necessary to care for that type of patient, with a greater value assigned to categories that require more resources.

● Stop and Think

Nathan Schnoor, an 84-year-old Medicare patient, was hospitalized at Bestcare Hospital for congestive heart failure. Medicare's ALOS for this DRG category was 21 days; however, at the end of this time, Nathan's condition had deteriorated. Bestcare staff informed Nathan's family that, under Medicare rules, he had to be discharged, and arrangements were made to transfer him to a nursing home. What are the ramifications of Medicare's PPS and the DRG structure in situations such as this?

MEDICARE'S TRANSITION TO RESOURCE-BASED RELATIVE VALUE SCALE

Beginning in January 1999, Medicare began a transition to RBRVS, and in January 2000, CMS implemented the resource-based professional liability insurance (PLI), formerly referred to as malpractice risk, relative value units (RVUs). With Medicare, the physician work component now accounts for an average of 52% of the total relative value for a service, whereas practice expense accounts for 44% and professional liability insurance 4% (as in the earlier example of CPT code 29530).

All three components of the relative value for a service—physician work RVUs, practice expense RVUs, and professional liability insurance RVUs—are factored by a corresponding adjustment for the locality. Geographic adjustments to Medicare payment amounts with the RBRVS were introduced in 1995. Such geographic adjustments were not part of the original RBRVS mandated by the 1985 legislation.

The 2006 Medicare Payment Schedule Conversion Factor was $37.8975. The general formula for calculating Medicare payment amounts with the RBRVS is expressed using the formula shown in Table 17-3.

To calculate payment for a CPT code, the conversion factor is multiplied by the sum of the RVUs for physician work, practice costs, and professional liability (malpractice) insurance (PLI). A **geographic practice cost index (GPCI)** is another factor considered in the formula. A GPCI

TABLE 17-3	Formula for Calculating Medicare Resource-Based Relative Value Scale

Work RVU × work GPCI
+ Practice expense (PE) RVU × PE GPCI
+ Malpractice (PLI) RVU × PLI GPCI

= Total RVU × \$37.8975 = payment

is used by Medicare to adjust for variance in operating costs of healthcare practices located in different parts of the United States. The Medicare RBRVS conversion factor completes the payment calculation. Medicare's payment for the example CPT code 29530 (strapping, knee), using a total RVU of 1.03, is approximately \$40, depending on geographic adjustments. Other insurance carriers may use Medicare's RBRVS with a different conversion factor to create physician fee schedules for their particular use.

Setting Medicare Payment Policy

Medicare payment rules are made by CMS, a federal agency headquartered in Baltimore, Maryland. The Medicare program is administered largely at the local and regional levels, however, by private insurance companies that contract with CMS to handle day-to-day billing and payment matters. CMS also administers and oversees the Medicaid program.

Medicare's Inpatient Hospital Prospective Payment System

The inpatient prospective payment system is the payment system whereby Medicare reimburses hospitals for providing inpatient care to beneficiaries. Under this system, which began in 1983, Medicare sets prices for more than 500 DRGs. The prospective payment price, also referred to as the DRG payment, covers all hospital costs for treating the patient during a specific inpatient stay, including the costs of all devices that are used. (Separate payment is made to physicians for the care they provide to patients during these inpatient admissions.) CMS adjusts DRG payments annually to reflect changes in hospital costs and changes in technology.

Medicare Long-Term Care Hospital Prospective Payment System

Under Medicare's PPS, long-term care hospitals (LTCHs) generally treat patients who require hospital-level care for an average of 25 days. The Balanced Budget Refinement Act of 1999 mandated a new discharge-based PPS for

Imagine This!

A GPCI is used by Medicare to adjust for variance in operating costs of medical practices located in different parts of the United States. Reimbursement to physicians for services performed under Medicare is governed by a formula that considers the product of three factors:
1. A nationally uniform RVU for the service
2. A GPCI value that adjusts each RVU component (work, practice expense, malpractice)
3. A nationally uniform conversion factor for the service

A conversion factor converts the relative values into payment amounts. For each physician fee schedule service, which is represented by an associated Health Care Common Procedure Coding System (HCPCS) code, there are three relative values:
1. An RVU for physician work
2. An RVU for practice expense
3. An RVU for malpractice expense

For each of these components, there is a GPCI that adjusts the RVU based on a practice's geographic location. GPCIs reflect the relative costs of practice expenses, malpractice insurance, and physician work in an area compared with the national average for each component. A computerized "GPCI Finder" software program can be used to help determine the correct GPCI values based on a practice's state, carrier, and locality.

Example: If a practice is located in Los Angeles, California, the GPCI values returned by the GPCI Finder are as follows:
Practice location—Los Angeles, CA
Work GPCI—1.056
Practice GPCI—1.139
Malpractice GPCI—0.955
Carrier/location—31146/18

The general formula for calculating the Medicare fee schedule amount for a given service in a given fee schedule area can be expressed as

$$\text{Payment} = [(\text{RVU work} \times \text{GPCI work}) + (\text{RVU practice expense} \times \text{GPCI practice expense}) + (\text{RVU malpractice} \times \text{GPCI malpractice})] \times \text{conversion factor}$$

So, the amount that Medicare would reimburse a physician (with a practice located in Los Angeles, CA) for a diagnostic colonoscopy (CPT/HCPCS 45378-53) would be calculated as

$$\$93.36 = [(0.96 \times 1.056) + (1.29 \times 1.139) + (0.07 \times 0.955)] \times 36.6137$$

http://www.mgma.com/research/gpci.cfm

LTCHs. This new payment system, referred to as the **LTCH PPS**, replaces the former fee-for-service or cost-based system. Congress provided further requirements for the LTCH PPS in the Medicare, Medicaid, and State Children's Health Insurance Programs Benefits Improvements and Protection Act of 2000. CMS published the Final Rule for the LTCH PPS on August 30, 2002.

The LTCH PPS uses long-term care (LTC)–DRGs as a patient classification system. Each patient stay is grouped into an LTC-DRG based on diagnoses (including secondary diagnoses), procedures performed, age, gender, and discharge status. Each LTC-DRG has a predetermined ALOS, or the typical length of stay for a patient classified to the LTC-DRG. Under the LTCH PPS, an LTCH receives payment for each Medicare patient based on the LTC-DRG to which that patient's stay is grouped. This grouping reflects the typical resources used for treating such a patient. Cases assigned to an LTC-DRG are paid according to the federal payment rate, including adjustments.

One type of case-level adjustment is a **short-stay outlier**. A short-stay outlier is an adjustment to the federal payment rate for LTCH stays that are considerably shorter than the ALOS for an LTC-DRG. Without this short-stay outlier adjustment, Medicare would be paying inappropriately for cases that did not receive a full episode of care at the LTCH. Cases qualify as a short-stay outlier when the length of stay is between 1 day and up to, and including, $\frac{5}{6}$ of the ALOS for the LTC-DRG to which the case is grouped. A length of stay that exceeds $\frac{5}{6}$ of the ALOS for the LTC-DRG is considered to have exceeded the short-stay outlier threshold. When a case exceeds the short-stay outlier threshold, Medicare pays a full LTC-DRG payment for that case.

☑ HIPAA Tip

HIPAA regulations do not apply to the format in which data are *stored*. Computer systems are free to use any data format of their choosing to store data. HIPAA applies only to the format in which data are *transmitted*.

OTHER REIMBURSEMENT SYSTEMS

After the prospective payment reimbursement systems proved successful and showed adequate care for patients, new offshoots appeared as different types of healthcare became prevalent. Two of these are the home health (HH) PPS and the inpatient rehabilitation facility (IRF) PPS.

Home Health Prospective Payment System

In 2000, the government began phasing in fixed payment for home health services, **HH PPS**. Determination of payment category depends on the Outcome and Assessment Information Set. This dataset includes coded information about the patient's diagnoses and functional status and includes information about the patient's outcome from services provided. There are currently 80 home health resource groups, and the home health agency receives a payment for each 60-day block of service.

Inpatient Rehabilitation Facility Prospective Payment System

In the Balanced Budget Act of 1997, Congress mandated that CMS implement a PPS for inpatient rehabilitation. CMS activated the **IRF PPS** in 2001. Reimbursement in the IRF PPS is based on the hospital stay, beginning with an admission to the rehabilitation hospital or unit and ending with discharge from that facility.

Under the IRF PPS methodology, each Medicare patient is assessed using an approved patient assessment instrument, which is used to classify each patient into a function-related group that is designed to reflect the resources required to treat the patient. Currently, there are 97 function-related groups in IRF PPS.

Reimbursement rates in IRF PPS are adjusted by an area wage index and updated for inflation. Payments are reduced for certain transfers and outliers, including cases with short stays, cases interrupted stays, and cases when the patient dies during the stay. Payments are increased for IRFs in rural areas, IRFs with a disproportionate share of low-income patients, and for certain high-cost cases.

SIGNIFICANCE OF REIMBURSEMENT SYSTEMS TO THE HEALTH INSURANCE PROFESSIONAL

A good deal of information has just been presented on various reimbursement systems with a focus mainly on PPS. What does all this information mean to the health insurance professional, and why is it significant? Being a successful health insurance professional does not stop with knowing how to complete and submit insurance claims. To function well on the job, an individual should have a working knowledge of each of the systems discussed in this chapter, what category of patients each applies to, how each is structured, how fees are established within each system, and what these fees are based on. There is a direct correlation between knowledge and capability and job prospects. The more informed a health insurance professional becomes, the better his or her employment prospects and job advancement.

Stop and Think

Megan Trimble and Bob Shackler are seeking employment after completing a medical insurance and billing program at a career school in their vicinity. Megan did her best to learn all she could about the various reimbursement systems, whereas Bob, considering the information insignificant for his career goals, disregarded it. What advantages might Megan have over Bob in their search for successful employment as health insurance professionals?

What Did You Learn?

1. On what principle is the PPS based?
2. What federal government legislation was responsible for the establishment of the PPS?
3. List the factors on which the DRG system is based.
4. What is a "cost outlier"?
5. The total RVU consists of what three components?
6. Name the six factors that define "work" in the RBRVS system.
7. What is the key piece of information that DRGs are based on?
8. Name the federal act that mandated APCs.
9. In what healthcare setting are RUGs?
10. What factors influence LTCH PPS payments?

PEER REVIEW ORGANIZATIONS AND PROSPECTIVE PAYMENT SYSTEM

A **peer review organization (PRO)** is an agency, typically composed of a group of practicing physicians and other healthcare professionals, paid by the federal government to evaluate the services provided by other practitioners and to monitor the quality of care given to patients. PROs were established by TEFRA to review quality of care and appropriateness of admissions, readmissions, and discharges for Medicare and Medicaid patients. These organizations are held responsible for maintaining and lowering admissions rates and reducing lengths of stay, while assuring adequate treatment. Sometimes, these organizations are called professional standards review organizations.

The basic responsibility of PROs is to ensure that Medicare hospital services are appropriate, necessary, and provided in the most cost-effective manner. The PROs have considerable power to force hospitals to comply with

HHS admission and quality standards. They may deny payment to hospitals where abusive practices are found and, in some instances, report such practices to HHS for further enforcement action. Congress required HHS to contract with PROs to monitor

- the validity of diagnostic information supplied by hospitals for payment purposes;
- the completeness, adequacy, and quality of care provided to Medicare beneficiaries;
- the appropriateness of admissions and discharges; and
- the appropriateness of care in outlier cases in which additional Medicare payments were made.

Not all PROs deal with healthcare. One of the largest and most complex PROs is the one used by the Internal Revenue Service to conduct audits through its Coordinated Examination Program. The Internal Revenue Service PRO, comprising teams of senior revenue agents and specialists including computer analysts, engineers, and economists, is the "watch dog" over the Coordinated Examination Program that audits taxpayers. For the purpose of relevancy, however, this section is limited to PROs as they apply primarily to government health programs, such as Medicare and Medicaid.

What Did You Learn?

1. What federal government act is responsible for the creation of PROs?
2. What are the responsibilities of a PRO?
3. Name two things that PROs monitor.

UNDERSTANDING COMPUTERIZED PATIENT ACCOUNTING SYSTEMS

In addition to learning about the various reimbursement systems related to medical billing and insurance, a well-rounded health insurance professional should be knowledgeable about computerized patient accounting systems. Chapter 16 discussed electronic data entry and submitting insurance claims electronically. To accomplish this, the healthcare office typically uses some kind of computerized patient accounting software. Reimbursement systems address the structure of various fee schedules and the structure and setting for each, whereas computerized patient accounting systems address receiving payment for professional services. Many different patient accounting systems are available today, and they all are capable of performing the following seven system functions:

1. Input and storage of patient demographic and insurance information
2. Transaction posting

3. Allocation of system control operations
4. Generating patient statements
5. Processing and submitting insurance claims
6. Managing and collecting delinquent accounts
7. Creating reports

Performing these seven functions in a systematic and timely manner is the key to effective and efficient patient accounting.

Chapter 14 suggested that a healthcare practice establish fair policies, practice sound accounting procedures, and maintain a well-trained staff. It is usually the responsibility of the physicians who run the practice to establish the practice's accounting policies and procedures. When the physicians have reached a consensus on these policies and procedures, they should meet with the staff and discuss how the procedures and policies are to be implemented and how to troubleshoot any potential problems that may arise. When a workable system has been established, the patient accounting policies and procedures should be documented. After this process is completed, it is a good idea for the staff to meet periodically to discuss suggested changes, updates, and revisions as necessary. Finally, patients must be informed, verbally or through practice brochures, about all established practice policies and procedures.

SELECTING THE RIGHT BILLING SYSTEM

To function efficiently and maximize collections, the practice should have a patient accounting system that fits their needs. When setting up a new healthcare practice or revamping an existing practice, when the policies and procedures have been established, the staff has been trained, and a method for informing patients has been established, the next step is selecting a patient accounting system that best fits the type of practice in question. Many factors need to be considered when deciding to purchase a new, or upgrade an old, software package to handle the practice's billing needs. The staff should take the time to do some homework when making this important decision because the billing system's capabilities create the framework for a satisfactory cash flow into the practice. Some important initial questions should be asked of any potential billing software and hardware seller to ensure that the practice is dealing with a reputable firm, including the following:

1. How long has the company been in business, and what is their history?
2. How long has the particular software package in question been on the market?
3. How many and what types of practices use their software?
4. Can client names be furnished for references?
5. Are software demo disks available?

6. What is the availability and accessibility of the software system's setup, training, and support?
7. What would it cost to get the system fully functional?
8. What hardware and networking requirements are recommended for optimal efficiency?

If the practice is upgrading from an older system, it also is important to find out if the new software would have the capability to import data from the previous billing system, and if so, what the cost for this service would be. In addition, it should be determined if such transfers would be successful, or is it likely that data sometimes would be lost or scrambled? In the case of the latter, it also would be necessary to know if the software company would furnish on-site technical support to "debug" the system.

Contrary to popular belief, the cost of a medical billing software system generally has no direct correlation with its capabilities or customer satisfaction ratings. The cost of software packages range from $2000 to $25,000 (and sometimes more), depending on the amenities that some companies offer in addition to their "basic package." Many medical billing software packages on the market today function well if managed by sufficiently trained personnel. It often takes several weeks of "trial and error" to get a new system running smoothly.

Some healthcare offices still depend solely on a manual patient accounting system, such as the still popular "one-write" method. Offices that use a computerized billing system that functions well are convinced, however, that the advantages far outweigh any disadvantages, such as computer "glitches" and occasional "down time." Today's medical billing software systems have built in capabilities that allow

• customized encounter form generation,
• appointment scheduling,
• electronic chart documentation,
• integrated test result reporting,
• creation and storage of multimedia patient documentation,
• electronic claims submission,
• electronic payment reconciliation,
• accounts receivable tracking, and
• internal collection modules.

All of these features provide efficiency, accountability, and oversight control that usually are not possible with a manual process. It is recommended, however, that to achieve optimal results from any computerized patient accounting system, the staff should allow adequate time for training and establish a suitable framework for monitoring the system for Health Insurance Portability and Accountability Act (HIPAA) compliance. Most software companies provide training sessions to assist the staff in learning how to use the system. *Remember:* Any computer system is only as good as the operators who input the data and the knowledge of the system's capabilities. It also is important to learn how to use all of the options that the billing system is capable of performing to use its full potential.

> **HIPAA Tip**
>
> HIPAA does not require patients to sign consent forms before physicians, hospitals, or ambulances can share information for treatment purposes as long as it pertains to the same case.

Managing Transactions

A successful healthcare practice must maintain control over the many transactions required in the process of providing quality services to patients. Whether the healthcare office is computerized or not, there are numerous transactions to handle throughout the day, such as

- posting and tracking patient charges,
- processing payments (cash, checks, or electronic funds transfers), and
- making adjustments to patient accounts.

Posting and Tracking Patient Charges

The typical process for posting and tracking patient charges is as follows. After the patient has completed the encounter, the health insurance professional enters the charge for the procedure or service on the patient's account ledger from the encounter form. This can be done either manually or using the computerized patient accounting software. Fig. 17-1 illustrates a typical software program screen showing a patient's charges and payments.

Code libraries that integrate with CPT and ICD-9-CM codes contained on peripheral electronic media (disk or CD-ROM) or that are integrated into the patient accounting software allow fast and accurate selection of applicable diagnostic and procedural coding. Most systems also allow the practice to set up specialty-specific or multiple "code sets" to streamline insurance submissions, facilitating billing the appropriate insurance carrier with the correct, carrier-specific codes.

Processing Payments

As with posting charges, all payments, whether they are in person, received in the mail, or electronic funds transfers, also must be posted to the patient's account. This task can be accomplished manually or by using the computerized patient accounting software. Fig. 17-2 shows how patient accounting software can track patient charges and remittance history.

Insurance Carrier Adjustments (Contractual Write-offs)

Contractual write-offs are used when some kind of contract or agreement exists between the provider and an insurance carrier whereby the provider agrees to accept the payer's allowed fee as payment in full for a particular service or procedure. If the patient has paid the yearly deductible and coinsurance, the provider cannot ask the patient to

File Edit Lists Activities Reports Graph HIPAA Programs Utilities
Patient Laura Roberts
Bill No. 1020
Date 01/24/2006
Provider JOHN
Bill To
Patient Yes
Federal Health Advocate Yes
Blue Cross No
Diagnosis
Start Date End Date Provider Billing Code M1 M2 M3 M4 POS Diagnosis Amount Units Extended
01/24/2006 JOHN VISA $50.00 1 ($50.00)
01/24/2006 JOHN ICHECK $25.00 1 ($25.00)
01/24/2006 JOHN ICHECK $31.61 1 ($31.61)
01/24/2006 JOHN 99381 $50.00 1 $50.00
01/24/2006 JOHN 46600 $32.86 1 $32.86
01/24/2006 JOHN 73620 $31.61 1 $31.61
01/24/2006 JOHN 99070 $25.00 1 $25.00
01/24/2006 JOHN 99381 $50.00 1 $50.00
Bill Patient
Co-pay/Deductible $0.00
Tax Rate
Primary Insurance
Bill Insurance Last Billed 01/04/2006
Resubmit Claim
Insurance Paid Status Pending
Secondary Insurance
Bill Insurance Last Billed
Resubmit Claim
Insurance Paid Status
Symptom Type
Symptom Date
Date of Last X-Ray
Referring Physician
Facility
Admitted
Discharged
Description Patient Payment - Visa/MasterCard
*Notes Thank you for your visit, and have a nice day!
Show Item Balances Show Bill Detail Tax:
Patient Resp. ($50.00)
Insurance Resp. $132.86
Bill Balance $82.86
Patient Balance $82.86
Family Balance $82.86
New Detail Billing... Line Detail... Print... Delete... Pay Item Visit... Help Close

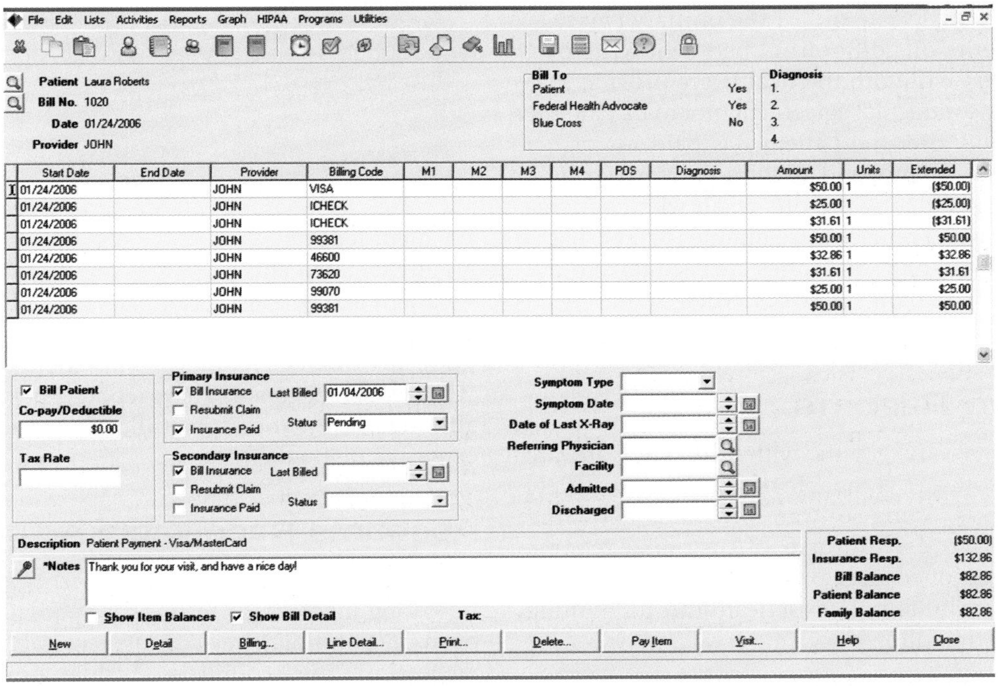

Fig. 17-1 Patient account.

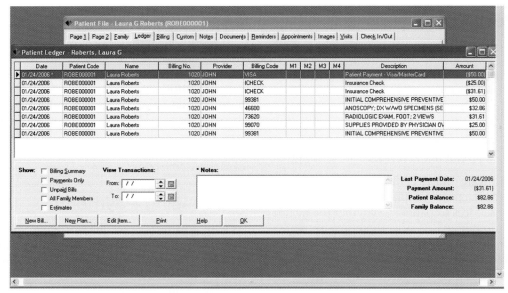

Fig. 17-2 Patient accounting software.

pay any difference between what is charged and what the insurance carrier allows.

The contractual write-off is the portion of the fee that the provider agrees does not have to be paid. This assumes there is no secondary insurance to which the provider can bill the unpaid (contract write-off) amount from the primary insurer. If there is secondary insurance, a claim (along with the explanation of benefits from the primary payer) should be submitted to the secondary carrier, and the remaining amount should be entered as the amount due from the secondary payer rather than recording it on the patient ledger as a contractual write-off for the primary payer.

Contractual write-offs differ from bad debt write-offs. With a contractual write-off, the healthcare provider has agreed, through a contractual agreement, not to be paid the remaining amount after the patient has paid his or her deductible and coinsurance and all third-party payers have paid their share. Bad debt write-offs result when patients (or third-party payers) refuse or are unable to pay what is owed. Bad debt write-offs sometimes are used to zero out the balance for a patient's services when it has been determined that the account is uncollectible.

GENERATING REPORTS

Reporting formats vary greatly with different software systems, but all software is capable of generating a variety of standard reports. Some software programs allow the healthcare practice to "self-format" or customize reports; however, this feature often adds to the cost. Typical reporting capabilities that are built in to most healthcare accounting software include the following:
• Patient day sheets
• Procedure day sheets

● Stop and Think

Grace Plummer, a 72-year-old patient, visited dermatologist Harold Grassley on November 17 for removal of a nonmalignant lesion on her left arm. The total fee for the procedure was $125. Dr. Grassley, a Medicare nonparticipating provider, received $85 from Medicare. Florence Martin, Dr. Grassley's health insurance professional, sent the Medicare remittance advice to Grace's Medicare secondary payer, Flatland Insurance Company, who paid $32. If Grace has met her Medicare deductible for the year, can Florence bill her for the $8 balance? Why or why not?

• Patient ledgers
• Patient statements
• Patient account aging
• Insurance claims submission aging reports
• Practice analysis reports
"One-write" systems also have report-generating capabilities, although the process is different and involves more extensive manual effort.

Accounts Receivable Aging Report

An **accounts receivable aging report** is a report showing how long invoices, or in this case patient accounts, have been outstanding. The accounts receivable aging report is an analysis of accounts receivables broken down into categories by length of time outstanding (Fig. 17-3).

Happy Valley Medical Clinic
Patient Aging by Date of Service
As of March 30, 2004
Show all data where the Date From is on or before 3/30/2004

Chart	Name		Current 0 - 30	Past 31 - 60	Past 61 - 90	Past 91 ---->	Total Balance
AGADW000	Dwight Again		130.00			86.00	216.00
Last Pmt: -200.00	On: 3/26/2004	434-5777					
AUSAN000	Andrew Austin		165.00				165.00
Last Pmt: 0.00	On:	767-2222					
BRIJA000	Jay Brimley					445.00	445.00
Last Pmt: -30.00	On: 10/23/2003	(222)342-3444					
BRISU000	Susan Brimley		8.00			32.00	40.00
Last Pmt: -30.00	On: 9/5/2003	(222)342-3444					
CATSA000	Sammy Catera					71.00	71.00
Last Pmt: 0.00	On:	227-7722					
DOEJA000	Jane S Doe		15.00			79.00	94.00
Last Pmt: 0.00	On: 3/11/2004	(480)999-9999					
JONSU001	Susan Jones					180.00	180.00
Last Pmt: 0.00	On:						
MARRO000	Roberto Marionellio					510.00	510.00
Last Pmt: 0.00	On:						
SIMTA000	Tanus J Simpson					456.00	456.00
Last Pmt: -10.00	On: 12/3/2002	(480)555-5555					
SMIJO000	John Smith					1,095.00	1,095.00
Last Pmt: 0.00	On:						
WAGJE000	Jeremy Wagnew					-1.00	-1.00
Last Pmt: -22.00	On: 8/22/2002	(121)419-7127					
YOUMI000	Michael C Youngblood					85.00	85.00
Last Pmt: 0.00	On:	(602)222-3333					
	Report Aging Totals		$318.00	$0.00	$0.00	$3,038.00	$3,356.00
	Percent of Aging Total		9.5 %	0.0 %	0.0 %	90.2 %	100.0 %

Fig. 17-3 Computer-generated accounts receivable report.

When analyzing a patient accounts receivable aging report, the total money owed that is 120 days old and older should be very small compared with the total accounts receivable. Most experts say that if 20% of the practice's unpaid revenues is 120 days old or older, steps should be taken to improve collections.

Insurance Claims Aging Report

A usable report for the health insurance professional is the insurance claims aging report. Chapter 15 discussed keeping a manual register or log of insurance claims submitted so that the health insurance professional can track claims, and no claim "falls between the cracks." This process can be done automatically with patient accounting software using report-generating features. Fig. 17-4 shows an example of a claims aging report sorted by payer.

Another useful report that can be computer generated is the one shown in Fig. 17-5. This report illustrates a list of patients whose claims have not been submitted yet. Computerized patient accounting software allows claims to be submitted in batches by payer or by date.

Practice Analysis Report

A practice analysis report allows the practice's business manager or accountant to evaluate the income flow for a particular time period, typically a month, a quarter, or a year. This report can be used to generate financial statements necessary for tax purposes, profit analysis, and future planning. A typical practice analysis report furnishes a breakdown of total charges, categorized specialty charges, total patient payments, insurance payments, and contractual adjustments (Fig. 17-6).

1500 A/R Aging All

SOFTAID DEMO DATA

03/19/2004 16:11:34

Status Carrier Code	Claim ID	Last Bill	Current	31 to 60	61 to 90
CLAIM STATUS: PRIMARY					
AETNA OF CALIFORNIA–AETNA5					
CLOONEY, GEORGE 58698775501	135741	03/05/2004	160.00	0.00	0.00
AETNA OF CALIFORNIA			**160.00**	**0.00**	**0.00**
HOME HEALTH AGENCY – AG					
CLOONEY, GEORGE 58698775501	135740	03/05/2004	60.00	0.00	0.00
HOME HEALTH AGENCY			**60.00**	**0.00**	**0.00**
BLUE CROSS BLUE SHIELD OF FLOR–BCBS					
CLOONEY, GEORGE 59709885501	135735	03/01/2004	160.00	0.00	0.00
CLOONEY, GEORGE 59709885501	135736	03/01/2004	240.00	0.00	0.00
CLOONEY, GEORGE 59709885501	135738	03/10/2004	80.00	0.00	0.00
CLOONEY, GEORGE 59709885501	135739	03/04/2004	113.00	0.00	0.00
BLUE CROSS BLUE SHIELD OF FLOR			**593.00**	**0.00**	**0.00**
TOTAL: PRIMARY			**813.00**	**0.00**	**0.00**
CLAIM STATUS: SECONDARY					
MEDICAID–MCD					
CLOONEY, GEORGE 58698775501	135737	03/03/2004	1,580.00	0.00	0.00
MEDICAID			**1,580.00**	**0.00**	**0.00**
TOTAL: SECONDARY			**1,580.00**	**0.00**	**0.00**

Current	31 to 60	61 to 90	91 to 120	> 120
2,393.00	0.00	0.00	0.00	0.00
100.00 %	0.00 %	0.00 %	0.00 %	0.00 %

Fig. 17-4 Claims aging report sorted by payer.

What Did You Learn?

1. List five functions most patient accounting software is capable of performing.
2. Name four important questions to ask a patient accounting software vendor.
3. What are three different ways a healthcare practice receives payment?
4. What is a "contractual write-off"?
5. List six different reports patient accounting software systems can generate.
6. What is the purpose of a practice analysis report?

HIPAA AND PRACTICE MANAGEMENT SOFTWARE

Today, many healthcare practices are computerized to some extent. The level of computerization may range from simple billing functions and patient scheduling to electronic healthcare records and entire practice management activities. HIPAA *does not* require healthcare practices to purchase computer systems. Some experts claim, however, that the installation of a HIPAA-compliant software system may help a practice reduce its administrative costs. Two of the principal areas

Happy Valley Medical Clinic
Primary Insurance Aging

Date of Service	Procedure	Current 0 - 30	Past 31 - 60	Past 61 - 90	Past 91 - 120	Past 121 ---->	Total Balance
Aetna (AET00)						Erik (602)333-3333	
SIMTA000 Tanus J Simpson						SSN:	
Claim: 1 Initial Billing Date: 12/3/2002 Last Billing Date: 10/30/2003 Policy: GG93-GXTA Group: 99999							
12/3/2002	43220	275.00					275.00
12/3/2002	71040	50.00					50.00
12/3/2002	81000	11.00					11.00
12/3/2002	99213	50.00					50.00
	Claim Totals:	386.00	0.00	0.00	0.00	0.00	386.00
Claim: 15 Initial Billing Date: 10/30/2003 Last Billing Date: 10/30/2003 Policy: GG93-GXTA Group: 99999							
10/25/2003	99213	60.00					60.00
10/25/2003	90707	10.00					10.00
	Claim Totals:	70.00	0.00	0.00	0.00	0.00	70.00
	Insurance Totals:	456.00	0.00	0.00	0.00	0.00	456.00
Cigna (CIG00)						Bill S. Preston 234-5678	
BRIJA000 Jay Brimley						SSN:	
Claim: 16 Initial Billing Date: 10/26/2003 Last Billing Date: 10/26/2003 Policy: 98547377 Group: 12d							
3/25/2002	99214	55.00					55.00
3/25/2002	97260	30.00					30.00
	Claim Totals:	85.00	0.00	0.00	0.00	0.00	85.00
	Insurance Totals:	85.00	0.00	0.00	0.00	0.00	85.00
U.S. Tricare (US000)							
YOUMI000 Michael C Youngblood						SSN:	
Claim: 17 Initial Billing Date: 10/26/2003 Last Billing Date: 10/26/2003 Policy: USAA236678 Group: 25BB							
8/22/2002	99213	60.00					60.00
8/22/2002	97128	15.00					15.00
8/22/2002	97010	10.00					10.00
	Claim Totals:	85.00	0.00	0.00	0.00	0.00	85.00
	Insurance Totals:	85.00	0.00	0.00	0.00	0.00	85.00
Report Aging Totals		$626.00	$0.00	$0.00	$0.00	$0.00	$626.00
Percent of Aging Total		100.0 %	0.0 %	0.0 %	0.0 %	0.0 %	100.0 %

Page 1

Fig. 17-5 List of patients whose claims have not been submitted yet.

Practice Analysis

Code	Description	Amount	Quantity	Average	Cost	Net
01	patient payment, cash	−8.00	1	−8.00		−8.00
02	patient payment, check	−15.00	1	−15.00		−15.00
03	insurance carrier payment	−154.00	2	−77.00		−154.00
04	insurance company adjustment	−10.00	1	−10.00		−10.00
06	OhioCare HMO Charge - $10	10.00	1	10.00		10.00
07	OhioCare HMO Charge - $15	15.00	1	15.00		15.00
29425	application of short leg cast, walking	30.00	1	30.00		30.00
50390	aspiration of renal cyst by needle	38.50	1	38.50		38.50
73510	hip x-ray, complete, two views	90.00	1	90.00		90.00
80019	19 clinical chemistry tests	80.00	1	80.00		80.00
84478	triglycerides test	50.00	2	25.00		50.00
90703	tetanus injection	20.00	1	20.00		20.00
92516	facial nerve function studies	125.00	1	125.00		125.00
96900	ultraviolet light treatment	23.50	1	23.50		23.50
99070	supplies and materials provided	20.00	1	20.00		20.00
99201	OF–new patient, problem focused	280.00	2	140.00		280.00
99211	OF–established patient, minimal	100.00	2	50.00		100.00
99212	OF–established patient, problem focused	200.00	5	40.00		200.00
99213	OF–established patient, expanded	300.00	3	100.00		300.00
99394	established patient, adolescent, per…	90.00	1	90.00	0.00	90.99

Total Procedure Charges	$1,472.00
Total Product Charges	$0.00
Total Inside Lab Charges	$0.00
Total Outside Lab Charges	$0.00
Total Insurance Payments	−$154.00
Total Cash Copayments	$0.00
Total Check Copayments	$0.00
Total Credit Card Copayments	$0.00
Total Patient Cash Payments	$0.00
Total Patient Check Payments	−$23.00
Total Credit Card Payments	$0.00
Total Deductibles	$0.00
Total Debit Adjustments	$0.00
Total Credit Adjustments	−$10.00
Total Medicare Debit Adjustments	$0.00
Total Medicare Credit Adjustments	$0.00
Net Effect on Accounts Receivable	$1,285.00

Fig. 17-6 Practice analysis report.

of a physician's practice affected by HIPAA are the practice's billing software and practice management software.

HIPAA includes rules related to the format of electronic transactions; protection of patient's privacy; ensuring the security of patients' health information; and defining universal identifiers for individuals, healthcare providers, and employers. The timeline for compliance for two components of HIPAA, the Transactions and Code Set Standard (Transaction Standards) and the Privacy Standards, took effect in October 2002 and April 2003.

According to the 2000 edition of *Guide to Medical Practice Software* (see References and Resources at the end of the chapter), there are more than 1500 active practice management software vendors. With this in mind, two questions arise:

 HIPAA Tip

Effective July 1, 2004, Medicare rejects electronic claims that have diagnosis codes, zip codes, or telephone numbers that are not HIPAA compliant. Medical facilities should ensure their billing systems are modified to generate electronic claims that pass Medicare's HIPAA compliancy edits for diagnosis codes, zip codes, and telephone numbers.

1. How does a healthcare practice evaluate its current software system for HIPAA compliance?
2. If a practice is in the market for a new software system, how should it evaluate various vendors in terms of HIPAA compliance?

It is important that the software vendor understands the requirements of HIPAA's Transaction Standards. The Transaction Standards has specified American National Standards Institute (ANSI) ASC X12 as the standard for electronic transactions, including billing, payment, eligibility verification, and preauthorization. This means that a physician must ensure the electronic claims sent to payers are in this ANSI ASC X12 format. According to HHS, there are approximately 400 different formats currently in place for electronic health transactions. Whether a practice is evaluating its current computer vendor or shopping for a new one, it should ensure that the vendor is not only aware of the Transaction Standards, but also is able to speak intelligently about or show how their systems are compliant with the Transaction Standards.

Imagine This!

Dr. Agussi uses a computer system that prepares claim information in an electronic file to be submitted to a claims clearinghouse. After the system prepares the electronic file, Dr. Agussi's health insurance professional, Angela Peters, uploads the file to the software provided by the clearinghouse. Later, Angela downloads an electronic remittance file. Dr. Agussi's software reads this file and automatically posts payment information. Dr. Agussi receives maximum value for his computer software if the electronic claim file prepared by the computer system and the electronic remittance file provided by the clearinghouse are in standard ANSI format. This is possible only if Dr. Agussi's system and the clearinghouse accept and submit standard transactions.

Dr. Benton uses a computer system that prepares claim information in an electronic file to be submitted *directly* to the payer. Franklin Zetta, Dr. Benton's health insurance professional, dials into the payer's system and uploads the electronic file. Later, Franklin dials back into the payer's system and downloads an electronic remittance file. Dr. Benton's software reads this file and automatically posts payment information. Dr. Benton's system and the payer must support standard transactions because Dr. Benton and the payer are transacting *directly* with each other.

A healthcare office gets maximum value from patient accounting software or a practice management system if it is able to prepare, send, receive, and process ANSI standard electronic transactions.

It also is important to ensure the vendor is able to assist the practice in complying with the HIPAA Privacy Rule. The Privacy Rule has imposed numerous requirements on healthcare providers and their practices. Before disclosing

a patient's protected health information (PHI) for the purposes of treatment, payment, or healthcare operations (TPO), a practice must obtain the patient's *consent*. In addition, the practice must obtain a patient's written *authorization* to use or disclose PHI for purposes other than TPO. A HIPAA-approved authorization form to release PHI is more detailed and specific than many generic authorizations and has a definite expiration date.

A computerized practice management system can alleviate potential administrative problems a healthcare practice may encounter in complying with the Privacy Rule with relative ease, often with just a few simple keystrokes or mouse clicks. Most practice management systems can provide various functions where PHI is concerned, such as

- tracking the date that the patient's consent to release PHI was obtained;
- maintaining electronic copies of the signed consent and authorization forms;
- tracking patient requests for restrictions on use and disclosure of PHI, whether the physician agreed to the request, and if so, retaining a copy of the modified consent;
- tracking whether and when the consent was revoked by the patient; and
- tracking when patient authorizations were obtained, what they were obtained for, and their expiration dates.

The Privacy Standards provide that a patient may request an accounting of all disclosures made by a **covered entity** (which includes healthcare plans, healthcare providers, and healthcare clearinghouses) within the preceding 6 years. The disclosure must include, among other items, the date, name and address (if available) of the person or entity that received the information, and a description of the PHI disclosed. Practice management software designed in compliance with HIPAA Privacy Standards makes all of this information available to the healthcare office by viewing the main "window" or connected "windows" related to that particular patient, rather than having to undertake a manual review of the hard copy of the file.

A software vendor is not *required* to provide all of these services. It is in the best interest of the healthcare facility to partner with a vendor who is willing to work with the practice in achieving HIPAA compliance, however.

If a practice contracts with an entity considered a **business associate**, as described by the Privacy Standards, the practice should ensure that the agreement between them includes certain protections as defined in the Privacy Standards. HIPAA defines a business associate as an individual or corporate "person" who

- performs on behalf of the covered entity any function or activity involving the use or disclosure of PHI and
- is *not* a member of the covered entity's workforce.

This definition includes a requirement that the business associate use appropriate safeguards to prevent use of disclosure of PHI other than as provided in the agreement.

If a healthcare practice finds that its current vendor is unable or unwilling to meet the HIPAA standards, it may be wise to begin shopping for a new vendor whose products and services can help the practice achieve HIPAA compliance.

What Did You Learn?

1. To what four areas of patient accounting software do HIPAA rules relate?
2. Why is it important that a software vendor understand HIPAA requirements?
3. What requirements has HIPAA imposed on healthcare practices that relate to patient privacy?
4. Name the three categories that constitute "covered entities."
5. List the two factors that define a "business associate."

SUMMARY CHECK POINTS

☑ There are basically four types of reimbursement:
- *Fee-for-service*—The healthcare provider charges a specific fee (typically the UCR fee) for each service rendered and is paid that fee by the patient or by the patient's insurance carrier.
- *Discounted fee-for-service*—The provider offers services at lower rates than UCR fees, such as when a provider is participating provider with a PPO and charges patients enrolled in that PPO lower rates in return for certain amenities from the PPO.
- *PPS*—Medicare's reimbursement system for inpatient hospital costs is based on predetermined factors and not on individual services. Rates are set at a level intended to cover operating costs for treating a typical inpatient in a given DRG. Payments for each hospital are adjusted for varying factors, such as differences in area wages, teaching activity, and care to the poor.
- *Capitation*—A common method of reimbursement used primarily by health maintenance organizations, the provider or healthcare facility is paid a fixed, per capita amount for each person enrolled in the plan without regard to the actual number or nature of services provided.

☑ PPS is a reimbursement system of predetermined prices that Medicare uses to compensate hospitals for inpatient and outpatient services, skilled nursing facilities, rehabilitation hospitals, and home health services. PPS rates are set at a level intended to cover operating costs for treating a typical inpatient in a given DRG.

☑ TEFRA, enacted by Congress in 1982, set limits on Medicare reimbursement that applied to stays in long term acute care hospitals. After TEFRA was passed, the fee-for-service–based payment system was replaced with the PPS. Congress adopted the PPS to regulate the amount of resources the federal government spends on medical care for the elderly and disabled. The Social Security Amendments of 1983 mandated the PPS for acute hospital care for Medicare patients. The system was intended to encourage hospitals to modify the way they deliver services.

☑ DRG is a system of classifying hospital inpatient cases into categories with similar use of the facility's resources. Under this system, a hospital is paid a predetermined, lump sum amount, regardless of the costs involved, for each Medicare patient treated and discharged.

☑ APC is a system designed to explain the amount and type of resources used in an outpatient encounter. Under the APC system, Medicare pays hospitals for treating patients in outpatient clinics and physicians for treating patients in their offices. Each procedure or treatment has an APC code. Services in each APC are similar clinically in terms of the resources they require. A fixed payment rate is established for each APC.

☑ RUGs are used to calculate reimbursement in a skilled nursing facility according to severity and level of care. Under Medicare's PPS, patients are classified into an RUG that determines how much Medicare would pay the skilled nursing facility per day for that patient.

☑ The responsibilities of a PRO as they relate to the PPS include the following:
- Evaluating services provided by practitioners and monitoring the quality of care given to patients
- Ensuring that Medicare hospital services are appropriate, necessary, and provided in the most cost-effective manner
- Monitoring the validity of diagnostic information supplied by hospitals for payment purposes
- Ensuring that the care provided to Medicare beneficiaries is complete, adequate, and of good quality

- Ascertaining the appropriateness of admissions and discharges
- Supervising the care in "outlier" cases in which additional Medicare payments were made

☑ PROs have the ability to force hospitals to comply with HHS admission and quality standards.

☑ Today's patient accounting software systems have the capability of performing many functions, including
- input and storage of patient demographic and insurance information,
- transaction posting,
- allocation of system control operations,
- generating patient statements,
- processing and submitting insurance claims,
- managing and collecting delinquent accounts, and
- creating reports.

☑ A *contractual write-off* is the process of adjusting or canceling the balance owing (often through a provider's contract agreement with the insuring party) on a patient's account after all deductibles, coinsurance amounts, and third-party payments have been made.

☑ Some advantages gained when a healthcare facility uses HIPAA-compliant software include the following:
- Transmits electronic claims in the correct ANSI format
- Protects patient privacy
- Ensures security of patients' health information
- Defines universal identifiers for individuals, healthcare providers, and employers
- Alleviates potential administrative problems using builtin privacy compliance functions
- Tracks and maintains electronic records of patient consents and authorizations.

CLOSING SCENARIO

Dave breathed a sigh of relief as they finished the chapter. "Now that wasn't so bad, was it?" teased Janetta. Grudgingly, Dave admitted that all the acronyms eventually made sense, and he was glad he had stuck with it. Dave believed he had a good grasp on how fees are calculated for the various healthcare settings. Empowered with this information, he believed he would be much more versatile as a health insurance professional. The information on patient accounting systems was "right down his alley," as he viewed himself as somewhat of a "computer guru," anyway. He and Janetta made a good team—she had helped him with the reimbursement issues, and he tutored her through the section on computerized office management. "This was great," exclaimed Janetta. "In a healthcare office, everyone works as a team, and this was good practice." Dave and Janetta feel confident that they are ready for new challenges in the ever-changing world of medical billing and health insurance.

WEBSITES TO EXPLORE

For live links to the following websites, please visit the Evolve® site at http://evolve.elsevier.com/Beik/today/

- To learn more about government acts regulating reimbursement systems, log on to the following website using "reimbursement systems" as your search words:
http://www.gpoaccess.gov/fr/index.html

- For additional information on RVS, explore the following websites:

http://www.cdc.gov/ (Centers for Disease Control and Prevention)
http://www.cms.hhs.gov/ (Centers for Medicare and Medicaid Services)

- For additional information on RBRVS, explore the following website:
http://www.ama-assn.org/ama/pub/category/10559.html

- For additional examples on calculating ALOS, log on to the following website and key "average length of stay in hospitals" in the advanced search box:
http://www.dsf.health.state.pa.us/health/

REFERENCES AND RESOURCES

Center for Health Policy Research, American Medical Association: The Impact of Medicare Payment Schedule Alternatives on Physicians. 1988, AMA.

Belli P: Reimbursement Systems: An Exploration of the Literature on Reimbursement Systems for Health Providers. 2000, World Bank, London.

Böhm-Bawerk E: Value and Price: An Extract, 2nd ed. South Holland, IL, 1973, Libertarian Press.

Hadley J, Berenson RA: Seeking the just price: constructing relative value scales and fee schedules. Ann Intern Med 106:461-466, 1987.

Hsiao WC, Braun P, Goldman P, et al: Resource Based Relative Values of Selected Medical and Surgical Procedures in Massachusetts: Final Report on Research Contract for Rate Setting Commission, Commonwealth of Massachusetts. Boston, 1985, Harvard School of Public Health.

Hsaio WC, Braun P, Becker ER, Thomas SR: The resource-based relative value scale: toward the development of an alternative physician payment system. JAMA 258:799-802, 1987.

Hsiao WC, Stasson W: Toward developing a relative value scale for medical and surgical services. Health Care Finance Rev 1:23-38, 1979.

Kirchner M: Will this formula change the way you get paid? Medical Economics 138-152, 1988.

Moorhead R: Here's what's wrong with the relative value scale. Presented at the 18th Annual Meeting of AAPS, Asheville, NC, October 12-14, 1961.

Orient JM: Physicians' pay targeted for "cost containment." AAPS News 43:1, 1987.

Sterling RB, 2000 Guide to Medical Practice Software, Harcourt, July 1999.

Hospital Billing and the UB-92

Chapter Outline

CHAPTER OBJECTIVES

After completion of this chapter, the student should be able to

- Explain the modern hospital system.
- State a major goal of today's healthcare system.
- Identify the major types of healthcare facilities.
- Discuss the legal and regulatory environment of today's hospitals.
- List the common hospital payers and know how to acquire their specific claims completion guidelines.
- Describe the UB-92 and its relation to the National Uniform Billing Committee.
- Discuss the structure and content of the hospital health record.
- State the initial step of the hospital billing process.
- Compare hospital billing and coding with that of a physician's office.
- Understand the importance of billing compliance.
- List some common hospital billing errors.
- Enumerate the advantages of submitting hospital claims electronically.
- Identify the components that compose a typical medical compliance program.
- Analyze the career opportunities in hospital billing.

CHAPTER TERMS

accreditation
Accreditation Association for Ambulatory Health Care (AAAHC)
activities of daily living
acute care
acute care facility
acute condition
ambulatory payment classifications (APCs)
ambulatory surgery centers
American Osteopathic Association (AOA) Commission on Osteopathic College Accreditation
benefit period
billing compliance
Blue Cross and Blue Shield member hospitals
carriers
case mix
cost sharing
covered entity
crosswalk
Defense Enrollment Eligibility Reporting System
diagnosis-related groups (DRGs)
electronic claims submission (ECS)
electronic medical records (EMRs)

electronic remittance notice (ERN)
Emergency Medical Treatment and Labor Act
emergent medical condition
form locators
for-profit hospitals
general hospital
governance
hospice
hospital outpatient prospective payment system
informed consent
intermediaries
Joint Commission on Accreditation of Healthcare Organizations (JCAHO)
licensed independent practitioners
long-term care facilities
medical ethics
National Committee for Quality Assurance (NCQA)
National Correct Coding Initiative
National Uniform Billing Committee (NUBC)
nonavailability statement (NAS)
outliers

pass-throughs
peer review
   organizations
per diems
principal diagnosis
Prospective Payment
   System (PPS)
registered health
   information
   technicians (RHITs)
respite care
routine charges

rubric
skilled nursing facility
   (SNF)
subacute care unit
surrogate
swing beds
UB-92
Utilization Review
   Accreditation
   Commission (URAC)
vertically integrated
   hospitals

OPENING SCENARIO

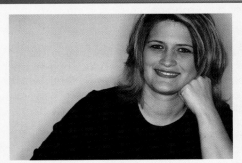

Brittany Weston has been employed as a health insurance professional in a two-physician practice for 5 years. Two years ago, she began taking evening classes at Deerfield Community College to become a health information technician. After graduating from Deerfield's accredited health information technician program, Brittany became eligible to write the registered health information technician (RHIT) examination. By passing this examination, Brittany is allowed to use the credentials RHIT. Brittany is required to obtain 20 continuing education hours every 2 years to maintain her credentials.

Brittany has now found new employment as an RHIT in the Health Information Management Department at Broadmoor Medical Center. One of the first things she learned during orientation at Broadmoor was the mission of the Health Information Management Department: total support of the facility's optimal standards for quality care and services by providing quality information. The functions of Broadmoor's Health Information Management team support administrative processes, billing through classification systems, medical education, research through data gathering and analysis, utilization, risk and quality management programs, legal requirements, data security, and release of information to authorized users.

Brittany realizes that her job duties as an RHIT will be different and perhaps more challenging that those of her former occupation. These duties include the following:

Compiling health information (e.g., reviewing, cataloging, and checking medical reports for completeness; organizing medical reports for placement in files; reviewing charts to ensure all reports and signatures are present)
Completing health information forms (e.g., preparing charts for new admissions, filling out forms, preparing requests for specific reports or certificates)
Compiling and filling out statistical reports, such as daily/monthly census, Medicaid days, admissions, discharges, or length of stay
Filing reports into health records, recording information in logs and files
Retrieving health information records in filing system
Providing information from health records after determining appropriateness of request
Coordinating health information records procedures with other departments

Brittany is looking forward to her new career as an RHIT. She hopes eventually to return to the classroom and acquire the necessary credentials in Health Information Management, which will allow her career aspirations to grow.

HOSPITAL VERSUS PHYSICIAN OFFICE BILLING AND CODING

Everything that we have discussed so far in this textbook has applied to billing, coding, and insurance claims processing for physicians' offices and clinics. This last chapter presents some basic information and guidelines regarding billing, coding, and general information concerning patient services in inpatient hospital facilities and other hospital-based healthcare. This chapter does not present enough detailed information necessary to become a hospital biller and coder. That amount of information would fill an entire textbook. Instead, this chapter provides an overview of the basics. If you find this information interesting, you may want to explore a career in hospital billing or health information management to a further degree.

MODERN HOSPITAL AND HEALTH SYSTEMS

The ideal modern hospital is a place where sick or injured individuals seek and receive care and, in the case of teaching hospitals, where clinical education is provided to the entire spectrum of healthcare professionals. Today's hospital provides continuing education for practicing physicians and increasingly serves the function of an institution of higher learning for entire neighborhoods, communities, and regions. In addition to its educational role, the modern hospital conducts investigational studies and research in medical sciences from clinical records and from its patients and basic research in science, physics, and chemistry.

The construction of today's modern hospital is regulated by federal laws, state health department policies, city ordinances, the standards of a private accrediting organization called the **Joint Commission on Accreditation of Healthcare Organizations (JCAHO)**, and national and local codes (e.g., building, fire protection, sanitation). These requirements safeguard patients' privacy and the safety and well-being of patients and staff. The popular ward concept of the mid 19th and early 20th centuries, where multiple patients were housed in one common area, is no longer permissible. Today, hospitals have mainly semiprivate and private rooms. Although permissible in most states, four-bed rooms are the exception.

The changing emphasis from inpatient to outpatient service and rapid advances in medical technology has caused new facility planning to focus on medical ancillary expansion and freestanding outpatient centers. Developing separate or freestanding buildings has allowed hospitals to minimize the financial impact of restrictive hospital building codes and regulations.

Beginning in the early 1990s, hospitals became part of the evolution toward **vertically integrated hospitals** (hospitals that provide all levels of healthcare) and other provider networks. It is predicted that inpatient care will

Imagine This!

When Brittany was going through her orientation, the presenter, the soon-to-be-retired health information manager, told the new recruits about the "ward system," which existed in the large teaching hospital where she was first employed. There were two large wards on each floor—medical was on the third floor, surgical was on the fourth floor, and so forth. The ward on the west end of the third floor was Ward M3A; the ward on the east end was Ward M3B. Each of these wards was a very large room with sometimes 30 beds. These beds were occupied by indigent or "state" patients, individuals who did not have insurance or the financial ability to pay for their healthcare. These patients wore dingy hospital gowns with their respective ward identification stenciled in large digits on the front so as to identify them if they wandered out of the ward.

Patients who had insurance or could pay for their care were housed on the second floor in private or semiprivate rooms and were attended by "staff" physicians. The patients in the wards were attended by medical students, interns, and residents who were overseen by staff physicians. The wards were not air-conditioned; they were crowded, malodorous, and noisy. Medical students acquired much of their medical education here, and it was common knowledge that patients were often used as "guinea pigs," more often than not to the amusement of the entire medical team.

The health information manager concluded, "Inpatient medical care as we know it today has improved 200-fold."

gradually diminish with continued advances in medicine, and hospitals, as we once knew them, are likely to continue downsizing. Simultaneously, ambulatory care in physicians' offices and clinics will increase. The hospital, particularly compared with its earliest days, will play a different role in the future as part of an integrated collection of providers and sites of care. For more information on the history of hospitals, refer to Websites to Explore at the end of this chapter.

EMERGING ISSUES

A goal of the entire healthcare system is to reduce costs and, at the same time, be more responsive to *customers,* a trendy designation being given to today's healthcare consumers (i.e., patients). The elderly are the heaviest users of healthcare services, and the percentage of elderly in the population is increasing significantly. Also affecting this scenario are the rapid advances in medical technology, often involving sophisticated techniques and equipment, which are making more diagnostic and treatment procedures available. Other emerging healthcare trends are as follows:

- Movement from hospital-based acute care to outpatient care
- Trend toward a more holistic, preventative, and continuous care of health and wellness
- Advent of Health Insurance Portability and Accountability Act (HIPAA) regulations addressing security and privacy of protected health information (PHI)
- Growing emphasis on security, especially in large public facilities, and the need to balance this with the desired openness to patients and visitors

What Did You Learn?

1. Describe a typical general hospital.
2. How are today's modern hospitals regulated?
3. What is meant by a "vertically integrated" hospital?
4. List at least three emerging healthcare trends.

COMMON HEALTHCARE FACILITIES

The best-known type of healthcare facility is the **general hospital**, which is set up to handle care of many kinds of disease and injury. It may be a single building or a campus and typically has an emergency department to deal with immediate threats to health and the capacity to dispatch emergency medical services. A general hospital is usually the major healthcare facility in a region, with large numbers of beds for intensive care and long-term care and specialized facilities for medical care, surgery, childbirth, and laboratories. Big cities may have several different hospitals of varying sizes and facilities. Large hospitals are often called medical centers and usually conduct operations in virtually every field of modern medicine. Types of specialized hospitals include trauma centers; children's hospitals; seniors' hospitals; and hospitals for dealing with specific medical needs, such as psychiatric problems, pulmonary diseases, and other specialized areas of care.

Some hospitals are affiliated with universities for medical research and the training of medical personnel. In the United States, many facilities are **for-profit hospitals**, meaning that monetary income is greater than expenses, whereas elsewhere in the world most hospitals are non-profit. Many hospitals have volunteer programs where individuals (usually students and senior citizens) provide various ancillary services.

A medical facility smaller than a hospital typically is referred to as a clinic and is often run by a government agency or a private partnership of physicians. Clinics generally provide only outpatient services.

ACUTE CARE FACILITIES

An **acute care facility** is what most individuals usually think of as a "hospital," although all services provided may not relate directly to an **acute condition** (where a patient's medical state has become unstable). This facility is equipped and staffed to respond immediately to a critical situation.

The Code of Federal Regulations [Title 29, Volume 2, revised July 1, 2002] defines an acute care hospital as:

Either a short term care hospital in which the average length of patient stay is less than thirty days, or a short term care hospital in which over 50% of all patients are admitted to units where the average length of patient stay is less than thirty days. Average length of stay shall be determined by reference to the most recent twelve month period preceding receipt of a representation petition for which data is readily available. The term "acute care hospital" shall include those hospitals operating as acute care facilities even if those hospitals provide such services as, for example, long term care, outpatient care, psychiatric care, or rehabilitative care, but shall exclude facilities that are primarily nursing homes, primarily psychiatric hospitals, or primarily rehabilitation hospitals.

Acute care facilities must be prepared and equipped to provide for the worst-case scenario. Whether a patient uses these services or not, equipment and staff must be in place and available, just in case. **Acute care** involves assessing and treating sudden or unexpected injuries and illnesses. Acute care facilities in general or specialty hospitals typically provide care for patients who have sustained life-threatening injuries or who have conditions that may lead to deteriorating health status. Increasingly, acute care and related services are provided within the complex environment of health systems. Saving lives and restoring health remain the primary objectives of acute care facilities, but hospitals and health systems also are expected to lead efforts to improve the health and well-being of their communities.

After a patient is discharged from the hospital, two different claims typically are generated—one from the hospital for institutional charges and the other from the physician for his or her professional services. As we learned in earlier chapters, physician services are submitted to the patient's insurance carrier using the CMS-1500 form. Hospital services are submitted using a nationally recognized billing form called the **UB-92** (short for uniform bill 1992), sometimes referred to as the CMS-1450 form. Also included in a later discussion is the UB-04, an updated version of the UB-92, which is tentatively scheduled to replace the UB-92 in 2007.

AMBULATORY SURGERY CENTERS

Ambulatory surgery centers (ASCs) are facilities where surgeries are performed that do not require hospital admission. They provide a cost-effective and convenient environment that may be less stressful than what many hospitals offer. Particular ASCs may perform surgeries in a variety of specialties or dedicate their services to one specialty, such as eye care or orthopedic services.

ASCs treat only patients who already have seen a healthcare provider, and the patient and the provider have selected surgery as an appropriate treatment. All ASCs must have at least one dedicated operating room and the equipment needed to perform surgery safely and ensure quality patient care. Physician offices and clinics that are not so equipped are not considered ASCs. Patients who elect to have surgery in an ASC arrive on the day of the procedure, have the surgery in a specially equipped operating room, and recover under the care of the nursing staff, all without a hospital admission.

ASCs are some of the most highly regulated healthcare facilities in the United States. Medicare has certified greater than 80% of these centers, and 43 states require ASCs to be licensed. These states also specify the criteria that ASCs must meet for licensure. States and Medicare survey ASCs regularly to verify that the established standards are being met. All accredited ASCs must meet specific standards that are evaluated during on-site inspections. In addition to state and federal inspections, many surgery centers choose to go through a voluntary accreditation process conducted by their peers. As a result, patients visiting accredited ASCs can rest assured that the centers provide the highest quality care.

OTHER TYPES OF HEALTHCARE FACILITIES

There are many other types of healthcare facilities besides acute care hospitals and ASCs (Fig. 18-1). Following is a brief discussion of a few of the more familiar types of facilities.

Subacute Care Facilities

The term "subacute" refers to healthcare that is received in a **skilled nursing facility (SNF)**. A **subacute care unit** is a comprehensive, highly specialized inpatient program designed for individuals who have had an acute event as a result of an illness, injury, or worsening (exacerbation) of a disease process. It specifies a level of maintenance care where there is no urgent or life-threatening condition that requires medical treatment. Subacute care may include long-term ventilator care or other procedures provided on a routine basis either at home or by trained staff at a SNF. This type of care often is seen as a bridge between the hospital's acute care units and facilities for patients who require ongoing medical care or who are still dependent on advanced medical technology.

In a subacute care facility, patients have the advantage of constant access to nursing care as they move toward

- Acute Care Facilities
- Ambulatory Surgical Centers
- Assisted Living Residences
- Assisted Living Residences: Residential Care Facilities-Mentally Ill
- Birth Centers
- Community Clinics & Emergency Centers
- Chiropractic Centers
- Community Mental Health Clinics Centers
- Comprehensive Outpatient Rehabilitation
- Designated Trauma Centers
- Free Standing End Stage Renal Disease Service
- Home/Community Based Services: Adult Day Programs
- Home/Community Based Services: Personal Care/Homemaker
- Home Health Agencies
- Hospices
- Hospitals (General, Psychiatric, Rehabilitation, Critical Access)
- Intermediate Care Facilities for Mentally Retarded
- Long-Term Care (Nursing Homes - Nursing Care) Facilities
- Physical Therapy: Outpatient
- Portable X-ray Services
- Residential Care Facilities - Developmentally Disabled
- Rural Health Clinics
- Skilled Nursing Facilities
- Sub-Acute Care Facilities
- Swing Bed Facilities

Fig. 18-1 List of healthcare facilities.

recovery and return to their home. Hospitals typically do not provide this type of care on an ongoing basis. If the physician determines that recuperative care is required after an acute hospitalization, the patient may be transferred to a facility that specializes in subacute services; however, a stay in a subacute care facility is generally short-term.

Skilled Nursing Facilities

A **SNF** is an institution or a distinct part of an institution that is licensed or approved under state or local law and is primarily engaged in providing skilled nursing care and related services as an SNF, extended care facility, or nursing care facility approved by JCAHO or the Bureau of Hospitals of the American Osteopathic Association (AOA), or as otherwise determined by the health plan to meet the reasonable standards applied by any of these authorities.

Previously referred to as nursing homes, SNFs have evolved in the services they provide. SNFs offer 24-hour skilled nursing care; rehabilitation services, such as physical, speech, and occupational therapy; assistance with personal care activities, such as eating, walking, toileting, and bathing; coordinated management of patient care; social services; and activities. Some SNFs offer specialized care programs for patients with Alzheimer's disease or other illnesses or short-term **respite care** for frail or disabled individuals when a family member requires a rest from providing care in the home. Respite care services provide individuals, such as family members, with temporary relief from tasks associated with caregiving. A crucial element of an SNF is periodic reviews by the Department of Social and Health Services.

Imagine This!

Broadmoor Respite Services offers a wide range of services to caregivers who require temporary relief from their responsibilities. These services include companion services, personal care, household assistance, and skilled nursing care to meet specific needs of patients with disabilities, patients with chronic or terminal illnesses, and the elderly. Broadmoor Respite Services provides overnight, weekend, and longer stays for individuals with Alzheimer's disease or a related dementia so that a caregiver can have longer periods of time off. The facility provides meals, helps with activities of daily living, and provides therapeutic activities to fit the needs of residents in a safe, supervised environment.

Long-Term Care Facilities

Long-term care facilities provide care for adults who are chronically ill or disabled and are no longer able to manage in independent living situations. Long-term care is the type of care that individuals may need when they no longer can perform **activities of daily living (ADL)** by themselves, such as bathing, eating, or getting dressed. It also includes the kind of care an individual would need if he or she had a severe cognitive impairment, such as Alzheimer's disease.

When we think of long-term care, we often think of nursing homes. Long-term care can be received in a variety of settings, however, including an individual's own home, assisted living facilities, adult day care centers, or hospice facilities. Long-term care is not the type of care that a patient would receive in the hospital or a physician's office. Long-term care does not refer to the medical care needed to get well from a sickness or an injury or short-term rehabilitation from an accident or recuperation from surgery.

Hospice

Hospice is not a specific place; it is a facility or service that provides care for terminally ill patients and support to their families, either directly or on a consulting basis with the patient's physician. Emphasis is on symptom control

and support before and after death. Hospice strives to meet each patient's unique physical, emotional, social, and spiritual needs and the special needs of the patient's family and close friends. The goals of hospice are to keep the patient as comfortable as possible by relieving pain and other discomforting symptoms, to prepare for a death that follows the wishes and needs of the patient, and to reassure the patient and loved ones by helping them to understand and manage what is happening. This support assists patients and families through the process of facing, understanding, and accepting death.

What Did You Learn?

1. Name three major types of healthcare facilities.
2. In what type of facility might an individual receive long-term care?
3. What is hospice?

LEGAL AND REGULATORY ENVIRONMENT

State and federal government, accrediting organizations, employers, and healthcare plans themselves have developed methods for ensuring quality in managed care plan systems. As physicians and healthcare consumers have become more aware of the need for protection against excessive managed care cost containment, many state governments have enacted laws designed to protect patient rights.

All acute care or general hospitals must be licensed by the particular state in which they are located to provide care within the minimum health and safety standards established by regulation and rule. The Department of Health and Human Services (HHS) enforces the standards by periodically conducting surveys of these facilities. Medicare pays for services provided by hospitals that voluntarily seek and are approved for certification by the Centers for Medicare and Medicaid Services (CMS). CMS contracts with HHS to evaluate compliance with the federal hospital regulations by periodically conducting surveys of these agencies.

A hospital may seek accreditation by nationally recognized accrediting agencies, such as JCAHO or AOA. Surveys conducted by JCAHO and AOA are based on guidelines developed by each of these organizations.

The federal **Emergency Medical Treatment and Labor Act (EMTLA)**, enacted by Congress as part of the Consolidate Omnibus Reconciliation Act of 1985, applies to all hospitals. This act requires that any hospital must respond to an individual's **emergent medical condition** (defined as the onset of a health condition that requires immediate medical attention) by determining the nature of the condition. If an emergent condition exists, it must be treated to the best of the facility's ability regardless of ability to pay. Patients then may be transferred as appropriate after stabilization of the condition.

● Stop and Think

After a fall from his bicycle on his way home from school, Bobby Thaddeus, an 8-year-old white boy, complained of pain in his right arm. His mother, fearing his arm might be fractured, brought Bobby to Meadville Hospital's emergency department. The emergency staff at Meadville refused to treat the child, advising Bobby's mother to take him to their family practitioner for treatment. A spokesman at Meadville defended the hospital's policy stating that it was put in place to curb misuse of emergency department services. Nonemergencies overload staff and facilities with routine medical problems that could be handled as well elsewhere. When routine injuries and illnesses are brought to the emergency department, they cause delayed treatment of true emergencies. Do you agree with the hospital's policy? Why or why not? Is Meadville violating the Emergency Medical Treatment and Active Labor Act in refusing to treat Bobby's injury?

ACCREDITATION

Accreditation is a voluntary process through which an organization is able to measure the quality of its services and performance against nationally recognized standards. It is the process by which a private or public agency evaluates and recognizes (certifies) an institution—in this case, hospitals—as fulfilling applicable standards. JCAHO evaluates whether hospitals, nursing homes, and managed care organizations meet certain specified requirements. The **Accreditation Association for Ambulatory Health Care (AAAHC)** and the National Committee for Quality Assurance (NCQA) assess and award compliance certifications to managed care organizations, including health maintenance organizations. Public agencies sometimes require accreditation by a private body as a condition of licensure or may accept accreditation as a substitute for their own inspection or certification programs. The next section discusses several of the more commonly known accreditation organizations.

Joint Commission on Accreditation of Healthcare Organizations

JCAHO is a private organization created in 1951 to provide voluntary accreditation to hospitals. JCAHO's purpose is to encourage the attainment of uniformly high standards of institutional medical care by establishing guidelines for the operation of hospitals and other health facilities. JCAHO conducts survey and accreditation programs.

In 1965, Congress passed amendments to the Social Security Act stating that hospitals accredited by JCAHO are "deemed" to be in compliance with most of Medicare's "Conditions of Participation for Hospitals" and are able to participate in Medicare and Medicaid. This means that by passing a JCAHO inspection, a hospital is eligible for millions of federal healthcare dollars. Additionally, many states rely on JCAHO accreditation as a substitute for their own inspection programs. Currently, JCAHO accredits more than 80% of U.S. hospitals and home health agencies, clinical laboratories, ambulatory surgical centers, and hospices.

In the past, hospitals had to request JCAHO to evaluate their facility for which they were charged a fee. Because JCAHO does not automatically renew accreditation, a full survey was required at least every 3 years. In 2004, JCAHO began using a new accreditation process called "Shared Visions–New Pathways." Beginning in 2006, all regular accreditation surveys will be conducted on an unannounced basis. The transition to unannounced surveys began with pilot tests conducted in volunteer organizations during 2004 and 2005.

American Osteopathic Association Commission on Osteopathic College Accreditation

The **AOA Commission on Osteopathic College Accreditation** serves the public by establishing, maintaining, and applying accreditation standards and procedures to ensure that academic quality and continuous quality improvement delivered by the College of Osteopathic Medicine (COM) reflect the evolving practice of osteopathic medicine. Accreditation of a COM means that it incorporates the science of medicine, the principles and practices of osteopathic manipulative medicine, the art of caring, and the power of touch within a curriculum that recognizes the interrelationship of structure and function for diagnostic and therapeutic purposes; recognizes the importance of addressing the body as a whole in disease and health; and recognizes the importance of homeostasis and self-regulation in the maintenance of health. Accreditation signifies that a COM has met or exceeded AOA standards for educational quality with respect to mission, goals, and objectives; governance, administration, and finance; facilities, equipment, and resources; faculty; student admissions, performance, and evaluation; preclinical and clinical curriculum; and research and scholarly activity.

National Committee for Quality Assurance

NCQA is an independent, nonprofit organization that performs quality-oriented accreditation reviews on health maintenance organizations and similar types of managed care plans. NCQA is governed by a board of directors that includes employers, consumer and labor representatives, health plans, policymakers, and physicians. The purpose of NCQA is to evaluate plans and to provide information that helps consumers and employers make informed decisions about purchasing health plan services. NCQA performs two distinct functions: One is the evaluation and accreditation of health plans; the other is performance measurement.

The NCQA accreditation process includes a comprehensive review of health plan structure, policies, procedures, systems, and records. The review includes an analysis of plan documents and an on-site inspection visit by a team of expert reviewers. Based on the review, plans are accorded one of several possible accreditation levels: excellent, commendable, accredited, or provisional accreditation. Plans that do not meet standards are denied accreditation status.

● Stop and Think

Elena Sanchez, a 42-year-old woman, lived in a large metropolitan area with several large and small hospitals. After a visit to her physician for complications of diabetes, her physician advised her that she should be admitted to one of the local hospitals for some tests and possible surgery. Elena asked the advice of her friend Teresa, a health information professional, how she should choose which hospital to go to. She preferred the one located in her neighborhood, Seacrest Memorial. Teresa told Elena that Secreast might not be the best choice because although it was handy, it was not accredited. Why might this be a concern for Elena?

Accreditation Association for Ambulatory Health Care

AAAHC was formed in 1979 to assist ambulatory healthcare organizations improve the quality of care provided to patients. The accreditation decision is based on a careful and reasonable assessment of an organization's compliance with applicable standards and adherence to the policies and procedures of AAAHC. AAAHC expects substantial compliance with all applicable standards, which is assessed through at least one of the following means:

- Documented evidence
- Answers to detailed questions concerning implementation
- On-site observations and interviews by surveyors

Utilization Review Accreditation Commission

The **Utilization Review Accreditation Commission (URAC)** is an independent, nonprofit organization. URAC's mission is to promote continuous improvement in the quality and efficiency of healthcare delivery by achieving a common understanding of excellence among purchasers, providers, and patients through the establishment of standards, programs of education and communication, and a process of accreditation. URAC is nationally recognized as a leader in quality improvement, reviewing and auditing a broad array of healthcare service functions and systems. Their accreditation activities cover health plans, preferred provider organizations, medical management systems, health technology services, health call centers, specialty care, workers' compensation, websites, and HIPAA privacy and security compliance.

PROFESSIONAL STANDARDS

Professional standards that govern U.S. hospitals typically are associated with an accrediting body, such as JCAHO, and differ from one organization to the next. JCAHO's Medical Staff Standard MS.6.9 requires "... hospitals to define (e.g., in a policy) the process for supervision of residents by **licensed independent practitioners** with appropriate clinical privileges." A licensed independent practitioner is defined as "any individual permitted by law and by the organization to provide care and services, without direction or supervision, within the scope of the individual's license and consistent with individually granted clinical privileges."

The standard also requires the medical staff to ensure that each resident is supervised in his or her patient care responsibilities by a licensed independent practitioner who has been granted clinical privileges through the medical staff process. Other issues to be addressed include providing medical staff with written descriptions of the role, responsibilities, and patient care activities of residents. In the written descriptions, hospitals must include the mechanisms by which the resident's supervisor and the graduate education program director are to make decisions about the resident's progressive involvement and independence in specific patient care activities. Finally, the rules require hospitals to identify in the medical staff rules, regulations, and policies individuals who may write patient care orders, the circumstances under which they may write such orders, and what entries must be countersigned by a supervising licensed independent practitioner.

GOVERNANCE

Governance, in its widest sense, refers to how any organization is run. With reference to healthcare facilities, it includes all the processes, systems, and controls that are used to safeguard the welfare of patients and the integrity of the institution. JCAHO's Revised Governance Standard GO.2 provides that in addition to providing for the effective functioning of activities related to delivering quality patient care, performance improvement, risk management, medical staff credentialing, and financial management, the governing body must provide for the effective functioning of professional graduate medical education programs (e.g., by adopting policies and bylaw provisions).

CONFIDENTIALITY AND PRIVACY

Most hospital accrediting organizations, specifically JCAHO, include strategies for accrediting a hospital on privacy and confidentiality issues that parallel the demands of HIPAA compliance. It is important for hospital staff to understand and abide by HIPAA's Privacy Standards, including such topics as

- who qualifies as "covered entities" under the Privacy Standards,
- what type of information is protected,
- what HIPAA's restrictions are on the use and disclosure of PHI,
- how the hospital follows the minimum necessary standard,
- how the hospital implements patient rights created by the Privacy Standards,
- what administrative requirements the HIPAA Privacy Standards impose,
- what business associates are and when the hospital needs contracts with them to disclose protected health information,
- what the HIPAA preemption provisions are, and
- what penalties HHS can impose for failing to comply with the HIPAA Privacy Standards.

 HIPAA Tip

HIPAA regulations state that hospitals are required by law to protect the privacy of health information that may reveal a patient's identity (referred to as PHI) and to provide the patient with a copy of a written notice that describes the health information privacy practices of the hospital.

A **covered entity** under HIPAA is a health plan, a healthcare clearinghouse, or a healthcare provider who transmits any health information in electronic form in connection with a transaction. The Privacy Rule requires a covered entity (in this case, the hospital) to make reasonable efforts to limit use, disclosure of, and requests for PHI to the minimum necessary to accomplish the intended purpose. The minimum necessary standard is intended to make

covered entities evaluate and enhance protections as needed to prevent unnecessary or inappropriate access to PHI. It is intended to reflect and be consistent with, not override, professional judgment and standards.

 HIPAA Tip

CMS has instructed its Medicare carriers and intermediaries to make free or low-cost software available to providers that would enable submission of HIPAA-compliant claims electronically.

The Privacy Rule is not intended to prohibit providers from talking to other providers and to their patients. The following practices are considered to be permissible, if reasonable precautions are taken to minimize the chance of inadvertent disclosures to others who may be nearby (e.g., using lowered voices, talking apart):
- Healthcare staff may orally coordinate services at hospital nursing stations.
- Nurses or other healthcare professionals may discuss a patient's condition over the phone with the patient, a provider, or a family member.
- A healthcare professional may discuss laboratory test results with a patient or other provider in a joint treatment area.
- Healthcare professionals may discuss a patient's condition during training rounds in an academic or training institution.

● Stop and Think

Elizabeth Cotter, a 74-year-old white woman, underwent a serious operation after experiencing a cardiac episode. After the surgery was completed, a nurse came to the reception area where Mrs. Cotter's family was waiting and informed them that although the procedure took longer than expected, Mrs. Cotter came through it okay and was in now in the recovery room. "You can see her as soon as she is transferred to her room, in about 30 minutes." Has there been a breach of patient confidentiality here? Why or why not?

After Mrs. Cotter returned to her room, her next-door neighbor telephoned the nurses' station to inquire as to her condition. The nurse informed the caller that although the procedure took longer than expected, and that it was "touch and go for a while," the patient was back in her room now and was expected to make a full recovery. Has there been a breach of confidentiality here? Why or why not?

FAIR TREATMENT OF PATIENTS

In Chapter 3, we learned about **medical ethics,** which are the moral principles that govern the practice of medicine by physicians and other healthcare practitioners. When dealing with patients or healthcare users, healthcare practitioners are governed by these ethical principles and the law. Breaches of ethical rules may result in disciplinary action by employers and professional bodies. Breaches of the law may result in similar disciplinary action and criminal or civil legal action against the healthcare practitioners concerned. Basic principles of medical ethics are usually regarded as

- showing respect for patient autonomy,
- not inflicting harm on patients,
- contributing to the welfare of patients, and
- providing justice and fair treatment of patients.

Ethical principles require healthcare practitioners to become advocates for their patients. The principle of justice or fairness requires medical personnel to ensure that their patients enjoy the constitutional right to equal treatment and freedom from unfair discrimination. The principle of autonomy requires medical personnel to ensure that their patients' constitutional and common law human rights to freedom and security of the individual are respected. This is safeguarded by the ethical and legal requirements of an informed consent. Respect of a patient's right to freedom of religion, beliefs, and opinions is legally required in terms of the U.S. Constitution. A patient's right to privacy is safeguarded by the ethical and legal rules regarding confidentiality. The principle of not inflicting harm requires medical personnel to ensure that their patients' constitutional human rights to dignity, life, emergency treatment, and an environment that is not harmful to health are upheld. The principle of contributing to the welfare of patients requires medical personnel to ensure that the constitutional imperative of medical malpractice and professional negligence are not allowed.

A breach of an ethical principle or of an ethical rule or regulation formally put into effect by a professional council may be used to establish medical malpractice or professional negligence, although the breach itself may not constitute a crime or civil wrong. For a civil wrong to be proved, it would have to be shown that the health professional's conduct was also a breach of a legal obligation.

☑ HIPAA Tip

A hospital billing department is prevented from answering questions from advocates or family members who work on a patient's behalf to help pay medical bills unless the patient has signed a written authorization directing billing department employees to do so.

Imagine This!

If a physician or other healthcare practitioner negligently causes the death of a patient by breaching an ethical rule, he or she may face a criminal charge of culpable homicide or a civil action by the deceased's dependents. Marcus Sherman, a 56-year-old man, saw Dr. Edmund Pithily because of rectal bleeding. Dr Pithily performed a limited sigmoidoscopy, which was negative. The patient continued to have rectal bleeding, but was repeatedly reassured by the physician that he was okay. Eighteen months later, after a 25-lb weight loss, he was admitted to a hospital for evaluation. He was found to have colon cancer with metastases to the liver. Despite all efforts to combat the spread of the disease, Mr. Sherman died. The physicians who reviewed his medical record judged that proper diagnostic management might have discovered the cancer when it was still curable. They attributed the advanced disease to substandard medical care. The event was considered adverse and due to negligence.

What Did You Learn?

1. What governing body licenses acute care and general hospitals?
2. List two nationally recognized organizations that play an important role in hospital accreditation.
3. What function does the Emergency Medical Treatment and Labor Act serve?
4. What is the purpose of accreditation?
5. What two distinct functions does NCQA perform?
6. What is URAC's "mission"?
7. What are the basic principles of medical ethics?

COMMON HOSPITAL PAYERS AND THEIR CLAIMS GUIDELINES

The major payers of hospital costs are much the same of those of physicians' offices and clinics. Government payers (Medicare, Medicaid, and TRICARE/CHAMPVA) typically have the largest share of claims, followed by Blue Cross and Blue Shield and managed care organizations. Other payers include private/commercial insurance companies, no-fault/liability, and workers' compensation. These shares differ, however, from state to state. As stated many times throughout this text, it is paramount for the health insurance professional to learn and follow the specific guidelines of each individual payer. Refer to specific corresponding chapters to learn more about these major payers.

MEDICARE

Medicare hospital claims are processed by nongovernment organizations or agencies that contract to serve as fiscal agents between providers (hospitals, physicians, and other healthcare providers) and the federal government. These claims processors are commonly referred to as **fiscal intermediaries** or **carriers**. They apply Medicare coverage rules to determine the appropriateness and medical necessity of claims.

Medicare fiscal intermediaries process Part A claims (hospital insurance) for institutional services, including inpatient hospital claims, SNF, home healthcare agencies, and hospice services. They also process hospital outpatient claims for Part B. Examples of intermediaries include Blue Cross and Blue Shield and other commercial insurance companies. Fiscal intermediaries are responsible for

- determining costs and reimbursement amounts,
- maintaining records,
- establishing controls,
- safeguarding against fraud and abuse or excess use,
- conducting reviews and audits,
- making the payments to providers for services, and
- assisting providers and beneficiaries as needed.

Medicare carriers handle Part B claims for services by physicians and medical suppliers. Their responsibilities include:

- determining charges allowed by Medicare,
- maintaining quality of performance records,
- assisting in fraud and abuse investigation,
- assisting suppliers and beneficiaries as needed, and
- making payments to physicians and suppliers for services that are covered under Part B.

Peer Review Organizations

Peer review organizations are groups of practicing healthcare professionals who are paid by the federal government to do the general overview of the care provided to Medicare beneficiaries in each state and to improve the quality of services. Peer review organizations act to educate and assist in the promotion of effective, efficient, and economical delivery of healthcare services to the Medicare population they serve. Peer review organizations are discussed in more detail in Chapter 9.

Keeping Current with Medicare

The Medicare Modernization Act of 2003 brought many new changes to the Medicare program. These new changes gave beneficiaries more choices in how they get their healthcare benefits, as follows:

- Medicare prescription drug plan (see Chapter 9), which began January 2006 (enrollment started in November 2005)
- New health plan choices, including Medicare Advantage health plans and regional preferred provider organization plans, which began in 2006
- New preventive benefits, first available January 1, 2005, including
  - cardiovascular screening blood tests,
  - diabetes screening tests, and
  - "welcome to Medicare" physical examination

Medicare Part A: Review

This chapter provides a quick review of the part of Medicare that deals with hospital insurance—Part A. Part A helps provide coverage for inpatient care in hospitals, including critical access hospitals, and SNF, but not care in custodial or long-term care facilities. Part A also helps cover hospice care and some home healthcare. Beneficiaries must meet certain conditions to obtain these benefits. Most individuals eligible for Medicare do not have to pay a monthly payment (premium) for Part A because they or a spouse paid Medicare taxes while employed. If Medicare beneficiaries do not get premium-free Part A, they may be able to buy it if

- they or their spouses are not entitled to Social Security because they did not work or did not pay Medicare taxes while working and are age 65 or older or
- they are disabled but no longer get free Part A because they returned to work.

What Medicare Part A Pays

All rules about how much Medicare Part A pays depend on how many days of inpatient care the beneficiary has during what is called a **benefit period**, or "spell of illness." The benefit period begins the day the individual enters the hospital or SNF as an inpatient and continues until he or she has been out of the hospital for 60 consecutive days. If the patient is in and out of the hospital or SNF several times but has not stayed out completely for 60 consecutive days, all inpatient bills for that time are figured as part of the same benefit period.

Medicare Part A pays only certain amounts of a hospital bill for any one benefit period, and the rules are slightly different depending on whether the care facility is a hospital, psychiatric hospital, or SNF, or whether care is received at home or through a hospice. Table 18-1 shows the 2006 Medicare Part A payment schedule.

How Medicare Part A Payments Are Calculated

Medicare payments are calculated using the **prospective payment system (PPS)**, which is Medicare's acute care

TABLE 18-1	2006 Medicare Payment Schedule		
Inpatient Hospital	**BENEFIT**	**MEDICARE PAYS**	**BENEFICIARY PAYS**
(Semi-private room, general nursing, misc. services)	First 60 days	All but $952	$952
	61st to 90th day	All but $238 per day	$238 per day
	91st to 150th day	All but $476 per day	$476 per day
	Beyond 150 days	Nothing	All charges
Skilled Nursing Facility Care			
(After hospital stay)	First 20 days	100% if approved	Nothing
	21st to 100th day	All but $119 per day	$119 per day
	Beyond 100 days	Nothing	All Charges
Home Health Care			
(Medically necessary skilled care, therapy)	Part-time care	100% is approved	Nothing
Hospice Care			
(for the terminally ill)	As long as doctor certifies need	All but limited costs for drugs & respite care	Limited costs for drugs & respite care
Blood	Blood	All but first 3 pints	First 3 pints
PART A MONTHLY PREMIUM (2006)			
40 quarters of Social Security work credit	Free		
30-39 quarters of Social Security work credits	$216		
< 30 quarters of Social Security work credits	$393		
PART B (2006)			
Deductible:	$124 per calendar year		
Premium:	$88.50 per month (deducted from beneficiaries Social Security check)		

payment method for inpatient care. PPS rates are set at a level intended to cover operating costs for treating a typical inpatient in a given **diagnosis-related group (DRG)**. DRG is a coding system that groups related diagnoses and their associated medical or surgical treatments. Payments for each hospital are adjusted for differences in area wages, teaching activity, care to the poor, and other factors. Hospitals also may receive additional payments to cover extra costs associated with **outliers** (atypical patients) in each DRG. The CMS uses the DRG system to determine the amount that Medicare would reimburse hospitals and other designated providers for the delivery of inpatient services. Each DRG corresponds to a specific patient condition, and each has a pre-established fixed amount that is paid for any patient in the DRG category. A lengthy discussion on the PPS and DRGs is presented in Chapter 17.

MEDICAID

Each state's Medicaid program determines the method it uses to pay for hospital inpatient services. Most states base reimbursement for hospital inpatient services on a PPS that includes DRGs and **per diems** (actual costs per day), and provide a single payment to the hospital with no

separate payment for specific services, such as imaging agents or other dugs and supplies. Some states use other reimbursement methods, including cost-based payments. Many Medicaid programs also adjust payments to reflect a hospital's **case mix** (reported data including patient demographic information, such as age, sex, county of residence, and race/ethnicity; diagnostic information; treatment information; disposition; total charges; and expected source of payment) or the intensity of care required by patients treated at the facility.

Medicaid reimbursement for outpatient services varies from state to state. Medicaid programs typically base hospital payments on state-specific fee schedules, preset per diem/ per-visit rates, or percentage of charges. There is a significant variation in Medicaid payment amounts among states; however, Medicaid programs typically pay less than other insurers.

Federal guidelines exist that affect Medicaid reimbursement. Title XIX of the Social Security Act requires that to receive federal matching funds, states must offer certain basic services to the categorically needy populations, which include
• inpatient hospital services,
• outpatient hospital services,
• prenatal care,

- physician services,
- nursing facility services for individuals age 21 or older,
- family planning services and supplies,
- rural health clinic services,
- home healthcare for individuals eligible for skilled nursing services,
- laboratory and x-ray services,
- pediatric and family nurse practitioner services,
- nurse-midwife services,
- certain federally qualified ambulatory and healthcare center services, and
- early and periodic screening, diagnostic, and treatment services for children younger than age 21.

Chapter 8 provides more detailed information on the Medicaid program.

TRICARE

Typically, patients covered under TRICARE are required to use a military treatment facility, if one is located near them. If a military treatment facility is unavailable or cannot provide the inpatient care needed, the patient must ask for a **nonavailability statement** (NAS). As discussed in Chapter 10, an NAS is certification from a military hospital stating that it cannot provide the necessary care. For all inpatient admissions covered by TRICARE (except bona fide emergencies), an NAS is required. An NAS is valid for a hospital admission that occurs within 30 calendar days after the NAS is issued. It remains valid from the date of admission until 15 days after discharge for any follow-up treatment that is related directly to the admission. It is usually the patient's responsibility to provide a copy of the NAS to the hospital and to each physician providing services to the patient. Each paper claim submitted to TRICARE must be accompanied by a copy of the NAS; hospital personnel should advise patients to keep the original copy of the NAS for their files and provide copies to the hospital and physician offices as necessary.

The NAS system is automated for facilities that use electronic claims submission. This means that, instead of paper copies of the NAS being mailed to the TRICARE carrier, the treating facility can enter the NAS electronically into the **Defense Enrollment Eligibility Reporting System (DEERS)** computer database.

An NAS is no longer required for outpatient procedures; however, to avoid claims rejection or delays, the patient or the treating facility should check with the TRICARE carrier for details on getting advance authorization before having any procedures done. Providers of care—whether or not they participate in TRICARE—are required to obtain these advance authorizations.

Inpatient TRICARE payments are calculated using the same PPS as Medicare, and the DRG-based payment is the TRICARE allowable charge regardless of the billed amount. TRICARE also uses the same conversion factors as Medicare; however, the formulas are not identical to the CMS, so the final calculation result may differ slightly from that calculated by Medicare. Reimbursement rates and methods are subject to change per Department of Defense guidelines.

TRICARE patients usually are required pay a portion of the bill (**cost sharing**) directly to the hospital at the time of discharge. Copies of the TRICARE Handbook should be available from the hospital admitting department or the patient financial services office. For more detailed information on TRICARE, refer to Chapter 10.

CHAMPVA

CHAMPVA uses the same DRG-based PPS as that used by TRICARE. As mentioned in the previous section, this reimbursement system is modeled on Medicare's PPS and applies to hospital inpatient services in all 50 states, the District of Columbia, and Puerto Rico. Current DRG weights and ratios are available in the TRICARE Reimbursement Manual. The manual also offers a DRG calculator.

Hospitals participating in Medicare must accept the CHAMPVA-determined allowable amount for inpatient services as payment in full. Although many of the procedures in the CHAMPVA DRG-based payment system are similar or identical to Medicare, the actual payment amounts, in some cases, are different. This is because the Medicare program is designed for a beneficiary population older than age 65, whereas many CHAMPVA beneficiaries are considerably younger than age 65 and generally healthier. Services such as obstetrics and pediatrics are rare for Medicare beneficiaries, but are common for CHAMPVA beneficiaries.

SNFs also are paid using the Medicare PPS. SNF PPS rates cover all routine, ancillary, and capital costs of covered SNF services. SNF admissions require preauthorization when TRICARE or CHAMPVA is the primary payer. SNF admissions for children younger than age 10 and critical access hospitals **swing beds** are exempt from SNF PPS and are reimbursed based on billed charges or negotiated rates. The swing bed concept allows a hospital to use their beds interchangeably for acute care or postacute care. A swing bed is a change in reimbursement status. The patient "swings" from receiving acute care services and reimbursement to receiving skilled nursing services and reimbursement.

As with most third-party payers, TRICARE and CHAMPVA reimbursement rates are subject to change on an annual basis. Health insurance professionals working in inpatient hospital facilities should keep a current TRICARE and CHAMPVA provider manual and a supply of reimbursement manuals on hand.

BLUE CROSS AND BLUE SHIELD

Inpatient hospitalization reimbursement for patients covered under Blue Cross and Blue Shield policies differ from region to region and depend on the benefit coverage outlined in the individual or group contract. With most Blue Cross and Blue Shield policies, coverage is provided for hospital charges for a semiprivate room and most other customary, or ancillary, inpatient services up to a specific number of days—typically 20. Patients usually must satisfy a deductible amount, which can be $50 to $5000, and pay a specific percentage, or copayment, of the charges—usually 10% to 20%—before reimbursement begins. Many Blue Cross and Blue Shield policies have an out-of-pocket limit that the patient is responsible for. This limit depends on the policy. Some policies also have a payment cap—a per-incident or a lifetime limit on reimbursement.

As with most third-party payers, preauthorization is necessary for inpatient hospitalization and some outpatient procedures and diagnostic testing. Although preauthorization is ultimately the patient's responsibility, most healthcare facilities are willing to make the necessary telephone call to obtain preauthorization for the required services. The telephone number to call for preauthorization is generally listed on the back of the patient's healthcare identification (ID) card. That is the main reason for making a photocopy of both sides of the ID card. As with other third-party payers, the health insurance professional should be aware of the guidelines of the Blue Cross and Blue Shield member organization before submitting claims.

Most hospitals in the United States are in the category of **Blue Cross and Blue Shield member hospitals**—that is, they have contracted as participating providers with the Blue Cross and Blue Shield member organization. Member hospitals must accept the Blue Cross and Blue Shield allowable fee as payment in full and, after the initial deductible and copayment are met, cannot bill the patient for any remaining charges. For nonmember hospitals—those that do not contract with Blue Cross and Blue Shield—reimbursement is affected. As with physician charges, nonparticipating hospitals can balance bill; that is, they can charge the patient for any charges above the allowable fee that Blue Cross and Blue Shield does not pay.

Blue Cross and Blue Shield fees for facility services are established using a variety of methods, as follows:
- Per case allowances (DRG or ambulatory payment classification [APC])
- Per diem allowances
- Percent of charges
- Resource-based relative value scale

See Chapter 17 for more details. The health insurance professional should refer to the provider payment manual or contact the particular carrier for the specific inpatient and outpatient fee calculations used for the facility in question.

PRIVATE INSURERS

Most private insurers negotiate contracts with facilities regarding hospital inpatient payment methods. These contracts typically are negotiated annually. Many private payers use the DRG system to reimburse hospital inpatient services. Other common payment arrangements used by private insurers are per diems, percentage of

allowable charges, and negotiated rates for specific treatments. Table 18-2 summarizes the payment mechanism by type of payer and setting of care.

What Did You Learn?

1. List the major hospital payers.
2. What are the responsibilities of Medicare Part A intermediaries?
3. Explain the functions of a peer review organization.
4. List the three major changes brought about through the Medicare Modernization Act of 2003.
5. How might individuals qualify for premium-free Medicare Part A benefits?
6. What benefits are included in Medicare Part A?
7. Many Medicaid programs adjust payments to reflect a hospital's case mix. What does this mean?
8. List the basic services states must offer Medicaid beneficiaries to receive federal matching funds.
9. What is a "nonavailability statement," and when is it applicable to inpatient care?
10. What reimbursement system does CHAMPVA use for inpatient charges?
11. Explain the "swing bed" concept.
12. List at least three methods by which Blue Cross and Blue Shield establishes reimbursement.

NATIONAL UNIFORM BILLING COMMITTEE AND THE UB-92

The American Hospital Association created the **National Uniform Billing Committee (NUBC)** in 1975. It includes the participation of all the major provider and payer organizations in the United States. The NUBC was formed to develop a single billing form and standard data set that could be used nationwide by institutional providers and payers for handling healthcare claims. The objective of NUBC is to achieve the goals of administrative simplification as outlined in HIPAA.

In 1982, after several years of discussion regarding technical data and policy issues, the NUBC voted to accept the UB-82 and its associated data manual for implementation as a national uniform billing form. Each of the represented organizations (including Medicare) expressed their support of the UB-82 data set.

DATA SPECIFICATIONS

In determining the data to be included in the UB-82, the NUBC attempted to balance the need for the information against the trouble created from providing that informa-

TABLE 18-2   Payment Mechanism by Type of Payer and Setting of Care

TYPE OF PAYER	FREESTANDING IMAGING CENTER/PHYSICIAN SERVICES	HOSPITAL OUTPATIENT DEPARTMENTS	HOSPITAL INPATIENT
Medicare	RBRVS physician fee schedule	APCs	DRGs
Private insurance	RBVS-based fee schedule	Percentage of charges	DRGs
	Other fee schedule	Negotiated rates	Per diems
	Discounted charges	Preset per diem/per visit rates	Percentage of charges
	Capitated rates		Negotiated rates
Medcaid	RBRVS-based fee schedule	State-specific fee schedule	DRGs
	Other fee schedule	Preset per diem/per visit rates	Per diems
		Percentage of charges	Cost based

tion. Basically, it applies HIPAA's administrative simplification principles. Data elements identified as necessary for claims processing in most cases are assigned designated spaces on the form. The designated spaces are referred to as **form locators**, and each one has a unique number. Other elements that occasionally are needed are incorporated into general fields that use assigned codes, codes and dates, and codes and amounts. This built-in flexibility of the data set is intended to promote the greatest use of the data set and to eliminate the need for attachments to the billing form. The data specifications manual seeks to identify the national requirements for preparing Medicare, Medicaid, military, Blue Cross and Blue Shield, and commercial insurance claims.

CREATION OF THE UB-92

When the NUBC established the UB-82 data set design and specifications, it also imposed an 8-year moratorium on changes to the structure of the data set design. In light of the expiration of the moratorium, the NUBC embarked on a process to evaluate how well the UB-82 data set performed. After several state surveys, the NUBC decided to implement improvements to the UB-82 design. Consequently, the UB-92 was created, incorporating the best of the UB-82 along with other changes that improved further on the previous data set design. These improvements reduced further the need for attachments. Today the UB-92 is the standard claim used for inpatient hospitalization (Fig. 18-2). Paper claims are still used in some small facilities; however, approximately 80% of all inpatient hospitalization episodes are submitted electronically.

Since the UB-92 became operational, NUBC's major role is to maintain the integrity of the data set. In addition, the NUBC serves as the forum for discussions that lead to mutually agreed-on data elements for the claim and data elements for other claim-related transactions.

Over the years, the uniform billing data set has become more than a billing instrument. It also is used by many other organizations, including public health and health researchers, as a tool to gauge the delivery of healthcare services to patients. The data set has broad policy implications for shaping the future of the U.S. healthcare delivery system.

THE UB-04

In February 2005, the NUBC approved the UB-04 (Fig. 18-3) as the replacement for the UB-92. Receivers (health plans and clearinghouses) have been notified that they need to be ready to receive the new UB-04 by March 1, 2007. Submitters (healthcare providers such as hospitals, SNFs, hospice, and other institutional claim filers) can use the UB-04 beginning March 1, 2007; however, they will have a transitional period between March 1, 2007, and May 22, 2007, where they can use the UB-04 or the UB-92. Starting May 23, 2007, all institutional paper claims must use the UB-04 because the UB-92 will no longer be acceptable after this date.

What Did You Learn?

1. What is the basic function and role of the NUBC?
2. Name the standard claim form used for inpatient hospitalization.
3. What are the designated spaces called on this universal claim form?
4. What other function does the uniform bill data set perform?

STRUCTURE AND CONTENT OF THE HOSPITAL HEALTH RECORD

Before we look at the UB-92 in depth, let's look at the structure and content of the typical hospital health record. The information included in a hospital health record is similar to that in a physician's office or medical clinic. It begins with demographic information—patient's name, address, age, sex, and occupation—collected on admission.

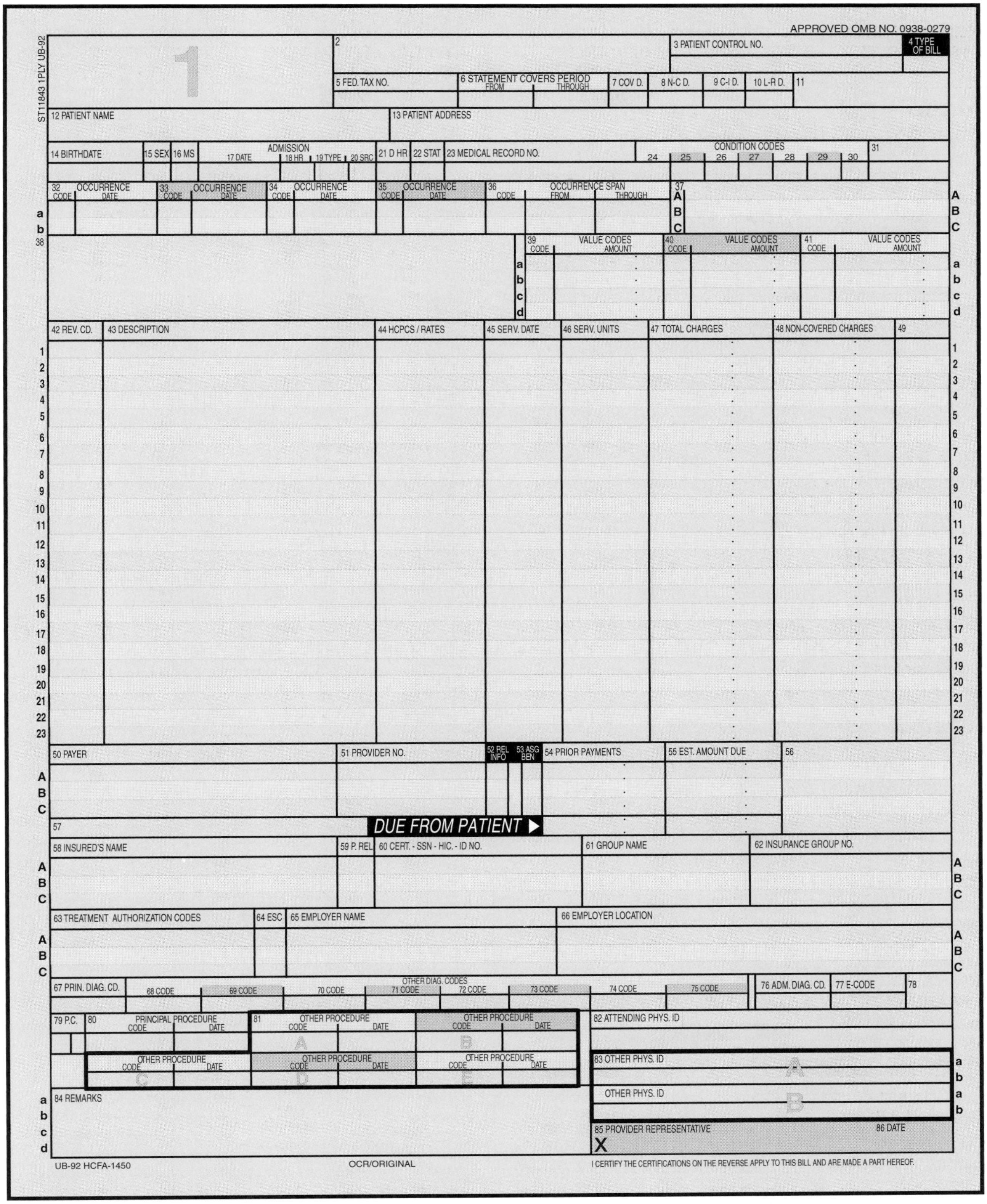
APPROVED OMB NO. 0938-0279

ST11843 1PLY UB-92

1 | 2 | 3 PATIENT CONTROL NO. | 4 TYPE OF BILL

5 FED. TAX NO. | 6 STATEMENT COVERS PERIOD FROM THROUGH | 7 COV D. | 8 N-C D. | 9 C-I D. | 10 L-R D. | 11

12 PATIENT NAME | 13 PATIENT ADDRESS

14 BIRTHDATE | 15 SEX | 16 MS | ADMISSION 17 DATE 18 HR 19 TYPE 20 SRC | 21 D HR | 22 STAT | 23 MEDICAL RECORD NO. | CONDITION CODES 24 25 26 27 28 29 30 | 31

32 OCCURRENCE CODE DATE | 33 OCCURRENCE CODE DATE | 34 OCCURRENCE CODE DATE | 35 OCCURRENCE CODE DATE | 36 OCCURRENCE SPAN CODE FROM THROUGH | 37 A B C

38 | 39 VALUE CODES CODE AMOUNT | 40 VALUE CODES CODE AMOUNT | 41 VALUE CODES CODE AMOUNT (a b c d)

42 REV. CD. | 43 DESCRIPTION | 44 HCPCS / RATES | 45 SERV. DATE | 46 SERV. UNITS | 47 TOTAL CHARGES | 48 NON-COVERED CHARGES | 49 (lines 1–23)

50 PAYER | 51 PROVIDER NO. | 52 REL INFO | 53 ASG BEN | 54 PRIOR PAYMENTS | 55 EST. AMOUNT DUE | 56 (A B C)

57 DUE FROM PATIENT ▶

58 INSURED'S NAME | 59 P. REL | 60 CERT. - SSN - HIC. - ID NO. | 61 GROUP NAME | 62 INSURANCE GROUP NO. (A B C)

63 TREATMENT AUTHORIZATION CODES | 64 ESC | 65 EMPLOYER NAME | 66 EMPLOYER LOCATION (A B C)

67 PRIN. DIAG. CD. | OTHER DIAG. CODES 68 CODE 69 CODE 70 CODE 71 CODE 72 CODE 73 CODE 74 CODE 75 CODE | 76 ADM. DIAG. CD. | 77 E-CODE | 78

79 P.C. | 80 PRINCIPAL PROCEDURE CODE DATE | 81 OTHER PROCEDURE CODE DATE (A) | OTHER PROCEDURE CODE DATE (B) | 82 ATTENDING PHYS. ID

OTHER PROCEDURE CODE DATE (C) | OTHER PROCEDURE CODE DATE (D) | OTHER PROCEDURE CODE DATE (E) | 83 OTHER PHYS. ID (A) | OTHER PHYS. ID (B)

84 REMARKS (a b c d) | 85 PROVIDER REPRESENTATIVE X | 86 DATE

UB-92 HCFA-1450 OCR/ORIGINAL I CERTIFY THE CERTIFICATIONS ON THE REVERSE APPLY TO THIS BILL AND ARE MADE A PART HEREOF.

Fig. 18-2 Blank UB-92 claim form.

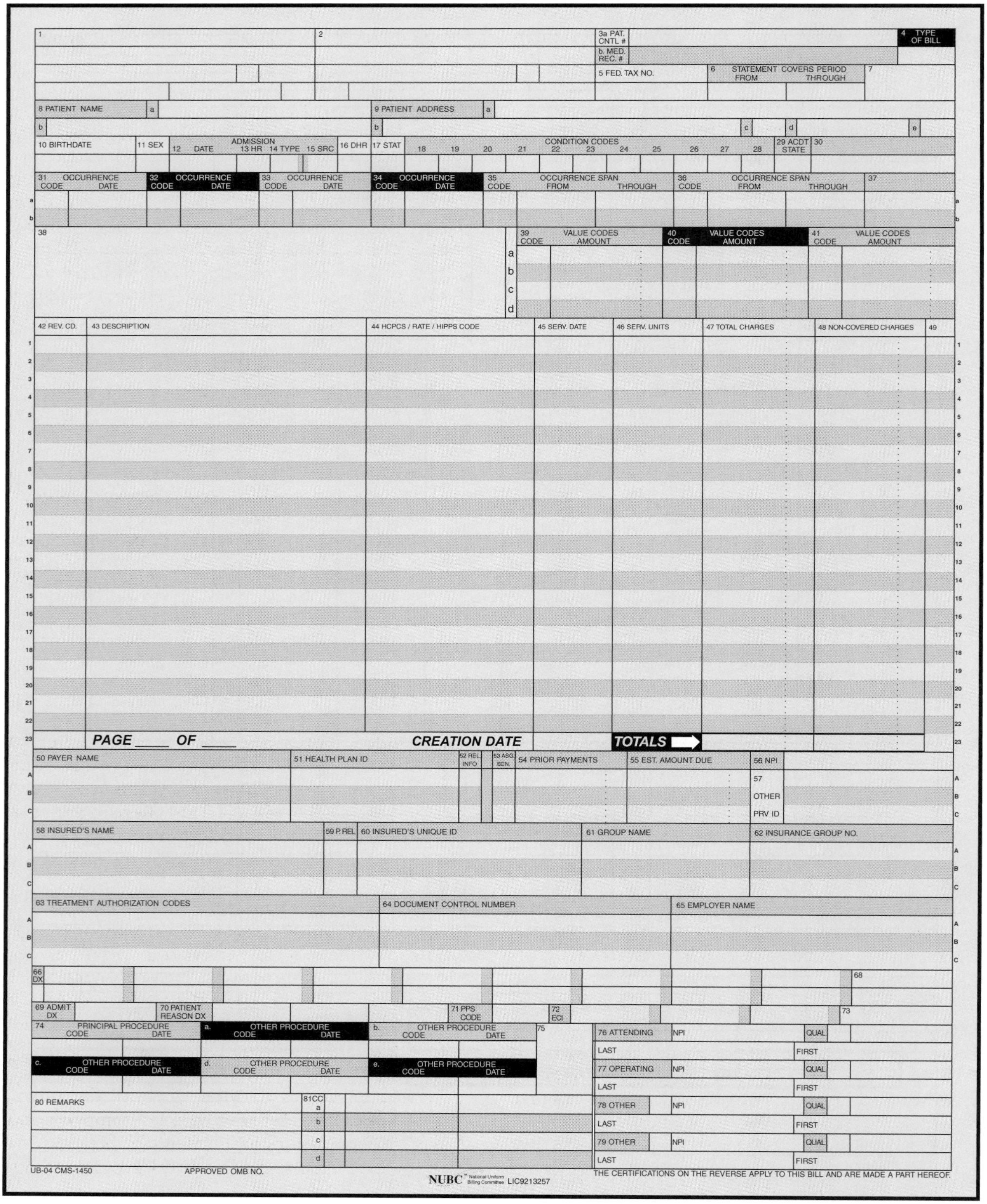
1
2
3a PAT. CNTL #
b. MED. REC. #
4 TYPE OF BILL
5 FED. TAX NO.
6 STATEMENT COVERS PERIOD FROM THROUGH
7
8 PATIENT NAME a b
9 PATIENT ADDRESS a b c d e
10 BIRTHDATE
11 SEX
ADMISSION 12 DATE 13 HR 14 TYPE 15 SRC
16 DHR
17 STAT
CONDITION CODES 18 19 20 21 22 23 24 25 26 27 28
29 ACDT STATE
30
31 OCCURRENCE CODE DATE
32 OCCURRENCE CODE DATE
33 OCCURRENCE CODE DATE
34 OCCURRENCE CODE DATE
35 CODE OCCURRENCE SPAN FROM THROUGH
36 CODE OCCURRENCE SPAN FROM THROUGH
37
38
39 VALUE CODES CODE AMOUNT
40 VALUE CODES CODE AMOUNT
41 VALUE CODES CODE AMOUNT
42 REV. CD.
43 DESCRIPTION
44 HCPCS / RATE / HIPPS CODE
45 SERV. DATE
46 SERV. UNITS
47 TOTAL CHARGES
48 NON-COVERED CHARGES
49
PAGE ____ OF ____
CREATION DATE
TOTALS
50 PAYER NAME
51 HEALTH PLAN ID
52 REL. INFO
53 ASG. BEN.
54 PRIOR PAYMENTS
55 EST. AMOUNT DUE
56 NPI
57 OTHER PRV ID
58 INSURED'S NAME
59 P. REL
60 INSURED'S UNIQUE ID
61 GROUP NAME
62 INSURANCE GROUP NO.
63 TREATMENT AUTHORIZATION CODES
64 DOCUMENT CONTROL NUMBER
65 EMPLOYER NAME
66 DX
67
68
69 ADMIT DX
70 PATIENT REASON DX
71 PPS CODE
72 ECI
73
74 PRINCIPAL PROCEDURE CODE DATE
a. OTHER PROCEDURE CODE DATE
b. OTHER PROCEDURE CODE DATE
75
76 ATTENDING NPI QUAL LAST FIRST
c. OTHER PROCEDURE CODE DATE
d. OTHER PROCEDURE CODE DATE
e. OTHER PROCEDURE CODE DATE
77 OPERATING NPI QUAL LAST FIRST
80 REMARKS
81CC a b c d
78 OTHER NPI QUAL LAST FIRST
79 OTHER NPI QUAL LAST FIRST
UB-04 CMS-1450
APPROVED OMB NO.
NUBC National Uniform Billing Committee LIC9213257
THE CERTIFICATIONS ON THE REVERSE APPLY TO THIS BILL AND ARE MADE A PART HEREOF.

Fig. 18-3 Example of the UB-04.

Every time a patient receives healthcare, a record is maintained of the observations, medical or surgical interventions, and treatment outcomes. This record includes information that the patient provides concerning his or her symptoms and medical history, the results of examinations, reports of x-rays and laboratory tests, diagnoses, and treatment plans. Medical records and health information technicians organize and evaluate these records for completeness and accuracy.

STANDARDS IN HOSPITAL ELECTRONIC MEDICAL RECORDS

An **electronic medical record (EMR)** is a computerized version of the paper medical record. Because hospitals in the United States increasingly are converting to EMRs, we should learn the background of hospital EMR standards. The American Society for Testing and Materials' (ASTM) Committee on Computerized Systems has been working on standards for the content and structure of hospital medical records for several years, and they have published a consensus standard on some aspects of this subject matter. ASTM represents the only standards-setting group that has focused on this issue. With input from the Computer-based Patient Record Institute, Inc. (CPRI), they have the formal standards responsibility for developing these content and structure standards.

STANDARD CODES AND TERMINOLOGY

Patient information for inpatient health records consists of many different kinds of data, including narrative progress notes, laboratory test results, radiology reports, history and physical examination reports, operative reports, and discharge summaries. Data come from many sites, including physician offices, hospitals, nursing facilities, public health departments, and pharmacies. Because various providers exist for each kind of data and site of care, standards for terminology are an essential requirement for a computer-based patient record that spans more than one provider's domain.

The important goal is to have an acceptable code system for each kind of data. It is unnecessary (and may not be desirable) to have all of the codes come from a single master code system because computers can integrate multiple code systems easily while avoiding collisions among assigned codes by adding a code source designation.

CPRI proposes that a first-stage computer-based patient record code system be created by using existing code systems to cover most of the patient data domains, including

- drugs,
- diagnoses,
- symptoms and findings,
- anatomic sites,
- microbes and etiologic agents,

- clinical observations,
- patient outcome variables and functional status,
- medical devices,
- units of measure,
- diagnostic study results,
- procedures, and
- interventions.

In addition to a universal coding system, there must be a common language of combining data structures and grammar so that meaningful coded messages can be sent between computer-based patient record systems. The federal government is working with CPRI and the ANSI Healthcare Informatics Planning Panel on arrangements that would make development of such a common language possible.

What Did You Learn?

1. What is an EMR?
2. List at least five items of *demographic* information that typically are collected when a patient is hospitalized.
3. What type of information does an inpatient health record consist of?
4. List the patient data domains used by the CPRI code system.

BILLING PROCESS

The hospital billing process begins when the patient registers for inpatient or outpatient admission. Although this procedure may differ from one institution to another, certain processes remain constant. Registration may be accomplished in person, by telephone, or via the Internet. At the time of registration, the patient typically must provide the following information:

- Full name and address
- Social Security number (*note:* some institutions are getting away from using Social Security numbers)
- Name of responsible party or emergency contact or both
- Insurance card information
- Name, address, and birth date of policy holder on insurance card (if different than patient)
- Name of employer (if applicable)
- Name and address of where to send the bill if the procedure is for liability or workers' compensation
- Details of accident or injury, if applicable

Fig. 18-4 is an example of a typical hospital admission form.

As we learned in previous chapters, preauthorization or precertification is necessary for all inpatient hospital admissions. In the case of emergency admission when preauthorization is impossible, most insurers allow 48 hours for notification of hospitalization.

A certain amount of patient education goes hand in hand with hospital admission. Hospital staff should inform patients of their rights and responsibilities. Typical patient responsibilities include an obligation to

- provide a complete medical history and any information pertaining to their health;
- be responsible for their actions if they refuse any treatment or do not follow physician's orders;

PRE-ADMISSION FORM

Please return this completed form in our SAE by post to The Lister Hospital, Chelsea Bridge Road, London SW1W 8RH, by fax to 020 7730 7208, or email from our web site www.thelisterhospital.com.

Ref No _____ Date of admission _____ Time _____

1) YOUR DETAILS

Surname _____ First Names _____

Sex: ☐ Male ☐ Female Date of Birth _____

Status: ☐ Married ☐ Single ☐ Widowed ☐ Other

Permanent Address _____

_____ Postcode _____

Day Telephone _____ Evening Telephone _____

Mobile Telephone _____

Country of residence _____ Nationality _____

Religion _____ Occupation _____

Allergies _____

Dietary needs _____

If you are currently staying in a hotel in the UK, please fill in your overseas address below:

_____

_____

2) NEXT OF KIN

Name _____ Relationship _____

Address _____

_____

_____ Telephone No _____

3) YOUR DOCTORS

Consultant _____

Address _____

_____

General Practitioner _____

Address _____

_____

Fig. 18-4 Typical hospital admission form.

---

4) PAYMENT DETAILS

Payment method: ☐ Health Insurance   ☐ Self Pay   ☐ Other (please specify)

_____

Insurance Company details/Name _____

_____

_____

Membership Number _____

We advise you to confirm cover with your insurance company prior to admission. If you have any doubts, contact the Reservations Department at The Lister Hospital on 020 7824 8679.

Self payment   ☐ Cash   ☐ Credit/Charge Card _____

Amount enclosed _____   Card Type /No _____

Expiry Date _____

Mailing Address (if different) _____

_____

TERMS OF ADMISSION

Patients' Valuables

Patients are advised not to bring valuables to the hospital. Where this is unavoidable, the patients should ensure that they are fully insured. The undersigned being the patient, acknowledges or, being a person other than the patient, acknowledges on the patient's behalf (and warrants that he/she is authorised to do so) that the hospital will have no liability whatsoever for any loss or damage to cash, valuables or personal effects which the patient or any other person brings into the hospital whether as a result of negligence or otherwise.

FINANCIAL AGREEMENT

I/We, the undersigned, undertake to HCA International Limited, that in consideration of its accepting me/the patient for treatment, I/we will pay for all services rendered and items supplied to the patient in accordance with the rates of charges, prices and terms of payment for the time being imposed.

Signature _____   Date _____
PATIENT/REPRESENTATIVE

Fig. 18-4—cont'd

- report perceived risks in their care and unexpected changes in their condition to the physician and other healthcare providers;
- report any perceived or identified safety issues related to their care or the physical environment to the physician or other healthcare providers;
- ask questions when they do not understand what they have been told about their care, or what they are expected to do regarding their care;
- ensure that the financial obligations of their hospital care are fulfilled as promptly as possible;
- follow hospital rules and regulations regarding patient care and conduct; and
- be considerate of the rights of other patients and hospital personnel.

INFORMED CONSENT

Informed consent is the process by which a fully informed patient can participate in choices about his or her healthcare. It originates from the legal and ethical rights patients have to direct what happens to their body and from the ethical duty of the physician to involve the patient in his or her healthcare.

The most important goal of informed consent is that the patient has an opportunity to be a knowledgeable participant in his or her healthcare decisions. Informed consent typically includes a discussion of the following elements:

- Nature of the decision or procedure
- Reasonable alternatives to the proposed intervention
- Relevant risks, benefits, and uncertainties related to each alternative

- Assessment of patient understanding
- Acceptance of the intervention by the patient

For the patient's consent to be valid, he or she must be considered competent to make the decision at hand, and this consent must be voluntary. Ideally, the physician should make it clear to the patient that he or she is participating in a decision, not merely signing a form. With this understanding, the informed consent process should be seen as an *invitation* to participate in healthcare decisions. The patient's understanding of what is about to take place is equally as important as the information provided; the discussion should be carried on in layperson's terms, and the patient's understanding should be assessed along the way.

If a patient is determined to be incapacitated or incompetent to make healthcare decisions in his or her best interest, a **surrogate** (someone with legal authority to take the patient's place) decision maker must speak for that patient. There is a specific hierarchy of appropriate decision makers defined by most state laws. If no appropriate surrogate decision maker is available, physicians are expected to act in the best interest of the patient until a surrogate is found or appointed.

HOSPITAL CHARGES

As with many aspects of healthcare, hospital charges vary from institution to institution and from one area of the United States to another. Hospitals that are part of healthcare systems and large hospitals often tend to have higher charges than independent and small hospitals. **For-profit hospitals** (hospitals that operate on the basis of making money) typically have the highest prices, whereas government hospitals have the lowest average charges.

● Stop and Think

Joseph Mason, a 68-year-old black man, was admitted to Broadmoor Medical Center with complaints of "tightness in his chest" and difficulty breathing. Dr. Ethan VanDerVoort, a cardiologist, visited Joseph in his hospital room and informed him that the results of his heart catheterization and other tests showed 80% blockage in a major artery of his heart. "We'll be putting a stint in the artery to open it up, allowing the blood to resume normal flow," Dr. VanDerVoort informed him. "Afterwards, you'll be as good as new." He patted the patient's arm and left the room.

Did Dr. VanDerVoort follow the rules of "informed consent" in this brief conversation with Mr. Mason? If not, what elements of a full informed consent scenario were ignored? How might Dr. VanDerVoort have approached this patient, as far as his planned remedy for his heart problem?

Every hospital inpatient incurs **routine charges**, such as room and board, medications, laboratory tests, x-rays (if applicable), and miscellaneous service charges. If surgery is involved, there are operating and recovery room charges and charges for supplies and equipment used. The anesthesiologist typically bills separately for anesthesia. Fig. 18-5 is an example of an inpatient encounter form.

Some hospitals, on request, provide an estimate of the charges that the patient is likely to incur for clear-cut procedures, such as uncomplicated hip replacement. It should be made clear to the patient, however, that these charges are merely estimates, and actual charges may be more or less, depending on the many extenuating circumstances. Some states, such as Washington, provide hospital user guides, where patients can search a database on the Internet for "average" charges for items and services provided by hospitals, based on the number of patients and total charges for that illness as reported in that particular region. Figures include charges for the hospital room, services ordered by a physician (e.g., x-rays and laboratory tests), and personal care items (e.g., hospital gowns). Physician fees are not included.

HOSPITAL CODING

Hospitals generate insurance claims for many third-party payers. To perform this task effectively, the health insurance professional or the health information technician must have expert knowledge of the coding and payment systems that these payers use. Hospital coding is similar to that which is done in a physician's office; however, some guidelines differ significantly.

MANUALS USED FOR CODING HOSPITAL CLAIMS

Hospital coders must use ICD-9 Volumes 1 and 2 for inpatient diagnostic coding and ICD-9 Volume 3 for inpatient procedural coding. Because hospital coders use a DRG Manual for assigning DRG codes on many claims (including Medicare), most hospitals use a computerized software program to determine DRG assignment.

ICD-9-CM Manual

We learned in Chapter 12 that the clinical modification of ICD-9 (ICD-9-CM Volumes 1 and 2) was adopted in the United States in 1979 for morbidity applications at the same time that ICD-9 (published by the World Health Organization [WHO]) was adopted for mortality data. In addition to its use in records and surveys, ICD-9-CM is used to classify diseases and health conditions on healthcare claims, and it is the basis for prospective payment to hospitals and certain other healthcare facilities and healthcare providers.

The United States also developed its own procedure coding system (ICD-9-CM Volume 3) for inpatient hospital services in the late 1970s to use with ICD-9-CM Volumes

PATIENT VISITS

X	DESCRIPTION	CODE	AMOUNT
	NEW PATIENT		
	Problem focused Hx	99201	
	Expanded prob/Focused Hx	99202	
	Detailed Hx	99203	
	Comp Hx/Moderate complex	99204	
	Comp Hx/High complex	99205	
	ESTABLISHED PATIENT		
	Minimal	99211	
	Problem focused Hx	99212	
	Expanded prob/Focused Hx	99213	
	Detailed Hx	99214	
	Comprehensive Hx	99215	
	CONSULTATION		
	Problem focused Hx	99241	
	Expanded prob/Focused Hx	99242	
	Detailed Hx	99243	
	Comp Hx/Moderate complex	99244	
	Comp Hx/High complex	99245	
	NURSE SPECIALIST		
	Computer analysis	99090	
	Group health ed	99078	
	Skills management (15 min.)	97535	
	PROCEDURES		
	Accucheck/One Touch	7182948	
	EKG w/interpretation	93000	
	IV infusion, up to 1 hr.	90780	
	IV infusion, each add'l hr.	90781	
	Immunization administration	90471	
	Two or more vaccines/toxoids	90472	
	Therapeutic/diagnostic injection	90782	
	Specify: med/dose		
	Injection of antibiotic	90788	
	Specify: med/dose		
	Occult blood (guaiac)	82270	
	ANS	95937	
	24 hour cardiac monitor	93230	
	Pap smear	88150	
	Thyroid fine needle asp. (proc.)	7190357	
	Group counseling, 30 min.	99411	
	Group counseling, 60 min.	99412	

PROCEDURES cont.

X	DESCRIPTION	CODE	ALPHA	AMOUNT
	Preventive counseling, 15 min.	99401		
	Preventive counseling, 30 min.	99402		
	Preventive counseling, 45 min.	99403		
	Preventive counseling, 60 min.	99404		
	DIABETES/LIPID			
	Cholesterol, HDL	7190053	HDL	
	C-peptide	7190219	CPEP	
	Glucose serum	7182947	GLU	
	HGB A1 C	7190057	HA1	
	Insulin	7190343	INS	
	Lipoprotein panel A	7175004		
	Micral, random	7190335	MLBU	
	Protein, urine 24 hr.	7195011	PROU	
	GONADAL			
	Estradiol	7190044	ESD	
	FSH	7190048	FSH	
	LH	7190069	LH	
	Progesterone	7190078	PROG	
	PSA	7190079	PSA	
	SHBG	7190622	SHBG	
	Testosterone	7190086	TEST	
	Testosterone, Free	7190322	FTES	
	PSA, Free	7184999		
	PROFILES			
	Basic metabolic panel	7180049	CH7	
	Comp. metabolic panel	7180054	CMP	
	Electrolyte panel	7180051	ELEC	
	Hepatic function panel	7180058	HFPA	
	Hepatitis panel	7180059		
	Lipid profile 2	7190257	LPP2	
	THYROID			
	Antimicrosomal antibody	7190213	TM	
	TSI	7190476	TSIG	
	Thyroglobulin	7190584	THY	
	T4 - Thyroxine	7190047	FT4	
	T3 uptake	7190292	TU	
	Total T3	7190095	T3 C	
	T3-Free	7190595	FT3	
	TSH (Thyroid stim hormone)	7190253	TSH	

CALCIUM/BONE/KIDNEY

X	DESCRIPTION	CODE	ALPHA	AMOUNT
	Calcium, ionized	7190821	ICAL	
	Calcium, serum	7190311	CAL	
	Calcium, urine 24 hr.	7190222	CALU	
	Creatinine, clearance ht. ___ wt. ___	7194754	CRCP	
	Microalbumin, urine 24 hr.	7190335	MLBT	
	Magnesium, serum	7190317	MAG	
	Parathyroid hormo	7190387	PTH	

ADRENAL/PITUITARY

X	DESCRIPTION	CODE	ALPHA	AMOUNT
	ACTH	7190005	ACTH	
	Aldosterone, serum	7190204	ALD	
	Androstenedione	7190336	AND	
	Cortisol, serum	7190032	COR	
	DHEA	7190341	DHEA	
	DHEA S serum	7190312	DHES	
	Human growth hormone	7190379	HGH	
	Prolactin	7190316	PRL	
	17OH Progesterone	7190479	HY17	
	17OH Pregnegalone	7190480	LONE	
	Urine catecholimine 24 hr.	7190021	CATU	
	Urine cortisol 24 hr.	7190033	CORU	
	Urine metanephrines 24 hr.	7194475	METU	
	Urine potassium 24 hr.	7190077	POTU	
	Urine sodium 24 hr.	7190261	SODU	
	Urine VMA 24 hr.	7190534	VMAU	

CHEMISTRY/HEMATOLOGY

X	DESCRIPTION	CODE	ALPHA	AMOUNT
	CBC w/diff & platelets	7190327	CBC1	
	Erthrocyte sed rate	7190330	ESR	
	Potassium, serum	7184813	POT	
	Urine culture	7190041	BACTI	
	Urinalysis, routine	7190334	URTN	
	Urinalysis, dipstick	7190384	URCH	
	Venipuncture	7190323	VENI	
	GGI	7184773		
	HCE	7190329		

AUTHORIZATION #
DIAGNOSIS
SPECIAL INSTRUCTIONS

REFERRING MD

Tax ID #	62-1162462
Previous bal.	
Amount paid	
Today's chrg	
Amount paid	
Total rec'd	
Balance due	

Physician signature: Date:

I authorize release of any medical information necessary to process this claim. I also authorize the direct payment of any benefits due me for the described services to ___ I understand I am financially responsible for paying any unpaid balance and will be responsible for the entire bill if this claim is not covered. **Medicare Patients:** The Medicare program requires that all diagnosis be ICD 9 coded. We are unable to provide this service to you at the time of your visit, and therefore, require that you permit us to file an insurance claim with your Medicare carrier.

Check one:
☐ Cash
☐ Check, M.O.# ___
☐ MC   ☐ VISA
☐ Care Card # ___

Patient (Beneficiary) signature: Date:

98381 7/99

Fig. 18-5 Example of an inpatient encounter form. (From Abdelhak M, Grostick S, Hanken MA, Jacobs E (editors): Health information: management of a strategic resource, ed 2, St Louis, 2001, Saunders.)

1 and 2 for coding diagnoses. This was necessary because the WHO had not yet produced a procedural coding system. As a result, since 1979, procedures performed in hospitals have been coded for hospital statistics and on hospital claims using ICD-9-CM Volume 3. The Current Procedural Terminology (CPT-4), developed and maintained by the American Medical Association, is used in the United States to code professional services on claims of physicians and other non-inpatient providers. All healthcare providers code diagnoses with ICD-9-CM Volumes 1 and 2.

When the inpatient PPS was implemented in 1983, ICD-9-CM Volumes 1, 2, and 3 were used as the basis for assigning cases to the DRGs. All diagnostic and procedural information was captured using ICD-9-CM. Because there had been radical changes and advances in healthcare since the implementation of ICD-9-CM, a need quickly arose to update and revise the system. This was particularly true for the procedure codes of the system, but users also wanted to update the diagnosis portion to attain greater clinical detail. An annual updating process was established through the ICD-9-CM Coordination and Maintenance Committee. Although this process continues to allow some addition of new conditions and procedures and expansion for greater detail, it uses a classification system that was developed nearly 30 years ago as its base.

Selecting the Principal Diagnosis

The health insurance professional or coder must identify key elements or words for possible use as the **principal diagnosis**. The principal diagnosis is defined in the Uniform Hospital Discharge Data Set (UHDDS) as *"that condition established after study to be chiefly responsible for occasioning the admission of the patient to the hospital for care."* The UHDDS definitions are used by hospitals to report inpatient data elements in a standardized manner. (These data elements and their definitions can be found in the July 31, 1985, *Federal Register* [Vol. 50, No. 147], pp. 31038-40.) Since that time, the application of the UHDDS definitions has been expanded to include all nonoutpatient settings (acute care, short-term care, long-term care, and psychiatric hospitals; home health agencies; rehabilitation facilities; nursing homes). In determining principal diagnosis, the coding conventions in the ICD-9-CM Volumes 1 and 2 take precedence over these official coding guidelines.

When more than one diagnosis meets the criteria for principal diagnosis, the coder should use the diagnosis that accounts for most of the services provided and code that as the primary diagnosis. When more than one condition is listed that pertains to similar and contrasting conditions, the coder should select the diagnosis that is

the condition that resulted in the admission and for which most of the services were provided. If one of the diagnoses is ruled out during the hospitalization, it should not be used for coding. When original treatment plans are not completed during the course of the encounter or admission, the reason for admission or encounter is still used as the principal or primary diagnosis.

Sometimes documentation describes symptoms, signs, and ill-defined conditions that are not linked to a specific disease. Some body system categories include codes for nonspecific conditions. The code for a breast lump is found in Volume 1 under "Genitourinary System," in the subcategory "Signs and symptoms in breast," and would be properly coded as 611.72, "Lump or mass in breast." Use these codes, rather than codes for more specific disorders, when the only facts you have are the patient's signs and symptoms. Table 18-3 provides a list of guidelines for coding inpatient hospital diagnoses.

The importance of consistent, complete documentation in the medical record cannot be overemphasized. Without such documentation the application of all coding guidelines is a difficult, if not impossible, task.

Coding Inpatient Hospital Procedures

As discussed previously, ICD-9-CM Volume 3 is used for coding and reporting inpatient hospital procedures. Volume 3 grew out of the procedural classifications developed in the early 1970s by an international committee sponsored by WHO. The current Volume 3 procedural coding process evolved from a 3-digit to 4-digit system necessitated by the demand for more specific clinical detail. The CMS maintains the Volume 3 codes, which include operative, diagnostic, and therapeutic procedures. Annual code revisions reflect the goal of a procedure coding system that can be used with equal efficiency in hospitals and in other primary

TABLE 18-3 Guidelines for Coding Inpatient Hospital Diagnoses

Select the diagnoses that require coding according to current coding and reporting requirements for inpatient services
Select the diagnoses that require coding according to current coding and reporting requirements for hospital-based outpatient services
Interpret conventions, formats, instructional notations, tables, and definitions of the classification system to select diagnoses, conditions, problems, or other reasons for the encounter that require coding
Sequence diagnoses and other reasons for the encounter according to notations and conventions of the classification system and standard data set definitions
Determine if signs, symptoms, or manifestations require separate code assignments
Determine if the diagnostic statement provided by the healthcare provider does not allow for more specific code assignments (e.g., 4th or 5th digit)
Recognize when the classification system does not provide a precise code for the condition documented (e.g., residual categories or nonclassified syndromes)
Assign supplementary codes to indicate reasons for the healthcare encounter other than illness or injury
Assign supplementary codes to indicate factors other than illness or injury that influence the patient's health status
Assign supplementary codes to indicate the external cause of an injury, adverse effect, or poisoning

care settings. Approximately 90% of the codes refer to surgical procedures with the remaining 10% accounting for other investigative and therapeutic procedures.

Format of Volume 3

Although Volume 3 may differ from publisher to publisher, most manuals offer the following features:
- Numeric listing is provided of all valid ICD-9-CM Volume 3 codes and their official, complete government descriptions.
- Each ICD-9-CM Volume 3 code is linked to all applicable CPT codes, which are printed with their official, complete American Medical Association descriptions.
- All ICD-9-CM Volume 3 codes are valid and of the highest level of specificity.
- The ICD-9-CM Volume 3 and CPT code sets are updated to include the current year's changes.

Fig. 18-6 shows a sample partial page from ICD-9-CM Volume 3.

Organization of Volume 3

The layout of ICD-9-CM Volume 3 procedure index is similar to the main sections of ICD-9-CM. It has an alphabetical index to procedures along with a numerical index. Volume 3 codes are presented in numeric order, and the section title from ICD-9-CM appears at the top of each page. The sections are organized by anatomy, rather than surgical specialty, as shown in Table 18-4.

The most important factor in ICD-9-CM procedure coding is understanding the rules. Only valid codes—codes that represent the highest level of specificity—are included in the **crosswalk**. A crosswalk is a table or search engine that maps the relationships and equivalencies between two or more data formats—in this case procedure codes. If you are seeking information about a code that is not at its highest level of specificity, you should look for your answer among all the valid codes within that **rubric** (grouping of numbers). If you are working with the invalid code 24.3, review 24.31, 24.32, and 24.39 for the best CPT crosswalk. In this frame of reference, a crosswalk translates the selected procedural codes for services provided by the physician in either the inpatient or the outpatient setting.

Using V and E Codes

V codes are used in all healthcare settings. They may be used as a first listed (principal diagnosis code in the inpatient setting) or secondary code, depending on the circumstances of the encounter. Certain V codes may be used only as first listed; others, only as secondary codes. V codes indicate a *reason* for an encounter. They are not procedure codes. A corresponding procedure code must accompany a V code to describe the procedure performed. The selection of the appropriate E code is guided by the Index to External Causes, which is located after the alphabetical index to diseases and by Inclusion and Exclusion notes in the Tabular List. An E code can never be a principal (first listed) diagnosis.

NEW HIPAA EDIT—ICD-9 PROCEDURE CODES

The new HIPAA edits check for the presence or absence of specific medical procedure codes reported at the claim level for inpatient or outpatient hospital services. These edits are being added to comply with the final HIPAA rule that named the ICD-9-CM Volume 3 Procedure Codes

---

INDEX TO PROCEDURES / Closure

Chondrectomy *(Continued)*
 hand and finger 80.94
 hip 80.95
 intervertebral cartilage - *see* category 80.5
 knee (semilunar cartilage) 80.6
 nasal (submucous) 21.5
 semilunar cartilage (knee) 80.6
 shoulder 80.91
 specified site NEC 80.99
 spine - *see* category 80.5
 wrist 80.93
Chondroplasty - *see* Arthroplasty
Chondrosternoplasty (for pectus excavatum repair) 34.74
Chondrotomy - *see also* Division, cartilage 80.40
 nasal 21.1
Chopart operation (midtarsal amputation) 84.12
Chordectomy, vocal 30.22
Chordotomy (spinothalamic) (anterior) (posterior) NEC 03.29
 percutaneous 03.21
 stereotactic 03.21

Clipping
 aneurysm (basilar) (carotid) (cerebellar) (cerebellopontine) (communicating artery) (vertebral) 39.51
 arteriovenous fistula 39.53
 frenulum, frenum
  labia (lips) 27.91
  lingual (tongue) 25.91
 tip of uvula 27.72
Clitoridectomy 71.4
Clitoridotomy 71.4
Clivogram 87.02
Closure - *see also* Repair
 abdominal wall 54.63
  delayed (granulating wound) 54.62
  secondary 54.61
  tertiary 54.62
 amputation stump, secondary 84.3
 aorticopulmonary fenestration (fistula) 39.59
 appendicostomy 47.92
 artificial opening
  bile duct 51.79
  bladder 57.82

Closure *(Continued)*
 fistula *(Continued)*
  aortoduodenal 39.59
  appendix 47.92
  biliary tract 51.79
  bladder NEC 57.84
  branchial cleft 29.52
  bronchocutaneous 33.42
  bronchoesophageal 33.42
  bronchomediastinal 34.73
  bronchopleural 34.73
  bronchopleurocutaneous 34.73
  bronchopleuromediastinal 34.73
  bronchovisceral 33.42
  bronchus 33.42
  cecosigmoidal 46.76
  cerebrospinal fluid 02.12
  cervicoaural 18.79
  cervicosigmoidal 67.62
  cervicovesical 57.84
  cervix 67.62
  cholecystocolic 51.93
  cholecystoduodenal 51.93
  cholecystoenteric 51.93

Fig. 18-6 Sample page from ICD-9 Volume 3

TABLE 18-4 Section of ICD-9-CM Volume 3 Showing Organization by Anatomy

Procedures and Interventions, NEC (00)
Operations on the Nervous System (01-05)
Operations on the Endocrine System (06-07)
Operations on the Eye (08-16)
Operations on the Ear (18-20)
Operations on the Nose, Mouth, and Pharynx (21-29)
Operations on the Respiratory System (30-34)
Operations on the Cardiovascular System (35-39)
Operations on the Hemic and Lymphatic System (40-41)
Operations on the Digestive System (42-54)
Operations on the Urinary System (55-59)
Operations on the Male Genital Organs (60-64)
Operations on the Female Genital Organs (65-71)
Obstetrical Procedures (72-75)
Operations on the Musculoskeletal System (76-84)
Operations on the Integumentary System (85-86)
Miscellaneous Diagnostic and Therapeutic Procedures
   (87-99)

(including *The Official ICD-9-CM Guidelines for Coding and Reporting*) as the HIPAA standard medical code set for inpatient hospital services, and the Healthcare Common Procedure Code System (HCPCS)/CPT codes as the HIPAA standard medical code set for physician services and other healthcare services (including outpatient hospital procedures).

NATIONAL CORRECT CODING INITIATIVE

In 1996, CMS implemented the **National Correct Coding Initiative** to control improper coding that leads to inappropriate increased payment for healthcare services. The HHS program uses Medicare guidelines. The agency uses National Correct Coding Initiative edits to evaluate billing of HCPCS codes by Medicare providers in post-payment review of providers' claims. Table 18-5 show commonly used insurer claim forms and coding systems by setting of care. For assistance in billing, providers may access the National Correct Coding Initiative Edit information online at the CMS website listed under Websites to Explore.

ICD-9-CM PROCEDURE CODES AND MEDICARE

ICD-9-CM procedure codes are required for inpatient hospital Part A claims only. HCPCS codes are used for reporting procedures on Part B and other claim types. Inpatient hospital claims require reporting the principal procedure if a significant procedure occurred during the hospitalization. The principal procedure is the procedure performed for definitive treatment, rather than for diagnostic or exploratory purposes, or that which was necessary to take care of a complication. It also is the procedure most closely related to the principal diagnosis. The principal procedure code shown on the billing form must be the full ICD-9-CM Volume 3 procedure code, including all 4-digit codes where applicable. Other procedure codes are reported using the full ICD-9-CM Volume 3 procedure codes, including all 4 digits where applicable. Five significant procedures other than the principal procedure may be reported on the form. ICD-9-CM diagnosis and procedure codes are available on the CMS website listed under Websites to Explore.

OUTPATIENT HOSPITAL CODING

Outpatient hospital coding includes ICD-9-CM Volume 1 and 2 codes, Volume 3 procedure codes, and CPT-4 codes when applicable. Table 18-6 lists the basic guidelines for coding outpatient hospital services.

Hospital Outpatient Prospective Payment System

In response to the rapidly increasing Medicare expenditures for outpatient services and large copayments being made by Medicare beneficiaries, Congress mandated that the CMS develop a **hospital outpatient prospective payment system** and reduce beneficiary copayments. This payment system was implemented August 1, 2000, and is used by CMS to reimburse for hospital outpatient services.

TABLE 18-5 Commonly Used Insurer Claim Forms and Coding Systems by Setting of Care

COMPONENTS OF CLAIMS	FREESTANDING IMAGING CENTER/PHYSICIAN SERVICES	HOSPITAL OUTPATIENT DEPARTMENTS	HOSPITAL INPATIENT
Claim form	CMS-1500	CMS-1450 (UB-92)	CMS-1450 (UB-92)
Patient diagnoses	ICD-9-CM	ICD-9-CM	ICD-9-CM
Procedures	CPT	CPT	ICD-9-CM
		Revenue	Revenue
Drugs, supplies, and certain contrast agents	HCPCS (when appropriate)	HCPCS (when appropriate) Revenue	Revenue

TABLE 18-6 Basic Guidelines for Coding Outpatient Hospital Services

The appropriate ICD-9-CM code or codes from 001.0-V84.8 must be used to identify diagnoses, symptoms, conditions, problems, complaints, or other reasons for the encounter/visit

For accurate reporting of ICD-9-CM diagnosis codes, the documentation should describe the patient's condition, using terminology that includes specific diagnoses and symptoms, problems, or reasons for the encounter. There are ICD-9-CM codes to describe all of these

Codes 001.0-999.9 frequently are used to describe the reason for the encounter. These codes are from the section of ICD-9-CM for the classification of diseases and injuries (e.g., infectious and parasitic diseases; neoplasms; symptoms, signs, and ill-defined conditions)

Codes that describe symptoms and signs, as opposed to diagnoses, are acceptable for reporting purposes when an established diagnosis has not been diagnosed (confirmed) by the physician. Chapter 16 of ICD-9-CM, Symptoms, Signs, and Ill-defined Conditions (codes 780.0-799.9), contain many, but not all, codes for symptoms

ICD-9-CM provides codes to deal with encounters for circumstances other than a disease or injury. The Supplementary Classification of Factors Influencing Health Status and Contact with Health Services (V01.0-V82.9) is provided to deal with occasions when circumstances other than a disease or injury are recorded as diagnosis or problems

ICD-9-CM is composed of codes with 3, 4, or 5 digits. Codes with 3 digits are included in ICD-9-CM as the heading of a category of codes that may be subdivided further by the use of 4th or 5th digits, which provide greater specificity. A 3-digit code is to be used only if it is not subdivided further. Where 4th-digit subcategories or 5th-digit subclassifications are provided, they must be assigned. A code is invalid if it has not been coded to the full number of digits required for that code

List first the ICD-9-CM code for the diagnosis, condition, problem, or other reason for encounter/visit shown in the medical record to be chiefly responsible for the services provided. List additional codes that describe any coexisting conditions

Do not code diagnoses documented as "probable," "suspected," "questionable," "rule out," or working diagnosis. Rather, code the condition to the highest degree of certainty for that encounter/visit, such as symptoms, signs, abnormal test results, or other reason for the visit. *Note:* This is contrary to the coding practices used by hospitals and medical record departments for coding the diagnosis of hospital inpatients

Chronic diseases treated on an ongoing basis may be coded and reported as many times as the patient receives treatment and care for the condition

Code all documented conditions that coexist at the time of the encounter/visit and require or affect patient care treatment or management. Do not code conditions that were treated previously and no longer exist. History codes (V10-V19) may be used as secondary codes if the historical condition or family history has an impact on current care or influences treatment

For patients receiving diagnostic services only during an encounter/visit, sequence first the diagnosis, condition, problem, or other reason for encounter/visit shown in the medical record to be chiefly responsible for the outpatient services provided during the encounter/visit. Codes for other diagnoses (e.g., chronic conditions) may be sequenced as additional diagnoses

For patients receiving therapeutic services only during an encounter/visit, sequence first the diagnosis, condition, problem, or other reason for encounter/visit shown in the medical record to be chiefly responsible for the outpatient services provided during the encounter/visit. Codes for other diagnoses (e.g., chronic conditions) may be sequenced as additional diagnoses. The only exception to this rule is that for patients receiving chemotherapy, radiation therapy, or rehabilitation, the appropriate V code for the service is listed first, and the code for the diagnosis or problem for which the service is being performed is listed second

For patients receiving preoperative evaluations only, sequence a code from category V72.8, other specified examinations, to describe the preoperative consultations. Assign a code for the condition to describe the reason for the surgery as an additional diagnosis. Code also any findings related to the preoperative evaluation

For ambulatory surgery, code the diagnosis for which the surgery was performed. If the postoperative diagnosis is known to be different from the preoperative diagnosis at the time the diagnosis is confirmed, select the postoperative diagnosis for coding because it is the most definitive

Ambulatory Payment Classification Coding

APC is the grouping system that the CMS developed for facility reimbursement of hospital outpatient services. This system of coding and reimbursement for services was introduced by Congress in the 1997 Balanced Budget Act and implemented by CMS in August 2000 in hospital outpatient settings. It is intended to simplify the outpatient hospital payment system, ensure the payment is adequate to compensate hospital costs, and implement deficit reduction goals of the CMS.

This is how the APC system works: All covered outpatient services are assigned to an APC group. Each group of procedure codes within an APC must be similar clinically and with regard to the use of resources. The payment rate associated with each APC is determined by multiplying the relative weight for the APC by a conversion factor, which translates the relative weights into dollar amounts. To account for geographic differences, the labor portion of the payment rate is adjusted by the hospital wage index. The hospital outpatient PPS allows for additional payments for certain **pass-throughs** and for outlier cases involving high-cost services. Pass-throughs are temporary payments for specified new technologies, drugs, devices, and biologics for which costs were unavailable when calculating APC payment rates. The APC payment rate is the total amount the hospital receives from Medicare and the beneficiary. These rates are updated annually and take effect in January of the following year.

On November 13, 2000, the *Federal Register* published the hospital outpatient PPS interim final rule (65 FR 67797). CMS publishes the Medicare Physician Fee Schedule and the Hospital Outpatient Prospective Payment System annually in the *Federal Register*. A website for accessing additional information regarding hospital outpatient PPS and APCs is listed under Websites to Explore.

What Did You Learn?

1. When does the hospital billing process begin?
2. List typical patient responsibilities for inpatient hospitalization.
3. Explain "informed consent."
4. What manuals are used for coding hospital claims?
5. Define "principal diagnosis."
6. How is the principal diagnosis determined?
7. What is the function of the National Correct Coding Initiative?
8. Where does one find the procedure codes used on inpatient claims?
9. What are APCs, and in what setting are they used?
10. Explain the term "pass-through" in the context it is used in this chapter.

HOSPITAL BILLING AND THE UB-92: UNDERSTANDING THE BASICS

The UB-92 form and instructions are used by institutional and other selected providers to complete a Medicare Part A paper claim for submission to Medicare fiscal intermediaries. The paper UB-92 (Form HCFA-1450) is neither a government-printed form nor distributed by the CMS. The form is, however, universally accepted by Medicare, Medicaid, and most third-party payers, as is the CMS-1500 form.

Billing compliance and an understanding of the UB-92 is more important now than ever before. The billing data that are being submitted to Medicare and other payers

are examined carefully for accuracy and completeness. It is crucial that the health insurance professional or the health information technician who is responsible for hospital billing thoroughly understands the instructions relating to the correct completion of the UB-92, possesses an insight as to how the data elements interact, and comprehends what the payers do with the data when they are adjudicating a claim. Data quality, coding, and billing compliance are important things to consider when submitting inpatient and outpatient claims. Staying abreast of current rules and regulations is a multidepartmental responsibility, as is staying on top of the *quality* of documentation, coding, and billing. Compliance cannot be viewed as a one-step process; it must be considered an ongoing effort by every member of the healthcare team.

STANDARD DATA ELEMENTS

The UB-92 and its predecessor the UB-82 have long been the standard for defining the core data content for billing and reporting of institutional health services. Based on that premise, a logical first step is to analyze the uniform bill content for reporting health services in an institutional setting. In the UB-92, 86 data elements contained in 86 different fields, referred to as form locators. These 86 data elements are generally grouped into the following 10 sections:

FLS 1-11—provider information
FLS 12-23—patient information
FLS 24-31—condition codes
FLS 32-38—occurrence codes and dates
FLS 39-41—value codes
FLS 42-49—revenue descriptions, codes, and charges
FLS 50-66—payer, insured, and employer information
FLS 67-81—diagnosis and procedure codes
FLS 82-83—attending physician information
FLS 84-86—remarks section

Each form locator has a specific format, such as numeric, alphabetic, alphanumeric, and text-based. Some of the form locators are not labeled because they are reserved for state or national assignment only and not intended for provider reporting. Tables 18-7 and 18-8 list the data elements for hospital claim forms and outpatient claim forms.

UB-92 CLAIM FORM COMPLETION GUIDELINES

CMS provides guidelines for completion of UB-92 paper claim form. Table 18-9 presents these step-by-step instructions. These instructions address all form locators required, or required if applicable, for providers who submit paper UB-92 claims. Fig. 18-7 shows a completed UB-92 claim for a Medicare Part A patient.

It is important to keep current with changes in claims completion guidelines including the UB-92. NUBC provides an informational website for keeping up to date. It is recommended that providers visit the site at least quarterly to learn

TABLE 18-7 — Standard Data Elements: Hospital Claim Forms

Patient Characteristics

Patient identifier (unique to each hospital or care facility)
Name (last, first, middle initial)
Address (street, city, state, Zip Code)
Date of birth
Gender
Marital status

Provider Characteristics

Hospital/facility identifier (unique)
Physician identifier (unique only for Medicare claims)
Diagnostic and treatment information
Admissions date
Admissions status
Admissions diagnosis code
Condition code
Diagnosis code
Description of service
Service date
Service units
Principal and other diagnoses (up to 6)
Principal and other procedures (up to 5)
Date of procedure
Emergency code

Insurance/Payment Information

Insurance group numbers (differ for each health plan)
Group name
Insured's name
Relationship to insured
Employer name
Employer location
Covered period
Treatment authorization codes
Payer
Total charges
Noncovered charges
Prior payments
Amount due from patient
Revenue codes
HCPCS/rates

Courtesy of U.S. Department of Health and Human Services, Centers for Medicare and Medicaid Services.

TABLE 18-8 — Standard Data Elements: Outpatient Claim Forms

Patient Characteristics

Patient identifier (Social Security number or other identifier)
Name (last, first, middle initial)
Address (street, city, state, Zip Code)
Date of birth
Gender
Marital status
Telephone number
Other health insurance coverage

Provider Characteristics

Physician identifier (tax identifier or other plan-specific identifier)
Physician's employer identification number

Diagnostic and Treatment Information

Date of encounter
Illness
Emergency
Admission and discharge dates
Diagnosis or nature of illness
Diagnosis code
Place of service
Procedure code
Description of services and supplies
Date patient able to return to work
Date of disability

Insurance/Payment Information

Payer's identifier (e.g., Medicare or Medicaid)
Group name
Insured's name
Insured's identification number
Insured's group number
Address and telephone number of insured
Relationship to insured
Employer name
Employer location
Covered period
Treatment authorization codes
Accept assignment
Total charges
Amount paid
Prior payments
Balance due

Courtesy of U.S. Department of Health and Human Services, Centers for Medicare and Medicaid Services.

about developments in billing and claims-related transactions. A subscriber's section provides users with current information about the latest deliberations and manual instructions. Refer to Websites to Explore for NUBC's Internet link.

What Did You Learn?

1. Why are billing compliance and an understanding of the UB-92 important?
2. List the three things the health insurance professional must understand about the UB-92.

COMMON HOSPITAL BILLING ERRORS

As with claims for physician services (the CMS-1500 form), errors are common when using the UB-92. By becoming aware of common errors, the health insurance profes-

TABLE 18-9 CMS Claims Completion Guidelines for the UB-92

FIELD	FIELD DESCRIPTION	FIELD TYPE	INSTRUCTIONS
1	Provider name, address, and telephone number	Required	Enter facility name with complete billing address and telephone number
2	Unlabeled field	Not required	Not applicable
3	Patient control number	Optional	Enter the unique number assigned by the facility or the patient
4	Type of bill	Required	Enter the 9-digit type of bill code, which provides specific information about the services rendered. Refer to Attachment B for valid codes
5	Federal tax number	Required	Enter the 9-digit employer identification number for the provider indicated in Box 1 assigned by the Internal Revenue Services
6	Statement covers period "from" and "through"	Required	Enter the beginning and ending dates of services for the period reflected on the claim in MM DD YY format
7	Covered days	Not required	Enter the number of inpatient days covered for the billing period noted in Field 6
8	Noncovered days	Not required	Enter the number of inpatient days not covered by the primary payer
9	Coinsurance days	Not required	Enter the number of inpatient Medicare days occurring after the 60th and before the 90th day in a single episode
10	Lifetime reserve days	Not required	Enter the number of lifetime reserve days used during the billing period noted on the claim
11	Unlabeled field	Not required	Not applicable
12	Patient's name (last name, first name, middle initial)	Required	Enter the patient name (last name, first name, and middle initial)
13	Patient's address	Required	Enter the complete mailing address of the patient. Include street number and name, PO box or rural route number, apartment number if applicable, city, state, and Zip Code
14	Birth date	Required	Enter the patient's birth date in MM DD YY format
15	Sex	Required	Enter the code for the gender status of the patient
16	Marital status	Required	Enter the code for the marital status of the patient on the date of the admission
17	Admission date	Required	Enter the original date the patient was admitted for care in MM DD YY format
18	Admission hour	Conditional	Enter the admission hour in Military Standard Time (e.g., 00:00 to 24:00), if applicable
19	Admission type	Conditional	Enter the code for the admission type, if applicable
20	Admission source	Conditional	Enter the appropriate admission source code. Then newborn coding structure for admission must be used when the admission type in Field 19 indicates 4. Refer to Attachment B for valid codes
21	Discharge hour	Conditional	Enter the hour at which the patient was discharged from inpatient care, if applicable
22	Patient status	Required	Enter the applicable code indicating the patient's disposition as of the ending date of service for the period of care
23	Medical record number	Optional	Enter the number assigned by the provider to the patient's medical or health record
24-30	Condition codes	Conditional	Enter a valid condition code if applicable
31	Unlabeled field	Not required	Not applicable
32a, b	Occurrence code and date	Conditional	Enter a valid occurrence code and date if applicable. Enter date in MM DD YY format
33a, b	Occurrence code and date	Conditional	Enter a valid occurrence code and date if applicable. Enter date in MM DD YY format

FIELD	FIELD DESCRIPTION	FIELD TYPE	INSTRUCTIONS
	TABLE 18-9 CMS Claims Completion Guidelines for the UB-92—cont'd		
34a, b	Occurrence code and date	Conditional	Enter a valid occurrence code and date if applicable. Enter date in MM DD YY format
35a, b	Occurrence code and date	Conditional	Enter a valid occurrence code and date if applicable. Enter date in MM DD YY format
36a, b	Occurrence code and date	Conditional	Enter a valid occurrence code and date if applicable. Enter date in MM DD YY format
37a-c	Unlabeled field	Not required	Not applicable
38	Responsible party name and address	Required	Enter the name and address of party responsible for payment of bill
39a-d	Value codes/amount	Conditional	Enter a valid value code and amount if applicable
40a-d	Value codes/amount	Conditional	Enter a valid value code and amount if applicable
41a-d	Value codes/amount	Conditional	Enter a valid value code and amount if applicable
42	Revenue code	Required	Enter the applicable revenue code for the services rendered. There are 23 lines available and should include the total line for revenue code 0001
43	Description	Optional	Enter the corresponding description of the revenue indicated in Field 43 lines 1-23
44	HCPCS/rates	Conditional	Enter a valid HCPCS or CPT procedure code for the ancillary services for outpatient or the accommodation rate for inpatient claims
45	Service date	Required	Enter the date the service was rendered in MM DD YY format
46	Service units	Required	Enter the service units for each service billed
47	Total charges	Required	Enter the amount equal to the per unit charge to the related revenue codes billed for the statement from and through dates. This amount includes the covered and noncovered charges
48	Noncovered charges	Conditional	Enter the total noncovered charges for the primary payer if applicable for service billed
49	Unlabeled field	Not required	Not applicable
50a-c	Payer	Required	Enter the names of primary, secondary, and tertiary payers as applicable. Provider should list multiple payers in priority sequence according to the priority the provider expects to receive payment from these payers
51a-c	Provider number	Conditional	Enter the number assigned to the provider by the payer indicated in Field 50, if known. Required if ValueOptions is primary, secondary, or tertiary payer
52a-c	Release of information certification indicator	Required	Enter the appropriate code denoting whether the provider has on file a signed statement from the beneficiary to release information. Refer to Attachment B for valid codes
53a-c	Assignment of benefits	Required	Enter the appropriate code to indicate whether the provider has a signed form authorizing the third-party insurer to pay the provider directly for the service rendered
54a-c	Prior payments	Conditional	Enter any prior payment amounts the facility has received toward payment of this bill for the payer indicated in Field 50 lines a-c
55a-c	Estimated amount due	Not required	Enter the estimated amount due from the payer indicated in Field 50 lines a-c
56	Unlabeled field	Not required	Not applicable
57	Unlabeled field	Not required	Not applicable
58a-c	Insured's name (last name, first name, middle initial)	Required	Enter the insured's name (last name, first name, and middle initial)

TABLE 18-9 CMS Claims Completion Guidelines for the UB-92—cont'd

FIELD	FIELD DESCRIPTION	FIELD TYPE	INSTRUCTIONS
59a-c	Patient's relationship to insured	Required	Enter the applicable code that indicates the relationship of the patient to the insured
60a-c	Certificate no.	Required	Enter the insured's identification number assigned by the payer organization
	Social Security number		Health insurance claim identification number
	Social Security number		Medicaid number
61a-c	Group name	Required	Enter the group or plan name of the primary, secondary, and tertiary payer through which the coverage is provided to the insured
62a-c	Insurance group number	Conditional	Enter the plan or group number for the primary, secondary, and tertiary payer through which the coverage is provided to the insured
63a-c	Treatment authorization codes	Optional	Enter the authorization number assigned by the payer indicated in Field 50 if known
64a-c	Employment status code	Optional	Enter the applicable code, which defines the employment status code of the insured indicated in Field 58a-c or employment status of the insured as indicated in Field 50. Refer to Attachment B for valid codes
65a-c	Employer name	Conditional	Enter the primary employer that provides the coverage for the insured indicated in Field 58.
66a-c	Employer location	Conditional	Enter the specific location of the primary insured individual identified in Field 58
67	Principal diagnosis	Required	Enter a valid ICD-9 diagnosis code (including 4th and 5th digits if applicable) that describes the principal diagnosis for services rendered
68-75	Other diagnosis code	Required	Enter a valid ICD-9 diagnosis code (including 4th and 5th digits if applicable) for any other conditions that exist for the services rendered
76	Admitting diagnosis code	Conditional	Enter a valid ICD-9 diagnosis code (including 4th and 5th digits if applicable) that describes the diagnosis at the time of admission
77	E-code	Not required	Enter a valid ICD-9 code (including 4th and 5th digits if applicable) for the external cause of injury, poisoning, or adverse effect
78	Unlabeled field	Not required	Not applicable
79	Procedure method used	Optional	Please denote the medical coding system used to complete the claim form
80	Principle procedure code/date	Required	Enter a valid ICD-9 code and date to identify the significant procedures performed during the statement from and through dates
81	Other procedure code/date	Conditional	Enter additional ICD-9 codes and dates to identify the significant procedures performed during the period covered by the bill
82	Attending physician identification	Required	Enter the name or assigned number of the licensed physician who has primary responsibility for the patient's care
83	Other physician identification number	Optional	Enter the name or the licensed physician who has primary responsibility for the patient's care
84	Remarks	Conditional	Enter "IOP" if billing for intensive outpatient programs. Enter any additional information pertaining to the third-party payer
85	Provider representative	Required	Enter the signature of an authorized representative noting the physician's certification is in effect. A stamp or facsimile of the provider's representative signature is acceptable
86	Date	Required	Enter the date the bill is submitted to the payer organization in MM DD YY format

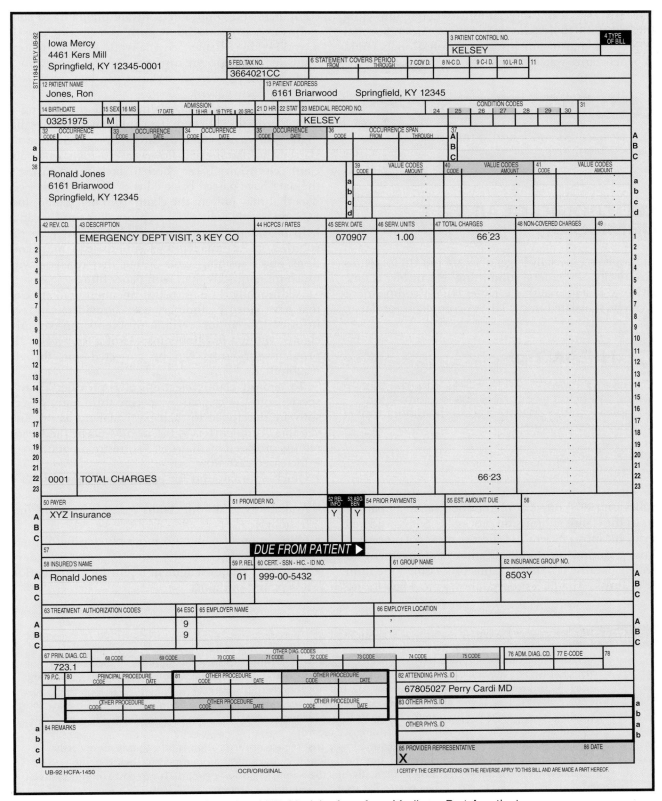

Fig. 18-7 Completed UB-92 claim form for a Medicare Part A patient.

sional can take extra precautions when completing claims. Table 18-10 lists the eight most common hospital billing errors that health insurance professionals could help beneficiaries watch for.

> ## What Did You Learn?
>
> List at least five common errors made on the UB-92 claim.

ELECTRONIC CLAIMS SUBMISSION

Most hospitals, especially larger ones, submit UB-92 claims electronically. Providers submitting electronic claims must do so in a format that is either HIPAA-compliant or that can be translated into a HIPAA-compliant format.

> **HIPAA Tip**
>
> Effective October 16, 2003, HIPAA requires that claims submitted electronically be in a format that complies with the appropriate standard adopted for national use.

As discussed in an earlier chapter, **electronic claim submission (ECS)** offers numerous benefits to all participants in the claims submission process. ECS is considered by many the most efficient and effective means of processing claims, ensuring swift adjudication and payment to providers because it reduces claims processing time from start to finish. The ECS process allows providers to use computers and applicable software programs to submit claims to a central location, such as a clearinghouse, via a World Wide Web interface. The World Wide Web interface sends the claims to the carrier system for processing. (In some instances, electronic claims can be sent *directly* to the third-party payer.)

With ECS, electronic claims avoid the sorting and keying process. The claim data are immediately available to the system. ECS not only can save providers time at the start of the claims cycle, however. Providers who submit claims electronically can check their claims to ensure that the data have passed basic edits or can determine claim data that may prevent the claim from being paid. Just as ECS can greatly reduce claims processing time, it can also help providers receive payment faster than with paper submission. As providers track submissions, make corrections, and resubmit claims online, they receive payment much more quickly than with paper filing.

Additionally, ECS provides an audit trail of claims that have failed preliminary edits. Providers can receive information about certain problems on submitted claims within a few hours instead of a few weeks. These problems or errors can be corrected and the claim resubmitted.

To submit claims electronically, providers may use special software created by specific third-party payers or software developed to their particular needs by outside vendors. Following is a list of advantages and various reports provided by many ECS software programs:

- Increased cash flow
- Quicker turnaround for payment compared with that of paper claims
- Availability to submit claims 7 days a week (including holidays)
- Elimination of paper, no more purchasing of the UB-92 forms
- Front end acknowledgment report for confirmation of acceptance of claims

	TABLE 18-10 Eight Common Billing Errors
1	*Duplicate billing:* Make sure you have not been charged twice for the same service, supplies, or medications
2	*Number of days in hospital:* Check the dates of your admission and discharge. Were you charged for the discharge day? Most hospitals charge for admission day, but not for day of discharge
3	*Incorrect room charges:* If you were in a semiprivate room, make sure you are not being charged for a private room
4	*Operating room time:* It is common for hospitals to bill for more operating room time than actually used. Compare the charge with your anesthesiologist's records.
5	*Upcoding:* Hospitals often shift the charge for a lower cost service or medication to one that is more costly (e.g., a physician orders a generic drug, but the patient is charged for a more expensive brand name)
6	*Keystroke error:* A computer operator accidentally hits the wrong key on a keyboard. It can cost you hundreds of dollars and result in an incorrect charge for a service you did not receive
7	*Canceled work:* Your physician ordered an expensive test, then cancelled it, but you were charged anyway
8	*Services never rendered:* Did you get every service, treatment, and medication for which you are being billed? Here's where your log comes in handy

Courtesy of bankrate.com.

- Availability of electronic remittance notice/advice (ERN/ERA) for faster posting of payments
- Availability of electronic funds transfer for paperless process
- Availability of electronic provider statistical and summary report
- Availability of electronic provider claims report
- Availability of electronic additional development requests

What Did You Learn?

1. Providers submitting electronic claims must do so in what type of format?
2. List six advantages provided by ECS.

HIPAA/HOSPITAL CONNECTION

HIPAA's Administrative Simplification and Compliance Act required providers, with limited exceptions, to submit all initial Medicare claims for reimbursement electronically on or after October 16, 2003. The act further prescribed that *"no payment may be made under Part A or Part B of the Medicare Program for any expenses incurred for items or services"* for which a claim is submitted in a nonelectronic form. Consequently, unless a provider fits one of the exceptions listed, any paper claims submitted to Medicare would not be paid. In addition, if it is determined that the provider is in violation of the statute or rule, it may be subject to claim denials, overpayment recoveries, and applicable interest on overpayments. The exceptions to this ECS requirement include the following:

- A small provider—a provider billing a Medicare fiscal intermediary that has fewer than 25 full-time equivalent employees or a physician, practitioner, or supplier with fewer than 10 full-time equivalent employees that bills a Medicare carrier
- A dentist
- A participant in a Medicare demonstration project in which paper claim filing is required because of the inability of the Applicable Implementation Guide, adopted under HIPAA, to report data essential for the demonstration
- A provider that conducts mass immunizations, such as flu injections, and may be permitted to submit paper roster bills
- A provider that submits claims when more than one other payer is responsible for payment before Medicare payment
- A provider that furnishes services only outside of the United States
- A provider experiencing a disruption in electricity and communication connections that are beyond its control
- A provider that can establish an "unusual circumstance" exists that precludes submission of claims electronically

Table 18-11 shows the data elements on the HIPAA X12N 837 institutional and professional healthcare claim forms that are required, but were not previously required on the electronic Part A (UB-92) formats and Medicare Part B (National Standard Format).

 HIPAA Tip

HIPAA standards allow the submission of paper-based claims and the use of paper-based remittances. HIPAA requires, however, that the electronic transaction and code set standards be followed whenever transactions are conducted electronically. Under the Administrative Simplification Compliance Act of 2001, physician practices with 10 or more full-time equivalent employees are required to submit Medicare claims electronically.

 HIPAA Tip

Hospitals can achieve HIPAA compliance successfully by meeting all of the government guidelines and requirements related to physical security, contingency plans, standard electronic transaction processes, integrity controls, and implementing the most advanced scenario of secure methods of data transmission and storage to ensure proper handling of patient accounts and other health-related information.

What Did You Learn?

1. What is HIPAA's rule on Medicare claims submission?
2. List the exceptions to this rule.

ANSI 835 ELECTRONIC REMITTANCE NOTICE

An **ERN** is an electronic data file that can be downloaded into a biller's computer via a modem. It is commonly referred to as the 835. The 835 shows claims that have been paid and the dollar amounts and shows claims denied with the reason for denial. This file is the same as the paper remittances suppliers receive through the mail.

After the 835 file has been downloaded, it must be run through a Paid File Reader to allow billers to view it in a readable format. This software may be purchased from a

> **TABLE 18-11** HIPAA (X12N 837) Institutional/Professional Health Care Claim Form Data Elements*

Part A 837

X12 837i transaction overhead information (ST, BHT, transmission type REF, HLs, and SE segments, along with numerous qualifiers)
Submitter identifier (837 overhead information)
Receiver name
Receiver identifier
Billing provider tax identification number or Social Security number (*note:* one of the following is required)
   Attending physician tax identification number or Social Security number
   Operating physician tax identification number or Social Security number
   Other provider tax identification number or Social Security number
Payer identifier
Explanation of benefits indicator
Provider or supplier signature indicator

Part B 837

Receiver name and ID
Submitter name
Submitter phone number
Billing provider tax identification number or Social Security number
Pay-to provider tax identification number or Social Security number
Rendering provider tax identification number or Social Security number

*Required data elements in the HIPAA X12N 837 institutional and professional health care transactions required on the UB92 (Part A) or National Standard Format (Part B) pre-HIPAA electronic formats.

software vendor, or an Electronic Media Claims (EMC) submitter could program their own software using the Implementation Guide and companion document (hipaa/code_sets.html#3). See Websites to Explore at the end of this chapter for more information on how the *835: Health Care Claim Payment/Advice Implementation Guide* may be downloaded and the *CMS 835 Companion Document*.

> ### What Did You Learn?
>
> 1. What is an ERN?
> 2. What does an 835 ERN show?

UNDERSTANDING THE FULL CIRCLE PROCESS: GUIDE TO MEDICAL COMPLIANCE

The creation of a compliance program is a major initiative of the Office of the Inspector General in its effort to engage the private healthcare community in preventing the submission of erroneous claims and in combating fraudulent conduct. In the past several years, the Office of the Inspector General has developed and issued compliance program guidelines directed at a variety of segments in the healthcare industry. The development of these types of compliance program guidelines is based on the belief that a healthcare provider can use internal controls to monitor adherence to applicable statutes, regulations, and program requirements more efficiently. A compliance program usually consists of the following elements:

- An internal compliance review or "legal audit" of the provider's operations (often focused in one or more targeted areas, such as billing practices)
- Identification of practices that are improper, illegal, or potentially abusive
- Drafting an appropriate code of conduct for management and staff
- Appointment of a compliance officer and compliance oversight committee
- Implementation of a hot line or some other manner of reporting mechanism
- Development and implementation of a training program for relevant staff
- Design of appropriate disciplinary sanctions for violations of the plan
- Securing continuing compliance through proper dissemination of new regulations and carrier or intermediary directives and statutes
- Periodic audits of the provider's practices and procedures to ensure continued compliance

Based on the success of this program, providers may wish to expand their compliance review to other areas as appropriate, such as Occupational Safety and Health Administration or Food and Drug Administration compliance.

 HIPAA Tip

It is recommended that hospitals periodically evaluate HIPAA rules to ensure that they are still in compliance. Experts suggest that administrative efficiencies gained from compliance in the long run will have a positive financial impact on hospitals and health systems.

A meaningful compliance plan addresses more than just billing procedures. Because this chapter focuses on hospital billing, however, we will take a closer look at **billing compliance**. Billing compliance begins with the gathering of complete and accurate information during the admission and registration interview. Most problems with claims originate in the claim development process: from the initial physician order, to the moment a patient presents in the facility, to the admission/registration process, to the clinical areas of patient care and the associated documentation, to coding, and finally to billing. A good comprehensive billing compliance program should provide hands-on admissions, registration, and billing personnel and others within the organization involved in the claims development process, with an appropriate level of information relating to the "full circle process" and instruction relating to compliance standards.

What Did You Learn?

1. What is the purpose of a medical compliance program?
2. List at least seven of the nine elements of a medical compliance program.
3. Where does billing compliance begin?
4. What three areas should be included in a comprehensive billing compliance program?

CAREER OPPORTUNITIES IN HOSPITAL BILLING

Medical records and health information technicians held nearly 150,000 jobs in 2002, and 37% of all jobs were in hospitals. The rest were mostly in offices of physicians, nursing care facilities, outpatient care centers, and home

healthcare services. Insurance firms that deal in health matters employ a few health information technicians to tabulate and analyze health information. Public health departments also hire technicians to supervise data collection from healthcare institutions and to assist in research.

TRAINING, OTHER QUALIFICATIONS, AND ADVANCEMENT

Medical records and health information technicians entering the field typically have an associate degree from a community college or career program. In addition to general education, coursework includes medical terminology, anatomy and physiology, legal aspects of health information, coding and abstraction of data, statistics, database management, quality improvement methods, and computer science. Applicants can improve their chances of admission into a program by taking biology, chemistry, health, and computer science courses in high school.

Hospitals sometimes advance promising health information clerks to jobs as medical records and health information technicians, although this practice may be less common in the future. Experienced medical records and health information technicians sometimes can advance in one of several ways—by specializing, furthering their education, or managing. Many senior technicians specialize in coding, particularly Medicare coding, or in cancer registry. More commonly, however, advancement requires 2 to 4 years of job experience, completion of a hospital's in-house training program, or acquiring specialized education or credentialing, such as certification in a health information management program.

Most employers prefer to hire **Registered Health Information Technicians (RHITs)**, who are required to pass a written examination offered by the American Health Information Management Association (AHIMA). To take the examination, an individual must graduate from a 2-year associate degree program accredited by the Commission on Accreditation of Allied Health Education Programs (CAAHEP) of the American Medical Association. Technicians trained in non–CAAHEP-accredited programs or on the job are not eligible to take the American Health Information Management Association examination. In 2003, CAAHEP accredited 182 programs for health information technicians. Technicians who specialize in coding may obtain voluntary certification.

In medical records and health information departments of large facilities, experienced technicians may advance to section supervisor, overseeing the work of the coding, correspondence, or discharge sections. Senior technicians with RHIT credentials may become director or assistant director of a medical records and health information department in a small facility. In larger institutions, the director is usually an administrator, with a bachelor's degree in medical records and health information administration.

JOB OUTLOOK

Job prospects are good. Employment of hospital billing specialists and medical records and health information technicians is expected to grow much faster than the average for all occupations through 2012, owing to rapid growth in the number of medical tests, treatments, and procedures that will be increasingly scrutinized by third-party payers, regulators, courts, and consumers.

Although employment growth in hospitals may not keep pace with growth in other healthcare industries, many new jobs nevertheless will be created. The fastest employment growth and the most new jobs are expected in offices of physicians, owing to increasing demand for detailed records, especially in large group practices. Rapid growth also is expected in nursing care facilities, home healthcare services, and outpatient care centers. Additional job openings will result from the need to replace technicians who retire or leave the occupation permanently (http://www.bls.gov/oco/ocos103.htm). Table 18-12 lists common certifications and their requirements and other career opportunities in hospital billing.

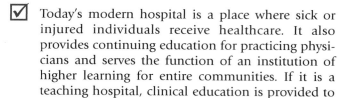

What Did You Learn?

1. What type of coursework should a student expect to complete when entering into a medical records or health information technologic field?
2. What are the career opportunities for health information clerks or technicians?
3. What is the job outlook?

SUMMARY CHECK POINTS

☑ Today's modern hospital is a place where sick or injured individuals receive healthcare. It also provides continuing education for practicing physicians and serves the function of an institution of higher learning for entire communities. If it is a teaching hospital, clinical education is provided to the entire spectrum of healthcare professionals. The hospital also might conduct investigational studies and perform research in medical sciences.

TABLE 18-12 **Certifications and Their Requirements and Other Career Opportunities in Hospital Billing**

Registered Health Information Administrator (RHIA)	Successful completion of an approved baccalaureate or post-baccalaureate program and pass a national RHIA certification examination
Registered Health Information Technician (RHIT)	Associate degree in an approved health information technology program and pass a national certification examination
Certified Coding Specialist (CCS)	Pass a national coding examination measuring medical terminology, disease processes, pharmacology, and the application of ICD-9-CM and CPT surgery coding systems
Certified Coding Specialist–Physician-based (CCS-P)	Pass a national coding examination measuring medical terminology, disease processes, pharmacology, and the application of ICD-9-CM, CPT, and HCPCS level II coding systems
Certified Coding Associate (CCA)	Pass a national coding examination measuring understanding of entry-level coding applications including medical terminology, disease processes, pharmacology, and ICD-9-CM and CPT medical record coding

Other Career Opportunities

Admissions coordinator
Discharge planner
Medical records clerk
Medical records technician
Medical secretary
Medical transcriptionist
Nutrition educator
Transplant coordinator
Tumor registrar
Unit coordinator

☑ A goal of the entire healthcare system is to reduce costs and, at the same time, be more responsive to customers (patients).

☑ The major types of healthcare facilities are as follows:
- Acute care facilities
- Subacute care facilities
- ASCs
- SNFs
- Long-term care facilities
- Hospice

☑ All acute care or general hospitals must be licensed by the state in which they are located to provide care within the minimum health and safety standards established by regulation and rule. HHS enforces the standards by periodically conducting surveys of these facilities. Hospitals may seek accreditation by nationally recognized accrediting agencies, such as JCAHO or AOA. Surveys conducted by JCAHO and AOA are based on guidelines developed by each of these organizations.

☑ Common hospital payers are as follows:
- Medicare
- Medicaid
- TRICARE/CHAMPVA
- Blue Cross and Blue Shield
- Private (commercial) insurers

☑ The health insurance professional must be aware of individual payer guidelines for accurate and timely claims completion. Current guidelines can be found on the payers' websites, or provider manuals may be acquired by contacting the payer or its fiscal intermediary/carrier.

☑ The UB-92 is the standard claim form used for inpatient hospitalization. Data elements necessary for claims processing in most cases are assigned designated spaces on the form called "form locators." There are 86 form locators, and each has a unique number. Applicable information is entered into these form locators using a numeric, alphabetic, alphanumeric, or text-based format. The UB-92 was created by the NUBC, whose objective was to develop a single billing form and standard data set that could be used nationwide by institutional providers and payers for handling healthcare claims, which would achieve the goals of administrative simplification as outlined by HIPAA.

☑ The information included in a hospital health record begins with demographic information—patient's name, address, age, sex, occupation—collected on admission. Every time a patient receives healthcare, a record is maintained of the observations, medical or surgical interventions, and treatment outcomes. This record includes information that the patient provides concerning his or her symptoms and medical history, the results of examinations, reports of x-rays and laboratory tests, diagnoses, and treatment plans.

☑ The hospital billing process begins when the patient registers for inpatient/outpatient admission. Hospital charges are recorded for room and board, each procedure performed, medications, laboratory tests, x-rays (if applicable), and miscellaneous service charges.

☑ Although hospital coding is similar to that done in a physician's office, there are some significant differences. Similar to physician's office coding, hospital coders must use the ICD-9-CM Volumes 1 and 2 for diagnostic coding; however, hospital coders use ICD-9-CM Volume 3 for procedure coding, rather than the CPT-4, which is used in physician offices. Additionally, hospital coders use the "principal diagnosis," which is defined as the condition determined to be chiefly responsible for the patient's admission to the facility. ICD-9-CM Volume 3 procedure codes are required for inpatient hospital Part A claims only. HCPCS codes are used for reporting procedures on Part B and other claim types. Outpatient hospital coding includes ICD-9-CM Volume 1 and 2 codes, Volume 3 procedure codes, and CPT-4 codes when applicable.

☑ The billing data that are being submitted to Medicare and other payers is examined carefully for accuracy and completeness. It is crucial that the health insurance professional who is responsible for hospital billing thoroughly understands the instructions relating to the correct completion of the UB-92, possesses an insight as to how the data elements interact, and comprehends what the payers do with the data when they are adjudicating a claim. Data quality, coding, and billing compliance are extremely important things to consider when submitting inpatient and outpatient claims. Staying abreast of current rules and regulations is a multidepartmental responsibility, as is staying on top of the *quality* of documentation, coding, and billing. Compliance cannot be viewed as a one-step process; it must be considered an ongoing effort by every member of the healthcare team.

☑ Common areas where overcharges and errors occur in hospital billing include the following:
- Duplicate billing
- Number of days in hospital
- Room charges
- Operating room time

- Upcoding
- Keystroke error/typographicals
- Canceled work
- Services not provided

☑ Advantages of submitting hospital claims using ECS include the following:
- Increased cash flow
- Quicker turnaround for payment compared with paper claims
- Availability to submit claims 7 days a week (including holidays)
- Elimination of paper, no more purchasing of the UB-92 forms
- Front End Acknowledgment Report—confirmation verifying the acceptance of claims
- Availability of ERN/ERA for faster posting of payments
- Availability of electronic funds transfer for paperless process
- Ability to generate a variety of reports

☑ A compliance program typically consists of the following elements:
- An internal compliance review or "legal audit" of the provider's operations (often focused in one or more targeted areas, such as billing practices)
- Identification of practices that are improper, illegal, or potentially abusive
- Drafting an appropriate code of conduct for management and staff
- Appointment of a compliance officer and compliance oversight committee
- Implementation of a hot line or some other manner of reporting mechanism

- Development and implementation of a training program for relevant staff
- Design of appropriate disciplinary sanctions for violations of the plan
- Securing continuing compliance through proper dissemination of new regulations and carrier or intermediary directives and statutes
- Periodic audits of the provider's practices and procedures to ensure continued compliance

☑ Many career opportunities fall under the umbrella of hospital billing. Careers that require completion of a specific program and successful passing of a certification examination include the following:
- Registered Health Information Administrator (RHIA)
- Registered Health Information Technician (RHIT)
- Certified Coding Specialist (CCS)
- Certified Coding Specialist–Physician-based (CCS-P)
- Certified Coding Associate (CCA)

☑ Other career opportunities that may or may not require special education or certification (or both) include the following:
- Admissions coordinator
- Discharge planner
- Medical records clerk
- Medical records technician
- Medical secretary
- Medical transcriptionist
- Nutrition educator
- Transplant coordinator
- Tumor registrar
- Unit coordinator

CLOSING SCENARIO

After working in Broadmoor Medical Center's Billing Department for several months, Brittany has learned the various stages of hospital billing. Previously, she worked in a small medical office where she was in charge of all billing and claims submission. At Broadmoor, a much larger facility, work is more specialized, and Brittany's tasks center around Medicare claims submissions.

The routine at Broadmoor is for new employees to learn the paper form of the UB-92 first, so as to understand what each "form locator" stands for and the information that goes in each one. The UB-92 was challenging at first, but with help from her coworkers, Brittany now feels comfortable with that phase of her job.

Broadmoor's Billing Department falls under the larger umbrella of the Health Information Management Department, which employs nearly 100 individuals. There are numerous opportunities for advancement within the Health Information Management Department, and after an employee has completed 6 months of orientation and training, he or she can apply for a position that offers better pay; however, a promotion comes with more responsibility. Brittany has decided to continue her education at Deerfield Community College and eventually acquire a bachelor's degree in health information management. She is confident that with all the job opportunities Broadmoor Medical Center offers, she will be able to achieve her long-term career goals at this medical facility.

WEBSITES TO EXPLORE

For live links to the following websites, please visit the Evolve® site at http://evolve.elsevier.com/Beik/today/

- The website for the CMS home page is http://www.cms.hhs.gov/

- For more information on TRICARE and CHAMPVA reimbursement, visit the following website and peruse the TRICARE Reimbursement Manual: www.tricare.osd.mil

- For a PowerPoint Presentation on TRICARE-for-Life, use the following URL: http://www.narmc.amedd.army.mil/kacc/Tricare/TFL_BRIEFING.pdf

- Refer to the CMS ICD-9-CM Official Guidelines for Coding and Reporting at http://www.cdc.gov/nchs/data/icd9/icdguide.pdf

- Additional websites for UB-92 claims information include UB-92 Valid Code Listing and Medicare Fiscal Intermediary Medicare UB-92 Manual http://www.dhs.state.mn.us/provider/training/tools/instruct-ub92.htm http://www.state.sd.us/social/Medical/provider/BillingCrossUB92.htm

- For more information on the NUBC and to keep up to date on UB-92 changes, log onto the following website http://www.nubc.org/index.html

- CMS has a Hospital Billing Manual you can study on the following URL http://www.cms.hhs.gov/manuals/10_hospital/ho255.asp

- ICD-9-CM diagnosis and procedure codes are available on the CMS website at http://cms.hhs.gov/paymentsystems/icd9/

- To see a copy of a blank UB-04 Form, log onto the following website http://www.nubc.org/public/whatsnew/UB-04Proofs.pdf

- To see the entire dialogue of the ASTM standard EMRs, use the following URL and key "E1384" in the site search http://www.astm.org/

- To learn more about Hospital Outpatient Prospective Payment System and APCs, explore the following website http://www.cms.hhs.gov/providers/hopps/2005p/1427p.asp

- For detailed information on the Medicare remittance advice, log onto the following website: http://www.cms.hhs.gov/medlearn/RA_Guide_05-27-05.pdf

- The *835: Health Care Claim Payment/Advice Implementation Guide* may be downloaded through http://www.wpc-edi.com

- The *CMS 835 Companion Document* is available at http://www.cignamedicare.com/

- HIPAA's transaction code sets can be located at http://www.cignamedicare.com/HIPAA/code_sets.html#3

- Peruse the following website for career opportunities in healthcare technology: http://www.ahima.org/careers/intro.html

Sample Blank CMS-1500 (12/90)

PLEASE
DO NOT
STAPLE
IN THIS
AREA

CARRIER

PICA		HEALTH INSURANCE CLAIM FORM	PICA	

1. MEDICARE   MEDICAID   CHAMPUS   CHAMPVA   GROUP HEALTH PLAN   FECA BLK LUNG   OTHER
(Medicare #)   (Medicaid #)   (Sponsor's SSN)   (VA File #)   (SSN or ID)   (SSN)   (ID)

1a. INSURED'S I.D. NUMBER   (FOR PROGRAM IN ITEM 1)

2. PATIENT'S NAME (Last Name, First Name, Middle Initial)

3. PATIENT'S BIRTH DATE   MM   DD   YY   SEX   M   F

4. INSURED'S NAME (Last Name, First Name, Middle Initial)

5. PATIENT'S ADDRESS (No., Street)

6. PATIENT RELATIONSHIP TO INSURED
Self   Spouse   Child   Other

7. INSURED'S ADDRESS (No., Street)

CITY   STATE

8. PATIENT STATUS
Single   Married   Other
Employed   Full-Time Student   Part-Time Student

CITY   STATE

ZIP CODE   TELEPHONE (Include Area Code) ( )

ZIP CODE   TELEPHONE (INCLUDE AREA CODE) ( )

9. OTHER INSURED'S NAME (Last Name, First Name, Middle Initial)

10. IS PATIENT'S CONDITION RELATED TO:

11. INSURED'S POLICY GROUP OR FECA NUMBER

a. OTHER INSURED'S POLICY OR GROUP NUMBER

a. EMPLOYMENT? (CURRENT OR PREVIOUS)
YES   NO

a. INSURED'S DATE OF BIRTH   MM   DD   YY   SEX   M   F

b. OTHER INSURED'S DATE OF BIRTH   MM   DD   YY   SEX   M   F

b. AUTO ACCIDENT?   PLACE (State)
YES   NO

b. EMPLOYER'S NAME OR SCHOOL NAME

c. EMPLOYER'S NAME OR SCHOOL NAME

c. OTHER ACCIDENT?
YES   NO

c. INSURANCE PLAN NAME OR PROGRAM NAME

d. INSURANCE PLAN NAME OR PROGRAM NAME

10d. RESERVED FOR LOCAL USE

d. IS THERE ANOTHER HEALTH BENEFIT PLAN?
YES   NO   *If yes,* return to and complete item 9 a-d.

READ BACK OF FORM BEFORE COMPLETING & SIGNING THIS FORM.
12. PATIENT'S OR AUTHORIZED PERSON'S SIGNATURE I authorize the release of any medical or other information necessary to process this claim. I also request payment of government benefits either to myself or to the party who accepts assignment below.

SIGNED _____ DATE _____

13. INSURED'S OR AUTHORIZED PERSON'S SIGNATURE I authorize payment of medical benefits to the undersigned physician or supplier for services described below.

SIGNED _____

14. DATE OF CURRENT: MM   DD   YY   ILLNESS (First symptom) OR INJURY (Accident) OR PREGNANCY(LMP)

15. IF PATIENT HAS HAD SAME OR SIMILAR ILLNESS. GIVE FIRST DATE   MM   DD   YY

16. DATES PATIENT UNABLE TO WORK IN CURRENT OCCUPATION   MM   DD   YY   FROM   TO   MM   DD   YY

17. NAME OF REFERRING PHYSICIAN OR OTHER SOURCE

17a. I.D. NUMBER OF REFERRING PHYSICIAN

18. HOSPITALIZATION DATES RELATED TO CURRENT SERVICES   MM   DD   YY   FROM   TO   MM   DD   YY

19. RESERVED FOR LOCAL USE

20. OUTSIDE LAB? $ CHARGES
YES   NO

21. DIAGNOSIS OR NATURE OF ILLNESS OR INJURY. (RELATE ITEMS 1,2,3 OR 4 TO ITEM 24E BY LINE)
1. _____   3. _____
2. _____   4. _____

22. MEDICAID RESUBMISSION CODE   ORIGINAL REF. NO.

23. PRIOR AUTHORIZATION NUMBER

24. A DATE(S) OF SERVICE		B Place of Service	C Type of Service	D PROCEDURES, SERVICES, OR SUPPLIES (Explain Unusual Circumstances) CPT/HCPCS MODIFIER	E DIAGNOSIS CODE	F $ CHARGES	G DAYS OR UNITS	H EPSDT Family Plan	I EMG	J COB	K RESERVED FOR LOCAL USE
From MM DD YY	To MM DD YY										
1											
2											
3											
4											
5											

25. FEDERAL TAX I.D. NUMBER   SSN   EIN

26. PATIENT'S ACCOUNT NO.

27. ACCEPT ASSIGNMENT? (For govt. claims, see back)
YES   NO

28. TOTAL CHARGE $

29. AMOUNT PAID $

30. BALANCE DUE $

31. SIGNATURE OF PHYSICIAN OR SUPPLIER INCLUDING DEGREES OR CREDENTIALS (I certify that the statements on the reverse apply to this bill and are made a part thereof.)
SIGNED _____ DATE _____

32. NAME AND ADDRESS OF FACILITY WHERE SERVICES WERE RENDERED (If other than home or office)

33. PHYSICIAN'S, SUPPLIER'S BILLING NAME, ADDRESS, ZIP CODE & PHONE #
PIN#   GRP#

(APPROVED BY AMA COUNCIL ON MEDICAL SERVICE 8/88)   **PLEASE PRINT OR TYPE**   APPROVED OMB-0938-0008 FORM CMS-1500 (12-90), FORM RRB-1500,
APPROVED OMB-1215-0055 FORM OWCP-1500, APPROVED OMB-0720-0001 (CHAMPUS)

PATIENT AND INSURED INFORMATION

PHYSICIAN OR SUPPLIER INFORMATION

Figure A-1 A sample CMS-1500 (12/90) form prior to the National Provider Identifier (NPI) updates.

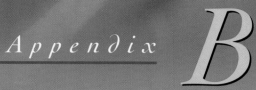

Sample Completed Claim Forms

BLUE CROSS AND BLUE SHIELD OF XY
PO BOX 1212
DUBUQUE XT 44444-1212

HEALTH INSURANCE CLAIM FORM

1. MEDICARE (Medicare #)	MEDICAID (Medicaid #)	TRICARE CHAMPUS (Sponsor's SSN)	CHAMPVA (Member ID#) [X]	GROUP HEALTH PLAN (SSN or ID)	FECA BLK LUNG (SSN)	OTHER (ID)	1a. INSURED'S I.D. NUMBER (For Program in Item 1) XQQ001BC1234

2. PATIENT'S NAME (Last Name, First Name, Middle Initial)	3. PATIENT'S BIRTH DATE	SEX	4. INSURED'S NAME (Last Name, First Name, Middle Initial)
BERTRAND MILDRED P	MM 03 DD 18 YY 1956	M F [X]	SAME

5. PATIENT'S ADDRESS (No., Street)
2001 WEST MAPLE STREET

6. PATIENT RELATIONSHIP TO INSURED
Self [X] Spouse Child Other

7. INSURED'S ADDRESS (No., Street)

CITY MIDDLETOWN   STATE XT

8. PATIENT STATUS
Single [X] Married Other

CITY   STATE

ZIP CODE 12345   TELEPHONE (Include Area Code) (555) 234 8888

Employed [X] Full-Time Student Part-Time Student

ZIP CODE   TELEPHONE (INCLUDE AREA CODE) ( )

9. OTHER INSURED'S NAME (Last Name, First Name, Middle Initial)

10. IS PATIENT'S CONDITION RELATED TO:

11. INSURED'S POLICY GROUP OR FECA NUMBER

a. OTHER INSURED'S POLICY OR GROUP NUMBER

a. EMPLOYMENT? (CURRENT OR PREVIOUS)
YES NO [X]

a. INSURED'S DATE OF BIRTH MM DD YY   SEX M F

b. OTHER INSURED'S DATE OF BIRTH MM DD YY   SEX M F

b. AUTO ACCIDENT?   PLACE (State)
YES NO [X]

b. EMPLOYER'S NAME OR SCHOOL NAME

c. EMPLOYER'S NAME OR SCHOOL NAME

c. OTHER ACCIDENT?
YES NO [X]

c. INSURANCE PLAN NAME OR PROGRAM NAME

d. INSURANCE PLAN NAME OR PROGRAM NAME

10d. RESERVED FOR LOCAL USE

d. IS THERE ANOTHER HEALTH BENEFIT PLAN?
YES NO [X] *If yes,* return to and complete item 9 a-d.

READ BACK OF FORM BEFORE COMPLETING & SIGNING THIS FORM.
12. PATIENT'S OR AUTHORIZED PERSON'S SIGNATURE I authorize the release of any medical or other information necessary to process this claim. I also request payment of government benefits either to myself or to the party who accepts assignment below.

SIGNED SIGNATURE ON FILE   DATE

13. INSURED'S OR AUTHORIZED PERSON'S SIGNATURE I authorize payment of medical benefits to the undersigned physician or supplier for services described below.

SIGNED

14. DATE OF CURRENT: ILLNESS (First symptom) OR INJURY (Accident) OR PREGNANCY(LMP)
MM 01 DD 21 YY XX

15. IF PATIENT HAS HAD SAME OR SIMILAR ILLNESS. GIVE FIRST DATE MM DD YY

16. DATES PATIENT UNABLE TO WORK IN CURRENT OCCUPATION
FROM MM DD YY   TO MM DD YY

17. NAME OF REFERRING PHYSICIAN OR OTHER SOURCE
R L JONES M D

17a.
17b. NPI 1234567890

18. HOSPITALIZATION DATES RELATED TO CURRENT SERVICES
FROM MM DD YY   TO MM DD YY

19. RESERVED FOR LOCAL USE

20. OUTSIDE LAB? $ CHARGES
YES NO [X]

21. DIAGNOSIS OR NATURE OF ILLNESS OR INJURY. (RELATE ITEMS 1,2,3 OR 4 TO ITEM 24E BY LINE)
1. 788 41
3.
2.
4.

22. MEDICAID RESUBMISSION CODE   ORIGINAL REF. NO.

23. PRIOR AUTHORIZATION NUMBER

24. A. DATE(S) OF SERVICE From MM DD YY	To MM DD YY	B. PLACE OF SERVICE	C. EMG	D. PROCEDURES, SERVICES, OR SUPPLIES (Explain Unusual Circumstances) CPT/HCPCS	MODIFIER	E. DIAGNOSIS POINTER	F. $ CHARGES	G. DAYS OR UNITS	H. EPSDT Family Plan	I. ID. QUAL.	J. RENDERING PROVIDER ID. #
1	01 24 XX	01 24 XX	11		99202		1	50 00	1		NPI	1234567890
2	01 24 XX	01 24 XX	11		81002		1	15 00	1		NPI	1234567890
3											NPI	
4											NPI	
5											NPI	
6											NPI	

25. FEDERAL TAX I.D. NUMBER   SSN EIN
42 1898989   [X]

26. PATIENT'S ACCOUNT NO.
3201

27. ACCEPT ASSIGNMENT? (For govt. claims, see back)
YES [X] NO

28. TOTAL CHARGE
$ 65 00

29. AMOUNT PAID
$

30. BALANCE DUE
$

31. SIGNATURE OF PHYSICIAN OR SUPPLIER INCLUDING DEGREES OR CREDENTIALS (I certify that the statements on the reverse apply to this bill and are made a part thereof.)
R L Jones MD
R L Jones
SIGNED   012520XX   DATE

32. SERVICE FACILITY LOCATION INFORMATION
BROADMOOR MEDICAL CLINIC
4353 PINE RIDGE DRIVE
MILTON XY 12345-0001
a. X100XX1000   b.

33. BILLING PROVIDER INFO & PH # (555) 6567890
BROADMOOR MEDICAL CLINIC
4353 PINE RIDGE DRIVE
MILTON XY 12345-0001
a. X100XX1000   b.

CARRIER | PATIENT AND INSURED INFORMATION | PHYSICIAN OR SUPPLIER INFORMATION

Figure B-1 (Bertrand): BCBS; no secondary.

Sample claim forms are for example only. Diagnostic and Procedural codes are subject to annual updates.

MEDICAID FISCAL INTERMEDIARY
STREET ADDRESS
CITY STATE AND ZIP

HEALTH INSURANCE CLAIM FORM

CARRIER

1. MEDICARE	MEDICAID	TRICARE CHAMPUS	CHAMPVA	GROUP HEALTH PLAN	FECA BLK LUNG	OTHER	1a. INSURED'S I.D. NUMBER	(For Program in Item 1)
☐ (Medicare #)	☒ (Medicaid #)	☐ (Sponsor's SSN)	☐ (Member ID#)	☐ (SSN or ID)	☐ (SSN)	☐ (ID)	92881044PL22	

2. PATIENT'S NAME (Last Name, First Name, Middle Initial)	3. PATIENT'S BIRTH DATE / SEX	4. INSURED'S NAME (Last Name, First Name, Middle Initial)
MARSALIS ELOISE A	MM 09 DD 08 YY 2000 M ☐ F ☒	

5. PATIENT'S ADDRESS (No., Street)	6. PATIENT RELATIONSHIP TO INSURED	7. INSURED'S ADDRESS (No., Street)
208 OAKLAWN LOT 402	Self ☐ Spouse ☐ Child ☐ Other ☐	

CITY	STATE	8. PATIENT STATUS	CITY	STATE
MILTON	XT	Single ☐ Married ☐ Other ☐		

ZIP CODE	TELEPHONE (Include Area Code)		ZIP CODE	TELEPHONE (INCLUDE AREA CODE)
12345	(555) 234 7112	Employed ☐ Full-Time Student ☐ Part-Time Student ☐		( )

9. OTHER INSURED'S NAME (Last Name, First Name, Middle Initial)	10. IS PATIENT'S CONDITION RELATED TO:	11. INSURED'S POLICY GROUP OR FECA NUMBER

a. OTHER INSURED'S POLICY OR GROUP NUMBER	a. EMPLOYMENT? (CURRENT OR PREVIOUS) ☐ YES ☒ NO	a. INSURED'S DATE OF BIRTH MM DD YY SEX M ☐ F ☐

b. OTHER INSURED'S DATE OF BIRTH MM DD YY SEX M ☐ F ☐	b. AUTO ACCIDENT? PLACE (State) ☐ YES ☒ NO	b. EMPLOYER'S NAME OR SCHOOL NAME

c. EMPLOYER'S NAME OR SCHOOL NAME	c. OTHER ACCIDENT? ☐ YES ☒ NO	c. INSURANCE PLAN NAME OR PROGRAM NAME

d. INSURANCE PLAN NAME OR PROGRAM NAME	10d. RESERVED FOR LOCAL USE	d. IS THERE ANOTHER HEALTH BENEFIT PLAN? ☐ YES ☐ NO *If yes*, return to and complete item 9 a-d.

READ BACK OF FORM BEFORE COMPLETING & SIGNING THIS FORM.

12. PATIENT'S OR AUTHORIZED PERSON'S SIGNATURE I authorize the release of any medical or other information necessary to process this claim. I also request payment of government benefits either to myself or to the party who accepts assignment below.

SIGNED _____ DATE _____

13. INSURED'S OR AUTHORIZED PERSON'S SIGNATURE I authorize payment of medical benefits to the undersigned physician or supplier for services described below.

SIGNED _____

PATIENT AND INSURED INFORMATION

14. DATE OF CURRENT: ILLNESS (First symptom) OR INJURY (Accident) OR PREGNANCY(LMP) MM DD YY	15. IF PATIENT HAS HAD SAME OR SIMILAR ILLNESS. GIVE FIRST DATE MM DD YY	16. DATES PATIENT UNABLE TO WORK IN CURRENT OCCUPATION FROM MM DD YY TO MM DD YY

17. NAME OF REFERRING PHYSICIAN OR OTHER SOURCE	17a.	18. HOSPITALIZATION DATES RELATED TO CURRENT SERVICES FROM MM DD YY TO MM DD YY
	17b. NPI	

19. RESERVED FOR LOCAL USE	20. OUTSIDE LAB? ☐ YES ☒ NO $ CHARGES

21. DIAGNOSIS OR NATURE OF ILLNESS OR INJURY. (RELATE ITEMS 1,2,3 OR 4 TO ITEM 24E BY LINE)

1. 308.1
2. _____ . _____
3. _____ . _____
4. _____ . _____

22. MEDICAID RESUBMISSION CODE _____ ORIGINAL REF. NO. _____

23. PRIOR AUTHORIZATION NUMBER

24. A. DATE(S) OF SERVICE From MM DD YY To MM DD YY	B. PLACE OF SERVICE	C. EMG	D. PROCEDURES, SERVICES, OR SUPPLIES (Explain Unusual Circumstances) CPT/HCPCS MODIFIER	E. DIAGNOSIS POINTER	F. $ CHARGES	G. DAYS OR UNITS	H. EPSDT Family Plan	I. ID. QUAL.	J. RENDERING PROVIDER ID. #
1	01 24 XX 01 24 XX	11		99213	1	75 00	1		NPI	1234567890
2									NPI	
3									NPI	
4									NPI	
5									NPI	
6									NPI	

25. FEDERAL TAX I.D. NUMBER SSN EIN	26. PATIENT'S ACCOUNT NO.	27. ACCEPT ASSIGNMENT? (For govt. claims, see back)	28. TOTAL CHARGE	29. AMOUNT PAID	30. BALANCE DUE
42 1898989 ☒	2644	☒ YES ☐ NO	$ 75 00	$ 00 00	$

31. SIGNATURE OF PHYSICIAN OR SUPPLIER INCLUDING DEGREES OR CREDENTIALS (I certify that the statements on the reverse apply to this bill and are made a part thereof.)	32. SERVICE FACILITY LOCATION INFORMATION	33. BILLING PROVIDER INFO & PH # (555) 6567890
R L Jones MD *R L Jones* SIGNED 012520XX DATE	BROADMOOR MEDICAL CLINIC 4353 PINE RIDGE DRIVE MILTON XY 12345-0001 a. X100XX1000 b.	BROADMOOR MEDICAL CLINIC 4353 PINE RIDGE DRIVE MILTON XY 12345-0001 a. X100XX1000 b.

PHYSICIAN OR SUPPLIER INFORMATION

Figure B-2 (Marsalis): Medicaid; no secondary.

MEDICARE CARRIER
STREET ADDRESS OR PO BOX NUMBER
CITY STATE ZIP

HEALTH INSURANCE CLAIM FORM

CARRIER

1. MEDICARE [X] (Medicare #)	MEDICAID [ ] (Medicaid #)	TRICARE CHAMPUS [ ] (Sponsor's SSN)	CHAMPVA [ ] (Member ID#)	GROUP HEALTH PLAN [ ] (SSN or ID)	FECA BLK LUNG [ ] (SSN)	OTHER [ ] (ID)	1a. INSURED'S I.D. NUMBER (For Program in Item 1)

181401234A

2. PATIENT'S NAME (Last Name, First Name, Middle Initial)

MARTINSON FREDERICK T

3. PATIENT'S BIRTH DATE
MM 10 | DD 18 | YY 1940   M [X]   F [ ]   SEX

4. INSURED'S NAME (Last Name, First Name, Middle Initial)

5. PATIENT'S ADDRESS (No., Street)

2300 PARNELL AVENUE

6. PATIENT RELATIONSHIP TO INSURED
Self [X] Spouse [ ] Child [ ] Other [ ]

7. INSURED'S ADDRESS (No., Street)

CITY **MELTON**   STATE **XT**

8. PATIENT STATUS
Single [ ] Married [X] Other [ ]
Employed [ ] Full-Time Student [ ] Part-Time Student [ ]

CITY   STATE

ZIP CODE **12345**   TELEPHONE (Include Area Code) **(555) 234 0001**

ZIP CODE   TELEPHONE (INCLUDE AREA CODE) **( )**

9. OTHER INSURED'S NAME (Last Name, First Name, Middle Initial)

10. IS PATIENT'S CONDITION RELATED TO:

11. INSURED'S POLICY GROUP OR FECA NUMBER

NONE

a. OTHER INSURED'S POLICY OR GROUP NUMBER

a. EMPLOYMENT? (CURRENT OR PREVIOUS)
YES [ ] NO [X]

a. INSURED'S DATE OF BIRTH MM | DD | YY   M [ ] F [ ] SEX

b. OTHER INSURED'S DATE OF BIRTH MM | DD | YY   M [ ] F [ ] SEX

b. AUTO ACCIDENT?   PLACE (State)
YES [ ] NO [X]

b. EMPLOYER'S NAME OR SCHOOL NAME

c. EMPLOYER'S NAME OR SCHOOL NAME

c. OTHER ACCIDENT?
YES [ ] NO [X]

c. INSURANCE PLAN NAME OR PROGRAM NAME

d. INSURANCE PLAN NAME OR PROGRAM NAME

10d. RESERVED FOR LOCAL USE

d. IS THERE ANOTHER HEALTH BENEFIT PLAN?
YES [ ] NO [ ] **If yes**, return to and complete item 9 a-d.

READ BACK OF FORM BEFORE COMPLETING & SIGNING THIS FORM.
12. PATIENT'S OR AUTHORIZED PERSON'S SIGNATURE I authorize the release of any medical or other information necessary to process this claim. I also request payment of government benefits either to myself or to the party who accepts assignment below.

SIGNED **SIGNATURE ON FILE** DATE ____

13. INSURED'S OR AUTHORIZED PERSON'S SIGNATURE I authorize payment of medical benefits to the undersigned physician or supplier for services described below.

SIGNED ____

PATIENT AND INSURED INFORMATION

14. DATE OF CURRENT: ILLNESS (First symptom) OR INJURY (Accident) OR PREGNANCY(LMP)
MM | DD | YY

15. IF PATIENT HAS HAD SAME OR SIMILAR ILLNESS. GIVE FIRST DATE MM | DD | YY

16. DATES PATIENT UNABLE TO WORK IN CURRENT OCCUPATION
FROM MM | DD | YY   TO MM | DD | YY

17. NAME OF REFERRING PHYSICIAN OR OTHER SOURCE
17a.
17b. NPI

18. HOSPITALIZATION DATES RELATED TO CURRENT SERVICES
FROM MM | DD | YY   TO MM | DD | YY

19. RESERVED FOR LOCAL USE

20. OUTSIDE LAB? $ CHARGES
YES [ ] NO [X]

21. DIAGNOSIS OR NATURE OF ILLNESS OR INJURY. (RELATE ITEMS 1,2,3 OR 4 TO ITEM 24E BY LINE)
1. 401.1
2. ___.___
3. ___.___
4. ___.___

22. MEDICAID RESUBMISSION CODE   ORIGINAL REF. NO.

23. PRIOR AUTHORIZATION NUMBER

24. A. DATE(S) OF SERVICE From MM DD YY	To MM DD YY	B. PLACE OF SERVICE	C. EMG	D. PROCEDURES, SERVICES, OR SUPPLIES (Explain Unusual Circumstances) CPT/HCPCS | MODIFIER	E. DIAGNOSIS POINTER	F. $ CHARGES	G. DAYS OR UNITS	H. EPSDT Family Plan	I. ID. QUAL.	J. RENDERING PROVIDER ID. #
1	01 25 XX	01 25 XX	11		99213	1	75 00	1		NPI	1234567890
2										NPI	
3										NPI	
4										NPI	
5										NPI	
6										NPI	

PHYSICIAN OR SUPPLIER INFORMATION

25. FEDERAL TAX I.D. NUMBER **42 1898989**   SSN [ ] EIN [X]

26. PATIENT'S ACCOUNT NO. **2774**

27. ACCEPT ASSIGNMENT? (For govt. claims, see back) YES [X] NO [ ]

28. TOTAL CHARGE $ **75 00**

29. AMOUNT PAID $ **00 00**

30. BALANCE DUE $

31. SIGNATURE OF PHYSICIAN OR SUPPLIER INCLUDING DEGREES OR CREDENTIALS (I certify that the statements on the reverse apply to this bill and are made a part thereof.)
R L Jones MD
R L Jones
SIGNED   DATE **012620XX**

32. SERVICE FACILITY LOCATION INFORMATION
**BROADMOOR MEDICAL CLINIC
4353 PINE RIDGE DRIVE
MILTON XY 12345-0001**
a. X100XX1000   b.

33. BILLING PROVIDER INFO & PH # **(555) 6567890**
**BROADMOOR MEDICAL CLINIC
4353 PINE RIDGE DRIVE
MILTON XY 12345-0001**
a. X100XX1000   b.

Figure B-3 (Martinson): Medicare (simple).

MEDICARE CARRIER
STREET ADDRESS OR PO BOX NUMBER
CITY STATE ZIP

HEALTH INSURANCE CLAIM FORM

1. MEDICARE	MEDICAID	TRICARE CHAMPUS	CHAMPVA	GROUP HEALTH PLAN	FECA BLK LUNG	OTHER	1a. INSURED'S I.D. NUMBER (For Program in Item 1)
X (Medicare #)	X (Medicaid #)	(Sponsor's SSN)	(Member ID#)	(SSN or ID)	(SSN)	(ID)	233991110D

2. PATIENT'S NAME (Last Name, First Name, Middle Initial)
ATKINSON PRICILLA M

3. PATIENT'S BIRTH DATE MM 11 DD 04 YY 1934 SEX M ☐ F X

4. INSURED'S NAME (Last Name, First Name, Middle Initial)

5. PATIENT'S ADDRESS (No., Street)
52 SUNSET CIRCLE

6. PATIENT RELATIONSHIP TO INSURED
Self X Spouse ☐ Child ☐ Other ☐

7. INSURED'S ADDRESS (No., Street)

CITY MILTON	STATE XT	8. PATIENT STATUS	CITY	STATE

8. PATIENT STATUS: Single X Married ☐ Other ☐

ZIP CODE 12345 **TELEPHONE (Include Area Code)** (555) 234 5454

Employed ☐ Full-Time Student ☐ Part-Time Student ☐

ZIP CODE **TELEPHONE (INCLUDE AREA CODE)** ( )

9. OTHER INSURED'S NAME (Last Name, First Name, Middle Initial)

10. IS PATIENT'S CONDITION RELATED TO:

11. INSURED'S POLICY GROUP OR FECA NUMBER
NONE

a. OTHER INSURED'S POLICY OR GROUP NUMBER

a. EMPLOYMENT? (CURRENT OR PREVIOUS) YES ☐ NO X

a. INSURED'S DATE OF BIRTH MM DD YY SEX M ☐ F ☐

b. OTHER INSURED'S DATE OF BIRTH MM DD YY SEX M ☐ F ☐

b. AUTO ACCIDENT? PLACE (State) YES ☐ NO X

b. EMPLOYER'S NAME OR SCHOOL NAME

c. EMPLOYER'S NAME OR SCHOOL NAME

c. OTHER ACCIDENT? YES ☐ NO X

c. INSURANCE PLAN NAME OR PROGRAM NAME

d. INSURANCE PLAN NAME OR PROGRAM NAME

10d. RESERVED FOR LOCAL USE
MCD00234MA16

d. IS THERE ANOTHER HEALTH BENEFIT PLAN? YES ☐ NO ☐ *If yes*, return to and complete item 9 a-d.

READ BACK OF FORM BEFORE COMPLETING & SIGNING THIS FORM.
12. PATIENT'S OR AUTHORIZED PERSON'S SIGNATURE I authorize the release of any medical or other information necessary to process this claim. I also request payment of government benefits either to myself or to the party who accepts assignment below.

SIGNED **SIGNATURE ON FILE** DATE

13. INSURED'S OR AUTHORIZED PERSON'S SIGNATURE I authorize payment of medical benefits to the undersigned physician or supplier for services described below.

SIGNED

14. DATE OF CURRENT: MM DD YY ILLNESS (First symptom) OR INJURY (Accident) OR PREGNANCY(LMP)

15. IF PATIENT HAS HAD SAME OR SIMILAR ILLNESS. GIVE FIRST DATE MM DD YY

16. DATES PATIENT UNABLE TO WORK IN CURRENT OCCUPATION FROM MM DD YY TO MM DD YY

17. NAME OF REFERRING PHYSICIAN OR OTHER SOURCE
R L JONES

17a.
17b. NPI 1234567890

18. HOSPITALIZATION DATES RELATED TO CURRENT SERVICES FROM MM DD YY TO MM DD YY

19. RESERVED FOR LOCAL USE

20. OUTSIDE LAB? YES ☐ NO X $ CHARGES

21. DIAGNOSIS OR NATURE OF ILLNESS OR INJURY. (RELATE ITEMS 1,2,3 OR 4 TO ITEM 24E BY LINE)
1. 714 .31
2. ___ . ___
3. ___ . ___
4. ___ . ___

22. MEDICAID RESUBMISSION CODE ORIGINAL REF. NO.

23. PRIOR AUTHORIZATION NUMBER

24. A. DATE(S) OF SERVICE From MM DD YY	To MM DD YY	B. PLACE OF SERVICE	C. EMG	D. PROCEDURES, SERVICES, OR SUPPLIES (Explain Unusual Circumstances) CPT/HCPCS MODIFIER	E. DIAGNOSIS POINTER	F. $ CHARGES	G. DAYS OR UNITS	H. EPSDT Family Plan	I. ID. QUAL.	J. RENDERING PROVIDER ID. #
1	01 24 XX	01 24 XX	11		99214	1	115 00	1		NPI	1234567890
2	01 24 XX	01 24 XX	11		J0800	1	25 00	1		NPI	1234567890
3										NPI	
4										NPI	
5										NPI	
6										NPI	

25. FEDERAL TAX I.D. NUMBER 42 1898989 SSN ☐ EIN X

26. PATIENT'S ACCOUNT NO. 2340

27. ACCEPT ASSIGNMENT? (For govt. claims, see back) YES X NO ☐

28. TOTAL CHARGE $ 140 00

29. AMOUNT PAID $ 00 00

30. BALANCE DUE $

31. SIGNATURE OF PHYSICIAN OR SUPPLIER INCLUDING DEGREES OR CREDENTIALS (I certify that the statements on the reverse apply to this bill and are made a part thereof.)
R L Jones MD
R L Jones
SIGNED 012520XX DATE

32. SERVICE FACILITY LOCATION INFORMATION
BROADMOOR MEDICAL CLINIC
4353 PINE RIDGE DRIVE
MILTON XY 12345-0001
a. X100XX1000 b.

33. BILLING PROVIDER INFO & PH # (555) 6567890
BROADMOOR MEDICAL CLINIC
4353 PINE RIDGE DRIVE
MILTON XY 12345-0001
a. X100XX1000 b.

Figure B-4 (Atkinson): Medicare/Medicaid.

MEDICARE CARRIER
STREET ADDRESS OR PO BOX NUMBER
CITY STATE ZIP

HEALTH INSURANCE CLAIM FORM

1. MEDICARE [X] (Medicare #)	MEDICAID [ ] (Medicaid #)	TRICARE CHAMPUS [ ] (Sponsor's SSN)	CHAMPVA [ ] (Member ID#)	GROUP HEALTH PLAN [X] (SSN or ID)	FECA BLK LUNG [ ] (SSN)	OTHER [ ] (ID)	1a. INSURED'S I.D. NUMBER (For Program in Item 1) 343668110A

2. PATIENT'S NAME (Last Name, First Name, Middle Initial)
FREEMAN OZWALD N

3. PATIENT'S BIRTH DATE MM 10 | DD 16 | YY 1933 SEX M [X] F [ ]

4. INSURED'S NAME (Last Name, First Name, Middle Initial)

5. PATIENT'S ADDRESS (No., Street)
1111 DOBSON CREEK ROAD

6. PATIENT RELATIONSHIP TO INSURED
Self [X] Spouse [ ] Child [ ] Other [ ]

7. INSURED'S ADDRESS (No., Street)

CITY **MILTON** STATE **XT**

8. PATIENT STATUS
Single [ ] Married [X] Other [ ]
Employed [ ] Full-Time Student [ ] Part-Time Student [ ]

CITY STATE

ZIP CODE **12345** TELEPHONE (Include Area Code) **(555) 234 3321**

ZIP CODE TELEPHONE (INCLUDE AREA CODE) ( )

9. OTHER INSURED'S NAME (Last Name, First Name, Middle Initial)
SAME

10. IS PATIENT'S CONDITION RELATED TO:

11. INSURED'S POLICY GROUP OR FECA NUMBER
NONE

a. OTHER INSURED'S POLICY OR GROUP NUMBER
MGAP 274805022F

a. EMPLOYMENT? (CURRENT OR PREVIOUS)
YES [ ] NO [X]

a. INSURED'S DATE OF BIRTH MM | DD | YY SEX M [ ] F [ ]

b. OTHER INSURED'S DATE OF BIRTH MM 10 | DD 16 | YY 1933 SEX M [X] F [ ]

b. AUTO ACCIDENT? PLACE (State)
YES [ ] NO [X]

b. EMPLOYER'S NAME OR SCHOOL NAME

c. EMPLOYER'S NAME OR SCHOOL NAME

c. OTHER ACCIDENT?
YES [ ] NO [X]

c. INSURANCE PLAN NAME OR PROGRAM NAME

d. INSURANCE PLAN NAME OR PROGRAM NAME
XT002245678

10d. RESERVED FOR LOCAL USE

d. IS THERE ANOTHER HEALTH BENEFIT PLAN?
YES [ ] NO [ ] If yes, return to and complete item 9 a-d.

READ BACK OF FORM BEFORE COMPLETING & SIGNING THIS FORM.
12. PATIENT'S OR AUTHORIZED PERSON'S SIGNATURE I authorize the release of any medical or other information necessary to process this claim. I also request payment of government benefits either to myself or to the party who accepts assignment below.

SIGNED **SIGNATURE ON FILE** DATE

13. INSURED'S OR AUTHORIZED PERSON'S SIGNATURE I authorize payment of medical benefits to the undersigned physician or supplier for services described below.

SIGNED

14. DATE OF CURRENT: ILLNESS (First symptom) OR INJURY (Accident) OR PREGNANCY(LMP) MM | DD | YY

15. IF PATIENT HAS HAD SAME OR SIMILAR ILLNESS. GIVE FIRST DATE MM | DD | YY

16. DATES PATIENT UNABLE TO WORK IN CURRENT OCCUPATION FROM MM | DD | YY TO MM | DD | YY

17. NAME OF REFERRING PHYSICIAN OR OTHER SOURCE
MARILOU LUCERO MD
17a.
17b. NPI **2907511822**

18. HOSPITALIZATION DATES RELATED TO CURRENT SERVICES FROM MM | DD | YY TO MM | DD | YY

19. RESERVED FOR LOCAL USE

20. OUTSIDE LAB? YES [ ] NO [X] $ CHARGES

21. DIAGNOSIS OR NATURE OF ILLNESS OR INJURY. (RELATE ITEMS 1,2,3 OR 4 TO ITEM 24E BY LINE)
1. 786.50
2.
3.
4.

22. MEDICAID RESUBMISSION CODE ORIGINAL REF. NO.

23. PRIOR AUTHORIZATION NUMBER

24. A. DATE(S) OF SERVICE From MM DD YY	To MM DD YY	B. PLACE OF SERVICE	C. EMG	D. PROCEDURES, SERVICES, OR SUPPLIES (Explain Unusual Circumstances) CPT/HCPCS	MODIFIER	E. DIAGNOSIS POINTER	F. $ CHARGES	G. DAYS OR UNITS	H. EPSDT Family Plan	I. ID. QUAL.	J. RENDERING PROVIDER ID. #
1	01 24 XX	01 24 XX	11		99214		1	115 00	1		NPI	2907511822
2	01 24 XX	01 24 XX	11		93350		1	175 00	1		NPI	2907511822
3	01 24 XX	01 24 XX	11		93017		1	55 00	1		NPI	2907511822
4											NPI	
5											NPI	
6											NPI	

25. FEDERAL TAX I.D. NUMBER **42 1898989** SSN [ ] EIN [X]

26. PATIENT'S ACCOUNT NO. **2544**

27. ACCEPT ASSIGNMENT? (For govt. claims, see back) [X] YES [ ] NO

28. TOTAL CHARGE $ **345 00**

29. AMOUNT PAID $ **00 00**

30. BALANCE DUE $

31. SIGNATURE OF PHYSICIAN OR SUPPLIER INCLUDING DEGREES OR CREDENTIALS (I certify that the statements on the reverse apply to this bill and are made a part thereof.)
Marilou Lucero
Marilou Lucero SIGNED 012520XX DATE

32. SERVICE FACILITY LOCATION INFORMATION
BROADMOOR MEDICAL CLINIC
4353 PINE RIDGE DRIVE
MILTON XY 12345-0001
a. X100XX1000 b.

33. BILLING PROVIDER INFO & PH # (555) 6567890
BROADMOOR MEDICAL CLINIC
4353 PINE RIDGE DRIVE
MILTON XY 12345-0001
a. X100XX1000 b.

Figure B-5 (Freeman): Medicare/Medigap.

EDU BENEFITS INC
15055 144TH AV SUITE 6B
GRANITE FALLS XT 34567

HEALTH INSURANCE CLAIM FORM

1. MEDICARE	MEDICAID	TRICARE CHAMPUS	CHAMPVA	GROUP HEALTH PLAN	FECA BLK LUNG	OTHER	1a. INSURED'S I.D. NUMBER (For Program in Item 1)
X (Medicare #)	(Medicaid #)	(Sponsor's SSN)	(Member ID#)	X (SSN or ID)	(SSN)	(ID)	222553320A

2. PATIENT'S NAME (Last Name, First Name, Middle Initial)
FRANKLIN ALMA L

3. PATIENT'S BIRTH DATE: 05 02 1941 SEX: F X

4. INSURED'S NAME (Last Name, First Name, Middle Initial)
FRANKLIN JOSEPH P

5. PATIENT'S ADDRESS (No., Street)
89 BRIDGEWAY
CITY: MILTON STATE: XT
ZIP CODE: 12345 TELEPHONE: (555) 234 1009

6. PATIENT RELATIONSHIP TO INSURED: Spouse X

7. INSURED'S ADDRESS (No., Street)
SAME

8. PATIENT STATUS: Married X ; Employed X

9. OTHER INSURED'S NAME

10. IS PATIENT'S CONDITION RELATED TO:
a. EMPLOYMENT? NO X
b. AUTO ACCIDENT? NO X
c. OTHER ACCIDENT? NO X

11. INSURED'S POLICY GROUP OR FECA NUMBER
XWT8739995
a. INSURED'S DATE OF BIRTH: 06 27 1938 M X
b. EMPLOYER'S NAME OR SCHOOL NAME
FLINT RIVER SCHOOL DISTRICT
c. INSURANCE PLAN NAME OR PROGRAM NAME
EDU BENEFITS INC
d. IS THERE ANOTHER HEALTH BENEFIT PLAN? NO

12. PATIENT'S SIGNATURE: SOF

13. INSURED'S SIGNATURE: SOF

14. DATE OF CURRENT: 01 16 XX
15. IF PATIENT HAS HAD SAME OR SIMILAR ILLNESS.
16. DATES PATIENT UNABLE TO WORK: FROM 01 16 XX TO 01 24 XX
17. NAME OF REFERRING PHYSICIAN: RONALD K PEPPERDINE MD
17b. NPI 3256654001
18. HOSPITALIZATION DATES
20. OUTSIDE LAB? NO X

21. DIAGNOSIS OR NATURE OF ILLNESS OR INJURY
1. 511.0

24. A. DATE(S) OF SERVICE From / To	B. PLACE	C. EMG	D. CPT/HCPCS	MODIFIER	E. DIAG PTR	F. $ CHARGES	G. UNITS	H.	I. QUAL	J. RENDERING PROVIDER ID #
01 20 XX 01 20 XX	11		99203		1	55 00	1		NPI	1234567890
01 20 XX 01 20 XX	11		71023		1	90 00	1		NPI	1234567890

25. FEDERAL TAX I.D. NUMBER: 42 1898989 X
26. PATIENT'S ACCOUNT NO.: 3322
27. ACCEPT ASSIGNMENT? YES X
28. TOTAL CHARGE: $145 00
29. AMOUNT PAID: $0 00
30. BALANCE DUE

31. SIGNATURE OF PHYSICIAN: R L Jones MD 012520XX
32. SERVICE FACILITY: BROADMOOR MEDICAL CLINIC, 4353 PINE RIDGE DRIVE, MILTON XY 12345-0001 a. X100XX1000
33. BILLING PROVIDER INFO & PH #: (555) 6567890 BROADMOOR MEDICAL CLINIC, 4353 PINE RIDGE DRIVE, MILTON XY 12345-0001 a. X100XX1000

Figure B-6 (Franklin): Group with Medicare Secondary.

TRICARE CARRIER NAME
STREET ADDRESS OR PO NUMBER
CITY STATE ZIP CODE

HEALTH INSURANCE CLAIM FORM

1. MEDICARE (Medicare #)	MEDICAID (Medicaid #)	TRICARE CHAMPUS [X] (Sponsor's SSN)	CHAMPVA (Member ID#)	GROUP HEALTH PLAN (SSN or ID)	FECA BLK LUNG (SSN)	OTHER (ID)	1a. INSURED'S I.D. NUMBER (For Program in Item 1) 321549876

2. PATIENT'S NAME (Last Name, First Name, Middle Initial) SINCLAIR EMILY J	3. PATIENT'S BIRTH DATE MM 04 DD 17 YY 2003 M SEX F [X]	4. INSURED'S NAME (Last Name, First Name, Middle Initial) SINCLAIR PARKER L

5. PATIENT'S ADDRESS (No., Street) 1344 ARGYLE COURT	6. PATIENT RELATIONSHIP TO INSURED Self [ ] Spouse [ ] Child [X] Other [ ]	7. INSURED'S ADDRESS (No., Street) APO 53555J

CITY MILTON	STATE XT	8. PATIENT STATUS Single [X] Married [ ] Other [ ]	CITY NEW YORK	STATE NY

ZIP CODE 12345	TELEPHONE (Include Area Code) (555) 234 4111	Employed [ ] Full-Time Student [ ] Part-Time Student [ ]	ZIP CODE 22222	TELEPHONE (INCLUDE AREA CODE) ( )

9. OTHER INSURED'S NAME (Last Name, First Name, Middle Initial)	10. IS PATIENT'S CONDITION RELATED TO:	11. INSURED'S POLICY GROUP OR FECA NUMBER

a. OTHER INSURED'S POLICY OR GROUP NUMBER	a. EMPLOYMENT? (CURRENT OR PREVIOUS) YES [ ] NO [X]	a. INSURED'S DATE OF BIRTH MM 10 DD 08 YY 1988 M [X] F SEX

b. OTHER INSURED'S DATE OF BIRTH MM DD YY SEX M F	b. AUTO ACCIDENT? PLACE (State) YES [ ] NO [X]	b. EMPLOYER'S NAME OR SCHOOL NAME

c. EMPLOYER'S NAME OR SCHOOL NAME	c. OTHER ACCIDENT? YES [ ] NO [X]	c. INSURANCE PLAN NAME OR PROGRAM NAME

d. INSURANCE PLAN NAME OR PROGRAM NAME	10d. RESERVED FOR LOCAL USE	d. IS THERE ANOTHER HEALTH BENEFIT PLAN? YES [ ] NO [X] If yes, return to and complete item 9 a-d.

READ BACK OF FORM BEFORE COMPLETING & SIGNING THIS FORM.

12. PATIENT'S OR AUTHORIZED PERSON'S SIGNATURE I authorize the release of any medical or other information necessary to process this claim. I also request payment of government benefits either to myself or to the party who accepts assignment below. SIGNED SIGNATURE ON FILE DATE	13. INSURED'S OR AUTHORIZED PERSON'S SIGNATURE I authorize payment of medical benefits to the undersigned physician or supplier for services described below. SIGNED

14. DATE OF CURRENT: MM 01 DD 24 YY XX ◄ ILLNESS (First symptom) OR INJURY (Accident) OR PREGNANCY(LMP)	15. IF PATIENT HAS HAD SAME OR SIMILAR ILLNESS. GIVE FIRST DATE MM DD YY	16. DATES PATIENT UNABLE TO WORK IN CURRENT OCCUPATION FROM MM DD YY TO MM DD YY

17. NAME OF REFERRING PHYSICIAN OR OTHER SOURCE MARILOU LUCERO MD	17a. 17b. NPI 2907511822	18. HOSPITALIZATION DATES RELATED TO CURRENT SERVICES FROM MM 01 DD 19 YY XX TO MM 01 DD 22 YY XX

19. RESERVED FOR LOCAL USE	20. OUTSIDE LAB? YES [ ] NO [X] $ CHARGES

21. DIAGNOSIS OR NATURE OF ILLNESS OR INJURY. (RELATE ITEMS 1,2,3 OR 4 TO ITEM 24E BY LINE) 1. 480 . 9 3. ___ . ___ 2. ___ . ___ 4. ___ . ___	22. MEDICAID RESUBMISSION CODE ORIGINAL REF. NO. 23. PRIOR AUTHORIZATION NUMBER 0221558766

24. A. DATE(S) OF SERVICE From MM DD YY	To MM DD YY	B. PLACE OF SERVICE	C. EMG	D. PROCEDURES, SERVICES, OR SUPPLIES (Explain Unusual Circumstances) CPT/HCPCS	MODIFIER	E. DIAGNOSIS POINTER	F. $ CHARGES	G. DAYS OR UNITS	H. EPSDT Family Plan	I. ID. QUAL.	J. RENDERING PROVIDER ID. #
1	01 19 XX	01 19 XX	21		99221		1	250 00	1		NPI	2907511822
2	01 20 XX	01 21 XX	21		99231		1	150 00	1		NPI	2907511822
3	01 22 XX	01 22 XX	21		99238		1	110 00	1		NPI	2907511822
4											NPI	
5											NPI	
6											NPI	

25. FEDERAL TAX I.D. NUMBER 42 1898989 SSN [ ] EIN [X]	26. PATIENT'S ACCOUNT NO. 2343	27. ACCEPT ASSIGNMENT? (For govt. claims, see back) [X] YES [ ] NO	28. TOTAL CHARGE $ 510 00	29. AMOUNT PAID $ 00 00	30. BALANCE DUE $

31. SIGNATURE OF PHYSICIAN OR SUPPLIER INCLUDING DEGREES OR CREDENTIALS (I certify that the statements on the reverse apply to this bill and are made a part thereof.) Marilou Lucero *Marilou Lucero* 012520XX SIGNED DATE	32. SERVICE FACILITY LOCATION INFORMATION BROADMOOR MEDICAL CLINIC 4353 PINE RIDGE DRIVE MILTON XY 12345-0001 a. X100XX1000 b.	33. BILLING PROVIDER INFO & PH # (555) 6567890 BROADMOOR MEDICAL CLINIC 4353 PINE RIDGE DRIVE MILTON XY 12345-0001 a. X100XX1000 b.

Figure B-7 (Sinclair): TRICARE Simple.

CARRIER

VA HEALTH ADMIN CENTER
PO BOX 65024
DENVER CO 80206-9024

HEALTH INSURANCE CLAIM FORM

1. MEDICARE	MEDICAID	TRICARE CHAMPUS	CHAMPVA	GROUP HEALTH PLAN	FECA BLK LUNG	OTHER	1a. INSURED'S I.D. NUMBER (For Program in Item 1)
(Medicare #)	(Medicaid #)	(Sponsor's SSN)	X (Member ID#)	(SSN or ID)	(SSN)	(ID)	223558890

2. PATIENT'S NAME (Last Name, First Name, Middle Initial)	3. PATIENT'S BIRTH DATE	SEX	4. INSURED'S NAME (Last Name, First Name, Middle Initial)
SALISBURY THEODORE V	MM 08 DD 11 YY 1957	M X F	SAME

5. PATIENT'S ADDRESS (No., Street)	6. PATIENT RELATIONSHIP TO INSURED	7. INSURED'S ADDRESS (No., Street)
2659 WEST LINCOLN	Self X Spouse Child Other	

CITY	STATE	8. PATIENT STATUS	CITY	STATE
MILTON	XT	Single Married Other X		

ZIP CODE	TELEPHONE (Include Area Code)		ZIP CODE	TELEPHONE (INCLUDE AREA CODE)
12345	(555) 234 3222	Employed Full-Time Student Part-Time Student		( )

9. OTHER INSURED'S NAME (Last Name, First Name, Middle Initial)	10. IS PATIENT'S CONDITION RELATED TO:	11. INSURED'S POLICY GROUP OR FECA NUMBER

a. OTHER INSURED'S POLICY OR GROUP NUMBER	a. EMPLOYMENT? (CURRENT OR PREVIOUS) YES X NO	a. INSURED'S DATE OF BIRTH MM DD YY SEX M F

b. OTHER INSURED'S DATE OF BIRTH MM DD YY SEX M F	b. AUTO ACCIDENT? YES X NO PLACE (State)	b. EMPLOYER'S NAME OR SCHOOL NAME USN RET

c. EMPLOYER'S NAME OR SCHOOL NAME	c. OTHER ACCIDENT? YES X NO	c. INSURANCE PLAN NAME OR PROGRAM NAME

d. INSURANCE PLAN NAME OR PROGRAM NAME	10d. RESERVED FOR LOCAL USE	d. IS THERE ANOTHER HEALTH BENEFIT PLAN? YES X NO If yes, return to and complete item 9 a-d.

READ BACK OF FORM BEFORE COMPLETING & SIGNING THIS FORM.

12. PATIENT'S OR AUTHORIZED PERSON'S SIGNATURE I authorize the release of any medical or other information necessary to process this claim. I also request payment of government benefits either to myself or to the party who accepts assignment below.

SIGNED SOF DATE _____

13. INSURED'S OR AUTHORIZED PERSON'S SIGNATURE I authorize payment of medical benefits to the undersigned physician or supplier for services described below.

SIGNED _____

14. DATE OF CURRENT: MM DD YY ◀ ILLNESS (First symptom) OR INJURY (Accident) OR PREGNANCY(LMP)	15. IF PATIENT HAS HAD SAME OR SIMILAR ILLNESS. GIVE FIRST DATE MM DD YY	16. DATES PATIENT UNABLE TO WORK IN CURRENT OCCUPATION FROM MM DD YY TO MM DD YY

17. NAME OF REFERRING PHYSICIAN OR OTHER SOURCE BENNETT V ASPELMYER PA	17a. 17b. NPI 8822343451	18. HOSPITALIZATION DATES RELATED TO CURRENT SERVICES FROM MM DD YY TO MM DD YY

19. RESERVED FOR LOCAL USE	20. OUTSIDE LAB? YES X NO $ CHARGES

21. DIAGNOSIS OR NATURE OF ILLNESS OR INJURY. (RELATE ITEMS 1,2,3 OR 4 TO ITEM 24E BY LINE)

1. 600 .20   3. ___ . ___

2. ___ . ___   4. ___ . ___

22. MEDICAID RESUBMISSION CODE   ORIGINAL REF. NO.

23. PRIOR AUTHORIZATION NUMBER

PHYSICIAN OR SUPPLIER INFORMATION

	24. A. DATE(S) OF SERVICE From MM DD YY	To MM DD YY	B. PLACE OF SERVICE	C. EMG	D. PROCEDURES, SERVICES, OR SUPPLIES (Explain Unusual Circumstances) CPT/HCPCS	MODIFIER	E. DIAGNOSIS POINTER	F. $ CHARGES	G. DAYS OR UNITS	H. EPSDT Family Plan	I. ID. QUAL.	J. RENDERING PROVIDER ID. #
1	01 23 XX	01 23 XX	21		52601		1	1200 00	1		NPI	1234567890
2											NPI	
3											NPI	
4											NPI	
5											NPI	
6											NPI	

25. FEDERAL TAX I.D. NUMBER SSN EIN	26. PATIENT'S ACCOUNT NO.	27. ACCEPT ASSIGNMENT? (For govt. claims, see back)	28. TOTAL CHARGE	29. AMOUNT PAID	30. BALANCE DUE
42 1898989 X	2466	X YES NO	$ 1200 00	$ 00 00	$

31. SIGNATURE OF PHYSICIAN OR SUPPLIER INCLUDING DEGREES OR CREDENTIALS (I certify that the statements on the reverse apply to this bill and are made a part thereof.) R L Jones MD R L Jones SIGNED 012520XX DATE	32. SERVICE FACILITY LOCATION INFORMATION BROADMOOR MEDICAL CLINIC 4353 PINE RIDGE DRIVE MILTON XY 12345-0001 a. X100XX1000 b.	33. BILLING PROVIDER INFO & PH # (555) 6567890 BROADMOOR MEDICAL CLINIC 4353 PINE RIDGE DRIVE MILTON XY 12345-0001 a. X100XX1000 b.

Figure B-8 (Salisbury): CHAMPVA.

WORKERS' COMP CARRIER
STREET ADDRESS OR PO BOX #
CITY, STATE, ZIP

HEALTH INSURANCE CLAIM FORM

1. MEDICARE	MEDICAID	TRICARE CHAMPUS	CHAMPVA	GROUP HEALTH PLAN	FECA BLK LUNG	OTHER	1a. INSURED'S I.D. NUMBER	(For Program in Item 1)
(Medicare #)	(Medicaid #)	(Sponsor's SSN)	(Member ID#)	(SSN or ID)	(SSN)	[X] (ID)	C94FPP29930	

2. PATIENT'S NAME (Last Name, First Name, Middle Initial)	3. PATIENT'S BIRTH DATE		SEX		4. INSURED'S NAME (Last Name, First Name, Middle Initial)
PORTER JAMES B	MM 03 DD 10 YY 1968	M [X]	F		COMPUTER SOLUTIONS LLC

5. PATIENT'S ADDRESS (No., Street)	6. PATIENT RELATIONSHIP TO INSURED	7. INSURED'S ADDRESS (No., Street)
23411 SOUTH 12TH AVENUE	Self [ ] Spouse [ ] Child [ ] Other [X]	4591 PRIME CIRCLE

CITY	STATE	8. PATIENT STATUS	CITY	STATE
DODGEVILLE	XT	Single [ ] Married [X] Other [ ]	LINCOLN	XT

ZIP CODE	TELEPHONE (Include Area Code)		ZIP CODE	TELEPHONE (INCLUDE AREA CODE)
12367	(555) 456 9981	Employed [X] Full-Time Student [ ] Part-Time Student [ ]	12470	(567) 822 0010

9. OTHER INSURED'S NAME (Last Name, First Name, Middle Initial)	10. IS PATIENT'S CONDITION RELATED TO:	11. INSURED'S POLICY GROUP OR FECA NUMBER
a. OTHER INSURED'S POLICY OR GROUP NUMBER	a. EMPLOYMENT? (CURRENT OR PREVIOUS) [X] YES [ ] NO	a. INSURED'S DATE OF BIRTH MM DD YY SEX M [ ] F [ ]
b. OTHER INSURED'S DATE OF BIRTH MM DD YY SEX M [ ] F [ ]	b. AUTO ACCIDENT? PLACE (State) [ ] YES [X] NO	b. EMPLOYER'S NAME OR SCHOOL NAME
c. EMPLOYER'S NAME OR SCHOOL NAME	c. OTHER ACCIDENT? [ ] YES [X] NO	c. INSURANCE PLAN NAME OR PROGRAM NAME
d. INSURANCE PLAN NAME OR PROGRAM NAME	10d. RESERVED FOR LOCAL USE	d. IS THERE ANOTHER HEALTH BENEFIT PLAN? [ ] YES [ ] NO If yes, return to and complete item 9 a-d.

READ BACK OF FORM BEFORE COMPLETING & SIGNING THIS FORM.
12. PATIENT'S OR AUTHORIZED PERSON'S SIGNATURE I authorize the release of any medical or other information necessary to process this claim. I also request payment of government benefits either to myself or to the party who accepts assignment below.

SIGNED _____ DATE _____

13. INSURED'S OR AUTHORIZED PERSON'S SIGNATURE I authorize payment of medical benefits to the undersigned physician or supplier for services described below.

SIGNED _____

14. DATE OF CURRENT: MM 01 DD 25 YY XX ◀ ILLNESS (First symptom) OR INJURY (Accident) OR PREGNANCY(LMP)	15. IF PATIENT HAS HAD SAME OR SIMILAR ILLNESS. GIVE FIRST DATE MM DD YY	16. DATES PATIENT UNABLE TO WORK IN CURRENT OCCUPATION FROM MM 01 DD 25 YY XX TO MM 02 DD 24 YY XX
17. NAME OF REFERRING PHYSICIAN OR OTHER SOURCE R L JONES MD	17a. / 17b. NPI 1234567890	18. HOSPITALIZATION DATES RELATED TO CURRENT SERVICES FROM MM DD YY TO MM DD YY
19. RESERVED FOR LOCAL USE		20. OUTSIDE LAB? [ ] YES [X] NO $ CHARGES

21. DIAGNOSIS OR NATURE OF ILLNESS OR INJURY. (RELATE ITEMS 1,2,3 OR 4 TO ITEM 24E BY LINE)

1. 354 . 0
2. ___ . ___
3. ___ . ___
4. ___ . ___

22. MEDICAID RESUBMISSION CODE   ORIGINAL REF. NO.

23. PRIOR AUTHORIZATION NUMBER

24. A. DATE(S) OF SERVICE From MM DD YY To MM DD YY	B. PLACE OF SERVICE	C. EMG	D. PROCEDURES, SERVICES, OR SUPPLIES (Explain Unusual Circumstances) CPT/HCPCS MODIFIER	E. DIAGNOSIS POINTER	F. $ CHARGES	G. DAYS OR UNITS	H. EPSDT Family Plan	I. ID. QUAL.	J. RENDERING PROVIDER ID. #
01 25 XX 01 25 XX	11		99213	1	75 00	1		NPI	1234567890
								NPI	
								NPI	
								NPI	
								NPI	
								NPI	

25. FEDERAL TAX I.D. NUMBER SSN EIN	26. PATIENT'S ACCOUNT NO.	27. ACCEPT ASSIGNMENT? (For govt. claims, see back)	28. TOTAL CHARGE	29. AMOUNT PAID	30. BALANCE DUE
42 1898989 [X]	3451	[X] YES [ ] NO	$ 75 00	$	$ 75 00

31. SIGNATURE OF PHYSICIAN OR SUPPLIER INCLUDING DEGREES OR CREDENTIALS (I certify that the statements on the reverse apply to this bill and are made a part thereof.) R L Jones MD *R L Jones* SIGNED 012520XX DATE	32. SERVICE FACILITY LOCATION INFORMATION BROADMOOR MEDICAL CLINIC 4353 PINE RIDGE DRIVE MILTON XY 12345-0001 a. X100XX1000 b.	33. BILLING PROVIDER INFO & PH # (555) 6567890 BROADMOOR MEDICAL CLINIC 4353 PINE RIDGE DRIVE MILTON XY 12345-0001 a. X100XX1000 b.

Figure B-9 (Porter): Workers' Compensation.

TANF Programs

State	Name
Alabama	FA (Family Assistance Program)
Alaska	ATAP (Alaska Temporary Assistance Program)
Arizona	EMPOWER (Employing and Moving People Off Welfare and Encouraging Responsibility)
Arkansas	TEA (Transitional Employment Assistance)
California	CALWORKS (California Work Opportunity and Responsibility to Kids)
Colorado	Colorado Works
Connecticut	JOBS FIRST
Delaware	ABC (A Better Chance)
Dist. of Col.	TANF
Florida	Welfare Transition Program
Georgia	TANF
Guam	TANF
Hawaii	TANF
Idaho	Temporary Assistance for Families in Idaho
Illinois	TANF
Indiana	TANF, cash assistance
	IMPACT (Indiana Manpower Placement and Comprehensive Training), TANF work program
Iowa	FIP (Family Investment Program)
Kansas	Kansas Works
Kentucky	K-TAP (Kentucky Transitional Assistance Program)
Louisiana	FITAP (Family Independence Temporary Assistance Program), cash assistance
	FIND Work (Family Independence Work Program), TANF work program
Maine	TANF, cash assistance
	ASPIRE (Additional Support for People in Retraining and Employment), TANF work program
Maryland	FIP (Family Investment Program)
Massachusetts	TAFDC (Transitional Aid to Families with Dependent Children), cash assistance
	ESP (Employment Services Program), TANF work program
Michigan	FIP (Family Independence Program)
Minnesota	MFIP (Minnesota Family Investment Program)
Mississippi	TANF
Missouri	Beyond Welfare
Montana	FAIM (Families Achieving Independence in Montana)
Nebraska	Employment First
Nevada	TANF
New Hampshire	FAP (Family Assistance Program), financial aid for work-exempt families
	NHEP (New Hampshire Employment Program), financial aid for work-mandated families
New Jersey	WFNJ (Work First New Jersey)

State	Name
New Mexico	NM Works
New York	FA (Family Assistance Program)
North Carolina	Work First
North Dakota	TEEM (Training, Employment, Education Management)
Ohio	OWF (Ohio Works First)
Oklahoma	TANF
Oregon	JOBS (Job Opportunities and Basic Skills Program)
Pennsylvania	Pennsylvania TANF
Puerto Rico	TANF
Rhode Island	FIP (Family Independence Program)
South Carolina	Family Independence
South Dakota	TANF
Tennessee	Families First
Texas	Texas Works (Department of Human Services), cash assistance Choices (Texas Workforce Commission), TANF work program
Utah	FEP (Family Employment Program)
Vermont	ANFC (Aid to Needy Families with Children), cash assistance Reach Up, TANF work program
Virgin Islands	(FIP) Family Improvement Program
Virginia	VIEW (Virginia Initiative for Employment, Not Welfare)
Washington	WorkFirst
West Virginia	West Virginia Works
Wisconsin	W-2 (Wisconsin Works)
Wyoming	POWER (Personal Opportunities With Employment Responsibility)

Index

J

Q

T

U